FIRST AID FOR THE® BASIC SCIENCES

General Principles

SENIOR EDITORS

TAO LE, MD, MHS
Assistant Clinical Professor
Chief, Section of Allergy and Clinical Immunology
Department of Medicine
University of Louisville

KENDALL KRAUSE, MD
Resident
Department of Emergency Medicine
Harvard Affiliated Emergency Medicine Residency

EDITORS

ELIZABETH EBY
Vanderbilt University School of Medicine
Class of 2009

JUSTIN P. FOX, MD
Resident
Department of Surgery
Wright State University

DANIELLE GUEZ
Yale University School of Medicine
Class of 2011

M. KENNEDY HALL
Albert Einstein College of Medicine
Class of 2009

SANDY MONG
Harvard Medical School
Class of 2009

KONSTANTINA M. VANEVSKI, MD
Senior Fellow
Department of Obstetrics and Gynecology
F. Edward Hébert School of Medicine Unifomed
Services University of the Health Sciences

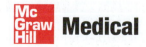
McGraw Hill **Medical**

New York   Chicago   San Francisco   Lisbon   London   Madrid   Mexico City
Milan   New Delhi   San Juan   Seoul   Singapore   Sydney   Toronto

The McGraw-Hill Companies

First Aid for the® Basic Sciences: General Principles

Disclosure: The opinions or assertions contained herein are the private views of the authors and are not to be construed as official or as reflecting the views of the Department of Defense, the United States Military, or the Department of Health and Human Services.

1 2 3 4 5 6 7 8 9 0   QPD/QPD 12 11 10 9 8

ISBN 978-0-07-154545-7
MHID 0-07-154545-X

NOTICE

Medicine is an ever-changing science. As new research and clinical experience broaden our knowledge, changes in treatment and drug therapy are required. The authors and the publisher of this work have checked with sources believed to be reliable in their efforts to provide information that is complete and generally in accord with the standards accepted at the time of publication. However, in view of the possibility of human error or changes in medical sciences, neither the authors nor the publisher nor any other party who has been involved in the preparation or publication of this work warrants that the information contained herein is in every respect accurate or complete, and they disclaim all responsibility for any errors or omissions or for the results obtained from use of the information contained in this work. Readers are encouraged to confirm the information contained herein with other sources. For example and in particular, readers are advised to check the product information sheet included in the package of each drug they plan to administer to be certain that the information contained in this work is accurate and that changes have not been made in the recommended dose or in the contraindications for administration. This recommendation is of particular importance in connection with new or infrequently used drugs.

This book was set in Electra LH by Rainbow Graphics.
The editor was Catherine A. Johnson.
The production supervisor was Phil Galea.
Project management was provided by Rainbow Graphics.

The illustration manager was Armen Ovsepyan.
The designer was Alan Barnett.
Quebecor Dubuque was printer and binder.
This book is printed on acid-free paper.

The following material was reproduced, with permission, from Le T, et al. *First Aid for the USMLE Step 1: 2008*, New York: McGraw-Hill, 2008:
Figures 1-3, 1-6, 1-7, 1-8, 1-19, 1-20, 1-22, 1-24, 1-25, 1-26, 1-27, 1-28, 1-30, 1-32, 1-33, 3-5, 3-7, 3-8, 3-9, 3-14, 3-15, 3-16, 3-17, 3-25, 3-27, 3-32, 3-34, 3-40, 3-42, 3-44, 3-45, 3-48, 3-49, 3-50, 3-52, 3-59, 3-70, 3-73, 3-101, 3-119, 3-120, 3-121, 3-122, 3-123, 4-3, 4-5, 4-6, 4-11, 4-25, 5-6, 5-7, 5-10, 5-37, 5-38, 5-40, 6-4, 6-5, 6-10, 6-11, 8-1, and 8-2; Tables 1-7, 3-20, 3-28, 4-7, 5-51, 6-6, 6-7, 6-10, and 6-12.

Cover images are modified and reproduced, with permission, from the following sources: Chandrasoma P, Taylor CR. Concise Pathology, 3rd ed. Originally published by Appleton & Lange. Copyright © 1998 by The McGraw-Hill Companies, Inc.; and Wolff K, Johnson RA, Suurmond D. *Fitzpatrick's Color Atlas & Synopsis of Clinical Dermatology*, 5th ed. New York: McGraw-Hill, 2005.

Library of Congress Cataloging-in-Publication Data

Le, Tao.
  First aid for the basic sciences. General principles / Tao T. Le, Kendall Krause.
     p. ; cm.
  Includes bibliographical references and index.
  ISBN-13: 978-0-07-154545-7 (pbk. : alk. paper)
  ISBN-10: 0-07-154545-X (alk. paper)
  1. Medical sciences—Outlines, syllabi, etc. 2. Medical sciences—Examinations, questions, etc. 3. Physicians—Licenses—United States—Examinations—Study guides. I. Krause, Kendall. II. Title. III. Title: General principles.
  [DNLM: 1. Biological Sciences—Outlines. 2. Medicine—Outlines. WB 18.2 L433f 2009]
  R834.5.L397 2009
  610.76—dc22
                                                                  2008044293

DEDICATION

To the contributors to this and future editions, who took time to share their
knowledge, insight, and humor for the benefit of students.

and

To our families, friends, and loved ones, who supported us
in the task of assembling this guide.

Contents

CONTRIBUTING AUTHORS

Kevan M. Akrami
Albert Einstein College of Medicine
Class of 2009

Ryan Patrick Bayley
Vanderbilt University School of Medicine
Class of 2008

Johnathan A. Bernard
Yale University School of Medicine
Harvard School of Public Health
Class of 2009

Melissa A Buryk, MD
Resident
Department of Pediatrics
Portsmouth Naval Medical Center

Trevor A. Crowell
Keck School of Medicine
University of Southern California
Class of 2008

Beverly (Ye) Du
Harvard Medical School
Class of 2009

Cicely Anne Dye
F. Edward Hérbert School of Medicine
Uniformed Services University of the Health Sciences
Class of 2009

Elizabeth Eby
Vanderbilt University School of Medicine
Class of 2009

Matthew C. Egalka, MD
Resident
Department of Pediatrics
Yale-New Haven Children's Hospital

Mary Evans, MD
Resident
Department of Internal Medicine
Boston Medical Center

Rolf Graning, MD
Uniformed Services University of the Health Sciences
Class of 2007

Britney L. Grayson
Vanderbilt University School of Medicine
Class of 2012

Alison Hanson
Vanderbilt University School of Medicine
Class of 2012

Nicole M. Hsu
F. Edward Hébert School of Medicine
Uniformed Services University of the Health Sciences
Class of 2009

Sean L. Jersey, MD
Flight Surgeon
99th Reconnaissance Squadron Air Force Base, California

Serge Kobsa
Yale University School of Medicine
Class of 2011

Pamela Landsteiner, MD
Transitional Resident
David Grant USAF Medical Center
Travis Air Force Base, California

Peter Liang
Harvard Medical School
Class of 2009

Joel Musee
Vanderbilt University School of Medicine
Class of 2013

Gregory Nelson, MD, MHS
Resident
Department of Orthopaedic Surgery
Barnes-Jewish Hospital
Washington University in St. Louis

Scott E. Potenta
Harvard Medical School
Class of 2011

Sofie Rahman
Vanderbilt University School of Medicine
Class of 2009

Rachel Reinert
Vanderbilt University School of Medicine
Class of 2013

Jakub Sroubek
Albert Einstein College of Medicine
Class of 2011

Brendon G. Tillman
F. Edward Hébert School of Medicine
Uniformed Services University of the Health Sciences
Class of 2009

Yolanda D. Tseng
Harvard Medical School
Class of 2009

Joshua Tyler, MD
Resident
Department of General Surgery
Brooke Army Medical Center

Eric Vaillant
Resident
University of California Davis Medical Center

Joshua J. Weaver, MD
Resident
Department of Neurology
New York Presbyterian /Weill Cornell

Cicely Williams
Yale University School of Medicine
Class of 2011

David Young
Vanderbilt University School of Medicine
Class of 2008

FACULTY REVIEWERS

Ronald Arky, MD
Charles S. Davidson Distinguished Professor of Medicine,
Brigham and Women's Hospital
Harvard Medical School

James B. Atkinson, MD, PhD
Professor
Department of Pathology
Vanderbilt University Medical Center

Susan J. Baserga, MD, PhD
Professor, Molecular Biophysics and Biochemistry, Genetics,
 Therapeutic Radiology
Yale University School of Medicine

Stephen C. Baum, MD
Professor of Medicine, Microbiology and Immunology
Albert Einstein College of Medicine

Douglas A. Berv, MD
Lecturer
Department of Psychiatry
Yale University School of Medicine

Jonathan Bogan, MD
Assistant Professor of Medicine and Cell Biology
Yale University School of Medicine

Florence M. Brown, MD
Assistant Professor of Medicine
Beth Israel-Deaconess Medical Center
Harvard Medical School

Yung-Chi "Tommy" Cheng, PhD
Henry Bronson Professor of Pharmacology
Yale University School of Medicine

Yoon Andrew Cho-Park, MD
Clinical Fellow in Neurology
Massachusetts General Hospital/Brigham and Women's Hospital
Harvard Medical School

Christoper Cimino, MD
Professor of Clinical Neurology
Albert Einstein College of Medicine

Celena Dancourt, MD
Chief Resident
Department of Psychiatry
Beth Israel Medical Center
Albert Einstein College of Medicine

Sachin Desai, MD
Clinical Fellow
Department of Pediatrics
Yale University School of Medicine

Jorg Dietrich, MD, PhD
Chief Resident
Department of Neurology
Massachusetts General Hospital/Brigham and Women's Hospital
Harvard Medical School

Eric Elster, MD
Assistant Professor of Surgery
Uniformed Services University of the Health Sciences

Susan Farrell, MD
Assistant Professor of Medicine
Brigham and Women's Hospital
Harvard Medical School

Dennis Finkielstein, MD
Assistant Professor of Medicine
Albert Einstein College of Medicine

David E. Golan, MD, PhD
Professor
Department of Biological Chemistry & Molecular Pharmacology
Harvard Medical School

Attilio V. Granata, MD, MBA
Associate Professor
Yale School of Medicine and Yale School of Public Health

Yvonne Grimm-Jorgensen, PhD
Assistant Professor
Department of Cell Biology
University of Connecticut Health Center

Mehrnaz Hojjati, MD
Assistant Professor
Department of Medicine
Medical School at the University of Minnesota

Paul D. Holtom, MD
Associate Professor of Medicine and Orthopedics
Keck School of Medicine of University of Southern California

Edmund G. Howe III, MD, JD
Professor of Psychiatry
Uniformed Services University of the Health Sciences

Anand D Jeyasekharan, MD, MBBS
Department of Oncology and Hutchison/MRC Research Centre
University of Cambridge

Shanta Kapadia, MD, MBBS
Lecturer
Department of Surgery
Yale School of Medicine

Joel Katz, MD
Assistant Professor of Medicine
Brigham and Women's Hospital
Harvard Medical School

George L. King, MD
Professor of Medicine
Brigham and Women's Hospital
Harvard Medical School

Philip Kingsley, MS
Assistant in Biochemistry
Vanderbilt University Medical Center

Michael Klompus, MD, PhD
Instructor
Department of Ambulatory Care and Prevention
Harvard Medical School

Fotios Koumpouras, MD
Assistant Professor of Medicine
University of Pittsburg School of Medicine

Patricia Kritek, MD
Instructor in Medicine
Brigham and Women's Hospital
Harvard Medical School

Jayde Kurland, MD
Staff Gastroenterologist
National Naval Medical Center

Joseph D. LaBarbera, PhD
Associate Professor
Department of Psychiatry
Vanderbilt University School of Medicine

John McArdle, MD
Assistant Professor of Medicine
Yale University School of Medicine

Cynthia Macri, MD
Assistant Professor, Obstetrics and Gynecology
Uniformed Services University of the Health Sciences

Jason B. Martin, MD
Division of Allergy, Pulmonary, and Critical Care
Department of Medicine
Vanderbilt University School of Medicine

Andrew Miller, DO
Senior Rheumatology Fellow
Vanderbilt University Medical Center

Tracey A. Milligan, MD, MS
Instructor in Neurology
Brigham and Women's Hospital
Harvard Medical School

Kenneth L. Muldrew, MD, MPH
Winchester Fellow in Clinical Microbiology
Department of Laboratory Medicine
Yale School of Medicine

Michael Parker, MD
Assistant Professor of Medicine
Beth Israel-Deaconess Hospital
Harvard Medical School

Jonathan P. Pearl, MD
Assistant Professor
Department of Surgery
Uniformed Services University of the Health Sciences

Cathleen C. Pettepher, PhD
Professor, Cancer Biology and Cell & Developmental Biology
Vanderbilt University School of Medicine

Staci E. Pollack, MD
Assistant Professor of Reproductive Endocrinology & Infertility
Department of Obstetrics, Gynecology & Women's Health
Albert Einstein College of Medicine

E. Matthew Ritter, MD
Assistant Professor of Surgery
Norman M. Rich Department of Surgery
Uniformed Services University of the Health Sciences

David H. Roberts, MD
Assistant Professor of Medicine
Beth Israel-Deaconess Medical Center
Harvard Medical School

Jeffrey J. Schwartz, MD
Associate Professor
Department of Anesthesiology
Yale University School of Medicine

Ravi Shah, MD
Resident in Internal Medicine
Massachusetts General Hospital

Keegan Smith, MD
Clinical Fellow
Division of Allergy, Pulmonary, and Critical Care Medicine
Vanderbilt University Medical Center

Darko Stefanovski, MSc
PhD Graduate Student; PIBBS (Physiology & Biophysics)
Keck School of Medicine of University of Southern California

Richard S. Stein, MD
Professor of Medicine
Vanderbilt University Medical Center

Howard M. Steinman, MD
Professor of Biochemistry
Albert Einstein College of Medicine

Srinivas Susarla, DMD
Clinical Fellow in Oral and Maxillofacial Surgery
Massachusetts General Hospital

Louise D. Teel, PhD
Research Assistant Professor
Department of Microbiology and Immunology
Uniformed Services University of the Health Sciences

Mark Thomas, MD
Associate Professor
Physical Medicine and Rehabilitation
Albert Einstein College of Medicine

Joseph I. Wolfsdorf, MB, BCh
Professor of Pediatrics
Children's Hospital
Harvard Medical School

Preface

With this first edition of *First Aid for the Basic Sciences: General Principles*, we continue our commitment to providing students with the most useful and up-to-date preparation guides for the USMLE Step 1. Both this text and its companion, *First Aid for the Basic Sciences: Organ Systems*, are designed to fill the need for a high-quality, in-depth, conceptually driven study guide for Step 1 of the USMLE. They are designed to be used either alone, or in conjunction with the original *First Aid for the USMLE Step 1*. In this way, students can tailor their own studying experience, calling on either book, according to their mastery of each subject.

These books would not have been possible without the help of the hundreds of students and faculty members who contributed their feedback and suggestions. We invite students and faculty to please share their thoughts and ideas to help us improve *First Aid for the Basic Sciences: General Principles*. (See How to Contribute, p. xiii.)

Tao Le
Louisville

Kendall Krause
Boston

Acknowledgments

This has been a collaborative project from the start. We gratefully acknowledge the thoughtful comments and advice of the residents, international medical graduates, and faculty who have supported the editors and authors in the development of *First Aid for the Basic Sciences: General Principles.*

We wish to extend a sincere and heartfelt thanks to our amazing editor, Isabel Nogueira, who truly was the backbone of this project. Without her enthusiasm and commitment, the publication of this project would not have been possible. For support and encouragement throughout the process, we are grateful to Thao Pham, Louise Petersen, and Selina Franklin.

Furthermore, we wish to give credit to our wonderful editors and authors, who worked tirelessly on the manuscript. We never cease to be amazed by their dedication, thoughtfulness, and creativity.

Thanks to Catherine Johnson and our publisher, McGraw-Hill, for their assistance and guidance. For outstanding editorial work, we thank Karla Schroeder, Michael Shelton, and Alison Kelley. A special thanks to Rainbow Graphics for remarkable production work.

Thanks to Peter Anderson of the Department of Pathology, University of Alabama at Birmingham, for use of images from the Pathology Education Instructional Resource Digital Library (http://peir.net). We also thank faculty at Uniformed Services University of the Health Sciences (USUHS) for use of their images.

Tao Le
Louisville

Kendall Krause
Boston

How to Contribute

To continue to produce a high-yield review source for the USMLE Step 1, you are invited to submit any suggestions or corrections. We also offer paid internships in medical education and publishing ranging from three months to one year (see below for details). Please send us your suggestions for:

- New facts, mnemonics, diagrams, and illustrations.
- High-yield topics that may reappear on future Step 1 exams
- Corrections and other suggestions

For each entry incorporated into the next edition, you will receive a $10 gift certificate, as well as personal acknowledgment in the next edition. Diagrams, tables, partial entries, updates, corrections, and study hints are also appreciated, and significant contributions will be compensated at the discretion of the authors. Also let us know about material in this edition that you feel is low yield and should be deleted.

The preferred way to submit entries, suggestions, or corrections is via our blog:

www.firstaidteam.com.

Otherwise, please send entries, neatly written or typed, or on disk (Microsoft Word), to:

First Aid Team
914 N. Dixie Avenue, Suite 100
Elizabethtown, KY 42701
Attention: First Aid General Principles

NOTE TO CONTRIBUTORS

All entries become property of the authors and are subject to editing and reviewing. Please verify all data and spellings carefully. In the event that similar or duplicate entries are received, only the first entry received will be used. Include a reference to a standard textbook to facilitate verification of the fact. Please follow the style, punctuation, and format of this edition if possible.

AUTHOR OPPORTUNITIES

The author team is pleased to offer opportunities in medical education and publishing to motivated medical students and physicians. Projects may range from three months (e.g., a summer) up to a full year. Participants will have an opportunity to author, edit, and earn academic credit on a wide variety of projects, including the popular *First Aid* series. English writing/editing experience, familiarity with Microsoft Word, and Internet access are required. Go to our blog **www.firstaidteam.com** to apply for an internship. A sample of your work or a proposal of a specific project is helpful.

CHAPTER 1

Anatomy and Histology

Cellular Anatomy and Histology

THE CELL

All living things, with the exception of viruses, are composed of cells. Cells, therefore, are considered the most basic unit of life. Each cell is a collection of diverse components; each component contributes to the integral biochemical processes that sustain the life of the organism. The most important eukaryotic cellular components will be covered in the following sections.

Plasma Membrane

Every eukaryotic cell is enveloped by an asymmetrical bilayer lipid membrane. This membrane consists primarily of two sheets of **phospholipids**, each one molecule thick. Phospholipids are **amphiphilic** (also referred to as amphipathic) molecules, containing both hydrophilic and hydrophobic regions (see Figure 1-1).

- The **hydrophilic** portions (i.e., phosphate groups) of the outer layer face the extracellular environment, and those of the inner layer face the cytoplasm.
- The **hydrophobic** portions of each layer (i.e., fatty acid chains) intermingle within the center of the membrane.

This bilayer membrane also contains **steroid** molecules (derived from cholesterol), glycolipids (fatty acids with sugar moieties), sphingolipids, proteins, and glycoproteins (proteins with sugar moieties). The cholesterol and glycolipid molecules alter the physical properties of the membrane (e.g., increase the melting point), in relative proportion to their presence. The proteins serve important specific roles in the transport and trafficking of nutrients across the membrane, signal transduction, and interactions between the cell and its environment.

The cell membrane performs the following functions:

- Enhancing cellular structural stability.
- Protecting internal organelles from the external environment.
- Regulating the internal environment (chemical and electrical potential).
- Enabling interactions with the external environment (e.g., signal transduction and cellular adhesion).

Nucleus and Nucleolus

The nucleus is the control center of the cell. The nucleus contains genetically encoded information, DNA, which directs the life processes of the cell. It is surrounded by two lipid bilayers: The inner membrane defines the boundaries of the nucleus, while the outer membrane is continuous with the **rough endoplasmic reticulum (RER)** (see Figure 1-2). In addition to DNA, the nucleus houses a number of important proteins that enable the maintenance (protection, repair, and replication), expression (transcription), and transportation of genetic material (DNA, RNA).

Most of the cell's **ribosomal RNA (rRNA)** is produced within the nucleus by the **nucleolus.** The rRNA then passes through the **nuclear pores** (transmembrane protein complexes that regulate trafficking across the nuclear membrane), to the cytosol, where it associates with the RER.

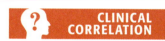

CLINICAL CORRELATION

Proteins comprise transmembrane transporters, ligand-receptor complexes, and ion channels; protein dysfunction underlies many diseases.

FLASH FORWARD

Genetic mutations may cause dysfunction of regulatory proteins, especially repair mechanisms, often leading to debilitating diseases, such as xeroderma pigmentosum.

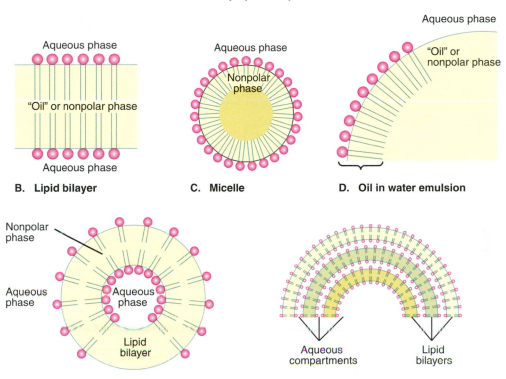

FIGURE 1-1. **Amphipathic lipids.** Formation of lipid membranes, micelles, emulsions, and liposomes from amphipathic lipids (e.g., phospholipids). (Modified, with permission, from Murray RK, Granner DK, Rodwell VW. *Harper's Illustrated Biochemistry*, 27th ed., New York: McGraw-Hill, 2006: 130.)

Rough Endoplasmic Reticulum and Ribosomes

As previously described, the RER is home to the majority of the cell's ribosomes (the many ribosomes studding the surface of the RER membrane give rise to its name). These rRNA doublets associate with **transfer RNA (tRNA)** to translate **messenger RNA (mRNA)** into amino acid sequences, and, eventually, proteins (see Figure 1-3). The RER functions primarily as the location for membrane and secretory protein production as well as protein modification (see Figure 1-2). The RER is most well developed in cell types that produce proteins for secretion (pancreatic acinar cells or plasma cells).

Smooth Endoplasmic Reticulum (SER)

The SER is the site of fatty acid and phospholipid production. Most eukaryotic cells have a relatively small SER, with some exceptions. For example, hepatocytes, constantly engaged in detoxifying hydrophobic compounds through conjugation and excretion, have well-developed SER.

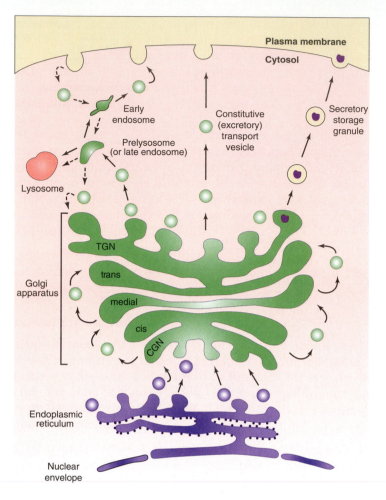

FIGURE 1-2. **Diagrammatic representation of the RER branch of protein sorting.** Newly synthesized proteins are inserted into the endoplasmic reticulum membrane or lumen from membrane-bound polyribosomes (small black circles studding the cytosolic face of the endoplasmic reticulum). Those proteins that are transported out of the endoplasmic reticulum (solid black arrows) do so from ribosome-free transitional elements. Such proteins may then pass through the various subcompartments of the Golgi until they reach the trans-Golgi network (TGN), the exit side of the Golgi. In the TGN, proteins are segregated and sorted. Secretory proteins accumulate in secretory storage granules from which they may be expelled, as shown in the upper right side of the figure. Proteins destined for the plasma membrane or those that are secreted in a constitutive manner are carried out to the cell surface in transport vesicles, as indicated in the upper middle area of the figure. Some proteins enter prelysosomes (late endosomes) and fuse with endosomes to form lysosomes, as depicted in the upper left corner of the figure. Retrieval from the Golgi apparatus to the endoplasmic reticulum is not considered in this scheme. CGN = cis-Golgi network; RER = rough endoplasmic reticulum. (Modified, with permission, from Murray RK, Granner DK, Rodwell VW. *Harper's Illustrated Biochemistry*, 27th ed. New York: McGraw-Hill, 2006: 508.)

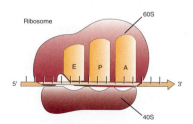

FIGURE 1-3. **Schematic representation of ribosomal RNA (rRNA).** Here, the 40S and 60S subunits of rRNA are shown, translating a portion of mRNA in the 5′ to 3′ direction. Many of these ribosomes are located within the membrane of the rough endoplasmic reticulum so that their initial protein product ends up within the lumen of the rough endoplasmic reticulum, where it undergoes further modification. E site = holds Empty tRNA as it Exits; P site = accommodates growing Peptide; A site = incoming Aminoacyl tRNA.

Golgi Apparatus

Shortly after being synthesized, proteins from the RER are packaged into transport vesicles and secreted from the RER. These vesicles travel to and fuse with the **Golgi vesicles.** Within the lumen of this organelle, secretory and membrane-bound proteins undergo modification. Depending on their final destination, these proteins may be modified in one of the three major regions or Golgi networks: **Cis (CGN), medial (MGN),** or **trans (TGN).** These proteins are then packaged in a second set of transport vesicles, which bud from the trans side, and are delivered to their target locations (e.g., organelle membranes, plasma membrane, and lysosomes; see Figures 1-2 and 1-4).

FUNCTIONS OF THE GOLGI APPARATUS

- Distributing proteins and lipids from the ER to the plasma membrane, lysosomes, and secretory vesicles.
- Modifying N-oligosaccharides on asparagines.
- Adding O-oligosaccharides to serine and threonine residues.
- Assembling proteoglycans from core proteins.
- Sulfating sugars in proteoglycans and tyrosine residues on proteins.
- Adding mannose-6-phosphate to specific proteins (targets the proteins to the lysosome).

Lysosomes

The lysosome is the **trash collector** of the cell. Bound by a single lipid bilayer, the lysosome is responsible for hydrolytic degradation of obsolete cellular components. Extracellular materials, ingested via endocytosis or phagocytosis, are enveloped in an endosome (temporary vesicle), which fuses with the lyso-

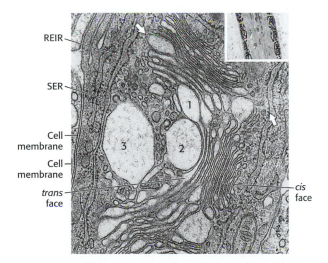

FIGURE 1-4. **Tunneling electron microscopy of Golgi apparatus.** The cis and trans faces of the Golgi apparatus are shown in relation to other important organelles, including the rough endoplasmic reticulum, smooth endoplasmic reticulum, and cell membrane. (SER = smooth endoplasmic reticulum; RER = rouch endoplasmic reticulum.) (Reproduced, with permission, from Junqueira LC, Carneiro J. *Basic Histology: Text and Atlas,* 11th ed. New York: McGraw-Hill, 2005: 36.)

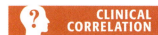

some, leading to enzymatic degradation of endosomal contents. Lysosomal enzymes (nucleases, proteases, and phosphatases) are activated at a pH below 4.8. To maintain this pH, the membrane of the lysosome contains a hydrogen ion pump, which hydrolyzes ATP to move protons against the concentration gradient.

Mitochondria

This is the primary site of **ATP** production in aerobic respiration. The proteins of the **outer membrane** enable the transport of large molecules (molecular weight ~ 10,000) for oxidative respiration. The **inner membrane**, separated from the outer by the **intermembranous** space, is highly selectively permeable (see Figure 1-5). While the inner membrane's surface area is greatly increased by numerous folds, known as **cristae**, its selectivity is maintained by transmembrane proteins. These proteins, comprising the electron transport chain, maintain a proton gradient between the intermembrane space and the lumen of the inner membrane. The role of the electron transport chain is to generate energy for storage in the bonds of ATP.

Microtubules and Cilia

These aggregate intracellular protein structures are important for cellular **support**, **rigidity**, and **locomotion**. Microtubules consist of α- and β-tubulin dimers, each bound to **two guanosine triphosphate** molecules. They combine to form cylindrical polymers of 24-nm diameter and variable lengths (see

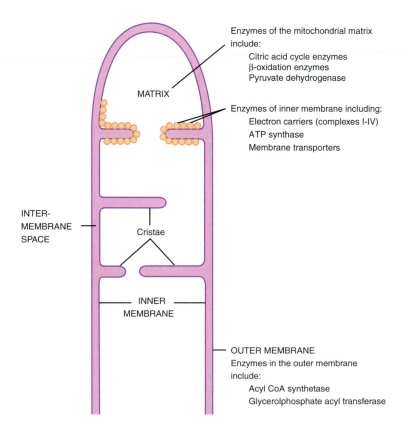

FIGURE 1-5. Structure of the mitochondrial membranes. In reality, the inner membrane contains many folds, or cristae. (Modified, with permission, from Murray RK, Granner DK, Rodwell VW. *Harper's Illustrated Biochemistry*, 27th ed. New York: McGraw-Hill, 2006: 101.)

Figure 1-6). Polymerization occurs slowly from the end of the microtubule, but depolymerization occurs rapidly.

Microtubules are incorporated into both flagella and **cilia.** Within cilia, the microtubules occur in pairs, known as **doublets.** A single cilium contains nine doublets around its circumference, each linked by an ATPase, **dynein** (Figure 1-6). These motile proteins, anchored to one doublet, move along the length of a neighboring doublet in a coordinated fashion, resulting in ciliary motion.

Epithelial Cell Junctions

These transmembrane proteins mediate intercellular interaction by providing cellular adhesion and cell signaling. Cellular adhesion and communication is vitally important to both the integrity and the function of an organ.

Organs and tissues exposed to the external environment are the most resilient. These tissues are referred to as **epithelial,** primarily due to their embryologic origin. The epithelial cells of these external tissues contain an array of **cell junctions** that mediate cellular adhesion and communication processes. There are five principal types of cell junctions: **Zona occludens (tight junctions), zona adherens (intermediate junctions), macula adherens (desmosomes), gap junctions (communicating junctions),** and **hemidesmosomes** (see Figure 1-7).

ZONA OCCLUDENS

Tight junctions, also referred to as occluding junctions have the following two primary functions:

- Determine epithelial cell polarity, separating the apical pole from the basolateral pole.
- Regulate passage of substances across the epithelial barrier (**paracellular transport**).

In a typical epithelial tissue, the membranes of adjacent cells meet at regular intervals to seal the inter- or paracellular space, thus surrounding the cell like a belt. These connections occur at the interaction of the junctional protein complex of neighboring cells. This complex is composed of the proteins **occludin,** a four-span transmembrane protein, and **claudin.**

ZONA ADHERENS

Intermediate junctions are located just below tight junctions, near the apical surface of an epithelial layer. Like the zona occludens, the zona adherens

Drugs that act on microtubules:

Drug	Disease
Mebendazole/ thiabendazole	Parasitic infections
Taxol	Breast cancer
Griseofulvin	Fungal infections
Vincristine/ vinblastine	Cancers
Colchicine	Gout

CLINICAL CORRELATION

A number of diseases arise from ineffective or insufficient ciliary motion.
Kartagener syndrome = dynein arm defect.
Cystic fibrosis = respiratory secretions that are too thick to be cleared by ciliary motion.

CLINICAL CORRELATION

Often, cells of adenocarcinomas lose their usual epithelial cell junctions, allowing them to infiltrate surrounding tissues and metastasize.

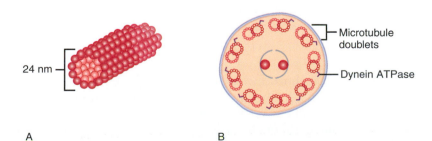

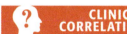

FIGURE 1-6. **Microtubules.** (A) Structure. The cylindrical structure of a microtubule is depicted as a circumferential array of 13 dimers of α- and β-tubulin. Each dimer binds two guanosine triphosphate molecules. (B) Ciliary structure. Nine microtubule doublets, circumferentially arranged, create motion via coordinated dynein ATP cleavage.

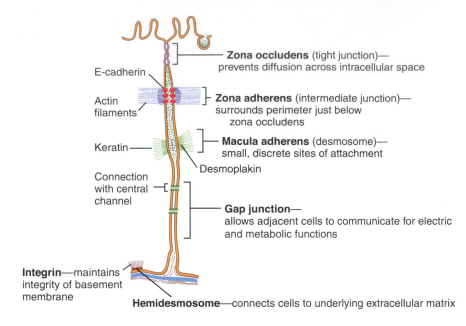

FIGURE 1-7. **Epithelial cell junctions.** Five types of epithelial cell junctions are depicted along with their supporting and component proteins.

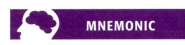

MNEMONIC

Cadherins are **C**alcium-dependent **ADHE**sion proteins.

occurs periodically along the circumference of the cell, in a belt-like distribution. Inside the cell, these transmembrane protein complexes are associated with actin microfilaments. Outside the cell, **cadherins** (see adjacent mnemonic) from adjacent cells use a calcium-dependent mechanism to span wider intercellular spaces than can the zona occludens.

Macula Adherens

As opposed to the belt-like distribution of the zona occludens and adherens, desmosomes resemble spot welds; single rivets erratically spaced below the apical surface of the epithelium. Intracellularly, they are associated with keratin intermediate filaments, providing strength and rigidity to the epithelial surface. This intercellular adhesion is also mediated by calcium-dependent cadherin interactions.

Gap Junctions

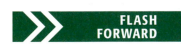

FLASH FORWARD

Gap junctions allow for "coupling" of cardiac myocytes, enabling the rapid transmission of electrical depolarization and coordinating contraction during the cardiac cycle.

These intercellular junctions allow for rapid transmission of biochemical information from one cell to the next (via chemical or electrical potential). A connexon is formed from a complex of six **connexin** proteins. Each single **connexon** exists as a hollow cylindrical structure spanning the plasma membrane. When a connexon of one cell is bound to a connexon of an adjacent cell, a gap junction is formed, creating an open channel for fluid and electrolyte transport across cell membranes.

Hemidesmosomes

These asymmetrical anchors provide epithelial adhesion to the underlying connective tissue layer, the **basal lamina.** The hemidesmosome contains **laminin 5** (instead of cadherins), an anchoring protein filament that binds the cell to the basal lamina. Although the intracellular portion structurally resembles that of the desmosome, none of the protein components are conserved, except for the cytoplasmic association with intermediate filaments.

HEMATOPOIESIS

Hematopoietic cells are primarily individual cells engaged in processes of cellular interaction, physiologic transport, and immune surveillance.

Blood

Blood is a connective tissue composed of cells suspended in a liquid phase. This liquid phase, which consists of water, proteins, and electrolytes is known as **plasma** or serum. The O_2-carrying red blood cells, known as **erythrocytes**, make up about 45% of blood by volume (this percentage is known as the **hematocrit**). Erythrocytes can be separated from white blood cells, or **leukocytes**, and **platelets** by centrifugation. The erythrocytes form the lowest layer, while the leukocytes and platelets form the next layer, also known as the **buffy coat**.

The Pluripotent Stem Cell

The hematopoietic stem cell is the grandfather of all major blood cells. These cells reside within the bone marrow, where **hematopoiesis** (blood cell differentiation) occurs. They are capable of asymmetric reproduction: Simultaneous self-renewal and differentiation.

- **Self-renewal**, integral to the maintenance of future hematopoietic potential, preserves the pool of stem cells.
- **Differentiation** leads to the production of specialized mature cells, necessary for carrying out the major functions of blood.

Two differentiated cell lines derive from the pluripotent stem cell: **Myeloid** and **lymphoid** (see Figure 1-8). These cells are considered **committed**; they have begun the process of differentiation, and no longer have the potential to become any blood cell. The myeloid lineage produces five colony-forming

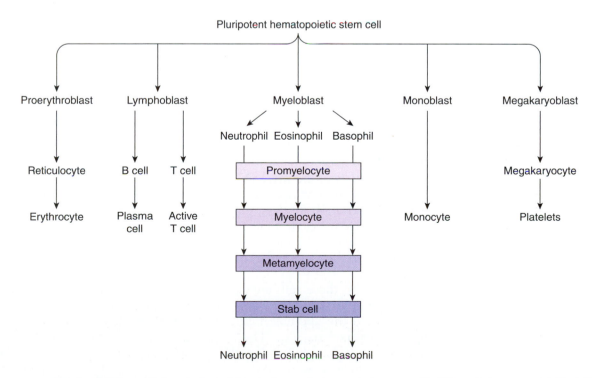

FIGURE 1-8. **Blood cell differentiation.** A chart of the pluripotent hematopoietic stem cell's differentiation potential. Each lineage is depicted as a separate column.

units (CFUs), each ending in a distinct mature cell: erythroid (producing erythrocytes), megakaryocyte (producing platelets), basophil, eosinophil, and granulocyte-macrophage (producing monocytes and neutrophils). The lymphoid lineage produces two cell lines: **T cells** and **B cells.**

Erythrocytes

Erythrocytes are nonnucleated biconcave disks designed for gas exchange. These cells measure 7.8 μm in diameter, and their biconcave shape increases their surface area for gas exchange. These cells lack organelles, which are jettisoned shortly after they enter the bloodstream. Instead, they contain only a plasma membrane, a cytoskeleton, hemoglobin, and glycolytic enzymes that help them survive via **anaerobic respiration** (90%) and the hexose monophosphate shunt (10%). This limits the red blood cell life span to approximately 120 days, after which they are typically removed via macrophages in the spleen. Mature erythrocytes are replaced by immature **reticulocytes**, which mature 1–2 days after entering the circulation. These precursors are active in protein metabolism because the mature red blood cells have expelled their nucleus and ribosomes. Reticulocytes are thereby distinguished from mature erythrocytes by their retained nucleus and slightly larger diameter.

Erythrocyte metabolism begins with the transport of glucose across the red cell membrane via the **GLUT1 transporter.** At this point, glycolytic enzymes produce ATP and lactic acid via anaerobic metabolism. Important aspects of erythrocyte metabolism are listed in Table 1-1.

Leukocytes

Leukopoiesis is the process by which white blood cells develop from hematopoietic stem cells. **Neutrophils** and **monocytes** develop through the granulocyte-macrophage CFU precursor. **Basophils** and **eosinophils** each have a lineage-specific CFU. Lymphocytes, although separate from myeloid cells, are also considered leukocytes, and arise from the lymphoid stem cell.

All leukocytes are involved in some aspect of the immune response:

- **Neutrophils** affect **nonspecific innate immunity** in the acute inflammatory response.
- **Basophils** mediate **allergic responses.**
- **Eosinophils** fight off **parasitic infections.**
- **Lymphocytes** are integral to both **innate** and **humoral immunity.**

NEUTROPHILS

These products of the myeloid lineage act as acute-phase granulocytes. They begin in the bone marrow as myeloid stem cells (see Figure 1-9) and mature over a period of 10–14 days, producing both primary and secondary granules (promyelocyte stage; see Figures 1-9, 1-10, and 1-11). Once mature, these leukocytes are vital to the success of the innate immune system and are especially prominent in the acute inflammatory response.

Histologically, these cells are distinguished by their large spherical size, multilobed nuclei, and **azurophilic** primary granules **(lysosomes).** These cells have earned the alternate name **polymorphonuclear cells** (**PMN**s) due to their multilobed nucleus. The key to their immune function, however, lies not in the nucleus, but in the ability of PMNs to phagocytose microbes and destroy them via **reactive oxygen species** (superoxide, hydrogen peroxide, peroxyl radicals, and hydroxyl radicals). Their azurophilic granules contain sev-

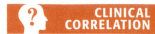

CLINICAL CORRELATION

Red cell cytoskeletal abnormalities (e.g., hereditary spherocytosis, elliptocytosis) and hemoglobinopathies (e.g., thalassemias, sickle cell anemia) cause significant morbidity and mortality.

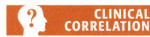

CLINICAL CORRELATION

Reticulocyte counts increase when the bone marrow increases production to replenish red cell levels in the blood in response to a bleed or hemolytic process.

KEY FACT

Leukos = Greek for white.
Cytos = Greek for cell.

TABLE 1-1.   Important Aspects of Red Blood Cell (RBC) Metabolism

The RBC is highly dependent upon glucose as its energy source; its membrane contains high-affinity glucose transporters.

Glycolysis, producing lactate, is the site of production of ATP.

Because there are no mitochondria in RBCs, there is no production of ATP by oxidative phosphorylation.

The RBC has a variety of transporters that maintain ionic and water balance.

Production of 2,3-bisphosphoglycerate, by reactions closely associated with glycolysis, is important in regulating the ability of Hb to transport O_2.

The pentose phosphate pathway is operative in the RBC (it metabolizes about 5%–10% of the total flux of glucose) and produces NADPH; hemolytic anemia due to a deficiency of the activity of glucose-6-phosphate dehydrogenase is common.

Reduced glutathione is important in the metabolism of the RBC, in part to counteract the action of potentially toxic peroxides; the RBC can synthesize glutathione and requires NADPH to return oxidized glutathione (G-S-S-G) to the reduced state.

The iron of Hb must be maintained in the ferrous state; ferric iron is reduced to the ferrous state by the action of an NADH-dependent methemoglobin reductase system involving cytochrome b5 and cytochrome b5 reductase.

Synthesis of glycogen, fatty acids, protein, and nucleic acids does not occur in the RBC; however, some lipids (e.g., cholesterol) in the RBC membrane can exchange with corresponding plasma lipids.

The RBC contains certain enzymes of nucleotide metabolism (e.g., adenosine deaminase, pyrimidine nucleotidase, adenylyl kinase); deficiencies of these enzymes are involved in some cases of hemolytic anemia.

When RBCs reach the end of their life span, the globin is degraded to amino acids (which are reused in the body), the iron is released from heme and also reused, and the tetrapyrrole component of heme is converted to bilirubin, which is mainly excreted into the bowel via the bile.

(Reprinted, with permission, from Murray RK, Granner DK, Rodwell VW. *Harper's Illustrated Biochemistry*, 27th ed. New York: McGraw-Hill, 2006: 619.)

eral enzymes, most notably **myeloperoxidase**, which produce O_2 radicals and direct the oxidative burst.

EOSINOPHILS

Eosinophils follow the same pattern of maturation as neutrophils, beginning in the bone marrow as eosinophilic CFUs. Eosinophils also contain azurophilic granules with myeloperoxidase. However, they differ in that they are larger cells with cationic proteins, such as **major basic protein** (antibacterial) and **eosinophilic cationic protein** (antiparasitic) within **acidophilic** granules. Once fully mature, eosinophils possess a large, bilobed nucleus and sparse endoplasmic reticulum and Golgi vesicles (see Figure 1-12).

 CLINICAL CORRELATION

Neutrophil dysfunction syndromes, such as Chédiak-Higashi syndrome (increased cytoplasmic granule fusion) and chronic granulomatous disease (decreased oxidative burst), lead to serious immunodeficiency.

Cell	Stage	Surface Markers[a]	Characteristics
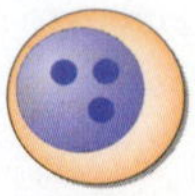	MYELOBLAST	CD33, CD13, CD15	Prominent nucleoli
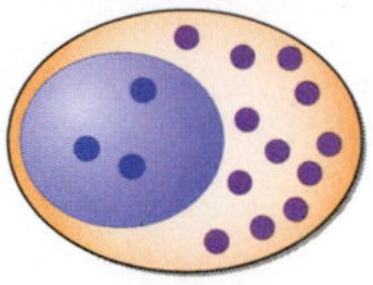	PROMYELOCYTE	CD33, CD13, CD15	Large cell Primary granules appear
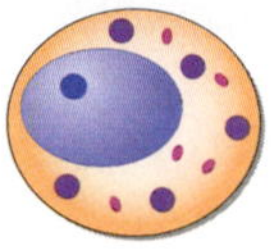	MYELOCYTE	CD33, CD13, CD15, CD14, CD11b	Secondary granules appear
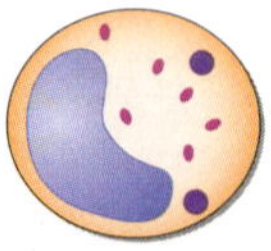	METAMYELOCYTE	CD33, CD13, CD15, CD14, CD11b	Kidney bean–shaped nucleus
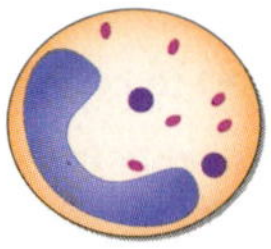	BAND FORM	CD33, CD13, CD15, CD14, CD11b CD10, CD16	Condensed, band–shaped nucleus
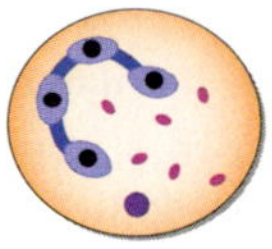	NEUTROPHIL	CD33, CD13, CD15, CD14, CD11b CD10, CD16	Condensed, multilobed nucleus

[a]CD= Cluster Determinant; ● Nucleolus; ● Primary granule; • Secondary granule.

FIGURE 1-9. **Schematic of neutrophil development stages.** TG-CSF (granulocyte colony-stimulating factor) and GM-CSF (granulocyte-macrophage colony-stimulating factor) are critical to this process. Identifying cellular characteristics and specific cell-surface markers are listed for each maturational stage. (Reproduced, with permission, from Fauci AS, Kasper DL, Braunwald E, et al., eds, *Harrison's Principles of Internal Medicine*, 17th ed, New York: McGraw-Hill, 2008.)

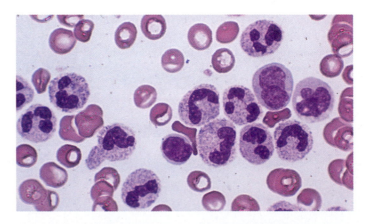

FIGURE 1-10. **Peripheral blood smear with neutrophilia.** This peripheral blood smear displays an extreme leukemoid reaction (neutrophilia). Most cells are band and segmented neutrophils. Two monocytes and a lymphocyte are also in the field. (Reproduced, with permission, from Lichtman MA, Beutler E, Kipps TJ, et al. *Williams Hematology*, 7th ed. New York: McGraw-Hill, 2006: Plate VIII-1.)

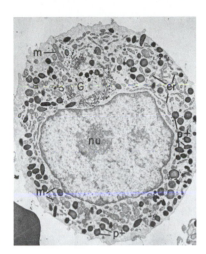
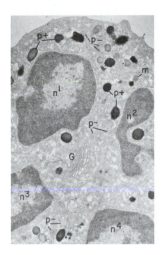

FIGURE 1-11. **Electron microscopy of neutrophils.** (A) Electron microscopy of neutrophil precursor and mature neutophil reacted for peroxidase. (B) Electron microscopy of a mature neutrophil from normal human marrow reacted for peroxidase. (Part A reproduced, with permission, from Lichtman MA, Beutler E, Kipps T, et al, *Williams Hematology*, 7th ed, New York: McGraw-Hill, 2006: 833. Part B reproduced, with permission, from Lichtman MA, Beutler E, Kipps T, et al, *Williams Hematology*, 7th ed, New York: McGraw-Hill, 2006: 833 and 835.)

BASOPHILS AND MAST CELLS

Distinguished by large, coarse, darkly staining granules, basophils produce peroxidase, **heparin**, and **histamine** (see Figure 1-13). Basophils also release **kallikrein**, which acts as an eosinophil chemoattractant during hypersensitivity reactions, such as contact allergies and skin allograft rejection. Because they share a great deal of structural similarities, basophils can be considered the bloodborne counterpart of the **mast cell**, which resides within tissues, near blood vessels. These cells, although similar to basophils, are typically larger and contain **serotonin** (i.e., **5-HT**), which basophils lack. Mast cells degranulate during the acute phase of inflammation, acting, via their released granule contents, on the nearby vasculature. This leads to vasodilation, fluid transudation, and swelling of interstitial tissues.

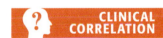

CLINICAL CORRELATION

Mast cells are an integral part of type I allergic reactions (think anaphylaxis), and they are what make allergy sufferers so miserable.

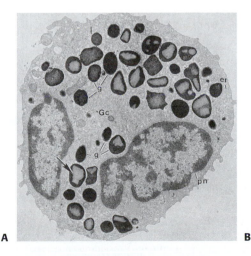
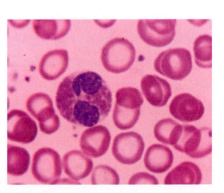

FIGURE 1-12. **Eosinophil microscopy.** (A) Human mature eosinophil incubated for peroxidase. (B) Light microscopy of a mature eosinophil. (Part A reproduced, with permission, from Lichtman MA, Beutler E, Kipps T, et al. *Williams Hematology*, 7th ed. New York: McGraw-Hill, 2006: 839. Part B adapted, with permission, from Lichtman MA, Shafer JA, Felgar RE, Wang N. *Lichtman's Atlas of Hematology*, New York: McGraw-Hill, 2007: Figure ll.D.2.)

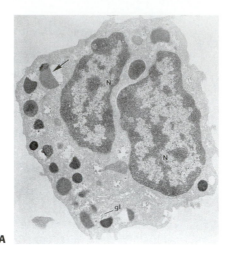

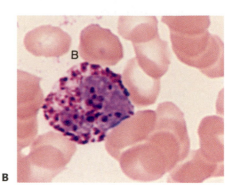

A **B**

FIGURE 1-13. **Basophil microscopy.** (A) Electron microscopy of a mature basophil from human blood reacted for peroxidase. (B) Light microscopy of a mature basophil. (Reproduced, with permission, from Lichtman MA, Beutler E, Kipps T, et al. *Williams Hematology*, 7th ed. New York, NY: McGraw-Hill, 2006: 840 [A] and Plate VII-4 [B].)

Monocyte Lineage

MONOCYTES

Monocytes are the myeloid precursor to the mononuclear phagocyte, the tissue macrophage. Morphologically, they appear as spherical cells with scattered small granules, akin to lysosomes. The blood monocyte is a large (10–18 μm), motile cell that marginates along the vessel wall in response to the expression of specific cell adhesion proteins. During an inflammatory response, these cell adhesion proteins (namely, platelet endothelial cell adhesion molecule, or **PECAM-1**) facilitate monocyte **diapedesis** (transmigration) across vessel walls into surrounding tissues. Once in close proximity to the inflammatory foci, the monocyte differentiates into a macrophage with increased phagocytic and lysosomal activity (see Figure 1-14).

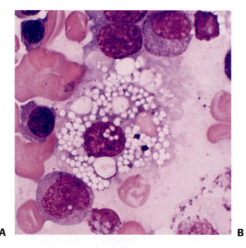

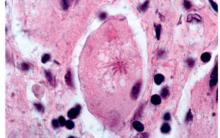

A **B**

FIGURE 1-14. **Macrophage microscopy.** (A) Active macrophage and (B) multinucleated giant cell. Seen here with the characteristic asteroid body in sarcoidosis. (Part A reproduced, with permission, from Lichtman MA, Beutler E, Kipps T, et al. *Williams Hematology*, 7th ed. New York: McGraw-Hill, 2006: Plate -IX-1. Part B image courtesy of PEIR Digital Library [http://peir.net].)

MACROPHAGES

During differentiation, monocyte cell volume and lysosome numbers increase. These lysosomes, which fuse with phagosomes, degrade ingested cellular and noncellular material. Macrophages (20–80 μm) also contain a large number of cell surface receptors. These differ, depending on the tissue in which the macrophage matures, contributing to the diversity of functions macrophages can perform (see Table 1-2).

As described in Table 1-2, several organs are involved in macrophage distribution. Similarly, connective tissues, such as the skin and bones, contain monocyte-derived cells that are structurally related to macrophages. These cells are typically derived from monocytes that have taken up residence in the tissue in question. Alternatively, monocytes can migrate into tissues during an acute inflammatory response, and there, transform into reactive macrophages to aid the innate immune system. Once out of the circulation, monocytes have a half-life of up to 70 hours. Their numbers within inflamed tissues begin to overcome those of neutrophils after approximately 12 hours.

MULTINUCLEATED GIANT CELLS

At sites of chronic inflammation, such as tuberculous lung tissue, macrophages sometimes fuse to produce multinucleated phagocytes (see Figure 1-14). These microbicidal cells can be produced in vitro via interferon-γ (IFN-γ) or interleukin-3 (IL-3) stimulation.

DENDRITIC CELLS

Antigen-presenting cells (**APCs**) are essential to the adaptive immune system. These monocyte-derived phagocytic cells take up antigens (primarily protein particles), process them, display them bound to the **major histocompatibility complex II (MHC II)** cell surface marker, and travel to lymph nodes, where

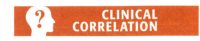

CLINICAL CORRELATION

Macrophage surface receptors can be stimulated by *Streptococcus pyogenes* superantigen, leading to massive cytokine release and tissue destruction (toxic shock syndrome).

TABLE 1-2. **Distribution of Mononuclear Phagocytes**

Marrow	Monoblasts, promonocytes, monocytes, macrophages
Blood	Monocytes
Body cavities	Pleural macrophages, peritoneal macrophages
Inflammatory tissues	Epithelioid cells, exude macrophages, multinucleate giant cells
Tissues	Liver (Kupffer cells), lung (alveolar macrophages), connective tissue (histiocytes), spleen (red pulp macrophages), lymph nodes, thymus, bone (osteoclasts), synovium (type A cells), mucosa-associated lymphoid tissue, gastrointestinal tract, genitourinary tract, endocrine organs, central nervous system (microglia), skin (dendritic cells)

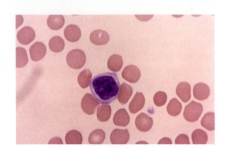

FIGURE 1-15. **Light microscopy of a lymphocyte from a blood smear.** Medium-sized agranular lymphocyte with a high nuclear to cytoplasmic ratio and an ill-defined chromatin pattern. (Adapted, with permission, from Lichtman MA, Shafer JA, Felgar RE, Wang N. *Lichtman's Atlas of Hematology.* New York: McGraw-Hill, 2007.)

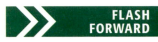
FLASH FORWARD

Dendritic cells are often the original effector of antigen presentation and initiation of humoral immunity.

they recruit other cells of the immune system into action. Dendritic cells are especially important in the initial exposure to a new antigen. Successful differentiation from monocytes depends on an endothelial cell signal that is secondary to foreign antigen exposure. In the absence of this second signal, these sensitized monocytes transform into macrophages.

Lymphocytes

Lymphocytes are easily distinguished from other leukocytes by their shared morphology (see Figures 1-15 and 1-16). After differentiating from lymphoblasts within the marrow, they migrate to the blood as spherical cells, 6–15 μm in diameter. Typically, the nucleus contains tightly packed chromatin, which stains a deep blue or purple and occupies approximately 90% of the cell cytoplasm.

As the primary actors in the adaptive immune response, lymphocytes undergo biochemical transformation into active immune cells via coordinated stimulatory signals. These activated lymphocytes then enter the cell cycle, produc-

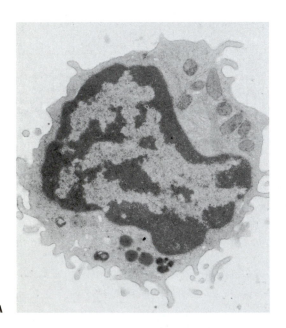

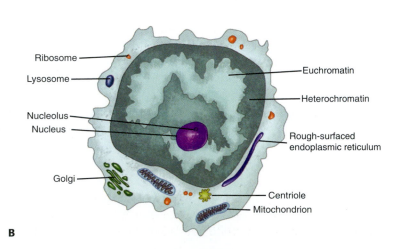

A   B

FIGURE 1-16. **(A) Electron micrograph of a normal human lymphocyte (× 12,000). (B) Diagrammatic representation of a normal lymphocyte with organelles labeled.** (Modified, with permission, from Lichtman MA, Beutler E, Kipps T, et al. *Williams Hematology,* 7th ed. New York: McGraw-Hill, 2006: 1024.)

ing a number of identical daughter cells. They eventually settle into G_0 as a memory cell while they await the next stimulation event. Alternatively, following replication, daughter cells can become terminally differentiated lymphocytes, primed for effector and secretory roles in immunologic defense of the host organism.

B Cells and Plasma Cells

B cells are the "long-range artillery" in the adaptive immune response. After the lymphoblast stage, the lymphocyte lineage diverges into B cells and T cells, each performing separate roles in the adaptive, or **humoral, immune response.** Once committed, B cells develop in the **B**one marrow and then migrate to other lymphoid organs. As they develop, B cells express immunoglobulins (IgM and IgD) on their surface, in association with costimulatory proteins. These **B-cell antigen receptor complexes** allow for the recognition of foreign antigens and subsequent activation of the B cell via phosphorylation of intracellular tyrosine domains. Downstream cell signaling leads to the expression of necessary genes for terminal differentiation to **plasma cells** that produce and secrete antibodies to aid the specific immune response. B cells that recognize self-antigens are triggered to undergo programmed cell death, or **apoptosis**, to reduce the chance of autoimmunity.

T Cells

"Infantry" of the adaptive immune response. During maturation in the Thymus, early T cells begin expressing several surface receptors simultaneously, including the thymic cell receptor (**TCR**), **CD4**, and **CD8.** If one of these CD receptors recognizes **receptors** of thymic APCs, either **MHC II** or **MHC I**, respectively, then this T cell is **positively selected**, proliferates, and matures. In this case, the T cell differentiates into either a **CD4+ helper T cell** or a **CD8+ cytotoxic T cell**, and no longer expresses the inactive receptor.

Helper T Cells

Two subtypes of T cells are derived from the CD4+ progenitor: T_H1 and T_H2. T_H1 responses occur in the presence of intracellular pathogens. In these instances, robust macrophage recruitment occurs in response to T_H1 IFN-γ release. Helminthic or **parasitic infections**, on the other hand, **drive T_H2-**mediated immune responses, with little macrophage involvement.

Helper T cells spring into action when they recognize foreign antigens bound to MHC II. Once activated, they secrete **cytokines**, chemical messengers that recruit and activate other immune effector cells. These cytokines, also called **interleukins**, specifically attract B cells, which, in turn, divide and differentiate into plasma cells. After the immune response is complete, some helper T cells become **memory cells**, quiescent immune cells that retain their specificity in case of rechallenge with the same antigen. The presence of memory cells increases the speed and efficiency of future immune responses.

Cytotoxic T Cells

CD8+ T cells also proliferate in response to cytokines; however, they only recognize antigens in association with class I MHC. These cells are actively involved in immune surveillance of intracellular pathogens.

FLASH FORWARD

Viruses, *Listeria*, malaria, *Rickettsia*, and *Chlamydia* are all intracellular pathogens capable of eliciting a T_H1 response.

KEY FACT

Helper T cells "help" by mediating the specificity of the adaptive immune response. They act as a messenger between APCs and B cells, triggering humoral immunity.

Every human cell contains MHC I, while only APCs contain MHC II.

- A cell infected by an intracellular pathogen (i.e., a virus) will process viral proteins and present them on the surface via MHC I.
- A roving CD8+ cell recognizes this signal and attaches to the infected cell via cell adhesion molecules.
- The activated cytolytic T cell releases **perforins**, which are proteins that form holes in the plasma membrane of targeted cells.

Cytolytic T cells also destroy target cells via the **Fas-Fas ligand** interaction.

- Activated CD8+ T cells express the Fas ligand on their surface.
- The interaction of Fas ligand with the Fas receptor of the infected cell leads to apoptosis.
- The intracellular pathogen is prevented from replicating, and the infection is cleared.

SUPPRESSOR T CELLS

These cells modulate helper T cell function and plasma cell differentiation. Through IFN-γ secretion, T_H1 cells stimulate the production of more T_H1 cells, while simultaneously suppressing the production of T_H2 cells. T_H2 cells can tip the scales of helper T populations toward more T_H2 cells via interleukin-4 (**IL-4**) production. In this way, the immune response reinforces itself, providing for maximum coordinated effectiveness. The type of pathogen initially triggering the immune response directs which response, T_H1 or T_H2, dominates.

KEY FACT

T_H1 cells are associated with **innate** immunity and **cytolytic** responses. T_H2 cells are associated with **humoral** immunity and **asthma.**

Gross Anatomy and Histology

ABDOMINAL WALL ANATOMY

Layers of the Abdominal Wall

The layers of the anterior abdominal wall, penetrated during surgical incision or sharp trauma, differ, depending on the location with respect to the midline and the umbilicus. They are listed in Table 1-3 and depicted in Figure 1-17.

In addition to the differences displayed in Table 1-8, the abdominal muscle aponeuroses composing the rectus sheath differ above and below the umbilicus. Above the umbilicus, the external oblique and anterior internal oblique aponeuroses are found anterior to the abdominis rectus muscle. The posterior rectus sheath is made of the posterior internal oblique and transverse abdominis aponeuroses. Below the umbilicus, the anterior rectus sheath is composed of all three abdominal muscle aponeuroses (external oblique, internal oblique, and transverse abdominis).

Inguinal Canal

The canal is an oblique, inferomedially directed channel, allowing the abdominal contents to traverse the abdominal wall to reach the scrotum and labia (see Figure 1-18). Lying superior and parallel to the **inguinal ligament**, the canal allows passage of the **round ligament** of the uterus in females and

TABLE 1-3. **Layers of the Abdominal Wall**

MIDLINE RELATION	UMBILICAL RELATION	LAYERS
Midline	Above or below	<ul><li>Skin</li><li>Subcutaneous tissue/Camper's fascia</li><li>Scarpa's fascia</li><li>Linea alba</li><li>Transversalis fascia</li><li>Parietal peritoneum</li></ul>
Anterolateral	Above or below	<ul><li>Skin</li><li>Subcutaneous tissue/Camper's fascia</li><li>Scarpa's fascia</li><li>Rectus sheath, composed of muscular aponeuroses</li><li>Transversalis fascia</li><li>Parietal peritoneum</li></ul>
Flank	Above or below	<ul><li>Skin</li><li>Subcutaneous tissue/Camper's fascia</li><li>Scarpa's fascia</li><li>External oblique muscle</li><li>Internal oblique muscle</li><li>Transverse abdominal muscle</li><li>Transversalis fascia</li><li>Parietal peritoneum</li></ul>

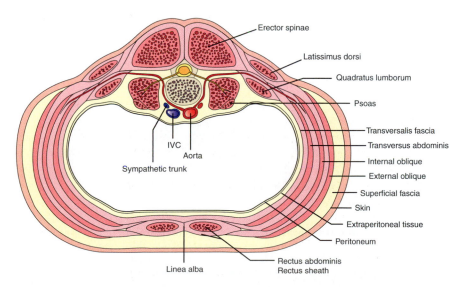

FIGURE 1-17. **Abdominal layers.** The major layers of the abdominal wall are shown, as well as the relation of several retroperitoneal structures.

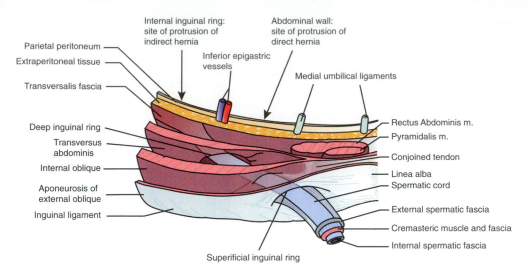

FIGURE 1-18. **Inguinal canal.** The location and contents of the inguinal canal, as well as the abdominal wall layers it traverses, are shown. Other important anatomic relations are also highlighted, including umbilical ligaments and inferior epigastric vessels.

the **spermatic cord** (ductus deferens and gonadal vessels) in males. The canal has two openings, the **internal** (or **deep**) and **external** (or **superficial**) **inguinal rings**. The transversalis fascia evaginates through the abdominal wall and continues as a covering of structures passing through the abdominal wall. The superficial ring is actually an opening through the external oblique aponeurosis.

Retroperitoneum

The posterior abdominal cavity contains several important structures situated between the parietal peritoneum and the posterior abdominal wall. This region, the retroperitoneum, contains portions of the gastrointestinal, genitourinary, endocrine, and cardiovascular systems (see Figure 1-19). The specific structures are listed below:

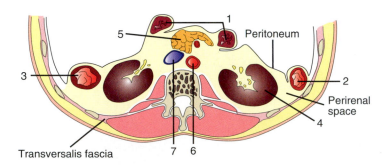

FIGURE 1-19. **Retroperitoneal structures.** The anatomic relations of important retroperitoneal structures are shown, including the duodenum (1; second, third, and fourth sections), descending colon (2), ascending colon (3), kidney and ureters (4), pancreas (5; head and neck), aorta (6), and inferior vena cava (7). The adrenal gland and rectum are not shown.

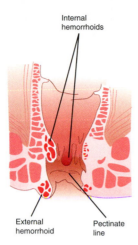

Internal
hemorrhoids

External
hemorrhoid

Pectinate
line

FIGURE 1-20. **Pectinate line.** A comparison of internal hemorrhoids (internal rectal vessels) and external hemorrhoids (external rectal vessels) is shown, highlighting their separation by the pectinate line. The endodermal and ectodermal origins of these structures underlie the anatomic distinction between them.

- Duodenum (second, third, and fourth parts)
- Ascending (right) colon
- Descending (left) colon
- Kidney
- Ureters
- Pancreas (head, neck, and body)
- Aorta
- IVC

The Pectinate Line

The pectinate line is where the ectoderm meets the mesoderm. In the developing embryo, the mesodermally derived hindgut fuses with the ectodermally derived external anal sphincter (see Figure 1-20). Tissues on each side of this boundary are fed by separate neurovascular sources (see Table 1-4).

TABLE 1-4. **Pectinate Line**

CHARACTERISTICS	ABOVE	BELOW
Cell types	Glandular epithelium.	Squamous cells.
Cancer type	Adenocarcinoma.	Squamous cell carcinoma.
Innervation	Visceral.	Somatic.
Hemorrhoids	Internal (painless).	External (painful).
Arterial supply	Superior rectal artery (branch of inferior mesenteric artery).	Inferior rectal artery (branch of inferior pudendal artery).
Venous drainage	Superior rectal vein → inferior mesenteric vein → portal system.	Inferior rectal vein → internal pudendal vein → internal iliac vein.

SPLENIC ANATOMY

The largest secondary lymphatic organ, the spleen, is located in the left superior flank. It is completely surrounded by peritoneum, except at its hilum, where the vasculature enters and exits. It is normally apposed to the underside of the diaphragm, where it rests against the posterior portions of ribs 9–11. Anterior to the spleen lies the stomach. Inferiorly lies the left colic flexure, and medially is the left kidney. The spleen is made up of two parenchymal tissues: **Red pulp** and **white pulp.** The red pulp aids the hematopoietic system by removing senescent and damaged erythrocytes from the circulation. The white pulp provides a location for the hematogenous activation of the humoral immune system.

Red Pulp

The **splenic sinusoids** make up an interconnected network of vascular channels. These are lined by elongated endothelial cells and a discontinuous basement membrane made of reticular fibers (see Figure 1-21). The walls separating the sinusoids are called **splenic cords.** The splenic cords contain plasma

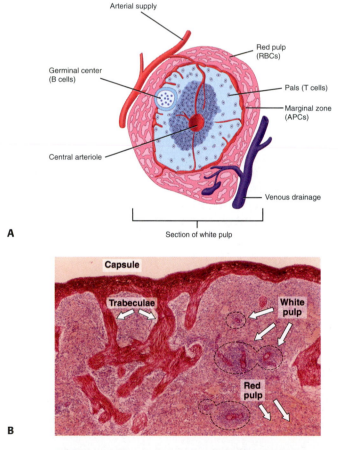

FIGURE 1-21. **Diagram and hisologic section depicting splenic sinusoids.** (A) Schematic diagram of splenic sinusoids. Here, the important regions of the splenic sinusoid are delineated. A central arteriole is surrounded by the T-cell periarterial lymphatic sheath, which is itself surrounded by B cells. A third concentric ring of tissue, the red pulp, contains antigen-presenting cells (APCs) and macrophages to aid in innate and humoral immunity. RBCs = red blood cells. (B) Section of spleen. The capsule is seen sending trabeculae to the interior of the organ. The red pulp occupies most of the microscopic field. Note the white pulp with its arterioles. Picrosirius stain. Low magnification. (Reproduced, with permission, from Junqueira LC, Carneiro J: *Basic Histology: Text and Atlas,* 11th ed. New York: McGraw-Hill, 2005.)

cells, macrophages, and blood cells supported by a connective tissue matrix. Macrophages adjacent to the sinusoids recognize opsonized bacteria, adherent antibodies, foreign antigens, and senescent red cells as they filter through the spleen.

White Pulp

The white pulp is made up of immunologic reinforcements. Arranged around a **central arteriole**, the white pulp contains immune cells in a specific orientation that facilitates immune activation via hematogenously delivered antigens. As an antigen enters the central arteriole, the vasculature branches into radial arterioles (emanating from the central arteriole like spokes of a wheel) and the antigen passes through a surrounding sheath of T cells. This region, known as the periarterial lymphatic sheath, allows for sampling of the arteriolar contents.

If an APC is present, it may activate a number of T cells, which then travel to the adjacent **lymphatic nodule** for B-cell activation. This process produces active germinal centers where B cells mature. Mature B cells, or plasma cells, defend the host via soluble immunoglobulins secreted into the circulation.

The radial arterioles, which branch from the central arteriole, empty their contents into the **marginal zone.** This region of sinusoids between the red pulp and white pulp contains a high concentration of phagocytic APCs (see Figure 1-21).

> **? CLINICAL CORRELATION**
>
> Disordered red cell removal occurs in sickle cell anemia, leading to autosplenectomy and immunodeficiency (against encapsulated bacteria).

THE LYMPHATIC SYSTEM

The Lymph Node

Like **little spleens** dispersed along the lymphatic system, these small secondary lymphatic organs aid regional adaptive immune responses by housing APCs, T cells, and B cells (see Table 1-5). Each node possesses multiple afferent lymphatic channels, which enter the node through its capsule near the cortex. The efferent lymphatics exit at the hilum, along with an artery and vein (see Figure 1-22). From the afferent lymphatics, antigens and APCs in the lymph enter the **medullary sinus.** There, free antigens meet macrophages for phagocytosis and presentation in association with MHC II for T-cell activation. Activated APCs bypass the adjacent **medullary cords** to reach the **para-**

> **≫ FLASH FORWARD**
>
> Acute lymphadenitis occurs when brisk germinal center expansion in response to a local bacterial infection (e.g., teeth or tonsils) leads to painfully swollen lymph nodes.

TABLE 1-5. Lymph Node Organization

REGION	DIVISIONS	CONTENTS AND FUNCTION
Cortex	Follicle (outer cortex)	▪ Primary follicles contain dormant B cells. ▪ Secondary follicles contain active germinal centers.
	Paracortex	▪ Helper T cells reside between follicles and the splenic medulla. ▪ High endothelial venules allow lymphocytes to enter circulation.
Medulla	Sinus	Reticular cells and macrophages communicate with efferent lymphatics.
	Cords	Closely packed lymphocytes and plasma cells.

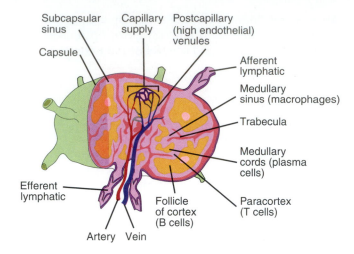

FIGURE 1-22. **Lymph node.** Schematic representation of the lymph node structure shows the major divisions of the node. The medulla consists of cords of plasma cells and sinuses of macrophages. The cortex consists of dormant and activated B-cell follicles, as well as a T-cell paracortex.

cortex, where T cells await stimulation. Activated T cells move to the adjacent **cortical follicle**, where B cells await costimulatory signals. Once activated, mature B cells travel back to the medullary cords, where they develop into plasma cells and secrete immunoglobulins into the adjacent vascular supply.

Lymphatics

As part of the cardiovascular system, the lymphatic vessels **drain interstitial fluid from surrounding tissues** (see Tables 1-6 and 1-7). They are also integral to the process of transporting fats and fat-soluble nutrients and facilitating the humoral immune response. Their role in immunity involves carrying foreign antigens and APCs to lymph nodes for T- and B-cell activation.

The lymph vessels are analogous to veins in their structure and organization. However, rather than originating from capillary systems, they begin as blind sacs. The walls of the lymphatic capillary are made up of a layer of loosely bound endothelial cells, lacking tight junctions and bound to an incomplete basal lamina. This allows fluid to enter the lumen via hydrostatic pressure. As distal lymphatic capillaries merge, they produce larger vessels containing valves, just like veins, that maintain the direction of flow. In addition to interstitial hydrostatic pressure, muscular contractions aid the flow of lymph.

During its course back to the systemic circulation, lymphatic fluid is filtered through lymph nodes for immune surveillance. The remaining lymph reaches the bloodstream via one of two major routes: The larger **thoracic duct** or the smaller **right lymphatic duct**.

TABLE 1-6. **Lymph Drainage Routes**

DRAINAGE ROUTE	ANATOMIC REGIONS DRAINED
Right lymphatic duct	Right arm, right half of head
Thoracic duct	All other regions

TABLE 1-7. Lymph Drainage Routes

ANATOMIC REGION	MAJOR LYMPH NODES
Head and neck	Submental, submandibular, retroauricular, parotid, occipital, superficial and deep cervical.
Breast	Axillary (pectoral, subscapular, humeral, apical, central) Parasternal, supra- and infraclavicular.
Gastrointestinal tract	Celiac, mesenteric, paracolic, and supraclavicular.
Gonads	Lumbar and preaortic.
Perineum	Superficial and deep inguinal.
Upper extremity	Cubital, humeral axillary, and deltopectoral.
Lower extremity	Superficial inguinal, external iliac, and deep inguinal.

PERIPHERAL NERVOUS SYSTEM

Nerve Cells

During embryonic development, **neural crest cells** migrate into the peripheral tissues, where they differentiate into **neurons** of the following tissues:

- Sensory neurons of the dorsal root ganglia.
- Neurons of the cranial nerve ganglia.
- Neurons of the autonomic system.
- Neurons of the myenteric plexus.

These neurons, the functional units of the peripheral nervous system, contain three major parts: The cell body (or **soma**), **dendrites**, and **axons**.

- The cell body houses the organelles (including the notable nucleus and the well-developed RER, referred to as the **Nissl body**).
- Dendrites are cytoplasmic processes arising from the soma that provide increased surface area for axonal synaptic connections, thus facilitating the reception and integration of information.
- Each neuron, in addition to multiple dendrites, has one axon, sprouting from the soma at the **axon hillock** and ending in a **synaptic terminal**, or **bouton.**

Because neurons are specialized for signal transduction, they can secrete several different **neurotransmitters.** These peptide molecules are produced in the RER, stored in secretory vesicles, transported through the axon along microtubules via molecular motors, and eventually released from the axon into the **synaptic cleft.** The synaptic cleft is the junction between the synaptic terminal and an adjacent cell. This vesicular secretion, which is triggered by a transmitted action potential, is the primary method of neural control.

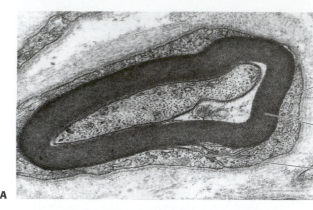

Schwann cell
cytoplasm

Myelin

Mesaxon

A

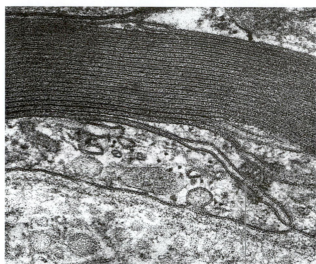

B

Outer mesaxon

FIGURE 1-23. **Electron micrographs of a myelinated nerve fiber.** (A) × 20,000. (B) × 80,000. (Reproduced, with permission, from Junqueira JC, Carneiro J. *Basic Histology: Text and Atlas*, 11th ed. New York: McGraw-Hill, 2005: 173.)

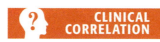

Myelin proteins can be highly antigenic, leading to autoimmune disorders, such as Guillain-Barré syndrome.

Neuroglia

The **Schwann cell**, also a descendent of neural crest cells, envelops neurons in cytoplasmic processes that wrap around the neuron several times. This encapsulation produces segments of **myelin sheathing** (see Figure 1-23) that extend from the axon hillock to the axon terminal. Between each segment is a naked region of the axon called the **node of Ranvier**; each myelinated segment is referred to as an **internode**.

Peripheral Nerve

Composed of multiple neuronal axons, Schwann cells, and protective connective tissues, the peripheral nerve carries impulses from the central nervous system to the most distal parts of the body, and everywhere in between. Although individual neurons are surrounded by Schwann cells, a nerve fiber is more complex (see Figure 1-24). The most external layer of a nerve, known as the **epineurium**, is a dense connective tissue layer that covers the entire nerve, including its vascular supply. Beneath this layer lie the vessels and the **perineurium**. The perineurium acts as a permeability barrier, regulating nutrient transport from capillaries to the nerve fibers below. The perineurium invests a number of nerve **fascicles**, bundles of individual nerves surrounded

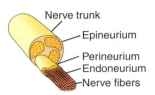

FIGURE 1-24.   **Peripheral nerve layers.**

by the **endoneurium**. This final connective tissue layer maintains the presence of Schwann cells, which create the **myelin sheaths** and **nodes of Ranvier**, necessary for fast neuronal conduction.

Dermatomes

Usually, successive spinal levels innervate successively caudal regions. Figure 1-25 displays the dermatomal organization of the body, as projected on the skin.

Brachial Plexus

The motor portions of spinal nerves are organized differently from the sensory neurons. Instead of clear divisions organized by spinal level that serve successively distal regions of the body, a great deal of mixing of neurons from each spinal level produces a single nerve supplying a specific muscle group. The upper extremity's **brachial plexus** is a prime example. As motor neurons exit the spinal column between C5 and T1, the ventral rami begin to exchange individual fibers. These rami are considered the **roots** of the brachial plexus (see Figure 1-26).

As the five roots reach the inferior portion of the neck, C5 and C6 unite to form the **superior trunk**, as C8 and T1 unite to form the **inferior trunk**, leaving C7 as the **middle trunk**. These three trunks pass beneath the clavicle, where they each split into **anterior** and **posterior divisions**. The anterior divisions of the superior and middle trunks merge to form the **lateral cord of**

KEY FACT

Following trauma, the perineurium must be repaired via microsurgery to ensure proper nerve regeneration and functional restoration.

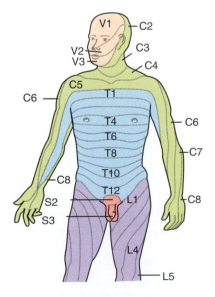

Important Dermatomes	
Forehead	V1
Nipples	T4
Umbilicus	T10
Anus	S5
Thumb	C6
Knee	L3/4
Great toe	L5

FIGURE 1-25.   **Landmark dermatomes.**

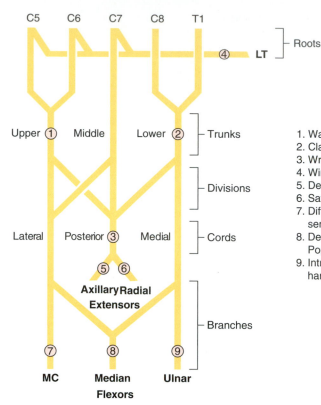

1. Waiter's tip (Erb's palsy)
2. Claw hand (Klumpke's palsy)
3. Wrist drop
4. Winged scapula
5. Deltoid paralysis
6. Saturday night palsy (wrist drop)
7. Difficulty flexing elbow, variable sensory loss
8. Decreased thumb function, Pope's blessing
9. Intrinsic muscles of hand, claw hand

FIGURE 1-26. Brachial plexus.

the brachial plexus, while the anterior division of the inferior trunk becomes the **medial cord.** Both of these cords will eventually supply the muscles of the anterior compartments of the arm. All three posterior divisions merge to form the **posterior cord,** which supplies the posterior compartments of the arm. From cords, the plexus divides further into its terminal infraclavicular **branches.** The major infraclavicular and supraclavicular nerve branches are listed in Table 1-8. Common injuries associated with the brachial plexus are listed in Table 1-9.

TABLE 1-8. Principal Branches of the Brachial Plexus

BRANCH	ROOT	INNERVATION
Long thoracic	Ventral rami of C5–C7	Serratus anterior.
Suprascapular	Superior trunk, C4–C6	Supraspinatus, infraspinatus.
Musculocutaneous	Lateral cord, C5–C7	Coracobrachialis, biceps brachii, brachialis.
Median	Medial and lateral cords, C6–T1	All forearm flexors (except flexor carpi ulnaris), abductor pollicis brevis, opponens pollicis, flexor pollicis longus, first and second lumbricals.
Ulnar	Medial cord, C7–T1	Flexor carpi ulnaris, flexor digitorum profundus, other intrisnsic hand muscles.
Axillary	Posterior cord, C5, C6	Teres minor, deltoid.
Radial	Posterior cord, C5–T1	Triceps brachii, brachioradialis, extensors.

TABLE 1-9. Common Brachial Plexus Injuries

Lesion Location	Syndrome	Deficits
Superior trunk C5/C6	Erb-Duchenne palsy ("waiter's tip").	▪ Abduction (deltoid). ▪ Lateral rotation (infraspinatus, teres minor). ▪ Supination (biceps).
Inferior trunk C8/T1	Interphalangeal joint extension and metacarpophalangeal joint flexion paralysis (full "claw hand").	Intrinsic muscles of hand, forearm flexors of hand.
Posterior cord C5/6/7/8	Axillary and radial nerve paralyses.	Same as for axillary and radial nerves.
Long thoracic nerve T1	Winged scapula.	Serratus anterior paralysis.
Axillary nerve	Deltoid paralysis.	Abduction.
Radial nerve	"Saturday night palsy."	Wrist drop (supinator, brachioradialis, triceps, extensors of wrist/fingers).
Musculocutaneous nerve	Biceps paralysis.	Elbow flexion, arm sensation.
Median nerve	"Pope's blessing" on making a fist.	Thumb abduction, thumb opposition, fourth/fifth digit extension.
Ulnar nerve	Fourth/fifth digit paralysis (partial "claw hand").	Grip strength, fourth/fifth digit flexion/extension, intrinsic muscles of hand.

THE INTEGUMENTARY SYSTEM

Skin

The skin has several functions:

- Mechanical protection
- Moisture retention
- Body temperature regulation
- Nonspecific immune defense
- Salt excretion
- Vitamin D synthesis
- Tactile sensation

The skin is composed of three layers: The **epidermis** (ectodermally derived), the **deep dermis** (endodermally derived), and the **hypodermis**, or subcutaneous tissues.

EPIDERMIS

The epidermis is predominantly made of **keratinocytes**, or epithelial cells named for the intermediate filament protein **keratin.** The epidermis is organized into five layers (see Figure 1-27).

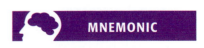

MNEMONIC

Layers of the epidermis:

Californians **L**ike **G**irls in **S**tring **B**ikinis.

Stratum **C**orneum
Stratum **L**ucidum
Stratum **G**ranulosum
Stratum **S**pinosum
Stratum **B**asalis

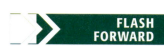

FIGURE 1-27. Epidermis layers.

The **stratum basalis** is composed of columnar keratinocytes bound to a basement membrane via hemidesmosomes. Cellular proliferation occurring at this level maintains the population of epidermal stem cells, replenishes sloughed skin cells, and contributes to epidermal wound healing. These columnar keratinocytes undergo a process of differentiation, during which time they become progressively flattened and superficially located. At the level of the **stratum spinosum**, keratinocytes have a flattened polygonal shape and an ovoid nucleus. By the time they reach the **stratum corneum**, they are completely flattened and lack nuclei.

The epidermis also contains other cell types: **melanocytes, Langerhans' cells**, and **Merkel cells.**

- Melanocytes, derived from the neural crest, produce **melanin**, a tyrosine derivative responsible for skin pigmentation.
- Langerhans' cells are bone marrow–derived dendritic cells residing in the skin. Once activated, they migrate to secondary lymph organs to present antigens to T cells.
- Merkel cells, found in the stratum basalis, contribute to the function of the numerous **mechanoreceptors** present in the epidermis. A myelinated sensory axon actually ends in an unmyelinated portion, called the **nerve plate**, which synapses on the Merkel cell. This synapse allows the Merkel cell to signal tactile sensation.

In addition to Merkel cells, two other specialized sensory structures exist within the body: **Meissner's corpuscles** in the dermis and **Pacinian corpuscles** in the deep tissues (see Figure 1-28).

DERMIS

The epidermis is anchored to its basement membrane by hemidesmosomes. Two indistinct layers, the **papillary layer** and the **reticular layer,** reside just below. The papillary layer (primarily loose connective tissue) consists of fibroblasts, collagen, and elastic fibers, while the reticular layer contains mostly collagen and elastic fibers.

SKIN APPENDAGES

Skin appendages (**hair follicles, sweat glands**, and **sebaceous glands**) are present in the dermis, as is the blood supply to the skin (see Figure 1-29). Hair shafts are made of hardened keratin, while the follicular bulb where the hair originates contains stem cells capable of repopulating the follicular shaft, or even the epidermis following injury. Sebaceous glands are oil-producing glands that actually empty their contents into the hair follicle, the tubular invagination that the hair shaft follows as it grows to the surface. Sweat glands occur in two forms. The **eccrine** sweat gland is a ubiquitous coiled

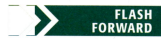

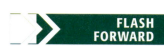
FLASH FORWARD

Autoantigens against cellular adhesion molecules lead to debilitating blistering diseases such as bullous pemphigoid.

FLASH FORWARD

A deficiency in **tyrosinase** leads to **albinism,** a congenital lack of melanin.

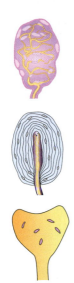

Meissner's - Small, encapsulated nerve endings found in the dermis of palms, soles, and digits of skin. Involved in light discriminatory touch of glabrous (hairless).

Pacinian - Large, encapsulated nerve endings found in deeper layers of skin at ligaments, joint capsules, serous membranes, and mesenteries. Involved in pressure, coarse touch, vibration, and tension.

Merkel's - Cup-shaped nerve endings (tactile disks) in dermis of fingertips, hair follicles, hard palate. Involved in light, and crude touch.

FIGURE 1-28. Sensory corpuscles.

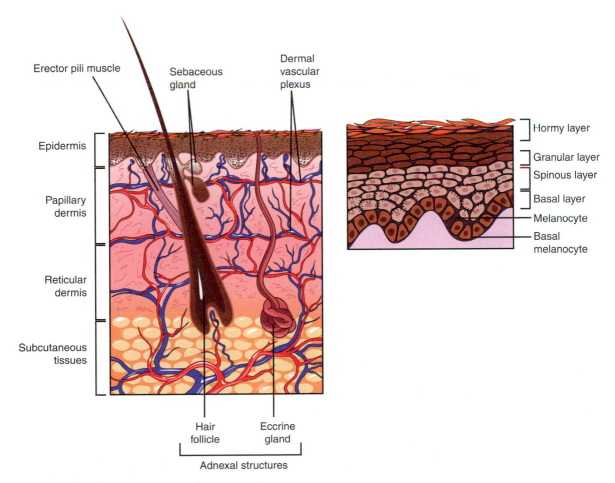

FIGURE 1-29. Skin appendages. The histologic schematic representation of skin (left) demonstrates a complex organization of cells, connective tissue, blood vessels, and adnexal structures. The drawing (upper right) depicts the orderly maturation of keratinocytes in the epidermis. The electron micrograph (lower right) shows details of the basement membrane, which is the interface between the epidermis and the dermis.

gland innervated by cholinergic nerves and used in temperature regulation. The **apocrine** glands, regulated by adrenergic stimuli, only become active following puberty. These coiled glands are found in the axilla, mons pubis, and circumanal regions.

THE RESPIRATORY SYSTEM

Respiratory Histology

Once air has traveled through the **air-conducting** channels (nasal cavities, nasopharynx, oropharynx, larynx, trachea, bronchi, and bronchioles), it enters the **respiratory tissues.** These include the respiratory bronchioles, alveolar ducts, alveolar sacs, and alveoli.

BRONCHI AND BRONCHIOLES

Except for their smallest divisions, these airways are involved in conducting inhaled air to the lung, rather than gas exchange. Primarily, the walls of the conducting airways contain a **pseudostratified columnar ciliated epithelium**, composed of three cell types:

- **Ciliated epithelial cells:** Coordinated ciliary motion helps to expel respiratory secretions that have collected pathogens and debris from inspired air.
- **Goblet cells:** Produce mucus and protect the airway and lung tissue from inspired particles.
- **Basal cells:** Provide structural support to the airway.

ALVEOLUS

Despite the many subdivisions of lung tissue, the basic functional unit is the alveolus. The lungs contain about 300 million alveoli, which increase the surface area for gas exchange to approximately 75 m². Each alveolar wall consists of two cell types, **type I** and **type II alveolar cells**, with each serving separate physiologic functions (see Figures 1-30 and 1-31).

Continuous with the low cuboidal epithelium of the adjacent respiratory bronchiole, 90% of the alveolar surface is covered with type I alveolar cells. This anatomic arrangement allows deoxygenated blood to come into close proximity with O_2 inhaled from the environment. In fact, the primary function of the type I alveolar cell, a simple squamous epithelial cell, is to form the first layer of the **air-blood barrier.** Below the type I cells lay a dual basal lamina and endothelial cells of the alveolar capillaries, completing a semipermeable barrier permissive of O_2 and CO_2 diffusion.

The type II alveolar cell, also known as the **Clara cell**, or **C cell**, is normally located at the angles formed by adjacent alveolar septa. Their primary function is the production of pulmonary surfactant. However, C cells also act as progenitors to the type I cell, differentiating, proliferating, and repopulating the alveolar surface during periods of injury and repair.

Lung Anatomy

The lungs are enveloped in serosal tissue, known as **pleura**, which has two layers. Apposed directly to the lung is the **visceral pleura.** The **parietal pleura** is adherent to the chest wall. Fluid within the potential space between the visceral and parietal pleura allows respiratory tissues to slide effortlessly as the lung expands.

KEY FACT

Type II pneumocytes are precursors to type I cells and produce surfactant.

FLASH FORWARD

Pulmonary surfactant reduces the surface tension at the air-fluid interface, thus decreasing the tendency for alveolar collapse.

FLASH FORWARD

Amniotic fluid surfactant levels can be used as a surrogate measure of fetal lung maturity. Steroids are given to premature infants to increase pneumocyte surfactant production.

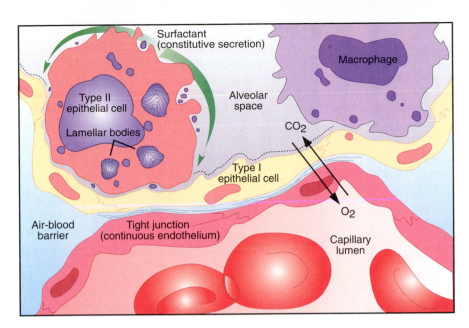

FIGURE 1-30. **Gas exchange barrier.** The thickness of the gas exchange barrier is highlighted, as well as the anatomic relations of important cell types: type I and type II epithelial cells, endothelial cells, macrophages, and red cells.

Each lung is divided into **lobes**, which are further divided into **bronchopulmonary segments.** Each bronchopulmonary segment corresponds to a branch of the **bronchial tree** that delivers O_2 to the lung. The right lung is composed of three lobes, and the left lung, two. However, the superior lobe of the left lung contains a region, the **lingula**, which is analogous to the right lung's middle lobe. The **cardiac notch**, into which the apex of the heart protrudes, replaces the middle lobe. The bronchial tree begins at the trachea, which branches into right and left **main stem bronchi.** The left is slightly longer, while the right makes a shallower angle (runs more vertically), with the trachea at its bifurcation.

The major vascular supply to each lung begins as a single branch of the **pulmonary artery** (carrying deoxygenated blood) and ends as two **pulmonary veins** (carrying oxygenated blood to the left atrium). Between these large ves-

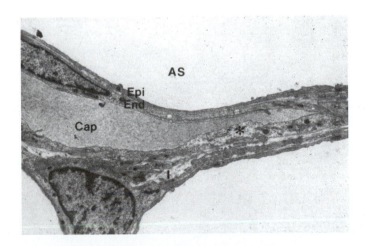

FIGURE 1-31. **Alveolar wall electron microscopy.** Electron microscopy shows a capillary lumen (Cap), an endothelial cell (End), a type I endothelial cell (Epi), and the alveolar space (AS). (Image courtesy of PEIR Digital Library [http://peir.net].)

sels, the vasculature branches into intrasegmental pulmonary arteries, which travel with branching airways. These end in capillary networks, within the alveolar septae, that facilitate gas exchange. In addition to the pulmonary vessels, the **bronchial circulation** aids in supporting the respiratory tissues. Originating from the aorta, blood from the bronchial circulation is dumped into the pulmonary venous circulation after passing through the lung. Although it is relatively deoxygenated, it mixes with recently oxygenated blood and is delivered to the left atrium.

ANATOMIC RELATIONS

The lungs reside within the rib cage, under the protection of the bony skeleton. The apices are at the level of the first rib, while the bases rest in the left and right costodiaphragmatic recesses. Along the midclavicular line, the lung can be auscultated from just above the clavicle to the seventh or eighth rib. Posteriorly, the lung extends more distally, deep into the costodiaphragmatic recess, at the 11th or 12th rib.

Within the chest, each of the three lung surfaces (**mediastinal**, **costal**, and **diaphragmatic**) is in close proximity to important structures.

- **Mediastinal surface:** Marks the lateral extent of the **mediastinum**, which houses the heart, great vessels, esophagus, trachea, thoracic duct, bronchial hilum, and hilar lymph nodes, as well as the vagus and phrenic nerves.
- **Costal surface:** Primarily contacts the inside of the chest wall. As mentioned previously, two layers of pleura exist between the functional lung tissue and chest wall.
- **Diaphragmatic surface:** The diaphragm, the major muscle of respiration, resides just below each lung.

The diaphragm, a thin sheet of muscle separating the thorax and abdomen, is innervated by the **phrenic nerves**, which originate from cervical roots C3, C4, and C5. A number of vital structures cross the diaphragm to pass from the thoracic to the abdominal cavity. In particular, the **aorta**, **esophagus**, and **inferior vena cava** (IVC) each pierce the diaphragm at different thoracic vertebral levels. The IVC, the most anterior of the three structures, crosses at the level of T8. The esophagus crosses at T10 and the aorta crosses at T12 (see Figure 1-32).

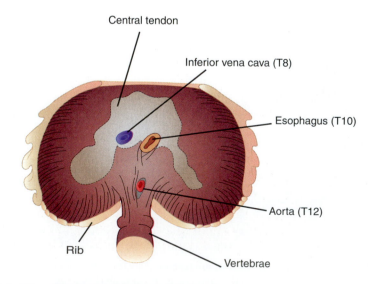

FIGURE 1-32. **Diaphragm structures.** Inferior view.

THE GASTROINTESTINAL SYSTEM

Small Intestinal Layers

The major organ of nutrient absorption from the gut, the small intestine is composed of several layers, each contributing to the coordination of digestion and transport.

- **Mucosa:** Absorption.
- **Submucosa:** Vascular and lymphatic supply.
- **Muscularis externa:** Mechanical mixing, dissociation, and propulsion.
- **Serosa:** Protection.

MUCOSA

The absorption barrier of the alimentary canal. Composed of polarized epithelial cells specialized in transport, the intestinal mucosa uses several molecular and structural adaptations that allow it to efficiently extract nutrients from digesting food.

Structurally, the mucosa has four adaptations that increase the absorptive surface area:

- **Plicae circulares** (circular folds, or **folds of Kerking**)
- **Intestinal villi**
- **Intestinal glands**
- **Microvilli** on the apical epithelium

A plicae circularis is a permanent folding of the mucosa and submucosa into the lumen of the intestine. Their distribution is not uniform throughout the intestine, but instead begins within the duodenum, peaks at the duodenojejunal junction, and ends at the mid-ileum. Intestinal villi, on the other hand, are near-uniform finger-like projections of the mucosa into the lumen. These projections extend deep into the mucosa, to the **muscularis mucosa**, the boundary between the mucosa and the submucosa and ending in **intestinal glands** known as **crypts of Lieberkühn**. These glands are not actually secretory glands, but rather exist to enhance absorption.

Finally, each **enterocyte**, or intestinal epithelial cell, contains microvilli on its apical border. This **brush border** increases the surface area approximately 30-fold. Microscopically, the microvillus contains a core of parallel cross-linked actin filaments bound to cytoskeletal proteins. The brush border is coated in a **glycocalyx**, a surface coat of glycoproteins excreted by columnar secretory **goblet cells.** In addition, the luminal membrane contains several intramembranous enzymes (e.g., maltase, lactase, enterokinase) integral to digestion and small molecule absorption. Intracytoplasmic enzymes break down absorbed di- and tripeptides.

SUBMUCOSA

The site of vascular and lymphatic supply to the intestine. This layer, composed of loose connective tissue, contains a vascular plexus that extends capillaries into the surrounding layers. The lymphatic drainage of the submucosa begins as blind-ended channels, known as **lacteals**, within the core of the intestinal villi. These lacteals empty into a submucosal lymphatic plexus that shuttles antigens to nearby lymphatic nodules and emulsified fat-soluble nutrients to the liver.

FLASH BACK

Molecularly, the intestinal epithelium employs cell adhesion molecules to determine polarity and maintain the physical barrier between the body and the intestinal lumen (external environment).

FLASH FORWARD

Defects in lactase activity lead to lactose intolerance. Loss of other intramembranous enzymes (e.g., enterocyte toxicity following chemotherapy) leads to osmotic diarrhea.

CLINICAL CORRELATION

Invasive adenocarcinomas that reach the submucosa are able to metastasize via the rich lymphatic and vascular plexus.

Within the **duodenum**, the submucosa contains **Brunner glands**, tubuloacinar mucus glands that produce an alkaline (pH ~ 9) secretion to neutralize acidified chyme from the stomach. Within the **ilium** reside the lymphatic nodules that provide immunologic surveillance to the intestines.

These nodules, also known as **Peyer's patches** or **gut-associated lymphoid tissue (GALT)**, contain a germinal center of B cells surrounded by specialized APCs: **M cells** and dendritic cells. Antigens enter the Peyer's patch through antigen presentation via M cells and dendritic cells. The B cells of the GALT germinal center are specialized; they produce a specific immunoglobulin, **IgA**, which can be secreted into the intestinal lumen to neutralize pathogens before they invade the epithelium.

The submucosa also houses one of the two neural plexus located within the small intestine. Considered part of the autonomic system, these neural networks receive a great deal of intrinsic input from the intestinal parenchyma. This allows the gut to operate nearly independently from the central nervous system, although its action can be modulated via extensive extrinsic neural input. Two networks control the activity of the small intestine: The submucosal **plexus of Meissner** and the **myenteric plexus of Auerbach.** They are extensively interconnected and probably equally modulate mucosal and muscular activity, coordinating action to maximize digestion.

MUSCULARIS EXTERNA

Intestinal motility is controlled by two layers of smooth muscle. One circular layer is surrounded by a second longitudinal layer (Auerbach's plexus resides between these two layers). Coordinated muscular contraction produces two types of mechanical results: **Propulsion** and **segmentation.**

FLASH FORWARD

Dysfunction of the plexus, due to either congenital absence (Hirschsprung's disease) or neurologic injury (diabetic neuropathy), leads to decreased intestinal motility.

- **Propulsion** occurs when proximal contraction is coordinated with distal relaxation. This leads to increased upstream pressure, which slowly propels food through the digestive system. Contraction of proximal sphincters ensures that the food bolus only moves distally.
- **Segmentation** occurs when a bolus of food is mechanically compressed and split into two portions as the lumen constricts near the bolus center, not merely proximal to it. If this contraction is not coordinated with distal relaxation, the bolus cannot be propelled forward. Instead, its contents are mixed by the muscular contractions.

SEROSA

The serosa is composed of visceral peritoneum covering the small intestine. It is lined by a simple squamous epithelium.

THE ADRENAL SYSTEM

Adrenal Gland

Situated atop the kidney, the adrenal gland has an outer **cortex** surrounding an inner **medulla.** The mesodermally derived cortex produces **steroid hormones**, while the neuroectodermally derived medulla produces **catecholamines.**

CORTEX

Three-story steroid hormone factory. Each of the three layers of the cortex (see Figure 1-33) expresses specific enzymes for producing steroid hormones built from a cholesterol precursor.

- **Zona glomerulosa:** The outermost layer, which produces salt-regulating **aldosterone.**
- **Zona fasciculata:** The middle layer, which produces the stress hormone **cortisol.**
- **Zona reticularis:** The innermost layer, which produces sex hormones **(androgens).**

The zona glomerulosa is a region of concentrically arranged secretory epithelial cells, surrounded by a vascularized stroma. Residing just below the protective fibrous capsule of the gland, these cells are marked by a well-developed SER producing the mineralocorticoid aldosterone. **Angiotensin II,** produced in the lung, can trigger both release of aldosterone and hypertrophy of the zona glomerulosa.

The functional distinctions between the zona fasciculata and zona reticularis are less well developed, as are their morphologic boundaries. These regions are often treated as a functional unit. The columns of polygonal cells in the zona fasciculata occupy the majority of the cortex. Fenestrated capillaries intersperse these fascicles, delivering **corticotropin (ACTH)** to regulate cortisol secretion back into the capillaries for systemic delivery. The zona reticularis, rather than forming columns or concentric circles, forms a network of cells, also surrounded by fenestrated capillaries for regulation by plasma ACTH.

MEDULLA

The adrenal medulla oversees the systemic stress response. **Epinephrine** and **norepinephrine** (NE), two tyrosine-derived chemical messengers of the systemic stress response, are produced here. Although NE is also released within

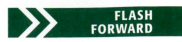

FLASH FORWARD

Deficiencies in enzymes of the adrenal gland lead to defects in physiology and sexual development.

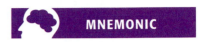

MNEMONIC

The **deeper** you go, the **sweeter** it gets:
Zona glomerulosa: **Salt** hormones (aldosterone)
Zona fasciculata: **Sugar** hormones (glucocorticoids)
Zona reticularis: **Sex** hormones (androgens)

FLASH FORWARD

Catecholamine breakdown products, vanillylmandelic acid (VMA) and metanephrine, can be measured in the urine to determine systemic catecholamine levels.

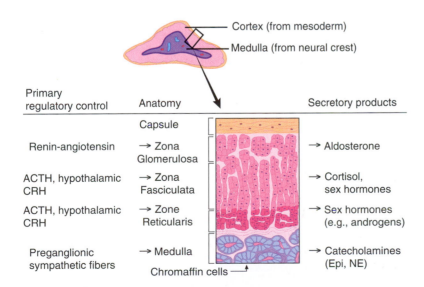

FIGURE 1-33. Schematic depiction of the cortex of the adrenal gland. ACTH = corticotropin; CRH = corticotropin-releasing hormone; Epi = epinephrine; NE = norepinephrine.

FLASH FORWARD

The most common tumors of the adrenal gland are adenomas from the cortex, neuroblastomas from medullary neural crest cells, and pheochromocytomas arising from the medullary chromaffin cells.

the synaptic cleft of adrenergic neurons, these catecholamines are released in bulk into the venous sinusoids of the medulla. In fact, the adrenal medulla, like the autonomic nervous system, is derived from the neuroectoderm. They also receive innervation from sympathetic presynaptic neurons, thus acting as a modified sympathetic postganglionic neuron.

The medullary secretory cells, **chromaffin cells**, synthesize either epinephrine (80%) or norepinephrine (20%), but not both. These secretory products are produced from tyrosine, rather than cholesterol, as in the cortex.

Behavioral Science

Epidemiology

Increasingly, emphasis has been placed on the concept of evidence-based medicine. Every year, more questions about the techniques used to conduct research and interpret basic tests appear on Step 1. An understanding of the methodology and interpretation of research studies and the significance of diagnostic test results is very helpful.

Common types of questions include:

- Given a description of the population studied and the methods used, what type of study is this?
- Given a description of the study population and the goals of the research, what type of study is most appropriate?
- Perform common calculations and understand the mathematical definitions and significance of terms such as "false-positive" and "false-negative."

STUDY METHODS

Studies can be divided into two types, purely observational and experimental. **Observational studies** look at events that will happen with little or no manipulation by the person performing the study. **Experimental studies** often require the person performing the study to assemble subjects, design a study protocol, and perform some type of intervention.

Observational Studies

CASE STUDY OR CASE SERIES

A written description of a patient or particular problem, generally used to document a unique manifestation of a disease, the first incidence of a new disease, or some clinical presentation that might be of interest to other physicians. A case series is simply a collection of case studies that document a similar patient presentation or disease manifestation.

Example: Case studies began to appear in the early 1980s that documented rare opportunistic infections in apparently healthy young patients. These were some of the earliest documentations of HIV/AIDS before the disease was recognized.

CROSS-SECTIONAL STUDY

Assesses a population of patients at a given point in time. It answers basic questions, such as, "In a given population, how many people have a disease?" or "How many people have risk factors in population X?" Think of a cross-sectional study as a large survey taken at a point in time.

Example: In the 1980s, some physicians noticed that hemophiliacs had a high incidence of AIDS. To determine how many hemophiliacs had HIV/AIDS in 1988, a cross-sectional study, or survey, could have been performed of this population to find that the number was over 50%.

CASE-CONTROL STUDY

Compares two groups of people: Those with a condition or disease versus similar persons without the condition or disease. Once a person with the condition is identified (a case), he or she is matched with a demographically similar person without the condition (control). The two groups are then compared for differences that may provide insight into possible causes or risk factors, as illustrated in Figure 2-1.

Example: To determine why some hemophiliacs contracted HIV/AIDS in the 1980s when many others did not, a case-control study was performed. A group of HIV-positive hemophiliacs was identified, and each case was matched to an age-, sex-, race-, and location-control hemophiliac who did not contract the disease. When the data were analyzed for differences between the two groups, it was found that the HIV-positive hemophiliacs were far more likely to have received more blood transfusions than the controls.

COHORT STUDY

Examines a large group and watches it evolve over time. Generally, at the outset, the participants do not have the condition or disease being studied. It is expected that some individuals in the study will develop the condition or complication being studied. This is shown in Figure 2-2.

Example: To determine the risk of HIV transmission in IV drug users, identify a cohort of HIV-negative IV drug users and follow them for 10 years.

Experimental Studies

CLINICAL TRIAL

A direct test of a drug, technique, or other intervention. Subjects are divided into at least two groups, with one group acting as a control that receives either a placebo or the current standard of care treatment. The other group is given the intervention being studied (see Figure 2-3). Often, such trials are double-blind, meaning that neither the subjects nor the experimenters know who is receiving the actual treatment and who is receiving the placebo.

Example: To test a new HIV drug, similar HIV subjects are recruited and divided randomly into treatment and placebo groups. Experimenters do not know who is receiving the actual drug versus the placebo. At the end of the experiment, the group assignment is revealed to allow for comparison of the outcomes.

 KEY FACT

In a case-control study, the cases already have a condition or illness, and controls are chosen **retrospectively**. In a cohort study, participants do not yet have a condition or illness; thus, they are observed **prospectively**.

 KEY FACT

The Framingham Heart Study is a very well-known cohort study that has followed the residents of Framingham, Massachusetts, for decades. Over 1000 papers on cardiac health have come out of this study.

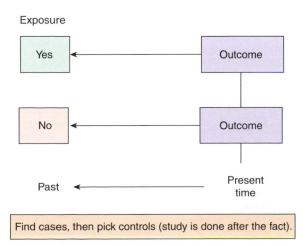

FIGURE 2-1.   Case-control study.

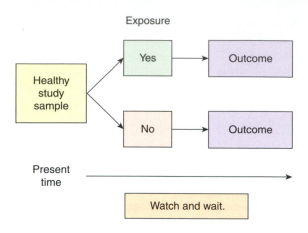

FIGURE 2-2. **Cohort study.**

CROSS-OVER STUDY

Participants are randomized into one of two treatment groups, with the control group often given a placebo. After the experiment is performed once, however, participants are switched, or crossed over, into the opposite treatment group and the experiment is run again. Thus each participant receives both treatments at different times and can act as his or her own control. In essence, this is a variation of a case-control study; it is illustrated in Figure 2-4.

Example: A drug that may temporarily raise CD4 T-cell counts in HIV-positive individuals is being tested. Half of the subjects are assigned to a treatment group the other half to a placebo group, and the effects are measured. Because the effect is not permanent, one could repeat the experiment with switched groups. One can compare each subject's response to the drug and the placebo.

META-ANALYSIS

Combines the data from many preexisting studies on the same topic to produce what is essentially one big study. It is not necessary to understand the statistical techniques for the USMLE.

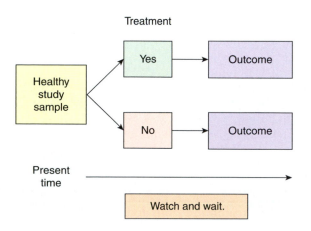

FIGURE 2-3. **Clinical trial.**

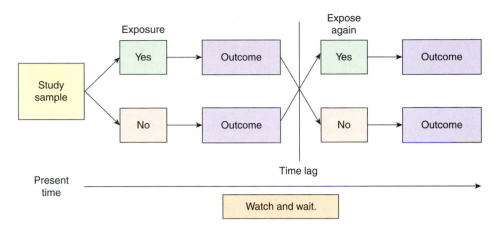

FIGURE 2-4.   Cross-over study.

Example: Many studies have assessed the effectiveness of treatments to prevent immunosuppression in HIV. However, no one study is large enough to state unequivocally that the treatment is truly effective. By combining the results of multiple studies, more definitive conclusions are possible.

Any time studies are combined, think meta-analysis. A meta-analysis is only as good as the studies it combines. Even when the studies are based on good data, it is hard to accurately combine studies because the methodology of each must be controlled.

All studies described above are compared in Table 2-1.

TABLE 2-1.   Comparison of Study Types

Case Studies/Case Series	Cross-Sectional Studies
▪ Easy.	▪ Fairly easy.
▪ Purely descriptive.	▪ Purely descriptive.
▪ Do not address causality.	▪ Do not address causality.
▪ Do NOT provide prevalence statistics or other epidemiologic data.	▪ DO NOT provide prevalence statistics or other epidemiologic data.
Case-Control Studies	**Cohort Studies**
▪ Retrospective.	▪ Prospective.
▪ Can be quick.	▪ Can take a long time.
▪ Do NOT provide prevalence statistics or other epidemiologic data.	▪ Do provide prevalence statistics or other epidemiologic data.
▪ Good for rare diseases.	▪ Not good for rare diseases.
Clinical Trials	**Cross-Over Studies**
▪ Good if effect is permanent.	▪ Good if the effect is temporary.
▪ Prone to bias.	▪ Prone to bias and unanticipated permanent effects.
▪ Gold standard if randomized and blinded.	

BIAS

In statistics, bias refers to any part of the study that **may inadvertently favor one outcome or result over another**. Bias is often unintentional, but has the potential to invalidate conclusions. It is possible to detect certain forms of bias by analyzing the study in question.

Types of Bias

CONFOUNDING BIAS

Can occur when one variable is closely related to another. If the researcher does not appreciate the relationship, the incorrect variable may be measured.

Example: A scientist notes that certain people stand outside every day during their breaks at work. He also notices that these same people often develop lung cancer. He collects data and finds that the more time one spends standing outside during work breaks, the more likely one is to develop lung cancer. He concludes that being outside causes lung cancer. In reality, of course, the people who stand outside a lot develop lung cancer because they smoke.

SAMPLING BIAS

Occurs when the sample of people chosen for the study (or one group within the study) is not representative of the pool from which they were chosen.

Example: To test a new treatment for diabetes, 1000 men over the age of 65 are enrolled in a study. The drug appears to be effective in controlling symptoms. However, when marketed to the general population, the results are less favorable because the original study excluded younger patients or females, who respond poorly to the medication.

RECALL BIAS

When people are asked to recall information retrospectively, they are often biased by knowledge gained after the fact, such as whether they received a placebo or a real drug.

Example: At the end of a study, a group of patients is told that they received the real drug and not a placebo. When asked if the drug worked, the patients are more likely to say "yes" if their personal bias going into the study was that the drug would work.

SELECTION BIAS

Occurs when either the subjects or the investigators choose how to group participants for the purposes of the study. In this situation, the distribution of subjects within the groups is often not random.

Example: Subjects with cancer are given the choice of receiving the standard chemotherapy treatment or an experimental treatment. The subjects with the advanced cancers disproportionately choose the experimental treatment because they know that the standard treatment is ineffective for late-stage cancer. Those receiving the experimental treatment might do worse on average, due not to the inherent ineffectiveness of the drug, but to the disproportionate number of very sick patients who chose this treatment.

LATE-LOOK BIAS

The results are recorded at the wrong time, skewing the outcomes.

Example: Persons with a certain stage of colon cancer have, on average, 5 months to live. Half are given an experimental treatment, and they are found to have lived an average of 3 months. The investigators conclude that the treatment actually shortens life expectancy by 2 months. However, they overlooked the fact that treatment itself took 3 months. In this situation, the treated group actually lived 1 month longer!

Reducing Bias

Two common ways to reduce bias include **blinding** and **randomization**.

BLINDING

Participants are not told which intervention they are receiving. Physicians performing the study may also be blinded, so that they do not know which intervention they are administering. In a double-blind study, neither party is aware who is receiving which intervention. Blinding **prevents recall bias**.

Example: A **placebo** is the classic way to blind participants in a study. A placebo is an inactive treatment that looks, tastes, and feels identical to the actual drug; thus, participants do not know which treatment they are receiving.

RANDOMIZATION

Participants are grouped randomly into study groups. Randomization **prevents selection bias**, because neither subjects nor study conductors are involved.

Example: After a pool of subjects for a study is chosen, the subjects are placed in the intervention group or the placebo group based on a coin toss. Potential differences between subjects that may skew results are more likely to be randomly distributed into both groups.

Prevalence, Incidence, and Duration

Prevalence is how many people in a sample group have a condition **at a certain point in time**. Often written as a ratio, such as "1 in 4 persons over the age of 40 has high cholesterol."

Incidence is how many people will **newly acquire** a condition in a given period, such as "1 in 50 per year."

Duration is how long a given condition lasts, on average.

These three terms are related by the formula:

$$\text{Incidence} \times \text{Duration} = \text{Prevalence}$$

Example: In a given population, 1 in 100 persons acquires a new plantar wart each year (incidence). On average, the wart will last two years (duration). Survey this population in any given year, and roughly 2 in 100 persons will have a plantar wart (Incidence × Duration = Prevalence).

Sensitivity, Specificity, and Predictive Value

When a patient is given a test for a condition, the test most often yields one of two results, positive or negative. However, no test is 100% accurate. Thus, there are four possibilities:

- **True-positive (TP)** is a positive test result in a person who has the condition.

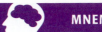

KEY FACT

Randomized, double-blind clinical trials are the gold standard for robust studies.

KEY FACT

For diseases with very short durations, incidence ≈ prevalence.

KEY FACT

Shorten the disease OR reduce the incidence to reduce the prevalence.

KEY FACT

Sensitivity = TP / (TP + FN)
Use sensitive tests to rule a
   condition out.

Specificity = TN / (TN + FP)
Specific tests are used to rule
   conditions **in** ("**SpIN**").

KEY FACT

Positive predictive value = TP /
   (TP + FP)
Negative predictive value = TN /
   (TN + FN)

KEY FACT

The lower the prevalence of a
disease, the lower the positive
predictive value, even if the test's
sensitivity and specificity are high!
Remember there can't be many
true-positives if there aren't many
patients.

- **False-positive (FP)** is a positive test result in a person who does not have the condition.
- **True-negative (TN)** is a negative test result in a person who does not have the condition.
- **False-negative (FN)** is a negative test result in a person who does have the condition.

True-positives and **false-negatives** actually have the condition being tested for. **True-negatives** and **false-positives** do not have the condition (see Figure 2-5).

These four outcomes for any test are used to calculate **sensitivity**, **specificity**, and **predictive values**.

Sensitivity is the percentage of positive test results (TP) among a population with the tested condition (TP + FN).

Specificity is the percentage of negative test results (TN) among a population without the tested condition (TN + FP).

Positive predictive value is the likelihood that a positive test result truly means that a patient has a given condition, i.e., the number of correct positive tests (TP) out of the total number of positive tests (TP + FP).

Negative predictive value is the likelihood that a negative test result truly means that a patient does not have a given condition, i.e., the number of correct negative tests (TN) out of the total number of negative tests (TN + FN).

The interrelationships between these values are depicted in Figure 2-6.

Steps to solve the common board questions related to sensitivity and specificity:

- Pick an easy number to use for the sample patient population (any number works).
- Use prevalence to calculate how many in the sample do and do not actually have the disease.
- For those who do have the disease, use the test's sensitivity to determine how many would test positive (true-positives) and how many would test negative (false-negatives).
- For those who do not have the disease, use specificity to calculate how many will test negative for the disease (true-negatives) and how many will test positive (false-positives).
- Calculate the positive predictive value by dividing the true-positives by all positive test results. Calculate the negative predictive value by dividing the true-negatives by all negative results.

	+ Test	**− Test**
Have the disease	True-positive	False-negative
Do not have the disease	False-positive	True-negative

FIGURE 2-5.   Positive and negative test results.

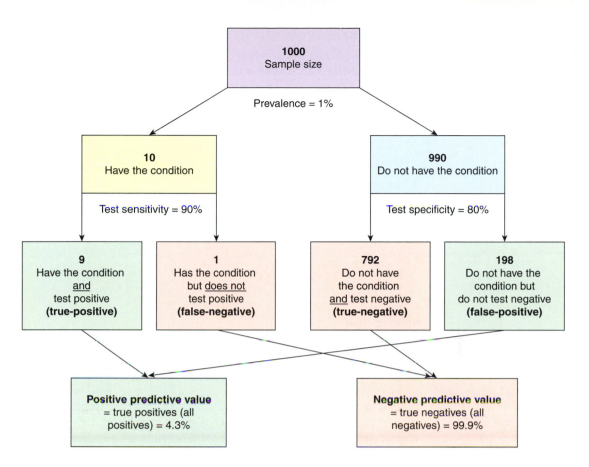

FIGURE 2-6.   **Integrating prevalence, sensitivity, specificity, and predictive values.**

Odds Ratio and Relative Risk

Odds ratios and **relative risk** express how much more likely something is to occur if a certain condition is met, such as a patient being exposed to an illness or receiving a particular treatment. These are calculated based on known outcomes, as in the example in Figure 2-7.

	Died	**Survived**
Exposed to pathogen	20 (A)	5 (B)
Not exposed to pathogen	10 (C)	20 (D)

FIGURE 2-7.   **Outcomes matrix for a patient exposed to a pathogen.**

ABSOLUTE RISK

Relative risks and odds ratios are calculated from the above type of chart using **absolute risk**, which is the likelihood of an outcome given a particular condition.

$$\text{Absolute Risk (of dying if exposed)} = A / (A + B)$$

$$\text{Absolute Risk (of dying if not exposed)} = C / (C + D)$$

ATTRIBUTABLE RISK

Absolute risk (if not exposed) demonstrates that some subjects will have the outcome being studied, even when the condition is not met. To calculate how much risk is actually due to the condition being studied, use **attributable risk**.

$$\text{Attributable Risk} = \text{Absolute Risk (if exposed)} - \text{Absolute Risk (if not exposed)}$$
$$= A / (A+B) - C / (C+D)$$

RELATIVE RISK

Absolute risk describes the likelihood of an outcome given a condition being met. **Relative risk** divides the likelihood (or percentage) of an outcome given a condition being met by the likelihood of the same outcome if the condition is not met.

$$\textbf{Relative Risk} \text{ is } (A/(A + B)) / (C/(C + D)).$$

In the example above, there is a 2.4 times greater chance of dying after being exposed to the pathogen versus not being exposed.

ODDS RATIO

This divides the odds of an outcome given a condition by the odds of the same outcome when the condition is not met.

$$\textbf{Odds Ratio} = (A / B) / (C / D)$$

In the example above, the odds of dying after being exposed to the pathogen are eight times higher than if not exposed.

KEY FACT

If the outcome investigated is very rare, odds ratio ≈ relative risk.

Studies that **create a sample population based on outcome,** such as case-control studies, must **use odds ratios.**

Studies that create a **sample population based on exposure or treatment,** such as a controlled trial or cohort study, can **use relative risk.**

Precision, Accuracy, and Error

Precision, accuracy, and **error** describe the quality of measurements, such as those produced by a laboratory test.

- **Precision** is the reproducibility of a measurement.
- **Accuracy** is how close a measurement is to the true value.
- **Systematic errors** are errors that **occur the same way every time** a measurement is taken. As a result, the measurements are wrong in the same way each time and thus are not accurate, but are precise.

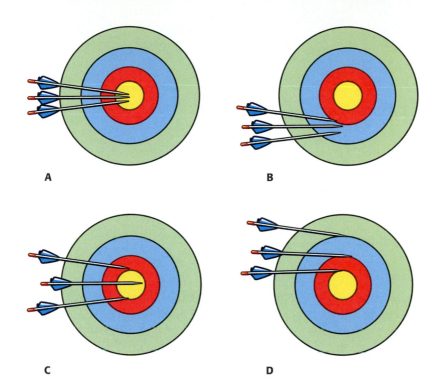

FIGURE 2-8.   Relationship of error to precision and accuracy. (A) High precision and high accuracy; low random error and low systematic error. (B) High precision, but low accuracy; low random error, but high systematic error. (C) Low precision, but high accuracy; high random error, but low systematic error. (D) Low precision and low accuracy; high random error and high systematic error.

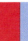 **Random error** is unavoidable error that is **different each time a measurement is taken.** This reduces precision. It also reduces accuracy if the amount of error is large.

These differences are shown in Figure 2-8.

KEY FACT

Systematic errors decrease **accuracy.** Random error decreases **precision.**

Disease Prevention

FORMS OF DISEASE PREVENTION

Public health officials try to limit disease through primary, secondary, or tertiary prevention.

Primary Disease Prevention

Primary disease prevention is a method used to stop the disease before it starts. For example, vaccination is used to build immunologic resistance and thus limit the infectivity and spread of a disease. Recently, a cervical cancer vaccine has been developed that prevents infection of certain serotypes of human papillomavirus (HPV), thereby reducing the rates of cervical cancer. Other vaccines (e.g., pneumococcal, tetanus, diphtheria, mumps-measles-rubella) fall under the heading of primary disease prevention because these interventions occur before the host has become diseased.

	"Truth" Disease	No disease
***Test result* Positive**	***a*** True-positive	***b*** False-positive
Negative	***c*** False-negative	***d*** True-negative

FIGURE 2-9. Diagnostic testing and disease state. (Modified, with permission, from Greenberg RS, Daniels SR, Flanders WD, et al. *Medical Epidemiology*, 4th ed. New York: McGraw-Hill, 2005: 94.)

Secondary Disease Prevention

Secondary disease prevention is the detection of the disease early in its course to reduce the associated morbidity and mortality. Examples of secondary disease prevention include cervical cancer screening through Pap smears, which detect HPV viral DNA, colonoscopy for the detection of colon cancers, and mammogram screening for the detection of breast cancers. Early detection can reduce the morbidity and mortality of the disease and also prevent epidemics.

Disease screening tests usually are very **sensitive** to retain a high true-positive rate, but may result in many false-positives (see Figure 2-9). **Sensitivity** is defined as the number or percentage of disease-positive individuals who have a positive test result. Because screening methods err on the side of including individuals with disease (remember, **sensitivity** rules people **in**), it may include false-positives (individuals who do not have the disease, but have a falsely positive test result).

$$\text{Sensitivity} = \text{True-positives} / (\text{true-positives} + \text{false-negatives}) \times 100$$
$$= a / (a + c) \times 100$$

$$\text{Specificity} = \text{True-negatives} / (\text{true-negatives} + \text{false-positives}) \times 100$$
$$= d / (d + b) \times 100$$

Tertiary Disease Prevention

Tertiary disease prevention aims to reduce the disability or morbidity resulting from disease. Examples include exogenous insulin for diabetes and surgical treatment of cancers. Tertiary disease prevention aims to treat the disease through available medical or surgical management.

REPORTING AND MONITORING DISEASE

Reportable Diseases

By reporting certain infectious diseases, public health officials can monitor, track, and try to control contagious diseases. **Reportable infectious diseases** are shown in Table 2-2.

TABLE 2-2.   Reportable Diseases

DISEASE	CAUSATIVE AGENT	COMMUNICABILITY
Acquired immune deficiency syndrome (AIDS)	HIV retrovirus	Spread by sexual contact, parental exposure, perinatal exposure.
Chickenpox	Varicella zoster virus (VZV)	Spread by inhalation of vesicles or close contact.
Gonorrhea	Gram-negative diplococcus *Neisseria gonorrhoeae*	Sexual contact.
Hepatitis A	Hepatitis A virus (HAV)	Fecal-oral route.
Hepatitis B	Hepatitis B virus (HBV)	Sexual contact, parental exposure.
Measles (rubeola)	Paramyxovirus	Inhalation of respiratory droplets.
Mumps	Paramyxovirus	Inhalation of respiratory droplets.
Rubella (German measles)	Togavirus	Inhalation of respiratory droplets.
Salmonella	Negative bacilli *Salmonella typhi*	Contaminated food or water.
Shigella	*Shigella dysenteriae*	Contaminated food.
Syphilis	Spirochete *Treponema pallidum*	Sexual contact, perinatal exposure.
Tuberculosis	*Mycobacterium tuberculosis*	Skin-to-skin contact and droplet transmission.

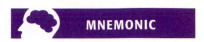

MNEMONIC

Be *A S-S-S-M-MART CHICKEN* or you're *GONe:*

Hep **B**
Hep **A**
Salmonella
Shigella
Syphilis
Measles
Mumps
AIDS
Rubella
Tuberculosis
CHICKENpox
GONorrhea

Medical Surveillance

The effort to continuously monitor and detect the occurrence of health-related events is known as medical surveillance. Through **medical surveillance**, it is possible to determine the **incidence rate** of disease (the rate of new disease in a given period), the number of deaths resulting from the disease (**case fatality**), the **mortality rate** (combination of incidence rate and case fatality), **rate ratios** (a ratio of the incidence rates of two different groups, resulting in a comparison of the rate of disease occurrence), and **mortality patterns**. Figures 2-10, 2-11, and 2-12 show examples of incidence rates, mortality rates or patterns, and rate ratios, respectively.

Despite the myriad of reportable diseases, infections do not account for the major leading causes of death in the United States (see Table 2-3).

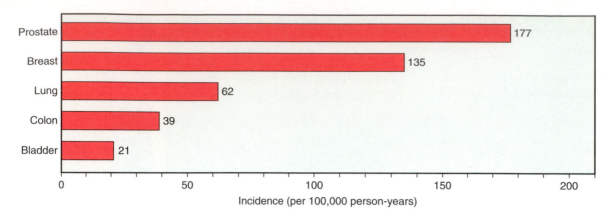

FIGURE 2-10. **Example of age-adjusted incidences rates.** Age-adjusted incidence rates of the leading cancers in men and women in the United States from 1996–2000. (Data from Ries LAG, Melbert D, Krapcho M, et al. SEER Cancer Statistics Review, 1975–2000. National Cancer Institute, 2003.) (Modified, with permission, from Greenberg RS, Daniels SR, Flanders WD. et al. *Medical Epidemiology*, 4th ed. New York: McGraw-Hill, 2005: 50.)

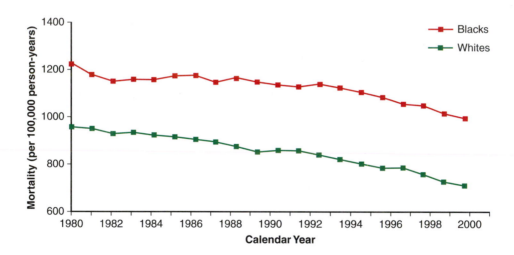

FIGURE 2-11. **Example of age-adjusted total mortality rates.** Age-adjusted total mortality rates by calendar year and race in the United States, 1980–2001. (Data from National Center for Health Statistics: National Vital Statistics Report, 2003.) (Modified, with permission, from Greenberg RS, Daniels SR, Flanders WD, et al. *Medical Epidemiology*, 4th ed. New York: McGraw-Hill, 2005: 58.)

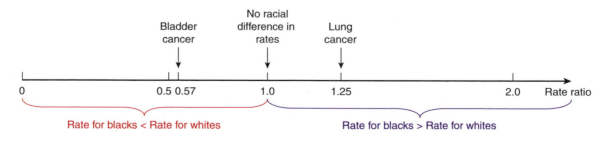

FIGURE 2-12. **Example of incidence rate ratio.** Schematic representation of black-to-white incidence rate ratio for cancers of the lung and bladder in the United States. (Data from Ries LAG, Melbert D, Krapcho M, et al. SEER Cancer Statistics Review, 1975–2000. National Cancer Institute, 2003.) (Modified, with permission, from Greenberg RS, Daniels SR, Flanders WD, et al, *Medical Epidemiology*, 4th ed, New York: McGraw-Hill, 2005: 52.)

TABLE 2-3. Leading Causes of Death in the United States by Age

Age Group	Leading Cause of Death
Infants	■ Congenital anomalies ■ Short gestation/low birth weight ■ Sudden infant death syndrome ■ Maternal complications ■ Respiratory distress syndrome
Age 1–14	■ Injuries ■ Cancer ■ Congenital anomalies ■ Homicide ■ Heart disease
Age 15–24	■ Injuries ■ Homicide ■ Suicide ■ Cancer ■ Heart disease
Age 25–64	■ Cancer ■ Heart disease ■ Injuries ■ Suicide ■ Stroke
Age 65+	■ Heart disease ■ Cancer ■ Stroke ■ COPD ■ Pneumonia ■ Influenza

GOVERNMENT FINANCING OF MEDICAL INSURANCE

Medical costs can be paid several ways: Out-of-pocket payments, individual private insurance, employment-based private insurance, or government financing. The two major types of government financing are Medicare and Medicaid (Figure 2-13).

Medicare and Medicaid

Medicare is a government-sponsored program financed through Social Security, federal taxes, and monthly premiums that provides financial coverage for hospital and physician services for persons 65 years and older. It consists of **Medicare Part A** and **Medicare Part B**.

MEDICARE PART A

Covers **certain costs for hospitalization, skilled nursing facilities, home health care, and hospice care**. The amount that Medicare Part A will reimburse varies with the length of stay at the facility.

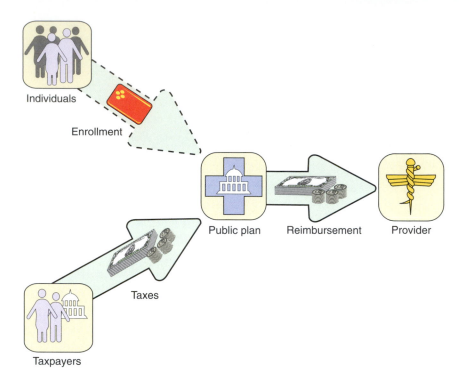

FIGURE 2-13. **Government-financed insurance.** Medicare and Medicaid are examples of government-financed insurance. (Modified, with permission, from Bodenheimer TX, Grumbach K. *Understanding Health Policy: A Clinical Approach,* 4th ed, New York: McGraw-Hill, 2005: 12.)

Example: For a hospitalization, Medicare Part A will pay for the first 60 days except a deductible per stay. After the first 60 days, Part A will cover all expenses except a daily deductible. Individuals older than 65 can enroll in Medicare Part A by paying a monthly premium. The program is also available to those who have chronic renal disease and are in need of dialysis or transplantation. It is also possible to enroll in Medicare Part A if a person is totally or permanently disabled. However, the individual must wait 24 months before enrollment.

MEDICARE PART B

Available for patients who elect to pay a separate Medicare Part B monthly premium. The rest of the program is financed through federal taxes. Medicare Part B covers **medical expenses to include physician services; physical, occupational, and speech therapy; medical equipment; diagnostic tests; and preventive care** (e.g., Pap smears, mammograms, vaccinations). Outpatient medications, along with eye, hearing, and dental services, are **NOT** covered.

MEDICAID

Medicaid is a state-sponsored program, although the federal government contributes 50%–80% of the funds (more money comes from the federal government in poorer states, as measured by per capita income). Medicaid provides **coverage for a number of services,** including **hospital fees, physician services, laboratory services, X-rays, prenatal care, preventive care, nursing home care, and home health services.** Requirements that need to be met to qualify for Medicaid vary from state to state. However, typically, they include low-income families with children, individuals (disabled, blind, or elderly) who receive cash assistance under the Supplemental Security Income (SSI) program, and pregnant women whose family income is less than or equal to 133% of the deferral poverty level.

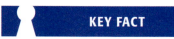

KEY FACT

Medi**CARE** takes **CARE** of the elderly.

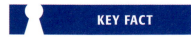

KEY FACT

Medic**AID** helps the state and federal government **AID** those in need.

Ethics

AUTONOMY

Patient autonomy is the right of patients to actively participate and make final medical decisions that affect their health. Autonomy and justice are the most deep-seated principle in bioethics (and in the U.S. legal system) in regards to medical decision-making. Autonomy means that people have **the right to choose** (accept or refuse) treatment.

For example, a police officer does not have the right to search an individual's home without a warrant. Similarly, a doctor does not have the right to perform a lung biopsy without the patient's consent.

- **Patients** have **the right to accept or refuse treatments** that the physician may recommend because the patient "owns" his or her body and therefore has the right to make his or her own choices regarding health care.
- **Physicians** have an **obligation to respect patients' autonomy**, and they must honor their preference for care.

A patient's autonomy can be **breached** under the following circumstances:

- The patient is infected with a highly infectious and dangerous disease (e.g., HIV).
- The patient has a greatly impaired decision-making capacity (e.g., a delusion impairing understanding of the decision).
- The patient's autonomy is legally waived by the U.S. government (e.g., epidemics).

Justice Cardozo established the legal medical autonomy standard in the *Schloendoff vs. Society of New York Hospital* (105 N.E. 92) **case in 1914**. The case involved a patient who consented to an examination of a fibroid tumor under ether, but explicitly denied consent for surgery. The surgeons performed the operation during the ether examination without her consent or knowledge.

Justice Cardozo stated, "Every human being of adult years and sound mind has a right to determine what shall be done with his own body; and a surgeon who performs an operation without his patient's consent, commits an assault, for which he is liable in damages."

- **This is true except** in cases of emergency, where the patient is unconscious, and situations in which it is necessary to take action before consent can be obtained (life-threatening events).

INFORMED CONSENT

Informed consent implies that the patient must have been fully informed of all options (benefits and risks) by the physician.

This legally requires the physician to:

- Discuss relevant information, including the risks and benefits of treatment, as well as the possible effect of no treatment.
- Obtain an agreement with the patient.
- Allow a patient's decision to be made free of coercion.

This principle is ethically rooted in the concept of respect for the patient's autonomy. Informed consent requires the presence of three related factors:

- The patient must have voluntarily chosen to seek treatment and must have the capacity to reasonably make decisions.
- The patient must receive full objective disclosure of all of the necessary information; however, recommendations and an assurance of full patient understanding about each choice should be made by the physician. In general, physicians should give patients the amount of information an average, reasonable patient would want.
- The idea is for the patient and physician to engage in a conversation where negotiation and conflict resolution of differences are welcomed to enhance patient autonomy.

For example, the patient should always feel free to obtain a second opinion.

- A decision and authorization from the patient are necessary to carry out the procedure, **unless the patient is a minor**, and therefore may not have decision-making capacity. This differs depending on the kind of decision being made.

Key facts to remember about informed consent:

- An exception to consent is made in the case of an emergency, where consent is **implied**.
- Consent is necessary for **each** specific procedure.
- The health care worker performing the procedure **should** be the one to obtain consent.
- Beneficence does **not** obviate the need for consent.
- Consent received via the telephone **is** legitimate, but must be documented.
- Pregnant women **can** refuse therapy for their fetus (once the child is born, lifesaving therapy cannot be refused).
- Decisions made by patients at a time when they were competent **continue** to be valid, even when they have lost the capacity to consent (i.e., loss of consciousness).
- A health care proxy, living will, or medical durable power of attorney is the best method to obtain consent (beforehand) from someone who has **lost** capacity.
- Informed consent must come from a parent, legal guardian, third-party court-appointed individual, or "substituted judgment" (an individual who ideally knows the patient well and can make decisions based on what he or she believes the patient would want). This prior preference may not be known for a **continuously** incompetent person (e.g., patients with severe Down's syndrome). Then the risk and benefits predominate.

INFORMED ASSENT

Informed assent consists of a **child's agreement** to medical procedures in the situation that he or she is not legally authorized or does not have the capacity to give consent competently (e.g., participation in clinical trials, terminal illness).

In line with the WHO Research Ethics Review Committee (ERC), the following recommendations must be honored:

- Before seeking consent and assent to involve children in research, it must be demonstrated that comparable research cannot be done with adults to the same effect and scientific impact.

- Researchers must obtain consent from a parent or guardian on an Informed Consent Form (ICF) for all children.
- Research supported by the WHO follows the **Convention on the Rights of the Child**, where "child" means "every human being below the age of eighteen years" unless under the law applicable to the child, majority age is attained earlier.
- Children should be provided with detailed information and a description of the research to be conducted, geared to the child's age, and should have their questions and concerns addressed. They have the right to express their agreement or lack of agreement to participate.
- Researchers should consider asking for assent from children over the age of 7 years, while taking assent from all children over the age of 12 years.
- Children express their agreement to participate on an informed assent form (IAF) written in age-appropriate language. This form is **in addition to**, and **does not replace**, parental consent on an ICF.
- **Assent that is denied by a child should be taken very seriously**.

DECISION-MAKING CAPACITY

Decision-making capacity is closely related to the concept of autonomy because autonomy is a necessary for appropriate medical decision-making.

The two key components of autonomy include:

- **Liberty**, which refers to one's freedom from controlling influences.
- **Agency**, which implies the individual's capacity to be intentional in his or her actions. If patients lack this capacity, they may be legally deemed **incompetent**.

Health care professionals are often faced with the difficult task of deeming a patient as having or not having the capacity to make decisions.

Example: A patient who is refusing psychiatric hospitalization will often need a psychiatrist to determine if the patient has the capacity to make medical decisions. This may be the case even when a patient is involuntarily hospitalized because he or she is a danger to self or others.

The components of legal competence generally include:

- The patient has the capacity to understand the material information.
- He or she can make a judgment about the information in light of his or her values.
- The patient intends a certain outcome.
- The patient is able to freely communicate his or her wish to caregivers or investigators.

While some ethical principles allow for individuals to fall anywhere on a spectrum, **competence is an "all or nothing" concept**. The patient is either competent or not. Thus, it is often a painstaking process to determine that a patient is indeed **incompetent**.

Several general standards must be met. They can be summarized as follows:

- The patient must have the ability to state a preference.
- The patient must have the ability to understand information and to appreciate the situation.
- The patient must have the ability to reason through a logical decision.

Case 1: Mrs. Jones is a 78-year-old woman with metastatic breast cancer who is intubated in the ICU. She can communicate through writing or pointing to a picture board. She is tired of heroic measures and wants to be at peace. She indicates her wish to withdraw respiratory support, but her husband knows that such an action will hasten her death.

- Although the husband is reluctant to follow her wishes, the principle of autonomy suggests that a **competent patient** such as his wife should be able to make her own decisions.

Case 2: Mr. Smith is an 82-year-old man with Alzheimer's disease who was recently diagnosed with lung cancer. His short-term memory and cognition are severely affected by his dementia, but he firmly states that he does not want chemotherapy when the doctor asks him about treatment options.

- **This patient may or may not be legally competent** to make medical decisions.
- **If he is not competent**, the decision about his treatment plan will depend on an advance directive or the statement of a person he has designated as having medical power of attorney, if he has done this before becoming incompetent.

ADVANCE DIRECTIVE

Advance directives are written while a person is competent and are used to direct future health care decisions. Thus, patients can maintain autonomy even when they lack legal competence.

Types of Advance Directives

There are two types of advance directives:

- **A living will** is a statement of exactly which procedures are acceptable or unacceptable, and under what circumstances.
- **Medical durable power of attorney** grants a specific surrogate person the authority to perform certain actions on behalf of the person who signs the document.

Case 2 continued: Mr. Smith never wrote an advance directive because he always thought he would "get around to it one day," but he never did. Fortunately, he **did appoint his son as having medical durable power of attorney** during the early, more lucid stages of his Alzheimer's dementia. The oncologists were able to call his son to ask for guidance in his father's care.

Oral versus Written Advance Directives

Oral advance directives are taken from an incompetent patient's previous oral statements. These should be written in the patient's chart whenever possible.

Example: A patient who watched her mother die after a prolonged period on a ventilator may have said to her family members that she would never want to be on a ventilator.

Recollecting this desire could act as an **oral advance directive** if the patient is incapacitated and faced with a similar situation.

Unfortunately, people can often misinterpret an incapacitated person's previous statements. Thus, the following criteria add more validity to oral statements:

- The patient is informed.
- The directive is specific.
- The patient makes a choice.
- The decision is repeated over time.

Written advance directives are preferred because they provide stronger evidence as to what the patient wants.

One source lists these **problems with advance directives:**

- Relatively few persons have them.
- Designated decision-makers may be unavailable or incompetent, or have a conflict of interest (e.g., inheritance).
- Some people change their treatment preferences, but do not change the legal document.
- State laws often severely restrict the use of advance directives.
- They leave no legal basis for health care providers to overturn instructions that turn out not to be in the patient's best medical interest, although the patient could not have reasonably anticipated this circumstance while competent.

Case 2: Mr. Smith's son had no written advance directive on which to base his decision regarding his father's chemotherapy. His mother suffered through chemotherapy for lung cancer, and he remembers that his father often remarked that he would rather die peacefully than endure chemotherapy.

- Although the son cannot be sure that his father understood the oncologist's question about treatment, he can confidently make a decision based on an oral advance directive from his father's previous aversion to chemotherapy.

BENEFICENCE

Beneficence is "**the principle of doing good**." Physicians have a special ethical responsibility to act in the patient's best interest. This is known as a **fiduciary** relationship because the physician has a commitment to the patient.

Patient autonomy may conflict with beneficence. If the patient makes an informed decision, then ultimately the patient has the right to decide what is in his or her best interest.

- The practice of doing whatever the physician feels is best for the patient without consideration of the patient's wishes is called **paternalism**. This old form of medical practice is no longer acceptable in most circumstances.

Case 3: An intern is riding the subway home after a long shift at the hospital. She witnesses one of her fellow passengers falling onto the floor because of a cardiac arrest.

- Although the exhausted intern is now off duty, she is **morally obligated** to help the unfortunate passenger **within the limits of her expertise and the established guidelines of care**. This obligation to act is often referred to as the "**good Samaritan principle**."

KEY FACT

Frakena's four general obligations for beneficence:
1. One ought not to inflict evil or harm (what is bad).
2. One ought to prevent evil or harm.
3. One ought to remove evil or harm.
4. One ought to promote or do good.

NONMALEFICENCE

The principal "**first do no harm**" is derived from *primum non nocere* in the Hippocratic oath. Nonetheless, if the benefits of an intervention outweigh the risks, ethically, the physician must act, as when there is an emergency.

Key issues that can be addressed by this principle include:

- Killing versus letting die.
- Intending versus foreseeing harmful outcomes.
- Withholding versus withdrawing life-sustaining treatment.
- Extraordinary versus ordinary circumstances.

Many of these issues center on the terminally ill and the seriously ill and injured.

CONFIDENTIALITY

Confidentiality in the medical setting refers to keeping secret any personal information a patient discloses to his or her physician. Clinicians must respect the patient's privacy and autonomy, thus building a doctor-patient relationship based on trust. Patients may specify any information that they would like the physician to share with their family; anything that is not so specified should be kept confidential.

Certain **exceptions exist to the rule of confidentiality.** Such exceptions include:

- The patient indicates that he or she may harm himself or someone else.

In the Tarasoff case, a jealous lover indicated to his therapist that he intended to shoot his flirtatious girlfriend. The therapist did not warn the girlfriend or her family out of respect for the patient's confidentiality. The man killed the girlfriend, and her family sued the University of California for her preventable death.

- The *Tarasoff* decision states that if a threat is revealed by a patient, a clinician must take some action, such as warning a threatened person of potential danger, regardless of the clinician's duty to confidentiality.
- Child abuse, spousal abuse, or elder abuse.
- Infectious diseases: The physician must report certain infectious diseases that pose significant public health risks. In addition, for some diseases, individuals at risk must be notified (i.e., sexual partners of someone newly diagnosed with HIV), an action referred to as "**contact tracing.**"
- Patients driving under the influence.
- Protection of individuals at risk for some harm that cannot be accomplished by some other means than by breaking confidentiality.
- Cases in which there is a reasonable chance that by breaking confidentiality the physician may be able to prevent some harm.

Case 4: A 47-year-old woman is diagnosed with metastatic breast cancer and is told she will probably not survive more than one year. She does not wish for her family to know about her disease or prognosis. The physician feels certain that the patient and her family will benefit by knowing the truth so that the family can support the patient and so they can make the most of their last months together.

KEY FACT

From the Hippocratic oath: "I will use treatment to help the sick according to my ability and judgment, but I will never use it to injure or wrong them."

KEY FACT

The *Tarasoff* case: This classic case took place in California in 1976. This case highlighted the limits of confidentiality and established that therapists are allowed to breach confidentiality if someone else is in danger.

KEY FACT

The suicidal or homicidal patient may be held against his or her will.

What should the physician do?

The physician **may certainly urge** the patient to consider informing her family, but the **physician should not break her confidence**.

MALPRACTICE

Medical malpractice is a civil suit that is taken out by patients or their family members against a physician due to some form of **negligence**, malfeasance, or nonfeasance by the physician or a direct subordinate that has caused some type of harm to the patient. Causes can be a direct act or an omission by the medical team that results in a deviation of the standard accepted practice and results in a negative consequence.

Four conditions must be met for the plaintiff (patient or family member) to prove that malpractice has occurred, which together are known as **the four D's of malpractice**.

1. **Duty:** The physician accepts a duty to the well-being of the patient when taking on the medical care of that patient.
2. **Dereliction:** This duty to the patient is not fulfilled when the accepted standards of medical care are not followed (resulting in a dereliction of one's duties).
3. **Damage:** Because of a dereliction of one's duty to the patient, a direct harm, or damage, occurs.
4. **Direct:** The dereliction of one's duty directly results in the damage that the patient has received.

Without the fulfillment of these four criteria, malpractice cannot be proven in a court of law, and the physician is **not legally liable** for the damages that the patient has received.

It must be remembered that accidents that can cause harm frequently occur. Not all of these accidents result in malpractice suits; however, as for a case to be made, all four conditions must have occurred.

Case 7: Samantha is an 8-year-old girl with a sore throat, fever, and painful submandibular lymph nodes. Her parents take her to the doctor's office, where Dr. Clark orders a rapid streptococcal throat swab, which is positive. **Samantha has never taken antibiotics before**, and Dr. Smith prescribes penicillin V 25 mg/kg PO BID for 10 days. The next morning, Samantha is taken to the emergency department by her parents and is in anaphylactic shock. Her parents sue Dr. Smith for malpractice.

- **Damage** was caused when Samantha took penicillin and had an allergic reaction.
- **Dr. Smith is found not guilty** because she was fulfilling her **duty** to the patient by treating her for streptococcal pharyngitis within the accepted medical guidelines.
- Therefore, there was no **dereliction** of duties that **directly** resulted in damage to the patient.

Statistics

MEASURES OF CENTRAL TENDENCY AND STATISTICAL DISTRIBUTION

Distribution is a term used to describe the **frequency** of observations in a population or data set as plotted on a graph.

Distribution of a set of observations is defined by the measures of central tendency:

- **Mean (arithmetic mean, or average)** is the most common measure of central tendency. It represents the ratio between the sum of all individual observations (**ΣX**) over the number of observations (**n**):

$$M = \Sigma X / n$$

  The mean, however, may not be an appropriate measure of central tendency for skewed distributions or in data sets which contain outliers.
- **Median (middle observation)** represents the **50th percentile of a distribution**, or the point at which half of the observations are smaller and half are larger. The median is often a more appropriate measure of central tendency for skewed distributions or in situations with large outliers.
- **Mode** represents the most common value in a distribution, and is commonly used for a large number of observations to identify the value that occurs most frequently.

All three are used for continuous data; the median may also be used for categorical data as well.

A **frequency curve** may be produced from the data set (see Figure 2-14).

Terms that describe the curves created include:

- **Gaussian:** Also known as a "normal," or "bell-shaped," curve. It indicates **symmetric distribution** of the observations.
  - The mean, median, and mode are identical.
- **Bimodal:** The curve produces two "peaks" due to two separate areas of increased frequency of data in the population or data set. These curves may indicate **symmetric** or **asymmetric distribution** of observations.

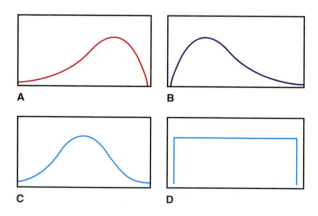

FIGURE 2-14. **Shapes of common distributions of observations.** (A) Negatively skewed. (B) Positively skewed. (C and D) Symmetric. (Modified, with permission, from Dawson B, Trapp RG, *Basic & Clinical Biostatistics*, 4th ed, New York: McGraw-Hill, 2004: 30.)

- **Positive skew: Asymmetric** curve with the tail on the **right** side of the graph. It indicates a large number of outlying values.
    - **Mean > median**
    - **Mean > mode**
- **Negative skew: Asymmetric** curve with the tail on the **left** side of the graph. It indicates a small number of outlying values.
    - **Mean < median**
    - **Mean < mode**

STATISTICAL HYPOTHESIS

A statistical hypothesis is a formal statement regarding the expected outcome of an experiment. There are two major types of hypothesis, differentiated by how the statement is framed:

- **Null hypothesis (H_0):** A statement that suggests that there is **no difference**, or association **between two or more variables**. In medicine, this normally relates to disease and risk factors. H_0 is tested for possible rejection under the assumption that the hypothesis is true.
- **Alternative hypothesis (H_1):** A statement that suggests that **there is an association between two or more variables**, and contrary to the null hypothesis, the observations are the result of a real effect.

Type I Error (α)

Type I error results when one states or determines that there **is** an effect or difference when in reality one does not exist. Stated another way, the **alternative** hypothesis is accepted when in actuality the **null** hypothesis is correct. Type I error is also known as a "**false-positive.**"

- This error is a **preset** level of significance, denoted as the Greek letter α, which is **defined as the probability of making a type I error.**
- The normal accepted α is usually < 0.5, which means that there is a less than 5% chance of making a type I error, or that the data will show something that **is not really there**.

Type II Error (β)

Type II error results when one states or determines that there **is not** an effect or difference when in reality one does exist. In other words, the **null** hypothesis is accepted when in actuality the **alternative** hypothesis is correct (see Figure 2-15). Type II error is also known as "**false-negative.**"

> **CLINICAL CORRELATION**
>
> An example of a null hypothesis is, "There is no association between sodium intake and hypertension."

> **CLINICAL CORRELATION**
>
> An example of an alternative (H_1) hypothesis is, "Increased sodium intake leads to increased blood pressure."

	Decision	
	Reject H_0	**Don't reject H_0**
H_0	Type I error	Right decision
Truth		
H_1	Right decision	Type II error

FIGURE 2-15. **Summary of possible results of any hypothesis test.**

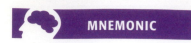

Power

Power is the probability of rejecting the null hypothesis when it is in fact false. The power can be manipulated based on sample size as well as the difference in compliance between sample groups. The power is calculated by subtracting the type II error (β) from 1.

$$\text{Power} = 1 - \beta$$

STANDARD DEVIATION VERSUS ERROR

Standard deviation is a statistical measurement that is used to describe the deviation, or variance, from the central tendency, or **mean**, within a statistical distribution (see Figure 2-16). It is used to describe the spread of values within a particular distribution.

All forms of measurement have some inherent error. For this reason, the **standard error of the mean** (SEM) is used to estimate the standard deviation of error in that particular method.

$$\text{SEM} = \sigma / \sqrt{n}$$

$$\sigma = \text{standard deviation}$$

$$n = \text{sample size}$$

Confidence Intervals

Confidence intervals essentially provide a range, with upper and lower limit values known as confidence limits, and can be used with any population parameter.

The confidence interval (CI) can be determined by using both the standard deviation and the SEM.

$$\text{CI} = \text{mean} \pm 1.96\,(\text{SEM}) \text{ or } \text{CI} = \text{mean} \pm 1.96\sigma$$

- If the CI includes zero, the null hypothesis is **accepted** (i.e., there is **no difference** between the variables).

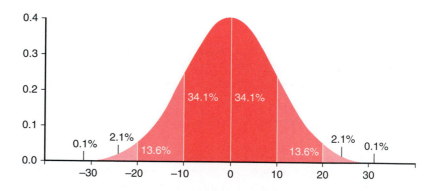

FIGURE 2-16. **Standard deviation.** Dark blue is less than one standard deviation from the mean. For the normal distribution, this accounts for about 68% of the set (dark blue), while two standard deviations from the mean (medium and dark blue) account for about 95%, and three standard deviations (light, medium, and dark blue) account for about 99.7%.

- If the CI does not contain zero, the null hypothesis is **rejected** and the alternative hypothesis is accepted (i.e., there **is a difference**, or association, between the variables).

Knowing the CI is important because it gives an estimate of how likely it is that a value is true. Thus, if a number falls between the upper and lower limits of a 95% confidence interval, one can be confident that the data are correct 95% of the time.

Example: Imagine a study in which a group of people in a certain town have their blood pressure measured several times over the course of a year (independent samples taken repeatedly from the same population). The results of the blood pressure measurements would be reported by giving a range. It is best to express this range as a CI because it tells readers that a value falling within that range was similar to the blood pressure of 95% of the patient population.

t-TEST, ANOVA, AND CHI-SQUARE (χ^2)

t-Test

The **t-test** is used to determine the difference between the mean values of two groups of observations. This test is based on the *t* distribution, which involves **degrees of freedom (df)**.

- For **groups with a large df** value, the *t* distribution is indistinguishable from the normal distribution.
- As the **df decreases**, the *t* distribution becomes increasingly spread out.
- The *t* distribution can be determined using a mathematical equation and correlated to a P value using the appropriate table.

ANOVA

ANOVA is used to determine the statistical difference between the means of three or more groups of observations.

Chi-Square (χ^2)

Chi-square is used to determine the statistical difference between two or more percentages or proportions of categorical outcomes (not mean values).

Correlation Coefficient

The **correlation coefficient (*r*)** is a numerical value that always falls between 1 and −1. It indicates the strength and direction of a linear relationship (correlation) between two or more different and independent variables. Values approaching 1, indicate a strong correlation between the variables. A value of 0 indicates no correlation, and values approaching −1 indicate an inverse relationship.

- The **coefficient of determination (R^2)** is the proportion of **variability** (or **sum of squares**) in a data set that is accounted for by a statistical model, using regression analysis. It helps to determine whether a linear relationship exists between the response variable and the "regressors."

If $R^2 = 1 \rightarrow$ there **is a linear relationship**, as explained by the fitted model.

If $R^2 = 0 \rightarrow$ there **is no linear relationship** between the response variable and regressors.

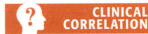

CLINICAL CORRELATION

A **t**-test would be useful when comparing the means of two groups (placebo versus treatment) to see if a statistical significance exists between the mean clinical outcomes of the two groups.

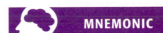

MNEMONIC

Mr. **T** is **mean**

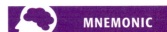

MNEMONIC

ANOVA = **AN**alysis **O**f **VA**riance of three or more variables.

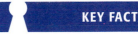

KEY FACT

χ^2 = compare percentages (%) or proportions.

CLINICAL CORRELATION

An example of the chi-square test is a clinical trial comparing a 28-day survival or treatment group versus a control group. The percentage of survivors versus controls can be compared using this test.

Life Cycle

DEVELOPMENT

APGAR Score

- The APGAR system is named after Dr. Virginia Apgar, a famous anesthesiologist. Each letter in APGAR stands for a sign assessed in newborns, as summarized in Table 2-4.
- The APGAR examination is fast, easy to use, and helpful for determining whether medical intervention, including resuscitation, is needed. However, it is not particularly accurate as a prognostic indicator.

SCORING

The APGAR score is determined at 1 and 5 minutes after birth. Reassessment may be performed after 5 minutes, and thereafter, if the APGAR score is abnormal.

- Each of the five signs is scored as 0, 1, or 2; the APGAR score is the sum of the five scores.
  - 8–10: Normal; however, a perfect score of 10 is not typically given.
  - 4–7: Some resuscitation may be needed.
  - 0–3: Immediate resuscitation is necessary. In general, a low score is related to inadequate ventilation, as opposed to cardiac pathology.

LOW BIRTH WEIGHT

Low birth weight (LBW) is defined as birth weight below 2500 g and is caused by premature birth or intrauterine growth restriction (IUGR). LBW infants are at increased risk for the following complications:

- **Sepsis:** With possible sequelae of septic shock and disseminated intravascular coagulation (DIC).
- **Infant respiratory distress syndrome:** Also known as **hyaline membrane disease**. In this disorder, the infant's lungs produce inadequate surfactant, a protein normally secreted by type II pneumocytes in mature lungs. Sur-

MNEMONIC

How **M**y **R**ecently **P**roduced (**G**ood) **B**aby **A**ppears:

Heart rate (pulse)
Movement (activity)
Response to **P**rovocation (**G**rimace)
Breathing (respiration)
Appearance

TABLE 2-4. APGAR Signs and Scoring Criteria

SIGN	0 POINTS	1 POINT	2 POINTS
Appearance (skin color)	Blue trunk, blue extremities	Pink trunk, blue extremities	Pink trunk, pink extremities
Pulse	Absent	< 100	≥ 100
Grimace (reflex irritability/response to stimulation)	No response	Grimace	Grimace and cough, pull away and/or sneeze
Activity (muscle tone)	None	Some	Active movement
Respiration	None	Weak, irregular	Strong, regular

factant (short for "surface active agent") facilitates inflation of alveoli and helps prevent alveolar collapse.

- **Necrotizing enterocolitis:** This is the most common neonatal gastrointestinal emergency; its etiology remains uncertain, but is thought to be multifactorial. Possibilities include immaturity of the intestinal mucosa, compromise of the intestinal blood supply, and the presence of abnormal bacteria.
- **Intraventricular hemorrhage:** This may result in long-term complications including cerebral palsy and delayed development.
- **Persistent pulmonary hypertension:** Also called **persistent fetal circulation**. Increased pressure in the pulmonary vasculature causes shunting of deoxygenated blood into the systemic circulation, resulting in hypoxemia.

REFLEXES OF THE NEWBORN

Infants exhibit characteristic reflexes at birth that fade and then vanish at certain points in development.

- **Moro:** Infant spreads, then unspreads the arms when startled. Generally disappears around three months; persists in certain conditions, such as cerebral palsy.
- **Babinski:** Toes fan upward upon plantar stimulation. Generally disappears around 12–14 months; persists in certain neurologic conditions.
- **Palmar:** Infant grasps objects that come in contact with the palm. Generally disappears around 2–3 months.
- **Rooting:** Nipple seeking. Generally disappears around 3–4 months.

INFANT DEPRIVATION

History. In the 1950s, psychologist Harry F. Harlow demonstrated that rhesus monkeys deprived of affection and physical contact developed abnormally. Later studies have suggested the existence of a similar phenomenon in humans: Long-term infant deprivation results in multiple long-term sequelae.

Major effects of long-term infant deprivation:

- **Illness:** Increased vulnerability to physical ailments.
- **Floppy:** Decreased muscle tone.
- **Wordless:** Language deficiencies.
- **Mistrust:** Difficulty in forming emotional bonds, sense of abandonment.
- **Thin:** Weight loss, failure to thrive.
- **Withdrawn:** Deficient socialization skills.
- **Anaclitic depression:** Relating to one person's physical and emotional dependence on another person (e.g., infant's dependence on mother).
  - The term "anaclitic" depression was used by Renee Spitz, a Hungarian-American psychoanalyst, to refer to the deteriorated psychological and physical health of infants who are separated from their caregivers and placed in cold, unstimulating institutional environments. Deprivation for longer than six months can lead to irreversible changes, such as withdrawn state, unresponsiveness, failure to thrive, and in severe cases, death.

CHILD ABUSE

Abuse of children by caregivers can be physical, emotional, or sexual; physical and sexual abuse are covered in Table 2-5. In addition, caregivers may commit neglect by failing to provide for a child's basic needs, such as food, clothing, and safety.

FLASH FORWARD

Infants born at 37–42 weeks' gestation are designated **term** infants; those born before 37 weeks' gestation are considered **premature.** An **LBW** infant need not be premature; he or she may have experienced IUGR or inappropriately low growth for gestational age.

MNEMONIC

My **B**aby's **P**rimary **R**eflexes:

Moro
Babinski
Palmar
Rooting

MNEMONIC

Infant **F**raught **W**ith **M**ajor **T**rouble **W**hen **D**eprived:

Illness
Floppy
Wordless
Mistrust
Thin
Withdrawn
Anaclitic **D**epression

TABLE 2-5.   **Characteristics of Child Abuse**

PHYSICAL ABUSE	SEXUAL ABUSE
Injuries intentionally caused by a caretaker that result in morbidity and mortality.	A child's involvement in an activity for purposes of adult sexual gratification.
Features include fractures visible on X-ray, cigarette burns, iron burns, subdural hematomas, bruises on the back, retinal hemorrhage, and psychiatric symptoms (e.g., anxiety, depression, withdrawal).	Features include genital/anal trauma, urinary tract infections (UTIs), sexually transmitted diseases (STDs), inappropriate social behavior for age (e.g., flirtatiousness in a young child), and psychiatric symptoms (e.g., anxiety, depression, withdrawal, discomfort around sexual impulses).
Abuser is usually female, young (below age 30), and the primary caregiver.	Abuser is usually male and known to the victim.
~ 3000 deaths annually in the United States; approximately half the children brought for physical abuse–related medical attention are under age 1.	Peak incidence at ages 9–12.

KEY FACT

In general, motor development proceeds cephalocaudally, from medial to lateral, and from proximal to distal. Ulnar precedes radial, grasp precedes release, and pronation precedes supination.

KEY FACT

In general, emotional differentiation proceeds as follows:
- Excitement → distress or delight at 2–3 weeks
- Distress → fear/anxiety and anger by 2–3 months
- Delight → joy and affection by 2–3 months

KEY FACT

Normal children progress at different rates, and variation may be considerable.

DEVELOPMENTAL MILESTONES

Developmental milestones are skill sets (described in Tables 2-6, 2-7, and 2-8) acquired by children at certain ages and are useful for determining whether a child is progressing at the expected rate. Variation among normal children can be considerable.

TABLE 2-6.   **Infant Developmental Milestones**

AGE	MOTOR MILESTONE	SOCIAL/COGNITIVE MILESTONE	LANGUAGE MILESTONE
3 months	Holds head up, Moro reflex disappears.	Social smile.	Begins babbling, turns head toward sound.
4–5 months	Rolls front to back, sits with support.	Recognizes people.	
7–9 months	Sits alone, transfers object from hand to hand.	Stranger anxiety, orients to voice.	Expresses joy and displeasure with voice.
12–14 months	Babinski reflex disappears.	Imitates gestures, finds hidden objects.	Says "Dada"/"Mama," tries to imitate words.
15 months	Walks alone.	Separation anxiety.	Speaks a few words.

TABLE 2-7.   **Toddler and Preschool Developmental Milestones**

AGE	MOTOR MILESTONE	SOCIAL/COGNITIVE MILESTONE	LANGUAGE MILESTONE
18 months	Stacks two blocks, runs while looking at ground.	Recognizes self in mirror or pictures, competes with other children for toys.	Speaks 8–10 words clearly, protests when frustrated.
2 years	Feeds self with spoon, stacks 3–4 blocks, walks backward.	Takes turns in play with other children, imitates parents.	Uses 2–3 word sentences, tries to hum or sing, listens to short rhymes.
3 years	Rides tricycle, copies line or circle, uses toilet with help.	Group play, knows first and last name.	Uses 3–5 word sentences, understands pronouns, asks short questions.
4 years	Simple drawings, hops on one foot, stacks 7–9 blocks, uses toilet alone.	Cooperative play, knows age, plays with imaginary objects.	Uses 5–6 word sentences, tells stories, uses past tense, enjoys rhyming.

NORMAL CHANGES OF AGING

As adults move from early to late adulthood, certain patterns of physiologic and psychological change are notable.

- Sexual changes (male): Slower erection and ejaculation; longer refractory periods.
- Sexual changes (female): Vaginal shortening, thinning, and dryness.
- Sleep pattern changes: Decreased rapid eye movement (REM) and slow-wave sleep, and increased sleep latency. The sleep period, or time from sleep onset to morning awakening, does not decrease. However, true sleep time does decrease due to increased awakening during the night.

TABLE 2-8.   **School Age and Adolescent Developmental Milestones**

AGE	PHYSICAL DEVELOPMENT	SOCIAL/COGNITIVE MILESTONE
6–11 years	Improving muscle coordination, maturation of eye function.	Development of conscience (superego), same-sex friends, identification with same-sex parent.
11 years (girls) 13 years (boys)	Development of secondary sex characteristics.	Abstract reasoning (formal operations), formation of personality, development of meta-cognition.

- Certain medical conditions become more common: Heart disease, some cancers, arthritis, hypertension, cataracts.
- Psychiatric problems, such as depression, are more common.
- Higher suicide rate.
- Thinking becomes less theoretical and more practical.

NORMAL GRIEF

Elisabeth Kübler-Ross defined the stages of grief in her landmark book, *On Death and Dying*. (Victims of physical or psychological trauma [e.g., rape] and various forms of personal loss may also experience these stages.) Although this order is typical, some individuals experience these stages in a different sequence. More than one stage may be present at a given time, and not all individuals experience all five stages.

- **Denial:** The reality of the loss is denied initially in an attempt to avoid emotional distress. One might understand the situation intellectually without experiencing the full emotional and psychological impact.
- **Anger:** Anger and resentfulness are experienced and possibly expressed toward the departed, family and friends, or caregivers. It is important for physicians to see the anger as normal and to not personalize it.
- **Bargaining:** The bereaved may try, in essence, to "make a deal," on the assumption that circumstances might improve if he or she alters his or her behavior or attitudes. In this stage, patients and family members may try excessively to be "good."
- **Despair** or **depression:** The loss is now acknowledged, with a passive, sad emotional response.
- **Acceptance:** One integrates the experience into his or her world and copes successfully.

Psychology

INTELLIGENCE QUOTIENT (IQ)

Intelligence testing originated in the early 20th century and was intended to identify intellectually deficient children who would benefit from enrollment in special education programs.

IQ is:

- Correlated with genetic factors.
- More highly correlated with educational achievement and socioeconomic status.
- Generally stable throughout life.

Commonly used IQ tests:

- **Stanford-Binet:** Tests verbal, spatial, and memory functions.
- **Wechsler Adult Intelligence Scale (WAIS):** Assesses verbal and nonverbal reasoning, as well as efficiency of processing of information.

FLASH FORWARD

Mental degeneration can be assessed by administering an IQ test and comparing the result with that expected for the patient's educational level and occupational achievement. Pathology may be harder to detect in individuals with a high baseline IQ, because their scores may appear normal despite a decline from their previous levels.

TABLE 2-9. Degrees of Mental Retardation and Corresponding IQ Ranges

DEGREE OF RETARDATION	IQ RANGE
Mild	55–69
Moderate	40–55
Severe	25–40
Profound	< 25

- **Wechsler Intelligence Scale for Children (WISC):** Similar to the WAIS, but created for children.
- **Wechsler Preschool and Primary Scale of Intelligence (WPPSI):** Used for preschoolers.

In addition to IQ tests, assessment of one's actual living skills is sometimes performed, and is required for the diagnosis of mental retardation. This refers to one's abilities in such areas as self-care, self-direction, social functioning, and communication. The Vineland Adaptive Behavioral Scale, which is based on information provided by a close observer, such as a parent or teacher, is one such test.

Interpretation of IQ tests:

- All major IQ tests use deviation IQs, measuring the degree to which an examinee deviates from the normal performance for his or her age.
- Mean = 100
- Standard deviation = 15
- Mental retardation is defined as an IQ less than 70 (greater than 2 SDs below the mean).
- Mental retardation comes in four degrees of severity, as described in Table 2-9.
- IQ tests are often administered with achievement testing to children who perform poorly in school. A specific learning disability is defined as past learning in reading, math, or writing that is significantly below expected for the person's IQ and cannot be accounted for by other factors, such as ill health or lack of educational opportunity.

KEY FACT

The mean IQ is 100, the standard deviation is 15, and mental retardation is defined as an IQ greater than 2 SDs below the mean.

ERIK ERIKSON'S PSYCHOSOCIAL DEVELOPMENT THEORY

Erikson's theory outlines eight stages through which a normal individual proceeds, as shown in Table 2-10. Each stage consists of a **basic crisis** that must be successfully overcome to proceed to the next stage. Although the stages correspond approximately to certain chronologic phases of life, the rate of progression varies among individuals.

TABLE 2-10. Erikson's Stages of Psychosocial Development

STAGE	BASIC CRISIS
Infancy	Trust versus mistrust
Early childhood	Autonomy versus shame and self-doubt
Play age	Initiative versus guilt
School age	Industry versus inferiority
Adolescence	Identity versus role confusion
Young adulthood	Intimacy versus isolation
Adulthood	Generativity versus stagnation
Late adulthood	Integrity versus despair

KEY FACT

- For cla**ss**ical conditioning, think **s**timulus: The goal is for a **new** stimulus to elicit the same desired response as an established stimulus (the unconditioned stimulus).
- For ope**r**ant conditioning, think **r**esponse: Reinforcements and punishments known to be effective are used to alter the frequency of voluntary behavior.

KEY FACT

All reinforcement of behavior increases the probability of such behavior in the future, and all punishment decreases the probability of such behavior.

KEY FACT

Reinforcement is most effective when presented in such a way that the individual can clearly perceive the connection between the behavior and the reinforcement. Thus, effective reinforcement generally occurs shortly following the behavior.

CONDITIONING

Conditioning is the alteration of behavior by consequences.

Classical Conditioning

Classical conditioning was first described by the Russian physiologist Ivan Pavlov. An **unconditioned stimulus (UCS)**, known to elicit a characteristic response (the **unconditioned response**, or **UCR**) is paired with a new, neutral stimulus (the **conditioned stimulus**, or **CS**) so that eventually the new stimulus alone elicits the same or a similar response. The response is known as the **conditioned response (CR)** when elicited by the CS alone. For the CS to effectively elicit a CR, it must precede the UCS during the conditioning phase.

Example: A young child naturally cries (UCR) in response to sharp pain (UCS). If the child is brought to a physician's office for a vaccination, sees the syringe, and immediately experiences sharp pain from the needle, the child will associate the needle with the pain and cry (CR) in response to the mere sight of the needle (CS), even before the vaccination is given.

Operant Conditioning

Operant conditioning was first described by B. F. Skinner, who observed that the likelihood of voluntary behavior is increased by subsequent **reinforcement** or decreased by subsequent **punishment**. Both reinforcement and punishment can be **positive** or **negative**.

- **Positive reinforcement**: A pleasant experience occurs (e.g., wages).
- **Negative reinforcement**: An unpleasant experience is removed (e.g., relief from household chores).
- **Positive punishment**: An unpleasant experience occurs (e.g., extra homework).
- **Negative punishment**: A pleasant experience is removed (e.g., loss of days off).

Beware of confusion between punishment and negative reinforcement. Any reinforcement, both positive and negative, encourages the reinforced behavior.

Extinction is the process by which a previously reinforced behavior is no longer reinforced, leading to its elimination. For example, in classical conditioning, visits to the doctor who no longer gives shots will lead to decreased association of the needle with pain. In operant conditioning, a rat that no longer receives food when pressing a bar will stop associating this behavior with food and stop responding. In other words, conditioned behavior can be unlearned as well as learned.

Reinforcement Schedules

The two main categories of reinforcement schedules are **ratio** and **interval**. In the ratio schedule, reinforcement occurs based on behavioral events, regardless of time intervals. In the interval schedule, reinforcement occurs based on time intervals, regardless of the frequency of behavioral events. In either category, reinforcement can be **fixed** or **variable**.

- **Fixed-ratio** schedule: Reinforcement occurs after a set number of behaviors. Example: Vending machines.
- **Variable-ratio** schedule: Reinforcement occurs after a varying number of behaviors. Example: Casino slot machines.
- **Fixed-interval** schedule: Reinforcement occurs after a set time interval (and a response on the part of the organism). Example: Timed pet feeders.
- **Variable-interval** schedule: Reinforcement occurs at varied times. Example: Pop quizzes.

EGO DEFENSE MECHANISMS

Ego defense mechanisms are the best-known work of Anna Freud, Sigmund Freud's daughter and a renowned psychoanalyst in her own right. Anna Freud,

KEY FACT

Classical conditioning causes a previously neutral stimulus to produce a characteristic (and preexisting) response. Operant conditioning uses effective reinforcement and punishment to alter voluntary behavior.

KEY FACT

Intermittent reinforcement is more resistant to extinction than is continuous reinforcement.

TABLE 2-11. Mature Defense Mechanisms

DEFENSE MECHANISM	DEFINITION	EXAMPLE
Altruism	Guilty feelings relieved by generosity and personal sacrifice.	Mafia boss making a large donation to charity.
Humor	Appreciation of the amusing aspects of an anxiety-inducing setting.	Nervous medical student joking about the boards.
Sublimation	Redirecting unacceptable impulses into more acceptable actions.	Joining the military out of a desire to kill.
Suppression	Voluntarily keeping a thought away from consciousness.	Refusing to think about getting revenge on someone.

like her father, believed strongly in the importance of unconscious drives in determining behavior, but also emphasized the importance of the ego, or executive decision-making, in the functioning of the person. One aspect thereof is the **ego defense mechanism**. These mechanisms are unconscious and act in response to psychological stress or threat. Some are mature (Table 2-11); others are immature (Table 2-12).

TABLE 2-12.   Immature Defense Mechanisms

DEFENSE MECHANISM	DEFINITION	EXAMPLE
Acting out	Unacceptable thoughts and feelings are expressed through actions.	Temper tantrums.
Dissociation	Avoidance of stress by a temporary drastic change in personality, memory, consciousness, or motor behavior.	Dissociative identity disorder (in extreme cases).
Denial	Pretending, believing, and/or acting as though an undesirable reality is nonexistent.	Common response in patients newly diagnosed with cancer or AIDS.
Displacement	Feelings one wishes to avoid are directed at a neutral party.	Man arguing with his wife after being reprimanded by his boss.
Fixation	Partially remaining at an age-inappropriate level of development.	Functional adult nibbling on her nails.
Identification	Learning unacceptable behavior from a model.	Abused child becoming an abuser.
Intellectualization	Focusing on the intellectual aspects of a situation to avoid anxiety.	Doing vigorous research on one's terminal disease to distract oneself from distress.
Isolation	Separation of feelings from ideas and events.	Attending a loved one's funeral without emotion.
Projection	Attributing an unacceptable impulse to an outside source rather than to oneself.	Man who wants another woman thinking that his wife is cheating on him.
Rationalization	Creating a logical argument to avoid blaming oneself.	A woman who is passed over for a desirable promotion saying that her current position is better.
Reaction formation	To avoid anxiety, acting the extreme opposite of an unacceptable manner.	Behaving obsequiously toward in-laws one strongly dislikes.
Regression	Abandoning a normal maturity level and going back to an earlier one.	Previously toilet-trained child wetting the bed.
Repression	Keeping anxiety-provoking thoughts and feelings from consciousness.	Involuntary or unconscious burying of memories of child abuse.
Splitting	Perceiving people as either all good or all bad.	Patient saying that all nurses are cold, but all doctors are friendly.

Biochemistry

Molecular Biology

NUCLEOTIDES

General Structure

Nucleotides are composed of three subunits (see Figure 3-1):

1. Pentose sugar
   - Ribose
   - Deoxyribose
2. Nitrogenous base
   - Purine
   - Pyrimidine
3. Phosphate group: Forms the linkages between nucleotides.

In contrast, a **nucleoside** is composed of only two units: a pentose sugar and a nitrogenous base. Nucleotides are linked by a **3′–5′ phosphodiester bond** (see Figure 3-2). By convention, DNA sequences are written from the 5′ end to the 3′ end.

PENTOSE SUGAR

Can be either **ribose**, which is found in RNA, or **2-deoxyribose**, which is found in DNA (see Figure 3-1). 2-Deoxyribose lacks a hydroxyl (–OH) group at the 2′ carbon (C2).

NITROGENOUS BASE

The two types differ by the number of rings composing the base.

Purines versus Pyrimidines

Each **purine** (adenine [A], guanine [G], xanthine, hypoxanthine, uric acid) is composed of two rings, whereas each **pyrimidine** (cytosine [C], uracil [U], thymine [T]) is composed of one ring (see Figure 3-3). Note that **uracil** is found only in RNA, whereas **thymine** is found only in DNA. All other bases are found in both RNA and DNA (see Table 3-1). The pyrimidines may be derived from one another: deaminating cytosine results in uracil. Adding a methyl group to uracil produces thymine.

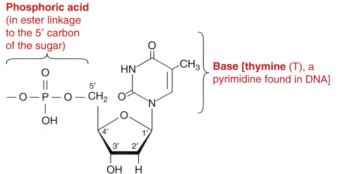
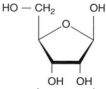

Phosphoric acid (in ester linkage to the 5′ carbon of the sugar)

Base [thymine (T), a pyrimidine found in DNA]

Pentose sugar (2-deoxyribose, found in DNA)

Ribose (pentose found in RNA; has ⁻OH at the 2′ position)

FIGURE 3-1. The general structure of nucleotides. Ribose and deoxyribose pentose sugars only differ at the 2′-carbon, in which deoxyribose lacks a hydroxyl (–OH) group.

FIGURE 3-2. **The phosphodiester bond links the 3′ end of a ribose sugar to the preceding sugar's 5′ carbon.** (Modified, with permission, from Murray RK. et al. *Harper's Illustrated Biochemistry*, 26th ed. New York: McGraw-Hill, 2003.)

- Substrates for DNA synthesis include: dATP, dGTP, dTTP, dCTP (d = deoxy).
- Substrates for RNA synthesis include: ATP, GTP, UTP, CTP.

Base Pairing

G-C bonds (3 H-bonds) are stronger than A-T bonds (2 H-bonds) (see Figure 3-4). Increased G-C content increases the **melting temperature** (T_m), which is the temperature at which half of the DNA base-pair hydrogen bonds are broken. Chargaff's rule also dictates that the G content equals the C content, and the A content equals the T content.

NUCLEOTIDE SYNTHESIS

Purine Nucleotide Synthesis

Occurs through either the de novo or the salvage pathway. De novo synthesis utilizes elemental precursors and is used primarily for rapidly dividing cells. The salvage pathway recycles the nucleosides and nitrogenous bases that are

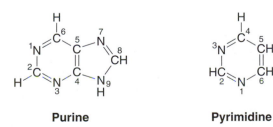

Purine   **Pyrimidine**

FIGURE 3-3. **Base structures of pyrimidines and purines.** (Modified, with permission, from Murray RK, Granner DK, Rodwell VW. *Harper's Illustrated Biochemistry*, 27th ed. New York: McGraw-Hill, 2006: 294.)

TABLE 3-1. Purines versus Pyrimidines

PURINES	PYRIMIDINES
Two rings.	One ring.
Adenine.	Cytosine.
Guanine.	Thymine (found only in DNA).
Xanthine, hypoxanthine, uric acid.	Uracil (found only in RNA).

released from degraded nucleic acids; it is considered the major route for synthesis in adults.

DE NOVO SYNTHESIS

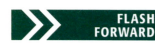

FLASH FORWARD

Allopurinol and 6-mercaptopurine are purine analogs that inhibit PRPP amidotransferase.

- Rate-limiting step by **glutamine PRPP (5-phosphoribosyl-1-pyrophosphate) amidotransferase.**
- PRPP amidotransferase is inhibited by downstream products (inosine monophosphate [IMP], guanosine monophosphate [GMP], adenosine monophosphate [AMP]) and purine analogs (allopurinol and 6-mercaptopurine).
- Required cofactors: tetrahydrofolate (THF), glutamine, glycine, aspartate.
- **Reciprocal substrate effect:** GTP and ATP are substrates in AMP and GMP synthesis, respectively. For example, $\downarrow$ GTP $\rightarrow$ $\downarrow$ AMP $\rightarrow$ $\downarrow$ ATP. This allows for balanced synthesis of adenine and guanine nucleotides.

PURINE SALVAGE PATHWAY (see Figure 3-5)

- Recycles ~90% of the preformed purines that are released when cells' nucleases degrade endogenous DNA and RNA and make new purine nucleotides.
- Catalyzed by **hypoxanthine phosphoribosyltransferase (HGPRT),** which is inhibited by IMP and GMP.
- Nitrogenous base (guanine, hypoxanthine) + PRPP $\rightarrow$ GMP/IMP + PP_i

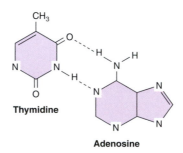

FIGURE 3-4. Hydrogen bonding between base pairs. (Modified, with permission, from Murray RK, Granner DK, Rodwell VW. *Harper's Illustrated Biochemistry*, 27th ed. New York: McGraw-Hill, 2006: 313.)

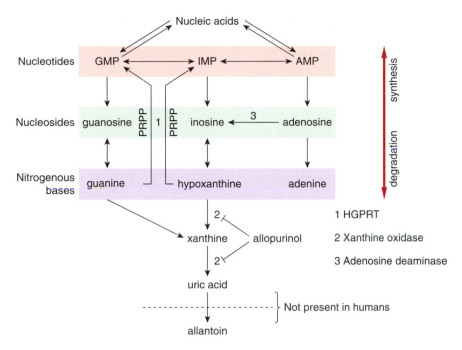

FIGURE 3-5. **Purine salvage pathway and deficiencies.** HGPRT = hypoxanthine phosphoribosyltransferase.

Purine Salvage Deficiencies

LESCH-NYHAN SYNDROME

X-linked recessive disorder of failed purine salvage due to the **absence of HGPRT**. HGPRT converts hypoxanthine → IMP and guanine → GMP. The inability to salvage purines leads to excess purine synthesis and consequent excess uric acid production.

PRESENTATION

Retardation, cerebral palsy, self-mutilation, aggression, gout, choreoathetosis, arthritis, nephropathy.

DIAGNOSIS

Orange crystals in diaper, difficulty with movement, self-injury, **hyperuricemia**.

TREATMENT

Allopurinol, which inhibits xanthine oxidase. Treatment does not ameliorate neurologic symptoms.

PROGNOSIS

Urate nephropathy, death in the first decade, usually as a result of renal failure.

GOUT

Disorder associated with **hyperuricemia**, due to either overproduction or underexcretion of uric acid. Uric acid is less soluble than hypoxanthine and xanthine, and, therefore, **sodium urate crystals** deposit in joints and soft tissues, leading to arthritis.

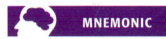

MNEMONIC

Lesch-**N**yhan **S**yndrome

Lacks
Nucleotide
Salvage (purine)

FLASH FORWARD

Differential diagnosis for increased uric acid and gout:
- Lesch-Nyhan, alcoholism, and G6PD.
- Alcoholism
- G6P deficiency, hereditary fructose intolerance, galactose 1P uridyl transferase deficiency—all disorders with increased accumulation of phosphorylated sugars, increased degradation products (e.g., AMP).

- **Primary gout:** Due to hyperuricemia without evident cause. Affected individuals may have a familial disposition. May occur in association with PRPP synthetase hyperactivity or HGPRT deficiency of Lesch-Nyhan syndrome; most common form.
- **Secondary (acquired) gout:** Uric acid overproduction can be caused by leukemia, myeloproliferative syndrome, multiple myeloma, hemolysis, neoplasia, psoriasis, and alcoholism and is more common in men. Secondary gout due to urate underexcretion can be caused by kidney disease and drugs such as aspirin, diuretics, and alcohol.

PRESENTATION

Monoarticular arthritis of distal joints (e.g., **podagra**—gout of the great toe), often with history of hyperuricemia for > 20–30 years, precipitated by a sudden change in urate levels (e.g., due to large meals, alcohol), eventually leads to nodular **tophi** (urate crystals surrounded by fibrous connective tissue) located around the joints and Achilles tendon.

DIAGNOSIS

Arthritis, hyperuricemia, detection of **negatively bifringent** crystals from articular tap.

TREATMENT

Normalize uric acid levels (allopurinol, probenecid for chronic gout), decrease pain and inflammation (colchicines, nonsteroidal anti-inflammatory drug [NSAIDs] for acute gout), avoid large meals and alcohol.

SEVERE COMBINED (T AND B) IMMUNODEFICIENCY (SCID)

Autosomal recessive disorder caused by a deficiency in **adenosine deaminase (ADA)**. Excess ATP and dATP causes an imbalance in the nucleotide pool via inhibition of **ribonucleotide reductase** (catalyzes ribose → deoxyribose). This prevents DNA synthesis and decreases the lymphocyte count. It is not understood why the enzyme deficiency devastates lymphocytes in particular.

PRESENTATION

Children recurrently infected with bacterial, protozoan, and viral pathogens, especially *Candida*, *Pneumocystis jiroveci*.

DIAGNOSIS

No plasma cells or B or T lymphocytes on complete blood count (CBC), no thymus.

TREATMENT

Gene therapy, bone marrow transplantation.

PROGNOSIS

Poor.

Pyrimidine Nucleotide Synthesis

Like purines, pyrimidine synthesis can occur through de novo synthesis or may be recycled through the salvage pathway. The salvage pathway relies on pyrimidine phosphoribosyl transferase enzyme, which is responsible for recycling orotic acid, uracil, and thymine, but not cytosine. De novo synthesis relies on a different set of enzymes.

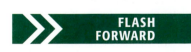

FLASH FORWARD

Chemotherapeutics exploit these pathways: Hydroxyurea inhibits ribonucleotide reductase; 5-fluorouracil (5-FU) inhibits thymidylate synthase; methotrexate and pyrimethamine inhibit dihydrofolate reductase.

HEREDITARY OROTIC ACIDURIA

Deficiency in orotate phosphoribosyl transferase and/or OMP decarboxylase (pyrimidine metabolism).

PRESENTATION

Retarded growth, severe anemia.

DIAGNOSIS

Low serum iron, leukopenia, megaloblastosis, white precipitate in urine.

TREATMENT

Synthetic cytidine or uridine given to maintain pyrimidine nucleotide levels for DNA and RNA synthesis.

NUCLEOTIDE DEGRADATION

Products of purine degradation include **uric acid**, which is excreted in urine. Pyrimidine degradation yields **β-amino acids, CO_2,** and **NH_4^+.** For example, thymine is degraded into β-aminoisobutyrate, CO_2, and NH_4^+. Since thymine degradation is the only source of β-aminoisobutyrate in urine, **urinary β-aminoisobutyrate levels** are often used as an **indicator of DNA turnover** (↑ in chemotherapy, radiation therapy).

DNA

DNA Synthesis

- Building blocks: Deoxyribonucleotides (dNTPs).
- **dADP, dGDP, dCDP, dUDP synthesis:** Depends on **ribonucleotide reductase** enzyme, which converts ADP, GDP, CDP, and UDP into dADP, dGDP, dCDP, and dUDP, respectively. **dATP,** an allosteric inhibitor, strictly regulates ribonucleotide reductase in order to control the overall supply of dNDPs.
- **dTDP synthesis: Thymidylate synthase** catalyzes the transfer of one carbon from N^5,N^{10}-methylene tetrahydrofolate (FH_4) to dUDP, yielding dTDP. The N^5, N^{10}-FH_4 coenzyme then must be regenerated by **dihydrofolate reductase,** which uses NADPH.

DNA Structure

The structure of DNA is characterized by its **polarity,** with a **5′ phosphate** end and a **3′ hydroxyl** end (see Figure 3-6). It is composed of two polynucleotide strands that run **antiparallel** to each other (i.e., in opposite directions). The two strands coil around a common axis to form a right-handed double helix (also called B-DNA). Rarely, there is also left-handed DNA, called Z-DNA. Nitrogenous bases sit inside the helix, whereas the phosphate and deoxyribose units sit outside. Each turn of the helix consists of 10 base pairs.

Organization of Eukaryotic DNA Supercoiling

DNA helices can be tightly or loosely wound, and the physical strain on the helix depends on the action of topoisomerases. Topoisomerases nick the helix at its sugar-phosphate backbone, rendering it either loosely wound (negatively supercoiled DNA) or overwound (positively supercoiled DNA).

FLASH FORWARD

Bacterial dihydrofolate reductase is inhibited by the antimetabolite trimethoprim. It is often used in combination with sulfonamides (e.g., sulfamethoxazole) to sequentially block folate synthesis.

KEY FACT

Conditions that lead to denaturation of the DNA helix: Heat, alkaline pH, formamide, and urea.

FLASH FORWARD

Quinolone antibiotics inhibit bacterial topoisomerase IV.

BUILDING BLOCKS OF DNA

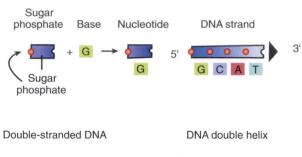

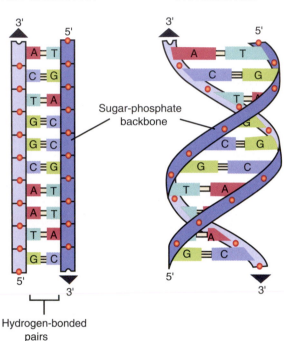

FIGURE 3-6. **Schematic representation of two complementary DNA sequences.**

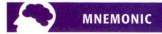
Nucleosome DNA is found associated with nucleoproteins as a protein-DNA complex (see Figure 3-7). Negatively charged DNA is looped twice around positively charged histones composed of H2A, H2B, H3, and H4 proteins. The DNA-covered octamer of histone proteins (**beads on a string**) forms a unit called a **nucleosome** (also called 10-nm fibers). H1 histone and linker DNA tie one nucleosome to the next; the nucleosomes, in aggregate, condense further to form the 30-nm fiber. The 30-nm fibers associate and loop around scaffolding proteins. During mitosis, DNA condenses to form chromosomes.

HETEROCHROMATIN

- Condensed.
- Transcriptionally inactive.
- Found in mitosis as well as interphase.

EUCHROMATIN

- Less condensed.
- Transcriptionally active.
- Includes the 10-nm and 30-nm fibers.

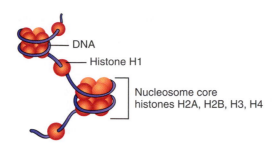

FIGURE 3-7. Chromatin structure and related proteins.

CHROMATIN STRUCTURE

Influenced by both **DNA methylation** and **histone acetylation**. Usually, inactive genes have increased amounts of methylated DNA. Acetylation of histone loosens the chromatin structure. Loosened DNA is more accessible, and more genes can be transcribed.

DNA Replication in Prokaryotes

SEMICONSERVATIVE REPLICATION (see Figure 3-8)

Each parent DNA strand serves as a template for the synthesis of one new daughter DNA strand. The resulting DNA molecule has one original parent strand and one newly synthesized strand.

SEPARATION OF TWO COMPLEMENTARY DNA STRANDS

Replication begins at a single, unique nucleotide sequence known as the **origin of replication**. A replication fork forms and marks a region of active synthesis. Replication is bidirectional with a leading and a discontinuous/lagging strand.

- Leading strand is replicated **in the direction** in which the replication fork is moving. Synthesized continuously.
- Lagging strand is copied **in the opposite direction** of the moving replication fork. Synthesized discontinuously. The short, discontinuous fragments are known as **Okazaki fragments**.
- Involves several other proteins (see Table 3-2).

 KEY FACT

Increased DNA methylation → *decreased* gene transcription
Increased histone acetylation → *increased* gene transcription

 CLINICAL CORRELATION

Antibodies against the SS-A and/or SS-B antigens are often present in Sjögren's syndrome.

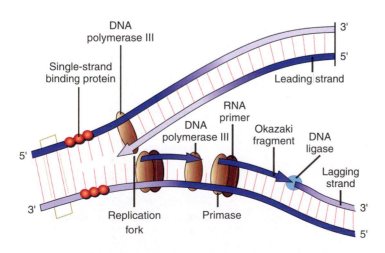

FIGURE 3-8. Prokaryotic DNA replication and DNA polymerases. DNA replication with the leading and lagging strands.

TABLE 3-2. Other Important Proteins Involved with Prokaryotic DNA Replication

PROTEIN	FUNCTION
DnaA protein	Binds to origin of replication and causes dsDNA to melt into a local region of ssDNA.
DNA helicase	Unwinds double helix. Requires energy (ATP).
Single-stranded DNA-binding (SS-B) protein	Binds and stabilizes ssDNA to prevent re-annealing.
RNA primase	Synthesizes 10 nucleotide primer.
DNA topoisomerase	Creates a nick in the helix to relieve the supercoils/strain imposed by DNA unwinding.

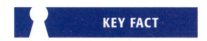

KEY FACT

DNA polymerase III has 5′ → 3′ polymerase activity and 3′ → 5′ exonuclease activity.

RNA Primer

Made by **primase;** necessary for DNA polymerase III to initiate replication.

Chain Elongation

Catalyzed by **DNA polymerase III,** which has both polymerase and proofreading functions.

- Elongates the DNA chain by adding deoxynucleotides (dNTPs) to the 3′-hydroxyl end of the RNA primer. Continues to add dNTPs from the **5′ → 3′ direction** until it reaches the primer of the preceding fragment.
- Proofreads each newly added nucleotide. Has **3′ → 5′ exonuclease activity.**

TABLE 3-3. Prokaryotic versus Eukaryotic DNA Replication

	PROKARYOTES	EUKARYOTES
DNA	Circular, small	Linear, long
Sites of replication	Only one (origin of replication, rich in AT base pairs), bound by DnaA proteins	Multiple sites that include a short sequence that is rich in AT base pairs (**consensus sequence**)
Primer synthesis	RNA primase	DNA polymerase α—primase activity, initiates DNA synthesis
Leading strand synthesis	DNA polymerase III (chain elongation, proofreading)	DNA polymerase α, δ—DNA elongation
Lagging strand synthesis	DNA polymerase I (degrades RNA primer)	DNA polymerase α, δ
DNA repair		DNA polymerase β, ε
Proofreading	DNA polymerase III	?DNA polymerase α
Mitochondrial DNA	N/A	DNA polymerase γ—replicates mitochondrial DNA
RNA primer removal	DNA polymerase I	RNase H

DNA POLYMERASE I

Degrades RNA primer. Has 5′ → 3′ exonuclease activity.

DNA LIGASE

Seals the remaining nick by creating a phosphodiester linkage.

Overall, eukaryotic DNA replication is similar to that of prokaryotic DNA synthesis, with several notable exceptions (see Table 3-3). Namely, replication begins at **consensus sequences** that are rich in A-T base pairs. Eukaryotic genome has multiple origins of replication. Eukaryotes have separate polymerases (α, β, γ, δ, ε) for synthesizing RNA primers, leading-strand DNA, lagging-strand DNA, mitochondrial DNA, and DNA repair (mutations and DNA repair are discussed later in the chapter).

RNA

Building blocks are ribonucleotides connected by phosphodiester bonds.

RNA versus DNA

RNA differs from DNA in the following ways:

- Smaller than DNA.
- Contains ribose sugar (deoxyribose in DNA) and uracil (thymine in DNA).
- Usually exists in single-strand form.

Types of RNA

There are three types of RNA, each with a specific function and location in the cell (see Table 3-4).

tRNA Structure

75–90 nucleotides in a cloverleaf form. Anticodon end is opposite the 3′ aminoacyl end. All tRNAs, both eukaryotic and prokaryotic, have CCA at the 3′ end, in addition to a high percentage of chemically modified bases. The amino acid is covalently bound to the 3′ end of the tRNA (see Figure 3-9). The anticodon of the tRNA is the same sequence as the DNA template strand (see Figure 3-10).

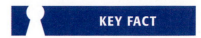

KEY FACT

DNA polymerase I excises RNA primer with 5′ → 3′ exonuclease.

KEY FACT

mRNA = largest type of RNA
rRNA = most abundant type of RNA
tRNA = smallest type of RNA

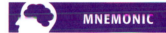

MNEMONIC

Massive (**m**RNA)
Rampant (**r**RNA)
Tiny (**t**RNA)

TABLE 3-4.   Comparison of the Three Types of RNA

RNA TYPE	FUNCTION	ABUNDANCE IN CELL (% OF TOTAL RNA)	NOTES
mRNA	Messenger—carries genetic information from nucleus to cytosol.	5	Largest type
rRNA	Ribosomal.	80	Most abundant type
tRNA	Transfer—serves as an adapter molecule that recognizes genetic code (the **codon**) that is carried by mRNA. A codon comprises three adjacent nucleotides that encodes one and only one amino acid. Carries and matches a specific amino acid that corresponds to the codon.	15	Smallest type

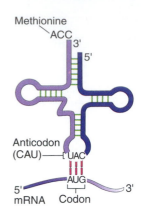

FIGURE 3-9. tRNA structure.

FEATURES OF THE GENETIC CODE

Central Dogma

The central dogma states that RNA is synthesized from a DNA template and protein is synthesized from an RNA template (see Figure 3-11).

DNA and RNA sequences are read in triplets (a **codon**), in which each codon encodes either an amino acid (61 possible codons) or a "stop" signal (UGA, UAA, UAG). The **start codon** AUG (or rarely GUG) is the mRNA initiation codon. It fixes the reading frame and encodes slightly different amino acids in prokaryotes versus eukaryotes (see Table 3-5). For both prokaryotes and eukaryotes, the genetic code is unambiguous, redundant, and (almost) universal.

UNAMBIGUOUS

1 codon → 1 amino acid.

DEGENERATE/REDUNDANT

More than 1 codon may code for the same amino acid (e.g., three codons encode for the same stop signal).

UNIVERSAL

Used by almost all known organisms with some exceptions (e.g., mitochondria, Archaebacteria, mycoplasma, and some yeasts).

DIRECTION OF DNA, RNA, AND PROTEIN SYNTHESIS

During DNA/RNA and protein synthesis, nucleotides and amino acids are always added in a set direction (see Table 3-6).

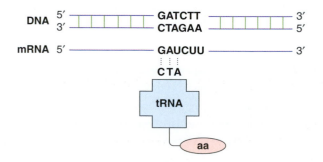

FIGURE 3-10. How the DNA template relates to mRNA and to the tRNA anticodon.

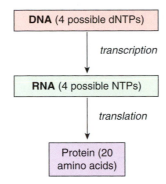

FIGURE 3-11. **The central dogma.** RNA is made from DNA, and protein is made from RNA.

TRANSCRIPTION

The DNA template is transcribed into RNA by RNA polymerase in a process similar to that of DNA replication/synthesis.

- RNA is composed of uracil (U) instead of thymine (T) bases. Therefore, in RNA, adenine (A) pairs with a uracil (U) instead of thymine (T).

The RNA immediately produced by RNA polymerase (before it undergoes modification) is known as the **primary transcript** or heterogeneous nuclear RNA (hnRNA).

- Eukaryotes modify hnRNA, but prokaryotes do not (see Table 3-7).
- Eukaryotes and prokaryotes possess different RNA polymerases.

Whereas prokaryotes have only one RNA polymerase that synthesizes all RNA types, eukaryotes have several, each of which is responsible for making mRNA, rRNA, and tRNA.

Transcription in Prokaryotes

In contrast to eukaryotes, prokaryotic RNA polymerase synthesizes all three types of RNA. It does not require a primer, and cannot proofread or correct mistakes. Structurally, it has two forms:

- **Core enzyme** composed of four subunits ($\alpha_2\beta\beta'$).
- **Holoenzyme,** a core enzyme with a sigma subunit that allows the enzyme to recognize promoter sequences.

Transcription occurs in three steps—initiation, elongation, and termination.

INITIATION

Sigma subunit of RNA polymerase recognizes promoter region of the sense strand of DNA, binds to DNA, and unwinds double helix. Upstream consensus sequences help the RNA pol find the promoter. This process is blocked by **rifampin.**

KEY FACT

DNA—A and **T** base pair
RNA—A and **U** base pair

KEY FACT

DNA polymerase has proofreading activity, but eukaryotic and prokaryotic RNA polymerases do not.

KEY FACT

Prokaryotes are unable to modify their primary transcript. One end of the mRNA can be translated, while the other end is still being transcribed!

TABLE 3-5. **Start Codon in Prokaryotes versus Eukaryotes**

Prokaryotes	AUG → formyl-methionine (f-met).
Eukaryotes	AUG → methionine (may be removed before translation is completed).

TABLE 3-6.   Direction of DNA, RNA, and Protein Synthesis

MOLECULE TYPE	DIRECTION OF SYNTHESIS	NOTES
DNA RNA	5′ End of nucleotide added to 3′-OH group of growing DNA/RNA (**5′ → 3′**).	5′ Triphosphate group is the energy source for the phosphodiester bond.
Protein	Amino acids linked N-terminus to C-terminus (**N → C**).	

ELONGATION

RNA grows as a polynucleotide chain from the 5′ end to the 3′ end. Meanwhile, RNA polymerase moves along the DNA template from the 3′ end to the 5′ end (see Figure 3-12). Blocked by **actinomycin D.**

TERMINATION

RNA polymerase and/or specific termination factors (e.g., rho factor in *Escherichia coli*) recognize special DNA sequences that cause their dissociation from the DNA template.

- Termination can be rho-dependent or independent.
  - Rho-dependent termination requires participation of a protein factor.
  - Rho-independent termination requires a specific secondary structure (a hairpin loop followed by a string of Us) in the newly synthesized RNA (see Figure 3-13).

Transcription in Eukaryotes

Transcription in eukaryotes involves both RNA polymerase and additional transcription factors that bind to DNA. Different RNA polymerases are required to synthesize different types of eukaryotic RNA (see Table 3-8).

TABLE 3-7.   Factors that Affect Modification of the Primary Transcript[a]

	POST-TRANSCRIPTIONAL MODIFICATION	
RNA TYPE	**PROKARYOTES**	**EUKARYOTES**
mRNA	No—identical with primary transcript	Yes
tRNA	Yes	Yes
rRNA	Yes	Yes

[a]Whether or not the primary transcript is modified depends on the RNA type (mRNA, tRNA, rRNA) and the organism (eukaryotes versus prokaryotes).

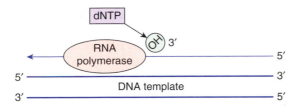

FIGURE 3-12. **Elongation step in transcription.** RNA synthesis occurs from 5' to 3', whereas the RNA polymerase moves along the DNA template in the 3' to 5' direction.

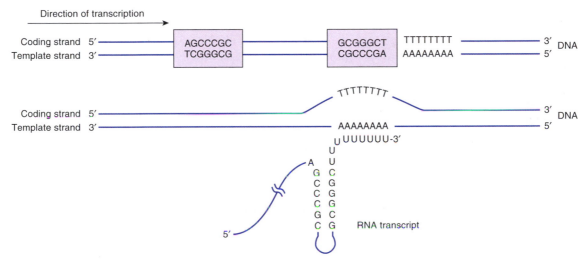

FIGURE 3-13. **Typical prokaryotic termination sequence.** (Modified, with permission, from Murray RK, Granner DK, Rodwell VW. *Harper's Illustrated Biochemistry*, 27th ed. New York: McGraw-Hill, 2006: 353.)

TABLE 3-8. **Eukaryotic RNA Polymerases and Their Function**

RNA POLYMERASE	RNA TYPE MADE	NOTES
RNA polymerase I	rRNA.	
RNA polymerase II	mRNA.	Cannot initiate transcription by itself, requires transcription factors.
RNA polymerase III	tRNA.	
Mitochondrial RNA polymerase	Transcribes RNA from mitochondrial genes.	Inhibited by rifampin, more closely resembles bacterial RNA polymerase than eukaryotic RNA polymerase.

TABLE 3-9. Types and Function of Post-transcriptional Modification

POST-TRANSCRIPTIONAL MODIFICATION	DESCRIPTION	FUNCTION
5′ Capping	7-Methyl-guanosine added to 5′ end of RNA.	Prevents mRNA degradation, allows translation (protein synthesis) to begin.
Poly-A tail	40–200 adenine nucleotides added to 3′ end of RNA by polyadenylate polymerase.	Stabilizes mRNA, facilitates exit from nucleus. Note: not all mRNAs have a poly-A tail (e.g., histone mRNAs).
RNA splicing	Performed by the spliceosome, which is composed of small nuclear ribonucleoprotein particles **(snRNP).** Binds the primary transcript at splice junctions flanked by GU-AG.	**Introns** (DNA sequences that do not code for protein) are removed and **exons** (coding sequences) are spliced together (see Figure 3-15). The excised intron is released as a lariat structure.

KEY FACT

In **eukaryotes**, RNA processing occurs in the nucleus.
In **prokaryotes**, RNA is not processed. The primary transcript is translated as soon as it is made.

MNEMONIC

INtrons stay **IN** the nucleus, whereas **EX**ons **EX**it and are **EX**pressed.

FLASH FORWARD

Defects in post-transcriptional RNA processing can cause pathology.
- Systemic lupus erythematosus is associated with the production of antibodies to host protein, including small nuclear ribonucleoprotein particles **(snRNPs).**
- 15% of genetic diseases result from defective RNA splicing (i.e., incorrect splicing of β-globin mRNA is responsible for some cases of β-thalassemia).

REGULATION OF GENE EXPRESSION AT THE LEVEL OF TRANSCRIPTION

Based on DNA sequences that may be located distant from, near, or within (e.g., in an intron, which is not expressed) the gene being regulated. These DNA sequences include:

- **Promoters:** In eukaryotes, includes a TATA sequence (the **TATA box**) and/or a CAAT sequence 25 and 70 base pairs, respectively, upstream of ATG start codon. Critical for initiation of transcription. Mutations may decrease the quantity of gene transcribed.
- **Enhancer:** Stretch of DNA that increases the rate of transcription when bound by transcription factors.
- **Silencer:** Stretch of DNA that decreases the rate of transcription when bound.

TRANSCRIPTION

Follows the same steps as prokaryotes (initiation, elongation, and termination), but requires different RNA polymerase machinery.

RNA PROCESSING

Unlike in prokaryotic mRNA, the primary transcript (hnRNA) is both spliced and modified with a 5′-cap and a 3′-tail before leaving the nucleus (see Table 3-9). The cap contains 7-methylguanine, which protects it against nuclear digestion and helps insure correct alignment of the RNA and ribosome for translation. The 3′ poly A tail protects the mRNA from exonucleases, allows it to be exported from the nucleus, and is important for translation. Splicing prevents translation of introns. Once modified, the RNA is known as mRNA (see Figure 3-14).

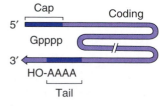

FIGURE 3-14. Structure of a typically processed mRNA in eukaryotes.

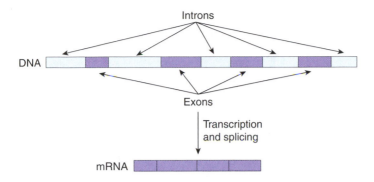

FIGURE 3-15. **Schematic representation of introns versus exons.**

TRANSLATION

Translation is the process by which mRNA base sequences are translated into an amino acid sequence and protein. It involves all three types of RNA; mRNA is the template for protein synthesis. tRNA contains a three-base anti-codon that hydrogen bonds to complementary bases in mRNA. Each tRNA molecule carries an amino acid that corresponds to its anticodon. rRNA—along with other proteins—composes the ribosomes. Ribosomes coordinate the interactions among mRNA, tRNA, and the enzymes necessary for protein synthesis.

Ribosomes

The site of protein synthesis. Composed of rRNA and protein. Consist of two subunits—one large, one small. The subunits in prokaryotes and eukaryotes differ in size (S values are usually not additive); eukaryotic ribosomes are larger.

	(Small subunit)		(Large subunit)		
Prokaryote ribosome:	30S	+	50S	=	70S
Eukaryote ribosome:	40S	+	60S	=	80S

tRNA STRUCTURE

Distinct structure designed to "translate" the mRNA sequence into the corresponding amino acid sequence (see Figure 3-10). tRNA is composed of 75–90 nucleotides in a cloverleaf form. The anticodon end is opposite the 3′ amino-acyl end and is antiparallel and complementary to the codon in mRNA (see Figure 3-9). All tRNAs—both eukaryotic and prokaryotic—have CCA at the 3′ end, in addition to a high percentage of chemically modified bases. The amino acid is covalently bound to the 3′ end of the RNA.

tRNA CHARGING

Requires aminoacyl-tRNA synthetase, ATP, and tRNA. Each amino acid has a specific synthetase that transfers energy from 1 ATP to the bond between the amino acid and the 3′ hydroxyl (OH) group of the appropriate tRNA (see Figure 3-16). This bond contains the energy that later forms the peptide bond when the amino acid is added to the growing peptide. If an amino acid is incorrectly paired with tRNA, aminoacyl-tRNA synthetase hydrolyzes the amino acid–tRNA bond.

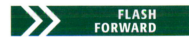

FLASH FORWARD

Buy **AT 30, CELL** AT **50.**

Certain antibiotics target the bacterial ribosome and disrupt translation.

Aminoglycosides and **T**etracycline inhibit the **30S** subunit.
Clindamycin, **C**hloramphenicol **E**rythromycin, and **l**incomycin inhibit the **50S** ribosome subunit.

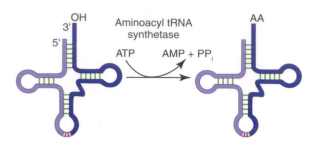

FIGURE 3-16. tRNA charging.

tRNA WOBBLE

The code for certain amino acids relies only on the base sequence of the first two nucleotides in the codon. As described earlier, often the same amino acid has multiple codons that differ in the third "wobble" position. Therefore, < 61 tRNAs are needed to translate all 61 codons.

Protein Synthesis

Proteins are assembled from the N- to the C-terminus, whereas the mRNA template is read from the 5′ to the 3′ end. The number of proteins that the mRNA can encode differs between prokaryotes and eukaryotes (see Table 3-10). mRNA from eukaryotes encodes for only one protein, whereas prokaryotic mRNA can encode several different proteins. Protein synthesis three steps followed by posttranslational modification(s).

INITIATION

In prokaryotes, the complex formed for initiation of translation consists of 30S ribosomal subunit, mRNA, f-Met tRNA, and three initiation factors. The formation of the initiation complex differs between prokaryotes and eukaryotes, as summarized in Table 3-11.

ELONGATION

Three-step cycle in which tRNA delivers the appropriate amino acid to the ribosome, the amino acid forms a peptide bond to the growing peptide chain, and the ribosome shifts one codon so that the next codon can be translated (see Figures 3-17 and 3-18).

- Aminoacyl-tRNA (charged tRNA) binds A site.
- Amino acid in A site forms peptide bond with peptide in P site. Reaction is catalyzed by peptidyl transferase and uses energy from the bond between the amino acid and tRNA. The peptide in the P site is effectively transferred to the amino acid–tRNA in the A site, leaving the tRNA in the P site empty.

TABLE 3-10. Prokaryotic versus Eukaryotic Translation

PROKARYOTE	EUKARYOTE
> 1 coding region **(polycistronic),** each of which is independently translated by ribosomes.	RNA encodes only 1 polypeptide chain **(monocistronic).**
Each region has its own initiation codon and produces a separate polypeptide. Thus, the mRNA may contain multiple proteins.	Each mRNA contains only 1 protein.

TABLE 3-11.   **Prokaryotic versus Eukaryotic Translation**

	PROKARYOTES	**EUKARYOTES**
Ribosomal binding	30S ribosomal subunit binds Shine-Dalgarno sequence, which is 6–10 nucleotides upstream (toward 5′ end) of AUG codon.	No Shine-Dalgarno sequence, 40S ribosomal subunit binds 5′ cap and moves down mRNA until it encounters AUG codon.
Initiator tRNA	fMet (methionine with a formyl group attached).	Met (methionine only)
Assembly of initiation complex	Facilitated by initiation factors (IF-1, IF-2, IF-3), 50S ribosomal subunit binds to make 70S complex.	Initiation factors (eIF, and at least 10 other factors).

- Ribosome translocates 1 codon (requires EF-2, GTP hydrolysis) toward the 3′ end of mRNA. Uncharged tRNA is now in the E site (where it exits), and tRNA with the growing peptide chain enters the P site.

TERMINATION

Occurs when one of three stop codons (UGA, UAA, UAG) is encountered. Peptide is released from ribosome via release factor (RF) protein and GTP.

POST-TRANSLATIONAL MODIFICATION

Modification may result in the removal of amino acids or addition of additional molecules to make protein active and/or properly tag the protein for proper transport to its final destination.

- **Trimming** removes portions of the peptide chain to make the protein active (i.e., zymogen, an inactive precursor of a secreted enzyme).
- Protein may be covalently modified through **phosphorylation** and **glycosylation**. Phosphorylation turns the protein on or off. Proteins that will be secreted or reside in the plasma membrane or lysosomes will be glycosylated in the endoplasmic reticulum (ER) and Golgi apparatus.

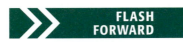

FLASH FORWARD

Drugs selective for prokaryotic protein synthesis machinery.

Drug	**Site of Action**
Tetracycline	Prevents initiation since charged tRNA cannot bind ribosome.
Streptomycin	Prevents initiation since code is misread.
Erythromycin	Inhibits translocation.

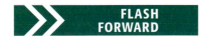

FLASH FORWARD

Many proteins of the coagulation cascade and enzymes involved in digestion (e.g., trypsinogen, pepsinogen) are zymogens.

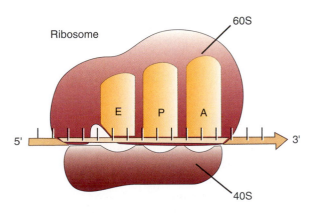

FIGURE 3-17.   **Schematic representation of eukaryotic ribosome and the sites involved in protein synthesis.** P (peptidyl) site initially binds initiator tRNA, later binds growing peptide chain. A (aminoacyl) site binds incoming tRNA molecule with activated amino acid (i.e., bound amino acid with high-energy bond). E site receives uncharged tRNA once amino acid has been added to polypeptide.

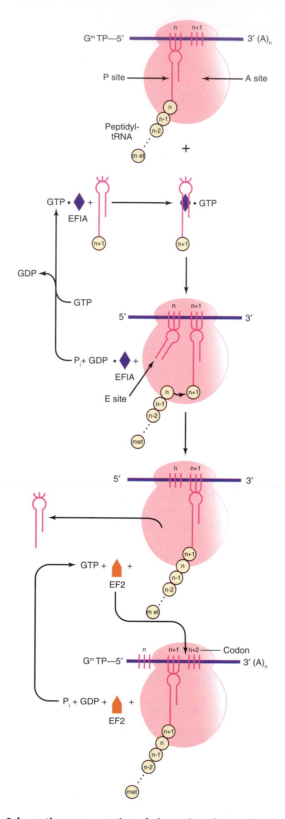

FIGURE 3-18. **Schematic representation of elongation phase of protein synthesis.** (Modified, with permission, from Murray RK, Granner DK, Rodwell VW. *Harper's Illustrated Biochemistry*, 27th ed. New York: McGraw-Hill, 2006: 375.)

Mutations and DNA Repair

DNA mutations and the intrinsic cellular mechanisms that act to minimize their occurrence play a very important role in health and disease. Not only do DNA mutations result in numerous pathologic conditions, they also form the basis for the evolution of novel traits in species.

DEFINITIONS

Mutation

A mutation is any change in the sequence of DNA base pairs that is permanent and arises by chance. To be considered a mutation, the change in the base-pair sequence must not be a result of recombination.

DNA Repair

Several molecular mechanisms exist to ensure that most changes in the DNA sequence are repaired and thus do not become permanent mutations. It is estimated that between 1000 and 1,000,000 DNA sequence damaging events occur in each cell every day. However, most of these are quickly corrected by one of the DNA repair mechanisms. Note that DNA repair is independent of the proofreading action of DNA polymerase during DNA replication.

Types of Mutations

Mutated DNA includes DNA in which one nucleotide has changed (point mutation) and DNA in which one or more nucleotides have been added or removed. Since the DNA code is read in triplets (a **codon**, three consecutive nucleotides, encodes an amino acid), adding or removing one or two nucleotides will cause a frame shift mutation. Point mutations lead to one of three outcomes: the identity of the amino acid is unchanged (silent mutation); the amino acid is changed to another amino acid (missense); or a stop signal is introduced (nonsense).

POINT MUTATIONS

Point mutations occur when a single DNA nucleotide base is replaced by a different nucleotide. These are also known as **substitutions**. Occasionally, single nucleotide deletions or insertions are also considered point mutations, but they cause reading frame shifts.

There are three types of point mutations: missense mutations, nonsense mutations, and silent mutations.

- **Missense mutations:** The replacement of a single nucleotide base with a different one, resulting in a change in the codon so that it codes for a different amino acid (see Figure 3-19B). These are common types of mutations and cause several genetic diseases.
- **Nonsense mutations:** Mutation causes premature introduction of a STOP codon (TAA, TAG, or TGA). This causes the translation of the mRNA to stop, resulting in a truncated protein (see Figure 3-19C).
- **Silent mutations:** Mutation results in the same amino acid as the original. Because the genetic code is redundant (i.e., several codons code for the same amino acid), in some cases a change in a single nucleotide base still codes for the same amino acid (see Figure 3-19D). Most often, this results from a base change in the **third** position of the codon (**wobble position**). The resulting protein is identical to the wild-type protein.

CLINICAL CORRELATION

In sickle cell anemia, a change in the sixth codon of the β-globin gene from A to T results in a modified hemoglobin structure. The result is hemoglobin S (sickle), which polymerizes under low-O_2 conditions, causing distortion of red blood cells and leading to the associated clinical phenotype.

CLINICAL CORRELATION

One of the mutations causing **cystic fibrosis (CF)** results when T is substituted for C at nucleotide 1609 of the **CFTR** gene. This converts a glutamine codon (CAG) to a STOP codon (TAG), thus stopping the translation of **CFTR** after the first 493 amino acids, instead of the normal 1480 (note: the most common CF-causing mutation [ΔF508], which accounts for about 66% of cases worldwide, is actually not a nonsense mutation).

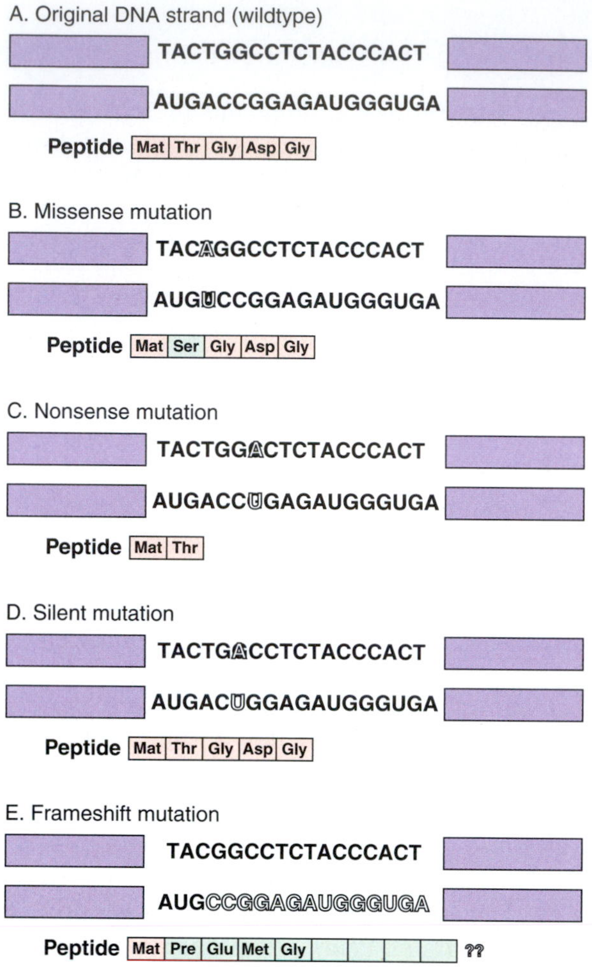

A. Original DNA strand (wildtype)

TACTGGCCTCTACCCACT

AUGACCGGAGAUGGGUGA

Peptide | Mat | Thr | Gly | Asp | Gly |

B. Missense mutation

TAC**A**GGCCTCTACCCACT

AUG**U**CCGGAGAUGGGUGA

Peptide | Mat | Ser | Gly | Asp | Gly |

C. Nonsense mutation

TACTGG**A**CTCTACCCACT

AUGACC**U**GAGAUGGGUGA

Peptide | Mat | Thr |

D. Silent mutation

TACTGA**C**CTCTACCCACT

AUGAC**U**GGAGAUGGGUGA

Peptide | Mat | Thr | Gly | Asp | Gly |

E. Frameshift mutation

TACGGCCTCTACCCACT

AUGCCGGAGAUGGGUGA

Peptide | Mat | Pre | Glu | Met | Gly | | | | ?? |

FIGURE 3-19. **Types of point mutations.** (A) Wild-type DNA sequence. (B) Missense mutation: a single amino acid is changed. (C) Nonsense mutation: the change results in a stop codon, truncating the protein. (D) Silent mutation: the change still codes for the same amino acid, and no changes are observed in the resulting protein. (E) Frameshift mutation: one base pair is deleted, causing all the subsequent codons to shift and resulting in a completely modified protein chain.

With respect to their biochemical origin, point mutations can be one of five types: transition, transversion, tautomerism, depurination, or deamination.

- **Transition:** A mutation in which a pyrimidine is replaced by a pyrimidine, or a purine by a purine. For example, a replacement of a G-C pair by an A-T pair would result in a transition.
- **Transversion:** A purine replaced by a pyrimidine or vice versa. An A-T pair replaced by either a T-A or C-G pair would be a transversion.
- **Tautomerism:** The modification of a base caused by migration of a proton or a hydrogen bond, which results in switching of an adjacent single and a double bond.
- **Depurination:** Caused by a spontaneous hydrolysis of a purine base (A or G), in such a way that its deoxyribose-phosphate backbone remains intact.
- **Deamination:** A spontaneous reaction that can result in the conversion of cytosine into uracil (C to U), 5-methylcytosine into thymine, or adenine into hypoxanthine (A to HX). Of note, the deamination of C to U is the only of these that can be corrected, since uracil can be recognized, whereas thymine and hypoxanthine are not detected as errant.

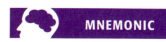

MNEMONIC

A **transition** is easy, **transversion** requires effort:

Transition: purine → purine; pyrimidine → pyrimidine.

Transversion: Substitute a purine for a pyrimidine or vice versa.

Insertions

Insertions are mutations in which one or several base pairs are added to the DNA sequence. Most commonly, insertions of short DNA fragments called **transposons** (or transposable elements) are responsible. Insertions may result from errors in DNA replication of nucleotide repeats. Insertions can result in frameshift mutations and splice site mutations.

FRAMESHIFT MUTATIONS

Because codons are always read in triplets, adding or deleting any number of bases that is not a multiple of three shifts the reading frame during translation and greatly alters the amino acid sequence of the protein (see Figure 3-19E).

SPLICE SITE MUTATIONS

At times, insertions of nucleotide bases in certain regions of a gene can alter the splicing of introns from the precursor mRNA. This results in mRNA that contains introns, resulting in significantly altered protein products.

Deletions

Deletions refer to the loss of one or several nucleotides from the DNA sequence. Much like insertions described above, they can result in frameshift mutations and splice site mutations. They are generally irreversible.

Amplifications

Amplifications are cellular events resulting in multiple copies of whole DNA segments, including all the genes located on them. Amplifications are usually caused by a disproportionately high level of DNA replication in a limited portion of the genome. In this manner, the multiplied genes are effectively amplified, leading to a higher number of copies of the encoded protein. This can alter the phenotype of the affected cell. For example, drug resistance in certain cancers is linked to amplifications of genes that confer resistance to chemotherapeutic agents by preventing their uptake into the cell.

Chromosomal Translocations

A chromosomal translocation is defined as an exchange of genetic material between two nonhomologous chromosomes.

- **Reciprocal (non-Robertsonian)** translocation: Results in a true exchange of DNA fragments between two chromosomes. This can lead to the formation of new fusion genes, or a changed level of expression of existing genes.
- **Robertsonian** translocation: A large fragment of a chromosome attaches to another chromosome, but no DNA is attached in return (see Figure 3-20). Common Robertsonian translocations are confined to the acrocentric chromosomes (those in which the centromere is located very near to one of the ends, e.g., 13, 14, 15, 21, and 22) because the short arms of these chromosomes contain no essential genetic material. A minority of cases of **Down's syndrome** are caused by the Robertsonian translocation of approximately one third of chromosome 21 on to chromosome 14.

Interstitial Deletions

Deletions of large DNA fragments on a single chromosome that results in the pairing of two genes that are not normally in sequence. Like chromosomal translocations, such events can lead to the formation of fusion oncogenes.

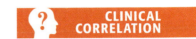

CLINICAL CORRELATION

A splice site mutation in the β-globin gene is responsible for certain cases of β-thalassemia.

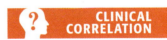

CLINICAL CORRELATION

The *bcr-abl* gene, associated with chronic myelogenous leukemia (CML), results from a translocation event between chromosomes 9 and 12 (Philadelphia chromosome).

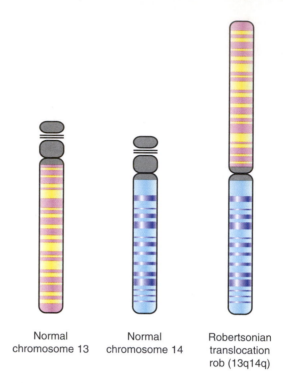

Normal chromosome 13   Normal chromosome 14   Robertsonian translocation rob (13q14q)

FIGURE 3-20. **Robertsonian chromosomal translocation.** A large fragment of a chromosome attaches to another chromosome, but no DNA is attached in return, resulting in the loss of a small amount of genetic material.

Chromosomal Inversions

Chromosomal inversions refer to a large segment of a single chromosome becoming reversed within the same chromosome, usually resulting from a rearrangement following chromosomal breakage. Similar to translocations and interstitial deletions, chromosomal inversions can create fusion genes.

ORIGINS OF MUTATIONS

Most mutations arise spontaneously, usually as a result either of errors in DNA replication (e.g., point mutations and amplifications) or random cellular events (including chromosomal translocations and inversions). However, many mutations are directly caused by specific agents, collectively known as **mutagens**. Some mutagens are external, whereas some are formed as by-products of cellular metabolism (e.g., reactive oxygen species [ROS]).

The type of cell in which a mutation arises is also important. When a mutation arises in a germ cell, it is termed a **germline mutation.** These mutations can be passed to the offspring. Conversely, a mutation in a somatic cell is termed a **somatic mutation** and cannot be passed on to offspring. However, somatic mutations are passed on to the somatic daughter cells of the organism (i.e., cancers resulting from somatic mutations).

MUTAGENS

These are agents that directly cause or increase the likelihood of changes in the DNA sequence. Innumerable mutagens have been identified, and novel ones are continually discovered. Mutagens generally fall into two categories: **chemical agents** and **ionizing radiation.** Because mutations often give rise to cancer, they are often also **carcinogens.**

Chemical Agents

ALKYLATING AGENTS

Chemical agents that transfer alkyl groups to other molecules, including DNA. Specifically, they cross-link guanine nucleotides in DNA, thus causing damage to the DNA that can lead to mutations in both replicating and nonreplicating cells. However, some alkylating agents are used as anticancer drugs because of their unique ability to introduce sufficient DNA damage to render a cell unable to divide. Examples of these chemotherapeutics include **cisplatin** and **carboplatin.**

BASE ANALOGS

Chemical agents that are similar to one of the four nucleotide bases found in DNA and can thus be incorrectly incorporated into DNA during replication. However, they differ enough chemically that they cause mismatch during base pairing, thus introducing mutations in daughter DNA strands. An example of a base analog is bromodeoxyuridine (**BrdU**), which researchers often use to identify dividing cells because it is incorporated into the DNA during replication.

Do not confuse base analogs with antimetabolites, which also share similarity with regularly occurring nucleotides, but upon incorporation into DNA, inhibit further replication. As a result, they can be considered competitive inhibitors of DNA replication and are used as anticancer chemotherapeutics.

METHYLATING AGENTS

Methylating agents, such as ethyl methanesulfonate (EMS), that introduce mutations by transferring methyl groups to DNA nucleotide bases. These substances are typically not used as anticancer agents because do not cause cell death.

DNA INTERCALATING AGENTS

Cause DNA damage by inserting themselves between two nucleotide base pairs. This physically interferes with DNA transcription and replication, leading to mutation events. Examples include **ethidium bromide,** a fluorescent DNA dye commonly used in research laboratories, and **aflatoxin,** a carcinogen produced by a fungus from the genus *Aspergillus.* Some DNA intercalating agents, such as **doxorubicin** and **daunorubicin,** are used as cancer chemotherapeutics. **Thalidomide,** a teratogen associated with numerous cases of phocomelia (very short or absent long bones and flipper-like appearance of hands and/or feet) in the 1960s, is also a DNA intercalating agent. It is now only used as a last resort anti-inflammatory agent in the treatment of erythema nodosum leprosum and sarcoidosis and as a salvage chemotherapeutic agent in patients with multiple myeloma.

DNA CROSS-LINKING AGENTS

These chemical agents act as mutagens by forming covalent bonds between nucleotide bases in DNA, therefore interfering with replication and transcription. A typical example is **platinum,** a derivative of which, **cisplatin,** is a chemotherapeutic agent commonly used in cancers.

REACTIVE OXYGEN SPECIES

ROS are free radicals, which are molecular species rendered highly reactive by the presence of unpaired electrons. They damage DNA by "stealing" electrons from DNA to become more stable. Examples include **superoxide,**

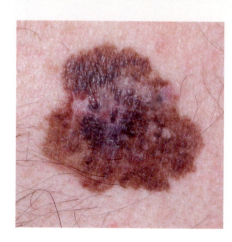

FIGURE 3-21. **Skin cancer.** Clinical appearance of malignant melanoma, a skin cancer caused by UV radiation, often a consequence of sun overexposure. (Reproduced with permission from Wolff K, Goldsmith LA, Katz SI, et al. *Fitzpatrick's Dermatology in General Medicine*, 7th ed. New York: McGraw-Hill, 2008.)

hydrogen peroxide, and **hydroxyl radicals.** These species are thought to be important in age-related cellular damage.

Ionizing Radiation

ULTRAVIOLET RADIATION

Ultraviolet (UV) radiation is a type of electromagnetic radiation with a shorter wavelength and higher energy than that of visible light. It causes DNA damage by inducing the formation of covalent bonds between adjacent thymine nucleotides, giving rise to bulky thymine dimers. This is the basis for increased risk of skin cancer resulting from sun overexposure (see Figure 3-21).

IONIZING RADIATION

Ionizing radiation, produced by radioactive materials, is electromagnetic radiation with energy high enough to ionize a molecule or atom by removing an electron from its orbit. This process causes significant DNA damage, resulting in mutations and eventual cell death. Although potentially very dangerous, this type of radiation can be used in targeted cancer treatment and radiography (X-rays).

DNA REPAIR

DNA repair mechanisms are responsible for minimizing the negative effects that DNA damage has on the cell. DNA damage occurs almost constantly in living cells. When DNA damage surpasses a certain threshold, either because there is too much accumulated damage or because DNA repair mechanisms are no longer effective, a cell can have one of the following three fates:

1. **Senescence:** A cell enters a dormant state that is irreversible, in which the main cellular processes and functions are suspended.
2. **Apoptosis:** A cell undergoes programmed cell death, or suicide, by activating specialized signal cascades.
3. **Cancer:** A cell starts undergoing unregulated cell division, resulting in neoplasia and tumor growth.

DNA repair is thus extremely important for proper functioning of cells and the organism as a whole. A number of specialized DNA repair mechanisms have evolved, and are discussed below (see Figure 3-22 for an overview).

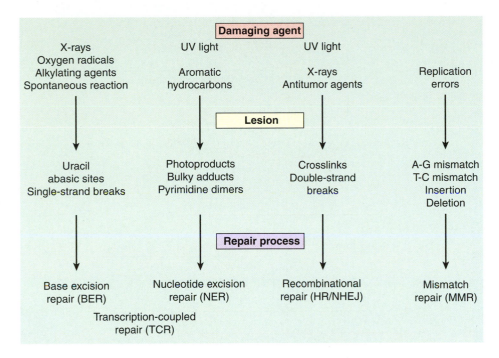

FIGURE 3-22. **DNA repair mechanisms.** Different agents cause a wide variety of DNA damage. Specialized mechanisms have evolved to repair this damage.

Direct Reversal

When specific DNA nucleotides are damaged by chemical modification, the resulting molecular species are specific to the nucleotide that was damaged. The cell can use this information to determine the original nucleotide and can directly reverse the damage using mechanisms specific to the type of damage. Examples include the repair of **UV light–induced thymine dimers.** Similarly, guanine bases that undergo methylation are repaired by methylguanine methyltransferase (**MGMT**). Certain cases of cytosine and adenine methylation are also repaired using direct reversal mechanisms.

Single-Strand Damage

When only one of the strands in the DNA double helix is damaged, the complementary base on the opposite strand can be used as a template for repair. Several DNA repair mechanisms rely on this principle.

BASE EXCISION REPAIR

When single nucleotides are damaged by alkylation, deamination, or oxidation reactions, two enzymes, **DNA glycosylase** and **AP** endonuclease remove and repair the damaged bases. Endonuclease nicks the phosphodiester bond next to the base, releases deoxyribose, and creates a gap. **DNA polymerase** then inserts the correct nucleotide in its place (based on the complementary base), and the nick is sealed by **DNA ligase.** The most common DNA damage is the deamination of cytosine to uracil.

NUCLEOTIDE EXCISION REPAIR (NER) (see Figure 3-23)

A set of mechanisms similar to base excision repair, but used to excise and replace longer stretches of nucleotides (2–30 bases). UV-damaged DNA: dimers form between adjacent pyrimidines (e.g., thymine), thus preventing DNA replication. **UV-specific endonuclease** (uvrABC excinuclease) recognizes the damaged base and makes a break several bases upstream (toward the 5′ side).

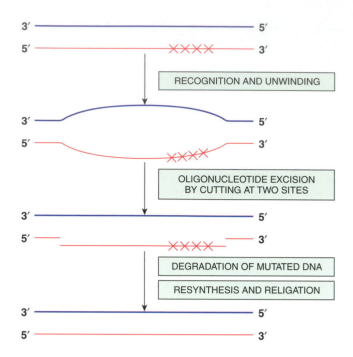

FIGURE 3-23. **Mechanism of nucleotide excision repair.** (Modified, with permission, from Murray RK, Granner DK, Rodwell VW. *Harper's Illustrated Biochemistry*, 27th ed. New York: McGraw-Hill, 2006: 345.)

Helicase removes the short stretch of nucleotides. The gap is filled in by DNA polymerase, and DNA ligase seals the nick.

MISMATCH REPAIR

Mismatch repair is used when there is an error in the pairing of nucleotides secondary to DNA replication or recombination. The base pair mismatch repair system detects errors that escaped proofreading during DNA replication.

- **Identify the mismatched strand:** In newly synthesized DNA, adenine residues in GATC sequence motifs have not yet been methylated. Thus, the DNA parent strand, but not the newly synthesized strand, is methylated.
- **Repair damaged DNA:** The mismatched strand is nicked with endonuclease and the mismatched base(s) is/are removed. The sister strand is used as a template, and DNA polymerase fills in the gap.

Double-Strand Breaks

The situation is distinctly different when both strands of the DNA double helix are broken. In this case, no direct template exists to guide the cell's repair process. Double-stranded breaks can be repaired by either homologous recombination (recombinatorial repair or crossing over) or nonhomologous end joining (NHEJ). In NHEJ, specific proteins bring the ends of two DNA fragments together. However, this is error prone and mutagenic.

NONHOMOLOGOUS END JOINING

When both strands of DNA are broken in a region that has not yet been replicated, there is truly no template for the cell to use to reconstruct the damaged DNA. However, because a complete break of the DNA double helix is highly deleterious for the cell, an attempt is made to fix the break using NHEJ. In this process, DNA ligase–containing complexes join the separated ends of the double helix, relying on microhomologies between the ends of the single-stranded fragments. However, by definition, NHEJ is always mutagenic.

RECOMBINATORIAL REPAIR

Sometimes a double-stranded break occurs during DNA replication. In this case, a fragment of the DNA has already been replicated and can serve as a template for the repair of the double-stranded break. Molecularly, the enzymatic complex involved in recombinatorial repair is similar to that involved in chromosomal crossover.

Translesion Synthesis

As a last resort, cells perform translesion synthesis as a means of continuing DNA replication. When DNA damage is extensive enough to prevent the replication machinery from advancing, special DNA polymerases repair the damaged DNA by inserting nucleotide bases. These nucleotide bases are not completely arbitrary, but they are also not based on a template. Therefore, translesion synthesis introduces mutations by necessity, but enables the cell to continue DNA replication.

CELL CYCLE CHECKPOINTS

When entering cell division or mitosis (M), the cell cycle enters the G_1 phase (growth phase 1). At this point, nonproliferating cells enter G_0, a quiescent phase, whereas active cells proceed to the synthesis (S) phase, which is characterized by DNA replication. Following the S phase is the G_2, or growth phase 2, a short period before the cell divides again (reenters the M phase).

Several checkpoints exist in the cell cycle for a damaged cell to prevent itself from proceeding to the next phase in the cycle (see Figure 3-24).

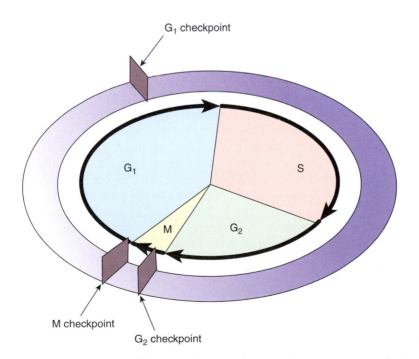

FIGURE 3-24. Cell cycle checkpoints. At several points during the cell cycle, a dividing cell ensures that multiple criteria are satisfied before proceeding with the cycle. Most notably, these include the G_1, G_2, and M (mitosis or anaphase) checkpoints.

G$_1$ Checkpoint

The first checkpoint takes place at the end of the G$_1$ phase. At this point, most eukaryotic cells decide whether to proceed with DNA replication (enter S phase) or become quiescent (enter the G$_0$ phase). The decision is made based on the availability of nutrients, the amount of DNA damage present, and surrounding conditions. This checkpoint is largely dependent on **p53** (a tumor suppressor protein), which can allow the cell to enter the S or the G$_0$ phases, or—if the amount of damage is too great—undergo apoptosis. Mutations in the *p53* gene are present in many cancers and are the basis for the **Li-Fraumeni syndrome**.

G$_2$ Checkpoint

The second crucial checkpoint occurs at the end of growth phase 2 (G$_2$) just before mitosis. This is the final checkpoint before the cell commits to division. Two crucial molecules, the maturation promoting factor (**MPF**) and a cyclin-dependent kinase (**CDK**), regulate this step.

M (Mitosis or Anaphase) Checkpoint

The final checkpoint in the cell cycle takes place in anaphase, when the action of Cdh1 triggers the destruction of **cyclins,** causing the cell to exit mitosis and initiate cytokinesis.

PATHOLOGY

Xeroderma Pigmentosum

CLINICAL FEATURES

Xeroderma pigmentosum (XP) is an autosomal recessive disorder caused by mutations that incapacitate the NER mechanism, rendering the cells unable to repair damage caused by UV radiation. Therefore, people with XP **cannot tolerate sunlight.**

Although patients are born with normal skin, the first signs of XP usually become apparent early in life (6 months of age) and include freckle-like increased pigmentation and diffuse erythema and scaling, especially in light-exposed areas. The second stage of disease usually involves the development of telangiectasias, skin atrophy, mottled irregular pigmentation, and other characteristics of poikiloderma. The final stage, which can occur in childhood, gives rise to malignancies, including malignant melanoma, squamous cell and basal cell carcinomas, and fibrosarcoma. In addition, patients exhibit generalized photosensitivity, photophobia, and conjunctivitis (80%). Neurologic problems are seen in approximately 20% of the patients and can include microcephaly, spasticity, hyporeflexia, ataxia, motor neuron signs, and mental retardation. These symptoms are related to the severity of the disease. Patients with XP are also more susceptible to infection.

CELLULAR CHARACTERISTICS

UV radiation causes DNA damage by inducing the formation of covalent bonds between adjacent thymine nucleotides, giving rise to bulky thymine dimers. Under normal circumstances, this damage is reversed by the **NER** mechanism. However, in XP, some of the proteins involved in NER are mutated, rendering the cell unable, or less able, to repair UV-induced damage. This leads to the accumulation of mutations and eventual development of skin cancers.

GENETICS

XP is an autosomal recessive disease caused by mutations in one of the seven identified XP repair genes (XPA through XPG). Seven subtypes of XP are recognized (XPA–XPG, respectively), and occur with different frequencies. Different subtypes differ in their severity and clinical manifestations. The overall incidence of the disease is about 1 in 250,000 except in Japan, where it is as high as 1 in 40,000.

TREATMENT AND PROGNOSIS

The only treatment for XP is the avoidance of sunlight. The main causes of mortality in XP are skin neoplasms, in particular, **malignant melanoma** and squamous cell carcinoma. Patients younger than 20 years have a 1000 times higher incidence of both melanoma and nonmelanoma, as compared to the general population. The average life span of a person with XP is reduced by about 40 years. Oral **retinoids** have been used to reduce the incidence of skin cancer, but they cause irreversible calcification of tendons and ligaments. **5-Fluorouracil** and topical **imiquimod** and **acitretin** have been used to treat keratoses. It has recently been discovered that topically applied bioengineered DNA repair enzymes lower the incidence of certain skin lesions during a year of treatment.

Cockayne's Syndrome

CLINICAL FEATURES

Cockayne's syndrome (CS), like XP, is an autosomal recessive disorder caused by mutations that affect the **NER** mechanism, thus rendering the cells unable to repair damage caused by UV radiation. However, unlike XP, skin malignancies are uncommon. CS is characterized by bird-like facies, progressive retinopathy, dwarfism, and photosensitivity. Patients tend to have large ears, a thin nose, and microcephaly, with deeply set eyes, short stature, and long limbs. Skin hyperpigmentation, telangiectasia, and erythema are also common. They exhibit premature signs of aging and progressive neurologic deterioration.

CELLULAR CHARACTERISTICS

The faulty NER mechanism leads to the inability of cells to repair DNA damage caused by exposure to UV light. This results in the accumulation of mutations and overall **accelerated aging of the cells**.

GENETICS

Both of the main types of CS are autosomal recessive and are involved in NER. The incidence of the disorder is less than 1 in 250,000. It affects both genders and all races equally.

TREATMENT AND PROGNOSIS

There is no cure for CS, and treatment is largely supportive. It involves protecting the patients from sun exposure, using sunscreen, and treating neurologic deficiencies that arise, such as deafness. CS-1, or classic CS usually presents in childhood, followed by progressive neurologic deterioration, with death typically occurring by the third decade. In contrast, CS-2 is a much more severe form of the disease and usually presents shortly after birth, with patients generally surviving to six or seven years of age.

Trichothiodystrophy

CLINICAL FEATURES

Trichothiodystrophy (TTD) is the rarest disorder arising from deficiencies in the NER mechanism. It is a heterogeneous group of autosomal recessive disorders characterized by sulfur-rich brittle hair and nails, photosensitive, dry, thickened, scaly skin ("fishskin") and both physical and mental retardation. Skin cancer is typically not associated with the disorder.

CELLULAR CHARACTERISTICS

As in XP and CS, deficiencies in numerous proteins involved in NER results in the accumulation of UV light-induced DNA damage.

GENETICS

TTD is an extremely rare disorder, with only over a dozen cases reported. The genetic abnormalities are heterogeneous, but all include genes involved in nucleotide exchange repair.

TREATMENT AND PROGNOSIS

No cure exists for TTD, and much like in other nucleotide exchange repair disorders, the treatment is largely supportive.

Fanconi's Anemia

CLINICAL FEATURES

Fanconi's anemia (FA) is an autosomal recessive disease characterized by **bone marrow failure and DNA repair defects.** Patients often develop pancytopenia as a consequence of **aplastic anemia,** leukemias, and solid tumors. In particular, liver, head and neck, esophageal, and vulvar cancers are very common. Newborns sometimes exhibit characteristic abnormalities, including genitourinary problems and poor growth. Pigmentation and **café-au-lait spots** are also often present. Symptoms of bone marrow failure include petechiae, bruises, pallor, fatigue, and infections.

CELLULAR CHARACTERISTICS

At least 11 genes are involved in the FA pathway. Mutations in any of these genes render cells more susceptible to damage by O_2-free radicals. These mutations also cause deficiencies in DNA repair mechanisms and interfere with cell cycle control. Hematopoietic cells are particularly affected, and the risk of malignancy is increased in many tissues.

GENETICS

FA is an autosomal recessive disorder that affects approximately 1 in 360,000 people worldwide; in Ashkenazi Jewish and Afrikaners populations, the incidence is approximately 10 times higher. The mutation can occur in any of the 11 genes involved in the pathway.

TREATMENT AND PROGNOSIS

There are no specific treatments for FA. The highest mortality and morbidity arise from bone marrow failure, leukemias, and solid cancers. Therefore, the treatments are focused on those specific clinical features.

Bloom Syndrome

CLINICAL FEATURES

Bloom syndrome (BS) is a rare autosomal recessive disorder characterized by growth delay (usually of prenatal onset), a significantly increased risk of malignancy (approximately 300-fold), and recurrent respiratory and gastrointestinal infections due to compromised immunity. Telangiectatic erythema is often seen in a butterfly facial distribution. (In fact, the disease is also known as congenital telangiectatic erythema.)

CELLULAR CHARACTERISTICS

The mutation causing BS affects a gene coding for a protein with a helicase activity thought to be involved in the maintenance of genomic stability. A significantly higher frequency of sister chromatid exchanges and chromosomal instability is also seen, and is thought to be due to consistent overproduction of superoxide radicals.

GENETICS

BS is an autosomal recessive disorder caused by a mutation in the *BLM* gene on chromosome 15. It is a very rare disorder (about 170 cases have been reported) that affects both sexes and all races, although it is somewhat more common in Ashkenazi Jews.

TREATMENT AND PROGNOSIS

Typically, there is no specific treatment for BS. Interventions are aimed at dealing with neoplasms, infection, and dermatologic manifestations. Sunscreen and sun avoidance are recommended. The highest risk of death is due to cancers, typically in the second and third decades of life.

Werner's Syndrome

CLINICAL FEATURES

Werner's syndrome (WS) is an autosomal recessive disease characterized by onset of accelerated aging, usually in the late teen years. The disease is also known as **progeria** of the adult. Affected individuals appear disproportionately aged, including thin, tight, scleroderma-like skin, muscle atrophy, wrinkling, hyperkeratosis, gray, thinning hair, and nail dystrophy. Cataracts, osteoporosis, neoplasias, diabetes mellitus, and arteriosclerosis are generally the sources of morbidity and mortality. Of note, development is typically normal in the first decade of life.

CELLULAR CHARACTERISTICS

The gene involved in WS codes for a DNA helicase involved in DNA repair mechanisms and general transcription and replication. WS particularly affects connective tissues, and overproduction of both collagen and collagenase has been reported. As in other diseases of this type, it is thought that the overall phenotype results from deficiencies in genome maintenance.

GENETICS

As noted, WS is a rare autosomal recessive disorder linked to a mutation in the WS gene, which codes for a helicase. It is estimated to affect 1 in 1,000,000 people. Even though no racial predilection is reported, more than 80% of the reported cases are found in Japan. It affects both men and women.

TREATMENT AND PROGNOSIS

There is no cure for WS, and the prognosis is grim. Treatments are aimed at conditions arising from the accelerated aging process, including cancers, diabetes mellitus, and arteriosclerotic complications. The mean survival for patients with WS is the middle of the fourth decade, with death usually resulting from malignancies and arteriosclerosis.

Ataxia-Telangiectasia

CLINICAL FEATURES

Ataxia-telangiectasia (AT) is a heterogeneous disease, typically characterized by progressive neurologic dysfunction, cerebellar ataxia, sinopulmonary infections, telangiectasias, increased risk of malignancy, and hypersensitivity to X-rays. Neurologically, it can progress to spinal muscular atrophy and peripheral neuropathies. Patients characteristically have dull, relaxed facies and oculomotor signs. About 30% of patients also have mild mental retardation. Skin and hair tend to show accelerated signs of aging.

CELLULAR CHARACTERISTICS

The protein affected by the AT mutation has been shown to be required for the maintenance of genome stability. Patients have higher frequencies of **chromosome and chromatid breaks and rearrangements,** disproportionately affecting chromosomes 7 and 14, which are responsible for T-cell receptor and immunoglobulin regulation.

GENETICS

Several genetic AT variants exist. The disease is inherited in an autosomal recessive pattern, and involves a mutation in the *ATM* gene (AT mutated), located on chromosome 11. It affects an estimated 1 in 100,000 people across all races and both sexes.

TREATMENT AND PROGNOSIS

The treatment in AT is aimed at controlling recurrent infections and malignancies. Supportive neurologic care is often required; the prognosis is very poor. Most patients survive until early or mid-adolescence, with the usual causes of death being bronchopulmonary infections and cancer.

Hereditary Nonpolyposis Colorectal Cancer

CLINICAL FEATURES

Affected individuals have a significantly increased risk of developing colorectal cancer in addition to other malignancies, such as cancers of the endometrium, ovary, stomach, and brain. Also known as Lynch syndrome, patients affected by this disorder have an **80% lifetime likelihood of developing colorectal cancer.** Female patients have an estimated 30%–50% chance of developing endometrial cancer.

CELLULAR CHARACTERISTICS

Several genes involved in the **mismatch DNA repair** pathway are involved in pathogenesis in HNPCC. This leads to significant **microsatellite instability** resulting in the accumulation of mutations that give rise to malignancies.

GENETICS

HNPCC is an **autosomal dominant** disorder. It is caused by mutations in a number of genes, most notably *MSH2, MLH1,* and *PMS2.* In addition, *ras*

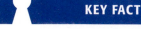
KEY FACT

Microsatellite instability is a change in the number of repeating units of microsatellites in germline alleles. Microsatellites are stretches of DNA made of short repeating motifs (usually between one and five bases in length).

gene mutations can be detected in the stool. HNPCC is thought to account for about 5% of all colorectal cancers.

TREATMENT AND PROGNOSIS

Treatment is focused on the prevention and treatment of colorectal malignancies or other cancers. Some affected individuals elect to undergo prophylactic colectomy or hysterectomy. Common screening for cancers, including colonoscopy, pelvic exam, and urine cytology are recommended. According to the most recent guidelines, colonoscopy should be performed every two years beginning at age 25, or five years younger than the age of the earliest diagnosis in the family, whichever is earlier. Beginning at age 40, colonoscopy should be performed annually.

Hereditary Breast Cancer

CLINICAL FEATURES

Patients affected with hereditary breast cancer have a 60% to 80% lifetime risk of developing breast cancer (compared with an average 11% lifetime risk in American women). Characteristically, there is a strong family history of breast cancer, and the patients often develop cancer at an early age. They may also develop bilateral disease. The malignancies disproportionately include **serous adenocarcinomas.** Patients with **BRCA2** mutations also have a significantly higher risk of developing ovarian, prostate, and pancreatic cancers.

CELLULAR CHARACTERISTICS

The genes involved in typical cases of hereditary breast cancer involve the DNA repair machinery. A higher frequency of $p53$ mutations is seen in affected patients.

GENETICS

Hereditary breast cancer is inherited as an **autosomal dominant** trait. It typically involves mutations of the **BRCA1** and **BRCA2** genes. Although it predominantly affects women, it is important to note that these mutations significantly increase the risk of breast tissue cancers in men as well. About 5% of all breast cancers are thought to be hereditary forms. Ashkenazi Jewish populations have increased frequencies of some common mutations in *BRCA1* and *BRCA2* genes.

TREATMENT AND PROGNOSIS

Primary interventions include breast cancer screening and mammography. Prophylactic mastectomy, oophorectomy, and chemoprevention remain controversial. The cancers are typically of higher histologic grade, and are also more likely to be estrogen receptor– and progesterone receptor–negative, which carries implications in treatment and prognosis.

Enzymes

GENERAL

Enzymes are biologic polymers that catalyze chemical reactions, allowing them to proceed at rates that are compatible with life as we know it.

Nomenclature

The suffix "-ase" **always** indicates an enzyme (e.g., DNA polymerase). Most enzyme names end with -ase.

Another common enzyme suffix is "-in" (e.g., fibrin).

Function

Enzymes allow nutrients to be absorbed and used by the body in many ways, as shown in Figure 3-25.

Activity

Many enzymes are dependent on the presence of a cofactor. A **cofactor** is a small molecule that binds to an enzyme, affording that enzyme catalytic activity. Without the cofactor, the enzyme is inert (i.e., it is an **apoenzyme**). All cofactors belong to one of two classes: metals (e.g., Mg^{2+}, Zn^{2+}) or small organic molecules (e.g., biotin, THF).

Many cofactors are derived from vitamins, for this reason, vitamin deficiencies can be devastating. However, not all symptoms of vitamin deficiencies result from the loss of enzymatic activity.

Vitamin deficiency → cofactor deficiency → certain holoenzymes are left unformed → cellular reactions cannot occur normally → disease states occur.

For example, vitamin B_1 (thiamine) deficiency → thiamine pyrophosphate (TPP) deficiency → pyruvate dehydrogenase, α-ketoglutarate dehydrogenase, and transketolase remain in their inactive, apoenzymatic forms → cells' ability to produce energy is drastically reduced → beriberi (neurologic dysfunction, cardiac dysfunction, weight loss).

THERMODYNAMICS

Enzyme activity can be quantified by several variables, as described in Table 3-12.

GIBBS' FREE ENERGY CHANGE

$$\Delta G = \Delta H - T\Delta S$$

ΔG represents the difference in free energy state between the products and the reactants in a reaction. Systems favor low-energy states. Thus, a reaction proceeds in the direction that decreases the system's free energy.

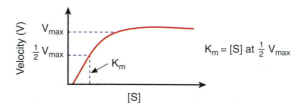

FIGURE 3-25.   **Enzyme functions.**

KEY FACT

Almost all enzymes are proteins. However, recent research has revealed that some RNA molecules can act as enzymes (known as ribo**zymes**).

KEY FACT

Apoenzyme + cofactor = holoenzyme.

KEY FACT

Enzymes do **not** affect ΔG. Therefore, they do **not** affect the direction, extent, or spontaneity of a reaction.

TABLE 3-12.   Thermodynamic Properties

	ΔG	ΔG$_{ACT}$	ΔH	ΔS
Represents	Change in free energy.	Free energy of activation.	Change in enthalpy (heat content).	Change in entropy.
Information given	Direction and extent of a reaction.	Rate of reaction.	Whether heat is given off or absorbed.	Level of disorder in a system.
Affect by enzymes	No.	Yes—they lower it, which increases the reaction rate.	No.	No.
If < 0	Exergonic reaction—will proceed spontaneously.	Does not occur.	Exothermic reaction—heat is given off.	Does not occur (except in isolated subsets of a system).
If it = 0	System is at equilibrium.	Does not occur.	No change in heat.	The components of the system have neither absorbed nor given off energy.
If > 0	Endergonic reaction—energy input necessary to drive reaction.	Energy of transition state—minimum energy required of reacting molecules for reaction to proceed.	Endothermic reaction—heat is absorbed.	Spontaneous reaction.

If the reaction, A + B → C + D, is characterized by ΔG = −3.0 kJ/mol, then by definition, the reverse reaction, C+D → A + B, is characterized by ΔG = +3.0 kJ/mol.

In this example, A + B → C + D is said to be **exergonic**. It proceeds spontaneously (i.e., no energy input is required to drive the reaction).

The reverse reaction, C + D → A + B is said to be **endergonic**. It does not proceed spontaneously but will occur if sufficient energy is added to the system.

For the reaction, A + B ⇄ C + D.

THE EQUILIBRIUM CONSTANT
K'_{eq} = [C] [D] / [A] [B]

K'_{eq} represents the ratio of the concentration of products to reactants when the reaction is at equilibrium (the rates of the forward and reverse reactions are equal, and there is no net change in the amounts of products or reactants).

When K'_{eq} > 1, the equilibrium lies to the right, and favors formation of products.

When K'_{eq} < 1, the equilibrium lies to the left and favors formation of reactants.

ΔG and K'_{eq} are related by the expression:

$$\Delta G = \Delta G^{o\prime} + RT \ln K'_{eq}$$

$\Delta G^{o\prime}$ represents the **standard free-energy change,** or the change in free energy when the concentration of the reactants and products are each 1.0 M and the pH is 7. R is the gas constant (8.31 J/mol/K, but do *not* memorize it), and T is the absolute temperature.

KINETICS

Many enzymes' kinetic properties can be explained by the Michaelis-Menten model. For the purposes of Step 1, you can assume Michaelis-Menten kinetics unless stated otherwise.

The Michaelis-Menten model states that:

$$E + S \underset{k_{-1}}{\overset{k_1}{\rightleftharpoons}} ES \overset{k_2}{\rightarrow} E + P$$

- E (enzyme) + S (substrate) must combine to form an ES (enzyme-substrate complex), which then proceeds to E + P (product).
- k_1 represents the rate of complex formation, while k_{-1} represents the rate of dissociation of the complex *back* to reactant.
- k_2 represents the rate of formation of product from the complex.

The concentration of enzyme-substrate complex is dependent on the rates of its formation (k_1) and dissociation (k_1 and k_2).

$$\text{ES formation} = k_1[E][S]$$

$$\text{ES breakdown} = (k_{-1} + k_2)\,[ES]$$

Assuming steady-state conditions for the complex,

$$k_1[E][S] = (k_{-1} + k_2)\,[ES]$$

or

$$[E][S] / [ES] = (k_{-1} + k_2) / k_1$$

The familiar Michaelis-Menten constant, K_M, combines all of the rate terms.

$$K_M = (k_{-1} + k_2) / k_1.$$

K_M compares the rate of breakdown of the complex with the rate of formation, thus representing the affinity that an enzyme and substrate have for each other.

The lower the K_m, the higher the affinity.

The higher the K_m, the lower the affinity.

The rate of the enzymatic reaction, V, is defined as the rate of formation of P.

$$V = k_2[ES].$$

TABLE 3-13. K_m Relationships

K_M	INDICATES	IMPLICATION	V
Low	Low k_1 or k_2 *or* High k_1	High enzyme-substrate affinity because ES state is preferred over E and S.	Fast
High	High k_1 or k_2 *or* Low k_1	Low enzyme-substrate affinity because E and S are preferred over ES state.	Slow

V, therefore, is directly related to [ES], and inversely related to K_M.

These relationships are summarized in Table 3-13 and are represented graphically in Figure 3-26.

As the substrate concentration increases, the rate of the reaction, V, increases. The asymptotic V_{max} occurs at the substrate concentration that saturates the enzyme's active sites. At this [S], adding more substrate will not increase the rate of the reaction because there are no additional sites for the formation of the ES complex. Often, the relationship between V and S is plotted reciprocally as a **Lineweaver-Burk plot** to obtain a linear plot, as shown in Figure 3-27.

Inhibitors are molecules that bind to an enzyme and decrease its activity.

Competitive inhibitors **compete** for the active site. They bind at the same site as the substrate, thus preventing the substrate from binding.

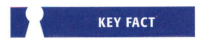

> **KEY FACT**
>
> Memorize the indications on these graphs. It will save you a lot of time during the exam.

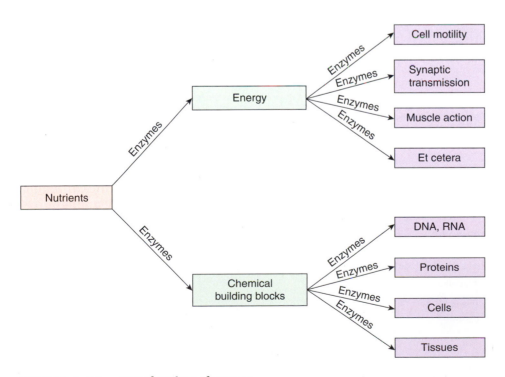

FIGURE 3-26.   Many functions of enzyme.

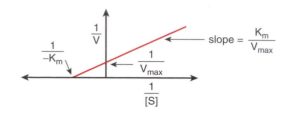

FIGURE 3-27. Lineweaver-Burk plot.

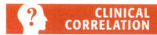
CLINICAL CORRELATION

Alcohol dehydrogenase catalyzes the conversion of methanol to formic acid and formaldehyde. The accumulation of these products causes blindness.

The antidote for methanol poisoning is ethanol administration. Ethanol **competitively inhibits** alcohol dehydrogenase by binding to the enzyme's active site and preventing the enzyme from binding to methanol. Inhibition of methanol binding prevents further accumulation of formic acid and formaldehyde by promoting the conversion of ethanol of nontoxic acetaldehyde.

Noncompetitive inhibitors bind at a site **distinct** from the active site. They reduce the enzyme's efficiency without affecting substrate binding. These differences are summarized in Table 3-14.

REGULATION

An enzyme's efficacy is regulated by many factors.

pH

The activity of enzymes is dependent on pH. Each enzyme has an optimal pH at which it is maximally active.

- The optimal pH varies by enzyme.
- The optimal pH often depends on the ionization state of the enzyme's side chain(s).
- The optimal pH often "makes sense" physiologically.
  - Pepsin is an enzyme that breaks down protein in the stomach. Its optimal pH is about 2, which corresponds to the stomach's acidic environment.

TABLE 3-14. Enzyme Inhibition

	COMPETITIVE INHIBITORS	WHY	NONCOMPETITIVE INHIBITORS	WHY
Resemble substrate	Yes	–	No	–
Overcome by increasing [S]	Yes	Greater probability that substrate, rather than inhibitor, will bind active site.	No	Inhibition is due to effect on enzyme alone, not enzyme-substrate interaction.
Bind active site	Yes	–	No	–
Effect on V_{max}	Unchanged	With maximal [S], inhibition is overcome.[a]	Down	Enzyme cannot function at maximal efficiency.
Effect on K_M	Up	Presence of inhibitor decreases the likelihood of enzyme-substrate binding (affinity of the enzyme for the substrate).	Unchanged	Inhibitor does not affect likelihood of enzyme-substrate binding since it binds to the enzyme at a separate site.

[a]Although V_{max} itself is unchanged, it occurs at a greater [S] than when no inhibitor is present.

Temperature

In general, as temperature increases, an enzyme's activity also increases (the heat increases the kinetic energy in the system). In biology lab, you probably incubated many enzymatic reactions at $37°C$ or higher. At these temperatures, the enzyme-catalyzed reactions occur much more rapidly than they would have occurred at room temperature ($22°C$).

- Above a certain temperature, enzymatic activity rapidly decreases. This is due to protein denaturation.
- Each enzyme has a different optimum temperature.

Concentration

- Increased enzyme concentration increases activity because more active sites are available for binding by reactants.
- Decreased enzyme concentration decreases activity because fewer active sites are available for binding by reactants.
- In the cell or the body, the concentration of any enzyme is determined by the relative rates of enzyme synthesis and enzyme degradation.
  - Enzyme synthesis may be increased in the presence of an inducer or decreased in the presence of a repressor.
  - Inducers and repressors act at the level of transcription by binding to DNA regulatory elements.
  - Enzyme degradation is mediated by ubiquitination, which tags proteins for destruction by the proteasome.

Covalent Modification

An enzyme's activity can be altered by the attachment or removal of other molecules. Such additions or subtractions may change the enzyme's structure or other properties, resulting in a change in enzyme activity.

Phosphorylation and Dephosphorylation

Each of these processes can increase *or* decrease enzymatic activity, depending on the particular enzyme.

- Phosphorylation occurs at serine, threonine, and tyrosine residues.
- Kinases are enzymes that catalyze phosphorylation.
- Phosphatases are enzymes that catalyze dephosphorylation.
  - **Acetylation** and **dephosphorylation** (e.g., COX-2)
  - **γ-Decarboxylation** (e.g., thrombin)
  - **ADP-ribosylation** (e.g., RNA polymerase)

Zymogens (Proenzymes)

Inactive precursors to enzymes that must be cleaved in some way to achieve their active form.

Example: The complement and coagulation cascades each consist of a chain of zymogens.

- Once activated, each zymogen cleaves and activates the next zymogen in the sequence.
- This mechanism allows large quantities of the complement and clotting proteins to be present at sites where they might be needed.
  - Because the factors are inactive, there is little risk of excessive immune response or thrombosis, respectively.
  - Because the factors are already synthesized and localized, the systems may be mobilized extremely quickly when needed.

FLASH FORWARD

Trypsin is a digestive enzyme that plays a major role in protein degradation. Its activity is controlled by the enzyme **enterokinase** (only expressed in the small intestine), which cleaves the zymogen trypsinogen to active trypsin.

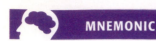

Allosteric Regulation

An enzyme's activity can be modified by the binding of a ligand to an allosteric site (a site **distinct from** the active site).

- The modulator may increase or decrease the enzyme's activity.
- The modulator may be the reactant or product itself, or it may be a distinct molecule.
- In many cases, the product of a reaction binds to its enzyme at an allosteric site to decrease further formation. This is a common mechanism of **feedback inhibition.**

The Cell

CELLULAR ORGANELLES AND FUNCTION

The **plasma membrane** is composed of a **lipid bilayer,** which separates the cytosol from the extracellular environment, maintains the structural integrity of the cell, and serves as an **impermeable barrier to water-soluble molecules** (see Figure 3-28). The lipid bilayer is a continuous double-sided membrane that is a dynamic, fluid structure. The membrane's fluidity allows movement of molecules laterally within a single membrane and can be influenced by the factors listed in Table 3-15.

There are two main functional groups within the lipid bilayer: **lipid molecules** and **membrane proteins.**

Lipids

Membrane lipids fall into the following three classes:

1. **Phospholipids:** The most abundant lipid molecules. Phospholipids are **amphipathic,** having both a **hydrophilic (polar) head group** and typically two **hydrophobic (nonpolar) tails** (see Figure 3-28). This amphipathic nature results in the spontaneous formation of a lipid bilayer when phospholipids are placed in an aqueous environment. There are four major phospholipids, arranged asymmetrically within the lipid bilayer (see Table

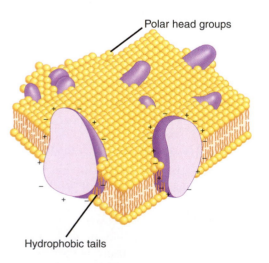

Polar head groups

Hydrophobic tails

FIGURE 3-28.   Plasma membrane structure.

TABLE 3-15.   **Factors that Affect Plasma Membrane Fluidity**

INCREASE MEMBRANE FLUIDITY	DECREASE MEMBRANE FLUIDITY
↑ Temperature.	↓ Temperature.
↑ Unsaturation of fatty acids (↑ no. of double bonds).	↓ Unsaturation of fatty acids (↓ no. of double bonds).
↓ Cholesterol content.	↑ Cholesterol content.

3-16). This asymmetry has many important functional consequences for the cell and, if altered, can trigger inflammatory reactions in surrounding cells.

2. **Cholesterol:** Decreases the fluidity of the membrane (see Table 3-15).
3. **Glycolipids:** Sugar-containing lipids found only on the outer membrane.

Proteins

The second major component of the lipid bilayer is proteins, which carry out most membrane functions. The plasma membrane contains two main types of proteins: peripheral membrane proteins and transmembrane proteins (see Figure 3-28).

PERIPHERAL MEMBRANE PROTEINS

- Are **hydrophilic** only.
- Bind to either the inner or outer membrane via noncovalent interactions with other membrane proteins.
- Do **not** extend into the hydrophobic interior of the membrane.

TRANSMEMBRANE PROTEINS

- Are **amphipathic** (have both hydrophobic and hydrophilic regions).
- Hydrophobic regions pass through the hydrophobic interior of the membrane and interact with the hydrophobic tails of the lipid molecules.
- Hydrophilic regions are exposed to water on both sides of the membrane.

Membrane proteins play many important roles in the plasma membrane, including functioning in transport and as receptors and enzymes.

TRANSPORT PROTEINS

Transmembrane proteins that allow small polar molecules (that would otherwise be inhibited by the hydrophobic interior of the plasma membrane) to cross the lipid bilayer. There are two main classes of transport proteins (see Figure 3-29):

- **Carrier proteins (transporters):** Undergo **conformational changes** to move specific molecules across the membrane.

KEY FACT

It requires **energy** to run **uphill = active transport**

It's **easy** to run **downhill** = no energy required for **passive transport**

TABLE 3-16.   **Membrane Location of the Four Major Phospholipids**

OUTER MEMBRANE	INNER MEMBRANE
Phosphatidylcholine	Phosphatidylethanolamine
Sphingomyelin	Phosphatidylserine

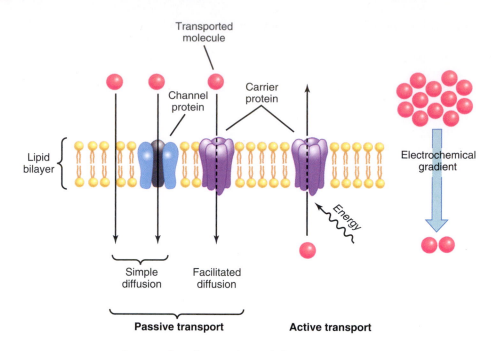

FIGURE 3-29. **Diagram of carrier proteins and channel proteins.**

- **Channel proteins (ion channels):** Form a narrow **hydrophilic pore** to allow passage of small inorganic ions.

Transport across the membrane can either be **active**, in which the solute is pumped **"uphill"** against its electrochemical gradient in an energy-dependent manner, or **passive**, in which the transport of a solute is driven by its electrochemical gradient **"downhill"** (see Figure 3-30). Active transport can be

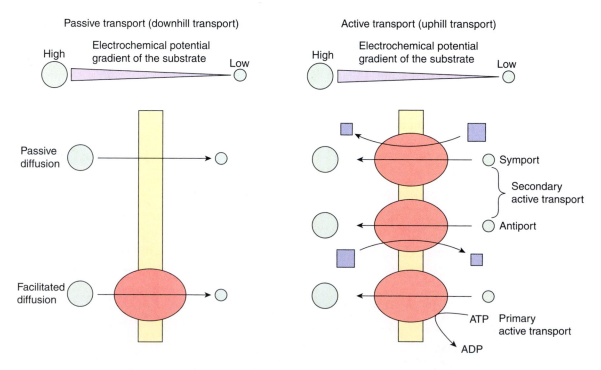

FIGURE 3-30. **Comparison of passive and active transport.**

driven either by ATP hydrolysis or by harnessing energy from the downhill flow of another solute. Transport via carrier proteins can be either active or passive, whereas transport by channel proteins is always passive.

CARRIER PROTEINS (TRANSPORTERS)

There are three types of carrier proteins, most of which use active transport mechanisms (see Figure 3-31):

- **Uniporters:** Transport a single solute from one side of the membrane to the other.
- **Symporters:** Transport two solutes across the membrane in the same direction.
- **Antiporters:** Transport two solutes across the membrane in opposite directions.

The most important carrier protein is the **Na⁺-K⁺ ATPase** or **Na⁺-K⁺ pump**, which is found in the basolateral membrane of nearly all cells. The Na⁺-K⁺ pump is an **antiporter** that utilizes the energy released from ATP hydrolysis to pump **three Na⁺ ions out of the cell** and **two K⁺ ions into the cell** with each cycle (see Figure 3-32). The transport cycle depends on the phosphorylation and dephosphorylation of the Na⁺-K⁺ pump.

CHANNEL PROTEINS (ION CHANNELS)

Form **small, highly selective hydrophilic pores** that allow the **passive transport of specific inorganic ions** (primarily Na^+, K^+, Ca^+, or Cl^-) down their

FLASH FORWARD

The Na⁺-K⁺ pump transports three positive ions out of the cell and only two positive ions into the cell, resulting in the creating of a relative negative charge inside the cell. This **electrical membrane potential** has many important functional consequences for the cell.

FLASH FORWARD

Ouabain and the **cardiac glycosides (digoxin and digitoxin)** both bind and inhibit the Na⁺-K⁺ ATPase by competing for sites with on the extracellular side of the pump. The binding of these inhibitors results in increased cardiac contractility (through a Ca²⁺-dependent mechanism).

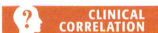

CLINICAL CORRELATION

The ABC transporter superfamily is a clinically important class of carrier proteins. This family includes:

- The **multidrug resistance (MDR) protein,** which harnesses the energy from ATP hydrolysis to pump hydrophobic drugs out of the cell. This protein is **overexpressed in many human cancer cells,** conferring chemotherapeutic drug resistance to these cells.
- The **CF protein,** which harnesses the energy from ATP hydrolysis to pump Cl⁻ ions out of the cell. CF results from a mutation in the CF gene on chromosome 7, which encodes the protein.

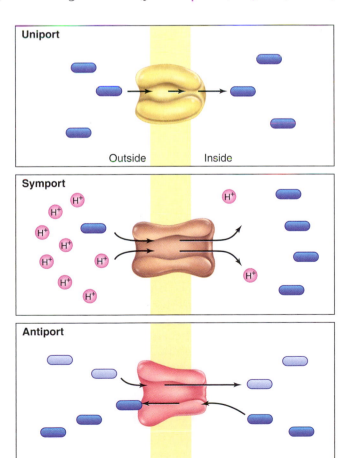

FIGURE 3-31. **Diagram of uniporters, symporters, and antiporters.**

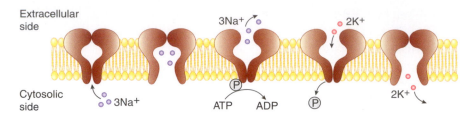

FIGURE 3-32. The Na+-K+ pump transport cycle.

electrochemical gradients. Transport across ion channels (which do not need to undergo a conformational change) is much faster than transport via carrier proteins. Ion channels are selectively opened and closed in response to different stimuli, which determines the specific ion channel type (see Figure 3-33):

- **Voltage stimulus** = voltage-gated ion channels
- **Mechanical stress stimulus** = mechanical-gated ion channels
- **Ligand binding stimulus** = ligand-gated ion channels

The activity of the majority of these channels is also regulated by protein phosphorylation and dephosphorylation.

The most common ion channels are the **K+ leak channels,** which are found in the plasma membrane of almost all animal cells. K+ leak channels are **open even when unstimulated or in a resting state,** which makes the plasma membrane much more permeable to K+ than to other ions. This K+-selective permeability plays a critical role in maintaining the membrane potential in nearly all cells.

G-Protein Coupled Receptors

In addition to transporting small molecules, membrane proteins can also function as receptors. **G-protein coupled receptors,** the most important class of cell membrane receptors, are proteins that traverse the plasma membrane seven times (**seven-pass receptors**). They are **coupled to trimeric GTP-binding proteins (G proteins),** which are composed of **three subunits: α, β, and γ.** The G proteins are found on the cytosolic face of the membrane and serve as relay molecules. G-protein coupled receptors have extremely diverse functions and respond to a vast array of stimuli. However, all G-protein coupled receptor signaling is transduced via a similar mechanism (see Figure 3-33).

When the receptor is **inactive,** the α subunit (active subunit) of the G protein is bound to **GDP.** When the receptor is **stimulated,** a change in conformation causes the α subunit to exchange GDP for **GTP,** thereby releasing itself from the βγ complex. Once released, it binds and activates target proteins. α Subunit activity is short-lived, however, because the **GTPase** quickly hydrolyzes GTP to GDP, resulting in its inactivation. The target proteins activated by the α subunit vary, depending on which of the three main types of G protein is involved.

- **Gs (stimulatory G protein)** = ↑ cAMP levels
- **Gi (inhibitory G protein)** = ↓ cAMP levels
- **Gq** = activates phospholipase C (**PLC**)

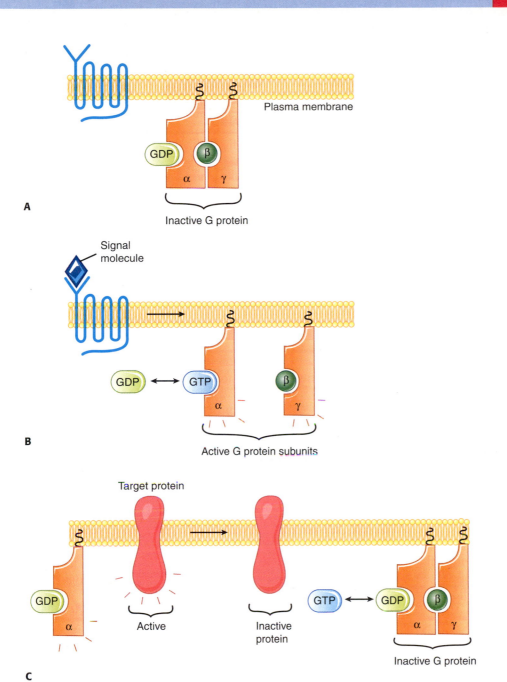

FIGURE 3-33. **G-protein coupled receptor signaling.**

Gₛ- AND Gᵢ-PROTEIN SIGNALING

Both the G_s and G_i proteins signal through the **adenylyl cyclase pathway.** Adenylyl cyclase is a plasma-membrane-bound enzyme that synthesizes cyclic AMP (cAMP) from ATP. Receptors coupled to G_s result in the **activation of adenylyl cyclase** and an **increase in cAMP.** Receptors coupled to G_i result in the **inhibition of adenylyl cyclase** and a **decrease in cAMP.**

Increased concentrations of cAMP (in the case of G_s) results in the activation of cAMP-dependent protein kinase **protein kinase A (PKA),** which phosphorylates certain intracellular protein targets to cause a specific cellu-

KEY FACT

$G_s \rightarrow \uparrow$ adenylyl cyclase $\rightarrow \uparrow$ cAMP $\rightarrow \uparrow$ PKA activity

$G_i \rightarrow \downarrow$ adenylyl cyclase $\rightarrow \downarrow$ cAMP $\rightarrow \downarrow$ PKA activity

Cholera toxin is an enzyme that catalyzes **ADP ribosylation of the α_s subunit.** This blocks GTPase activity so it is continuously bound to GTP and therefore continuously active. The resulting activation of adenylyl cyclase causes large effluxes of Na^+ and water into the gut lumen, resulting in **severe diarrhea.**

Pertussis toxin is an enzyme that catalyzes the **ADP ribosylation of the α_i subunit,** blocking its dissociation from the $\beta_i\gamma_l$ complex so it is unable to inhibit adenylyl cyclase. Thus, adenylyl cyclase is permanently activated resulting in **whooping cough.**

KEY FACT

$G_q \rightarrow \uparrow$ PLC activity $\rightarrow$ PIP$_2$ $\rightarrow$ IP$_3$ + DAG
IP$_3 \rightarrow \uparrow$ Ca^{2+} $\rightarrow \uparrow$ cAM-kinase activity
DAG $\rightarrow \uparrow$ PKC activity

lar response. A protein phosphatase dephosphorylates the protein targets, thus turning off their activity.

In G_i-protein signaling, the activated α_i subunit inhibits adenylyl cyclase, resulting in decreased cAMP and decreased PKA activity. Although this does elicit a cellular response, it is thought that the main effect of G_i signaling is the activation of K^+ ion channels via the $\beta_i\gamma_l$ complex, which allows K^+ to flow into the cell.

G_Q-Protein Signaling

Occurs via the **phospholipase C (PLC) pathway.** Phospholipase C is a plasma membrane–bound enzyme that, when activated, cleaves the inositol phospholipid **phosphatidylinositol 4,5-bisphosphate (PIP$_2$),** which is present in the inner leaflet of the plasma membrane in small amounts (see discussion of plasma membranes earlier under The Cell). This cleavage results in the formation of **inositol 1,4,5-triphosphate (IP$_3$)** and **diacylglycerol (DAG).** IP$_3$ causes **Ca^{2+}release from the ER,** which activates the **Ca^{2+}/calmodulin-dependent protein kinase (or cAM-kinase).** cAM-kinase then phosphorylates certain intracellular proteins, resulting in a specific cellular response. DAG activates **protein kinase C (PKC)** directly, which also phosphorylates certain intracellular proteins, resulting in a specific cellular response (see Figure 3-34).

Connective Tissue

CLASSIFICATION

One of the four basic tissue types, connective tissue serves as the structural support and internal framework of the body. There are many types of connective tissue (i.e., bone, ligaments, tendons, cartilage, adipose tissue, and aponeuroses), but they all contain the same basic structural components: **few cells** and a large amount of **extracellular matrix (ECM)** that includes **ground substance and fibers.** Adult connective tissue can be classified based on the composition and function of each tissue type:

G protein-linked 2nd messengers

FIGURE 3-34. G-protein coupled receptor summary.

Composition

- **Loose connective tissue:** Loosely arranged fibers, abundant cells, and ground substance (i.e., lamina propria).
- **Dense irregular connective tissue:** Irregularly arranged collagen fibers and few cells (i.e., reticular layer of the dermis).
- **Dense regular connective tissue:** Densely packed parallel fibers with few cells packed in between (i.e., tendons, ligaments, aponeuroses).

Function

- **Structural:** Forms capsules around organs or adipose tissue that fills the spaces between organs.
- **Support:** Hard connective tissue with fibrous components arranged in parallel arrays (i.e., bone, cartilage).
- **Nutrition.**
- **Defense:** The presence of phagocytic cells (i.e., macrophages) and immunocompetent cells (i.e., plasma cells and eosinophils) in the ECM are part of the body's defense mechanism against foreign objects.

GROUND SUBSTANCE

Ground substance is a viscous, clear substance that occupies the space between the cells and fibers within connective tissue. Ground substance contains three main types of macromolecules:

- Proteogylcans
- Glycoproteins
- Fibrous proteins

The fibrous proteins and glycoproteins are embedded in a proteoglycan gel, where they form an extensive **ECM** that serves both structural and adhesive functions.

Proteoglycans

Large macromolecules consisting of a **core protein** that is covalently attached to approximately 100 **glycosaminoglycan (GAGs)** molecules and a **linker protein**, which binds hyaluronic acid (HA) and strengthens its interaction with the proteoglycan molecule (see Figure 3-35). Proteoglycans are very large, highly negatively charged macromolecules that attract water into the ground substance, giving it a gel-like consistency. This highly hydrated gel is able to resist compressive forces while allowing diffusion of O_2 and nutrients between the blood and tissue cells.

Glycosaminoglycans (GAGs)

Long polysaccharide chains composed of repeating disaccharide units. One of the disaccharide units is always an **amino sugar** (N-acetylglucosamine or N-acetylgalactosamine), which is most often **sulfated (SO_4^{2-})**. The second sugar is usually an **uronic acid** (glucuronic or iduronic). GAGs are the most negatively charged molecules produced by animal cells because of the sulfate and carboxyl groups present on most of their sugars. These highly negatively charged molecules are essential for maintaining the high water content present in ground substance. Five types of GAGs are found in the human body (see Table 3-17).

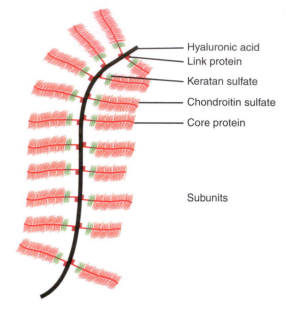

FIGURE 3-35. Proteoglycan structure.

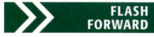
FLASH FORWARD

Alport syndrome results from a **mutation** in the α5 chain of type **IV collagen,** which destroys the ability of the glomerular basement membrane to properly filter blood in the kidney. Patients with Alport's syndrome suffer from **kidney failure, nerve deafness,** and **ocular disorders** (all places where the α5 chain of type IV collagen are found.)

FLASH FORWARD

Bullous pemphigoid is an **autoimmune disorder** in which an **IgG antibody** against the **epidermal basement membrane** is produced resulting in destruction of the basement membrane and **subepidermal bullae.**

Glycoproteins

Large, multidomain proteins that help organize the ECM and attach it to surrounding cells. There are two main glycoproteins: **fibronectin** and **laminin,** both of which are present in the **basal lamina** of cells.

BASAL LAMINA (BASEMENT MEMBRANE)

Specialized ECM that underlies all epithelial cells and surrounds individual muscle, fat, and Schwann cells. It separates the cells from the underlying connective tissue, serves as a filter in the renal glomerulus, and functions as a scaffold during tissue regeneration/wound healing. The basal lamina is synthesized by the cells that rest on it and contains the following elements:

- Fibronectin
- Laminin
- Heparan sulfate
- Type IV collagen

TABLE 3-17. Glycosaminoglycans

GAG	LOCATION
Hyaluronic acid	Most connective tissues binds to the link protein of many proteoglycans to form proteoglycan aggregates.
Chondroitin sulfate	Cartilage and bone; heart valves.
Keratan sulfate	Cartilage, bone, cornea, and intervertebral disk.
Dermatan sulfate	Dermis of skin, blood vessels, and heart valves.
Heparan sulfate	Basal lamina, lung, and liver.

FIBRONECTIN

A dimer composed of two large subunits bound together by disulfide bridges that each contain domains specialized for binding a specific molecule (i.e., integrins, collagen, or heparan) or cells. Fibronectin helps cells attach to the extracellular matrix via its different binding domains.

LAMININ

Composed of three long polypeptide chains (α, β, γ) arranged in the shape of an asymmetric cross. Individual laminin molecules self-assemble and form extensive networks that bind to type IV collagen and form the major structural framework of basement membranes. Laminin also contains many functional domains that bind other ECM components and cell surface receptors, thus linking cells with the ECM.

FIBERS

Fibers are present in varying amounts based on the structural and functional needs of the connective tissue type. **All fibers are produced by fibroblasts** present in the connective tissue and are composed of long peptide chains. There are three types of connective tissue fibers:

- Collagen fibers
- Reticular fibers
- Elastic fibers

Collagen Fibers

Composed of collagen, the most abundant protein in the human body. Collagen fibers are flexible and provide high tensile strength to tissues. Collagen consists of **three polypeptide chains (α chains)** wound around each other to form a long, stiff **triple helical structure** (see Figure 3-36). Collagen is **glycine and proline rich**, with glycine present every third amino acid. The repeating amino acid sequence found in collagen is thus **gly-X-Y**, in which X and Y can be any amino acid (but X is commonly proline and Y is commonly hydroxyproline). This sequence is absolutely critical for triple-helix formation.

The α chains in each collagen molecule are not the same. They range in size from 600 to 3000 amino acids. At present, at least 42 types of α chains encoded by different genes have been identified, and 27 different types of collagen have been categorized based on their distinct α chain compositions. Depending on the specific type of collagen molecule, it may consist of three identical α chains (homotrimeric) or consist of two or three genetically

KEY FACT

Collagen amino acid sequence = **Gly-X-Y**

MNEMONIC

Type **I**: B**ONE**
Type **II**: car**TWO**lage
Type **IV**: Under the **floor** (basement membrane)

FLASH FORWARD

During **wound healing, type III collagen** is laid down first in **granulation tissue.** As healing progresses, fibroblasts secrete **type I collagen,** which **eventually replaces type III collagen in late wound repair.**

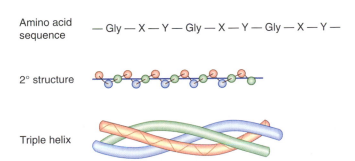

Amino acid sequence — Gly — X — Y — Gly — X — Y — Gly — X — Y —

2° structure

Triple helix

FIGURE 3-36. **Structure of a collagen molecule.** (Modified, with permission, from Murray RK, Granner DK, Rodwell VW. *Harper's Illustrated Biochemistry*, 27th ed. New York, NY: McGraw-Hill; 2006: 39.)

TABLE 3-18.   Collagen Types, Composition, and Location

TYPE	COMPOSITION[a]	LOCATION
I	$[\alpha 1(I)]_2, \alpha 2(I)$	Most abundant (90%). **Bone,** tendon, skin, dentin, fascia, cornea, late wound repair.
II	$[\alpha 1(II)]_3$	**Cartilage,** vitreous body, nucleus pulposus.
III (Reticulin)	$[\alpha 1(III)]_3$	Skin, **blood vessels,** uterus, fetal tissue, **granulation tissue.**
IV	$[\alpha 1(IV)]_2, [\alpha 2(IV)]$	**Basal lamina** (basement membrane); kidney, glomeruli, lens capsule.
X	$[\alpha 1(X)]_3$	Epiphyseal plate.

[a]The Roman numerals simply indicate the chronological order of discovery and that each α chain has a unique structure that differs from the α chains with different numerals.

KEY FACT

**Wound healing: Type III →
Type I**

Three: owie (just scraped your knee).
One: it's all done.

distinct α chains (heterotrimeric). The most important collagen types are described in Table 3-18.

COLLAGEN SYNTHESIS

Connective tissue cells or fibroblasts produce the majority of the collagen fibers. The biosynthesis process involves a series of both intra- and extracellular events (see Figure 3-37).

INTRACELLULAR EVENTS

- Uptake of amino acids (proline, lysine, etc.) by endocytosis.
- Formation of α chains (preprocollagen) mRNA in nucleus.
- Nuclear export of preprocollagen mRNA followed by entry into the rough ER (RER).
- Synthesis of preprocollagen α chains with registration sequences by ribosomes within the RER.
- Hydroxylation of proline and lysine within the RER catalyzed by peptidyl proline hydroxylase and peptidyl lysine hydroxylase. *This step requires vitamin C.*
- Glycosylation of hydroxylysine residues within the RER.
- Formation of α chain triple helix (procollagen) within the RER.
- Addition of carbohydrates within the Golgi network.
- Packaging into vesicles and movement to the plasma membrane.
- Exocytosis of procollagen.

EXTRACELLULAR EVENTS

- Cleavage of registration sequences of procollagen to form tropocollagen by procollagen peptidases.
- Self-assembly of tropocollagen into fibrils.
- Cross-linking of adjacent tropocollagen molecules catalyzed by lysyl oxidase.

CLINICAL CONSIDERATIONS

Many disorders are associated with defects in collagen synthesis:

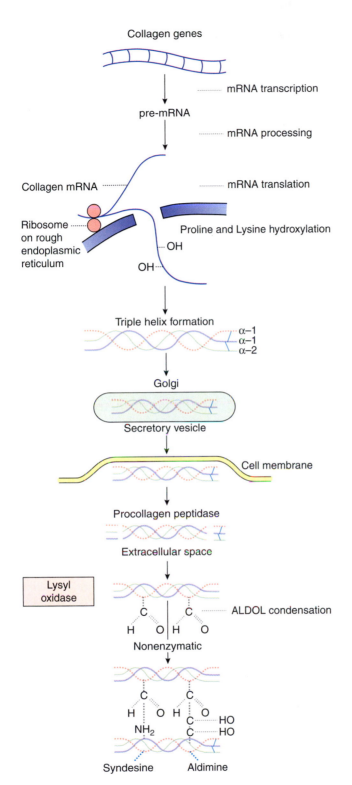

FIGURE 3-37.   Collagen synthesis. (Modified, with permission, from Brunicardi FC, Andersen DK, Billiar TR, et al. *Schwartz's Principles of Surgery*, 8th ed. New York: McGraw-Hill, 2007: 227.)

SCURVY

Vitamin C deficiency resulting in the inability to hydroxylate proline and lysine residues in α-chain polypeptides of collagen molecules (**Step 5 above**). This results in **weakening of the capillaries** and the following complications:

- Ulceration of gums.
- Tissue hemorrhage.
- Anemia.
- Poor wound healing.
- Loose teeth (due to loss of periodontal ligaments).
- Impaired bone formation (in infants).

OSTEOGENESIS IMPERFECTA (OI)

Primarily an **autosomal dominant** disorder caused by a **variety of gene defects** leading to either **less collagen or less functional collagen** than normal (with the same amount of collagen present). Both conditions result in **weak or brittle bones.** The incidence is approximately 1:10,000 individuals. There are four types of OI, each with a range of symptoms. Type II is fatal in utero or in the neonatal period. The most common characteristics are:

- **Multiple fractures with minimal trauma** (may occur during the birthing process and is often confused with child abuse).
- **Blue sclerae** (due to the translucency of the connective tissue over the choroids).
- **Hearing loss** (abnormal middle ear bones).
- **Dental Imperfections** (due to lack of dentition).

EHLERS-DANLOS SYNDROME

Group of rare genetic disorders resulting in **defective collagen synthesis.** There are over 10 types with the disease severity ranging from mild to life-threatening, depending on the specific mutation. The most common symptoms are:

- Hyperextensible skin.
- Bleeding tendency (easy bruising), associated with berry aneurysms.
- Hypermobile joints.

Reticular Fibers

Type III collagen fibrils arranged in a mesh-like pattern provide a supporting framework for cells in various tissues and organs. Reticular fibers contain a higher content of sugar groups (6%–12% compared with 1% in collagen fibers) and are easily identified by the periodic acid–Schiff (PAS) stain. They are also recognized with silver stains and are thus termed **argyrophilic** (silver loving) (see Figure 3-38). Networks of reticular fibers are found in loose connective tissue in the space between the epithelia and connective tissue, as well as around adipocytes, small blood vessels, nerves, and muscle cells. Reticular fibers are also found in the stroma of hemopoietic, lymphatic, and endocrine tissues.

Elastic Fibers

Allow tissues to stretch and distend. Elastic fibers are found in skin, vertebral ligaments (ligamenta flava of the vertebral column and ligamentum nuchae of the neck), the vocal folds of the larynx, and elastic arteries.

Elastic fibers consist of two structural components: elastin and surrounding fibrillin microfibrils.

ELASTIN

Highly hydrophobic protein that, like collagen, is rich in proline and glycine. However, unlike collagen, elastin is poor in hydroxyproline and lacks hydroxylysine. The glycine molecules are randomly distributed allowing for random

---

CLINICAL CORRELATION

Defect in collagen synthesis
- Collagen has three polypeptide chains that form a triple helix. Chains are made up of glycine-X-Y repeats.
- Point mutation in glycine prevents the formation of a triple helix.

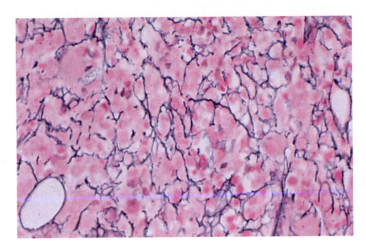

FIGURE 3-38.   **Reticular fibers (silver stain).** (Reproduced, with permission, from Lichtman MA, Beutler E, Kipps TJ, et al. *Williams Hematology*, 7th ed. New York: McGraw-Hill, 2007: Plate XIV-12.)

coiling of its fibers Elastin is produced by fibroblasts and smooth muscle cells, and its synthesis parallels collagen production. In fact, both processes can occur simultaneously within the same cell. Elastin synthesis entails two main steps:

1. **Secretion of tropoelastin** (elastin precursor).
2. **Cross-linking of tropoelastin** molecules via their two unique amino acids **desmosine and isodesmosine** to form extensive networks of elastin fibers and sheets.

Single elastin polypeptides adopt a loose "random coil" conformation when relaxed. When individual elastin proteins are cross-linked into an elastic fiber network, their collective random coil properties allow the network to stretch and recoil like a rubber band.

FIBRILLIN-I

Glycoprotein that forms fine microfibrils. Fibrillin microfibrils are formed first during elastic fiber genesis; elastin is then deposited on to the surface of the microfibrils. Elastin-associated fibrillin microfibrils play a major role in organizing elastin into fibers.

CLINICAL CONSIDERATION—MARFAN'S SYNDROME

Relatively common (1:3–5000) **autosomal dominant** connective tissue disorder caused by a **mutation in the fibrillin gene (*FBN1*).** Individuals with Marfan's syndrome have an absence of elastin-associated fibrillin microfibrils, resulting in the formation of **abnormal elastic tissue.** The severity of the disease varies; affected individuals may die young or live essentially normal lives. Common symptoms include:

- **Bone elongation** (tall individuals with long, thin limbs).
- **Spider-like fingers** (arachnodactyly).
- **Hypermobile joints.**
- **Lens dislocation** (glaucoma and retinal detachment also common).
- **Cardiac abnormalities** (mitral valve prolapse is very common).
- **Aortic rupture—most common cause of death** (due to loss of elastic fibers in tunica media).

CELLS

Two different cell populations are found within connective tissue:

- Resident cells
- Transient cells

Resident Cells

Relatively stable, permanent residents of connective tissue. These cells remain in the connective tissue and include:

- **Fibroblasts and myofibroblasts** (primary cells involved in collagen and ground substance secretion).
- **Macrophages** (arise from migrating monocytes).
- **Adipose cells.**
- **Mast cells** (arise from stem cells in the bone marrow).
- **Mesenchymal cells.**

Transient Cells

Wandering cells that have migrated into the connective tissue from the blood in response to specific stimuli (usually during inflammation). This population is not normally found in connective tissue and is composed of cells involved in the immune response:

- Lymphocytes
- Plasma cells
- Neutrophils
- Eosinophils
- Basophils
- Monocytes

Homeostasis and Metabolism

Various processes contribute to the maintenance of the living cell's needs for energy, structure, and waste removal. These systems are intricate and interdependent, as summarized in Figure 3-39.

Metabolism converts four classes of substrate into energy or other usable products. These substrates include:

- Carbohydrates
- Lipids and fatty acids
- Proteins and amino acids
- Nucleotides

CARBOHYDRATE METABOLISM

A process by which carbohydrates are broken down into water and carbon dioxide, accompanied by the generation of energy, mainly in the form of **adenosine triphosphate (ATP)**. The overall reaction is very simple.

$$C_6H_{12}O_6 + 9O_2 \rightarrow 6H_2O + 6CO_2$$

However, the process is complicated by its relation to other metabolic cycles, namely, the fatty acid cycle, the urea cycle, Kreb's cycle (TCA cycle), and the HMP shunt.

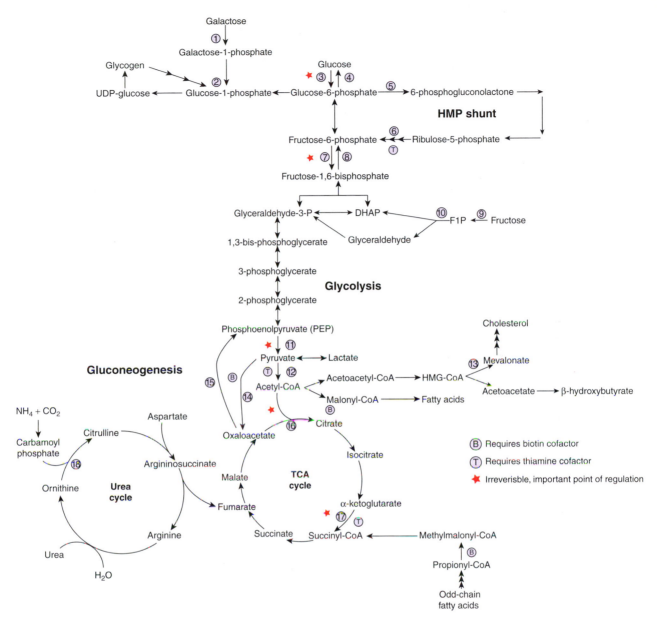

FIGURE 3-39.   **Metabolic pathways.** (1) Galactokinase (mild galactosemia); (2) Galactose-1-phosphate uridyltransferase; (severe galactosemia); (3) Hexokinase/glucokinase; (4) Glucose-6-phosphatase (von Gierke's); (5) Glucose-6-phosphate dehydrogenase (G6PD); (6) Transketolase; (7) Phosphofructokinase; (8) Fructose-1,6-bisphosphatase; (9) Fructokinase (essential fructosuria); (10) Aldolase B (fructose intolerance); (11) Pyruvate kinase; (12) Pyruvate dehydrogenase; (13) HMG-CoA reductase; (14) Pyruvate carboxylase; (15) PEP carboxykinase; (16) Citrate synthase; (17) a-ketoglutarate dehydrogenase; (18) Ornithine transcarbamylase.

Intake and Absorption

- Digestion of carbohydrates begins in the mouth and ends in the small intestine with absorption of the breakdown products. **Polysaccharides** (starch) and **oligosaccharides** (sucrose and lactose) are converted into **disaccharides** and **monosaccharides.**
- The monosaccharides are absorbed via transporters and carried to the liver through the portal vein.
- Ultimately, these are oxidized, stored as glycogen, transformed to fat (triglycerides), or transported as glucose via the circulation.

Glycolysis

FUNCTION

Initial step in the metabolism of glucose to produce energy for the cell.

LOCATION

Cytoplasm of all cells that utilize glucose.

REACTANTS

One molecule glucose.

PRODUCTS

Two molecules pyruvate, two ATP, two NADH.

CYCLE

See Figure 3-40.

REGULATION

Phosphorylation of glucose to glucose-6-phosphate blocks its ability to diffuse across the cell membrane, **trapping** it within the cell. Two kinases in the cytosol are involved. The process consumes one molecule of ATP per molecule of glucose phosphorylated.

- **Hexokinase:** Ubiquitous, nonspecific (phosphorylates many different six carbon sugars), low K_m (easily saturable), feedback inhibited by glucose-6-phosphate.
- **Glucokinase:** Mainly in the liver, very specific for glucose, high K_m (not easily saturable), feedback inhibited by fructose-6-phosphate (the product of the subsequent step in glycolysis).
- **Pyruvate dehydrogenase:** Converts pyruvate to acetyl-CoA, which enters the Kreb's cycle, an irreversible and important regulatory step.

PATHOPHYSIOLOGY

Deficiencies of any of the glycolytic enzymes can lead to episodes of hemolysis because red blood cells (RBCs) depend solely on glycolysis for their energy needs. These deficiencies are exacerbated by certain drugs (sulfa drugs, antimalarial agents). The most common such disorder is glucose-6-phosphate dehydrogenase (**G6PD**) deficiency. Its role is illustrated in Figures 3-41 and 3-42.

G6PD deficiency is especially prominent in the African-American community, although variants are also seen in Mediterranean and Asian populations. It is an X-linked recessive disorder; the defective allele is carried by 10% of American blacks. The disease manifests in a milder fashion in women than in men. The RBC is protected from oxidative stress by glutathione (GSH). Since the regeneration of GSH is dependent on NADPH production and thus the HMP shunt, G6PD leads to denaturation of hemoglobin, resulting in the formation of Heinz bodies in the RBCs affected individuals. **Favism** is a similar condition seen in individuals of Mediterranean origin. G6PD is exacerbated by consumption of fava beans (common in Mediterranean diets), usually within 24–48 hours after consumption. Other characteristics of glycolytic enzyme deficiencies are summarized in Table 3-19.

◄◄ FLASH BACK

A kinase is an enzyme that phosphorylates a substrate.

KEY FACT

G6PD is the most common glycolytic deficiency (90% of all cases) and leads to hemolytic anemia.

Pyruvate kinase deficiency is the second most common deficiency (9% of all cases) and leads to hemolysis.

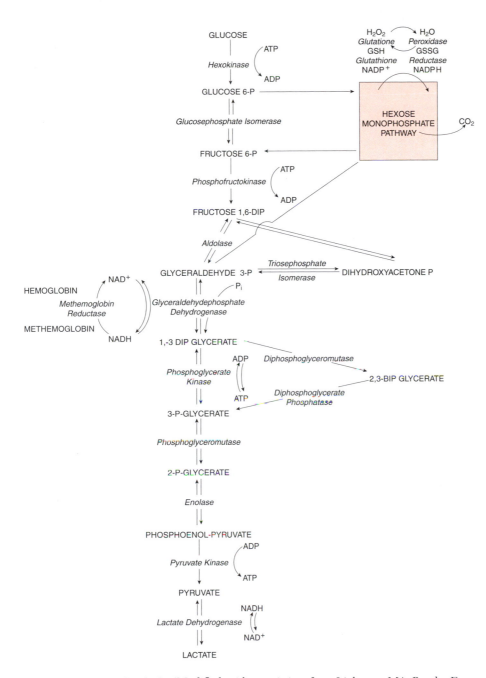

FIGURE 3-40. **Glycolysis.** (Modified, with permission, from Lichtman MA, Beutler E, Kipps TJ, et al. *William Hematology*, 7th ed. New York: McGraw-Hill, 2006: 605.)

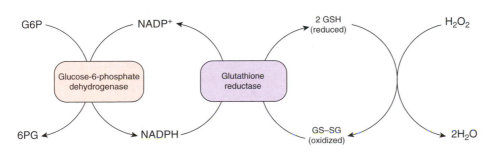

FIGURE 3-41. **Role of glucose-6-phosphate dehydrogenase.**

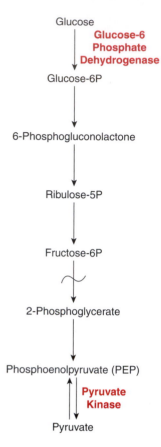

FIGURE 3-42.   **Glycolysis flow chart highlighting deficiencies and diseases.**

Kreb's (TCA) Cycle

FUNCTION

Production of high-energy electron carriers for ATP generation in the mitochondria; completes metabolism of glucose (final common pathway).

LOCATION

Mitochondria.

TABLE 3-19.   **Enzyme Deficiencies in Glycolysis**

	GLYCOLYTIC ENZYME DEFICIENCY	PYRUVATE DEHYDROGENASE DEFICIENCY
Affected cells	RBCs (no mitochondria depend solely on glycolysis).	All cells with mitochondria.
Clinical symptoms	Hemolytic anemia.	Neurologic defects.
Treatment	Avoid fava beans, sulfa drugs such as sulfamethoxazole, anti-malarials and similar drugs that induce oxidative stress (doxorubicin).	Increase intake of ketogenic nutrients (fat, amino acids lycine and leucine).

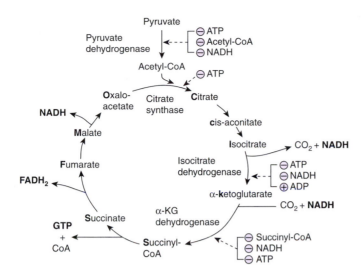

FIGURE 3-43.   Kreb's (TCA) cycle.

REACTANTS

Pyruvate is chief substrate. Proteins and fats enter the cycle after being converted to acetyl-CoA.

PRODUCTS

Three NADH, one $FADH_2$, two CO_2, and one GTP. This is equivalent to 12 ATP per acetyl-CoA.

CYCLE

Summarized in Figure 3-43.

REGULATION

The cycle is controlled at three major steps:

- Acetyl-CoA + OAA → citrate, catalyzed by citrate synthase (allosterically inhibited by ATP).
- Isocitrate → α-ketoglutarate, controlled by isocitrate dehydrogenase (activated by ADP and inhibited by ATP and NADH).
- α-Ketoglutarate → succinyl-CoA, controlled by α-ketoglutarate dehydrogenase (inhibited by succinyl-CoA and NADH).

Electron Transport Chain and Oxidative Phosphorylation

FUNCTION

High-energy electrons from NADH and $FADH_2$ are transduced to ATP.

LOCATION

Mitochondria.

REACTANTS

High-energy electrons from NADH and $FADH_2$, O_2. Since NADH and $FADH_2$ cannot physically cross the mitochondrial membrane, the electrons are shuttled into mitochondria by organ-specific shuttles.

- **Glycerol phosphate shuttle** → ubiquitous; transfers NADH electrons to mitochondrial $FADH_2$.
- **Malate-aspartate shuttle** → found in muscle, liver, and heart; transfers NADH electrons to mitochondrial NADH.

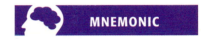

MNEMONIC

TCA intermediates—

Can **I** **K**eep **S**elling **S**ex **F**or **M**oney, **O**fficer?
Citrate
Isocitrate
α-**K**etoglutarate
Succinyl-CoA
Succinate
Fumarate
Malate
Oxaloacetate

PRODUCTS

ATP and H_2O.

CYCLE

Summarized in Figure 3-44.

Pentose Phosphate Pathway (HMP Shunt)

FUNCTION

Shunts glucose-6-phosphate to form ribulose-5-phosphate for nucleotide synthesis. Generates NADPH as a reducing equivalent for GSH/GSSG (the premier antioxidant system in the cell) and NADPH for steroid and fatty acid biosynthesis.

LOCATION

Cytoplasm of all cells.

REACTANTS

Glucose-6-phosphate.

PRODUCTS

NADPH, which is used in steroid and fatty acid biosynthesis and regeneration of GSH in the GSH/GSSG antioxidant system. Ribose-5-phosphate, CO_2.

CYCLE

Summarized in Figures 3-45 and 3-46.

REGULATION

The reaction consists of two parts:

- The first irreversible step is catalyzed by G6PD to produce NADPH from glucose-6-phosphate (this step is oxidative).
- The second, reversible, step isomerizes the sugars so they can re-enter glycolysis. This step is nonoxidative.

PATHOPHYSIOLOGY

G6PD deficiency has a high prevalence among African-Americans.

Fructose Metabolism

FUNCTION

Converts dietary fructose into a substrate for glycolysis.

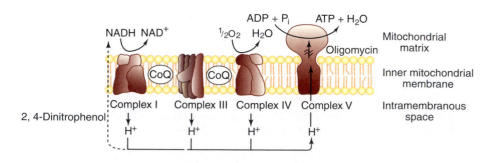

FIGURE 3-44.   **Electron transport chain and oxidative phosphorylation.**

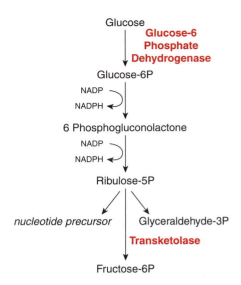

FIGURE 3-45. Pentose phosphate pathway (HMP shunt).

LOCATION

Muscle, kidney, and liver.

REACTANTS

Fructose and ATP.

PRODUCTS

Glyceraldehyde-3 phosphate.

CYCLE

See Figure 3-47.

- Dietary sucrose is broken down by sucrase in the small intestine to fructose and glucose.
- Fructose is phosphorylated by hexokinase to fructose-6-phoshate in muscle and kidney.
- In the liver, fructose is converted to fructose-1-phosphate by fructokinase.
- Fructose-1-phosphate aldolase converts fructose-1-phosphate to dihydroxy-acetone phosphate (DHAP) and glyceraldehyde. DHAP can be combined with glyceraldehyde and converted to glyceraldehyde-3-phosphate, which can enter glycolysis.

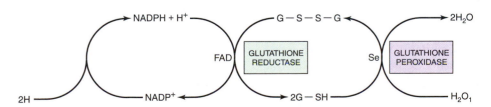

FIGURE 3-46. **Pentose phosphate pathway (HMP shunt).** (Modified, with permission, from Murray RK, Granner DK, Rodwell VW, *Harper's Illustrated Biochemistry*, 27th ed, New York: McGraw-Hill, 2006: 181.)

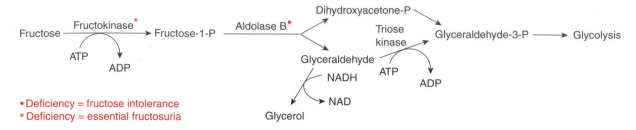

FIGURE 3-47. **Fructose metabolism in the liver.**

PATHOPHYSIOLOGY

- Deficiencies in fructokinase are benign, leading to **fructosuria** (essential fructosuria).
- Fructose-1-phosphate aldolase deficiency leads to **hereditary fructose intolerance,** characterized by severe hypoglycemia upon sucrose or fructose ingestion).

Galactose Metabolism

FUNCTION

Converts dietary galactose (from lactose) to a form that can enter glycolysis.

LOCATION

Kidney, liver, and brain.

REACTANTS

Galactose and ATP.

PRODUCTS

Glucose-1-phosphate.

CYCLE

See Figure 3-48.

- Dietary lactose is broken down in the small intestine by lactase to galactose and glucose.
- Galactose is phosphorylated by galactokinase to galactose-1-phosphate.
- Galactose-1-phosphate is converted by galactose-1-phosphate uridyl transferase to glucose-1-phosphate.

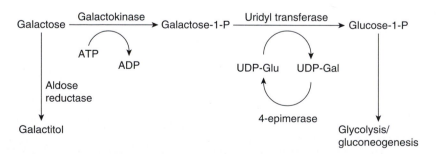

FIGURE 3-48. **Galactose metabolism.**

PATHOPHYSIOLOGY

- Deficiencies in galactokinase lead to **galactosemia** and early cataract formation.
- Deficiencies in galactose-1-phosphate uridyl transferase lead to severe galactosemia with growth and mental retardation and possibly early death.

Anaerobic Metabolism and Cori's Cycle

FUNCTION

Shuttles lactate from muscle into the liver, allowing muscle to function anaerobically when energy requirements exceed oxygen consumption.

LOCATION

Muscle and liver.

REACTANTS

Anaerobic metabolism uses glucose. The Cori cycle begins with lactate and consumes six ATP.

PRODUCTS

Anaerobic metabolism produces two net ATP and two pyruvate per glucose molecule. Lactate is converted to glucose in the Cori cycle.

CYCLE

See Figure 3-49.

Gluconeogenesis

FUNCTION

Generates glucose from glycolysis, fatty acid, or TCA (Kreb's) cycle intermediates.

LOCATION

Cytoplasm and mitochondria of kidney, liver, and intestinal epithelium.

REACTANTS

Pyruvate.

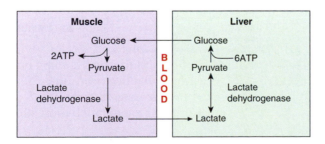

FIGURE 3-49. **Cori cycle.** Transfers excess reducing equivalents from RBCs and muscle to liver, allowing muscle to function anaerobically (net 2 ATP).

PRODUCTS

Glucose.

CYCLE

See Figure 3-50.

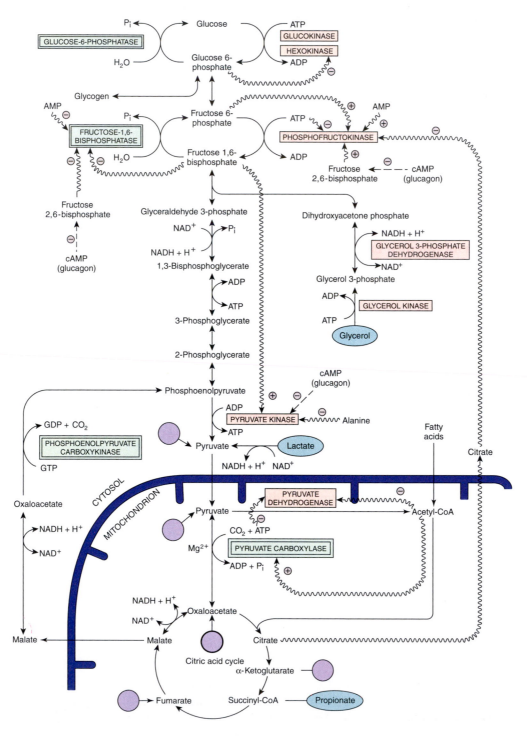

FIGURE 3-50. Gluconeogenesis. (Modified, with permission, from Murray RK, Granner DK, Rodwell VW. *Harper's Illustrated Biochemistry*, 27th ed. New York: McGraw-Hill, 2006: 168.)

REGULATION

Although some of the steps in glycolysis and the TCA cycle are irreversible, they can be bypassed by the use of ATP or GTP and four enzymes, found only in the kidney, liver, and intestinal epithelium.

- Pyruvate carboxylase converts pyruvate → oxaloacetate (OAA).
- PEP (phosphoenolpyruvate) carboxykinase converts OAA → PEP.
- Fructose-1,6-bisphosphatase converts fructose-1,6-bisphoshate → fructose-6-phosphate.
- Glucose-6-phosphatase converts glucose-6-phosphatase → glucose.

Glycogen Metabolism

FUNCTION

Helps maintain glucose homeostasis by forming (**glycogenesis**) or breaking down (**glycogenolysis**) glycogen. Crucial for the storage of energy derived from carbohydrate metabolism.

LOCATION

Glycogenesis—liver and muscle. Glycogen*olysis*—heart, liver, and muscle.

REACTANTS

Glucose/glycogen.

PRODUCTS

Glycogen/glucose.

GLYCOGENESIS

Glucose is catabolized to glycogen, its insoluble storage form. Mainly stored in the liver and muscle tissue.

$$\text{Glucose} \xrightarrow{1} \text{uridine diphosphate-glucose} \xrightarrow{2} \text{chains with 1–4 linkages} \rightarrow \text{complex with 1–6 linkages (ultimate storage form)}$$

1. glycogen synthase
2. aminotransglycosylase

GLYCOGENOLYSIS

Release of glucose from glycogen stores.

$$\text{Glycogen} \xrightarrow{1} \text{glucose-1-phosphate} \xrightarrow{2} \text{glucose-6-phosphate}$$

1. phosphorylase
2. phosphoglucomutase

REGULATION

These opposing processes are regulated by the hormones insulin and glucagon. **Insulin** promotes the removal of glucose from the bloodstream, thereby increasing **glycogenesis** and decreasing glycogenolysis. Glucagon does the opposite.

TABLE 3-20.   Glycogen Storage Diseases

TYPE	DISEASE	ENZYME	TISSUE	CLINICAL FEATURES
I	Von Gierke's disease	Glucose-6-phosphatase.	Liver and kidney.	Severe fasting hypoglycemia. Lactic acidosis. Hepatomegaly (100%). Short stature (90%). Delayed puberty. Bleeding diathesis (especially epistaxis). Hepatic adenomas (75%), renal failure and gout in 20s and 30s.
II	Pompe's disease	α-1,4-glucosidase (acid maltase).	All organs (enzyme is in lysosomes).	Progressive muscle weakness. Breathing and feeding difficulties. Hyporeflexia or areflexia due to glycogen accumulation in spinal motor neurons. Cardiomegaly leading to congestive heart failure and death before the age of 2.
III	Cori's disease	Debranching enzyme (α-1,6-glucosidase).	Muscle and liver.	Similar to type I without lactic acidosis. ▪ Hypoglycemia. ▪ Hepatomegaly. ▪ Delayed (ultimately normal) growth. Symptoms, including hepatomegaly, usually regress in adulthood.
V	McArdle's disease	Myophosphorylase.	Muscle.	Muscle weakness and cramps after exercise. Myoglobinuria (burgundy urine) after exercise.

PATHOPHYSIOLOGY

There are 12 types of glycogen storage diseases. All result in abnormal glycogen metabolism and an accumulation of glycogen within cells. See Table 3-20 for the most common types and Table 3-21 for a summary of the metabolic cycles and pathways.

Urea Cycle

FUNCTION

Excretion of NH_4^+ from amino acid metabolism; accounts for 90% of nitrogen in urine.

LOCATION

Mitochondria and cytoplasm.

REACTANTS

CO_2 and NH_4^+.

PRODUCTS

Urea and fumarate (fumarate enters the TCA).

CYCLE

See Figure 3-51.

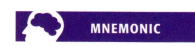

MNEMONIC

Urea cycle—

Oridinarily, **C**areless **C**rappers **A**re **A**lso **F**rivolou**s A**bout **U**rination:

Ornithine
Carbamoyl phosphate
Citruline
Aspartate
Argininosuccinate
Fumarate
Fumarate
Arginine
Urea

TABLE 3-21. **Summary of Metabolic Cycles and Pathways**

CYCLE/PATHWAY	FUNCTION	LOCATION	REACTANTS	PRODUCTS
Glycolysis	Break down of sugars for Kreb's cycle.	Cytoplasm of cells that use glucose.	Glucose.	2 Pyruvate, 2 ATP and 2 NADH.
Kreb's cycle/ TCA cycle	Production of high-energy electron carriers for the ATP generation mitochondria.	Mitochondria.	Pyruvate (alternatively, fats and proteins after conversion to acetyl-CoA).	3 NADH, 1 $FADH_2$, 2 CO_2, 1 GTP. All equivalent to 12 ATP per acetyl-CoA.
Electron transport chain/oxidative phosphorylation	Transduction of high-energy e- from NADH and $FADH_2$ to ATP.	Mitochondria.	NADH, $FADH_2$ and O_2 as the final electron acceptor.	ATP and H_2O.
Pentose phosphate pathway (Hexose monophosphate shunt)	1. Shunts glucose-6-phosphate to form ribulose-5—for nucleotide synthesis. 2. Generation of NADPH for: ■ Regeneration of GSH in the GSH/GSSG antioxidant system vi. ■ Steroid and fatty acid biosynthesis.	Cytoplasm.	Glucose-6-phosphate.	Ribulose-5-phosphate, NADPH, and CO_2.
Fructose pathway	Converts fructose to substrate for glycolysis.	Muscle, kidney, and liver.	Fructose.	Glyceraldehyde-3-phosphate.
Galactose pathway	Converts galactose to substrate for glycolysis.	Kidney, liver and brain.	Galactose and ATP.	
Cori's cycle/anaerobic metabolism	Cori's cycle shuttles lactate from anaerobic metabolism in muscle to liver.	Shuttles lactate from muscle to liver.	Lactate and 6 ATP.	Glucose.
Gluconeogenesis	Generates glucose from glycolysis intermediates, fatty acid or Kreb's cycle.	Cytoplasm and mitochondria of kidney and liver, interstitial epithelium.	All substrates end up as pyruvate/phosphoenolpyruvate → converted to glucose.	Glucose.
Glycogen metabolism	Maintains glucose homeostasis.	Glycogenesis (muscle and liver), glycogenolysis (heart, muscle, and liver).	Glycogen/ glucose.	Glycogen/glucose.
Urea cycle	Excretion of NH_4^+ from amino acid metabolism.	Partly in the mitochondria and partly in the cytoplasm.	CO_2 and NH_4^+.	Urea and fumarate (enters TCA).

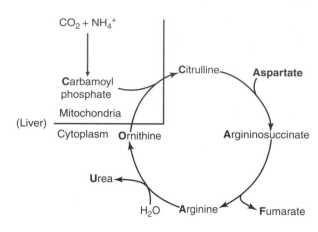

FIGURE 3-51. **Urea cycle.**

Amino Acids

AMINO ACID METABOLISM

Metabolism is a key process in the human body as it provides the energy required to maintain the body's organization. Metabolism utilizes various chemical reactions to extract energy and building blocks from food. Amino acids are extensively used in the synthesis of new proteins (e.g., enzymes, hormones, growth factors) and can also be used as an energy source.

AMINO ACID STRUCTURE

Amino acids consist of a carboxylic acid, an amine group, and a characteristic functional side group (see Figure 3-52).

Acidic Amino Acids

Aspartic acid and glutamic acid contain an additional carboxylic acid group and are negatively charged at physiologic pH (7.4).

Basic Amino Acids

Arginine, lysine, and histidine are polar and very hydrophilic. At physiologic pH (7.4), arginine and lysine are positively charged, whereas histidine has no

MNEMONIC

Aspartic **ACID** and Glutamic **ACID** are the **acidic** amino acids.

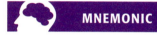

KEY FACT

All acidic and basic amino acids are polar, but not all polar amino acids are acidic or basic.

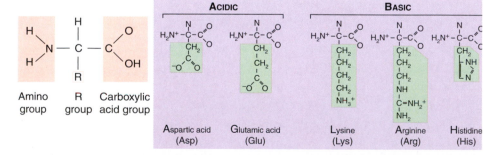

FIGURE 3-52. **Amino acid structure.** An amino acid consists of three main groups (1) an amine group, (2) a functional side group, and (3) a carboxylic acid group. At physiologic pH, acidic amino acids are negatively charged, whereas basic amino acids, with the exception of the histidine, have a net positive charge.

net charge. Arginine is the most basic amino acid and is found in high concentrations along with lysine bound to negatively charged DNA in histones, the major component of chromatin.

THE AMINO ACID POOL

Amino acids are continually being used to synthesize proteins, and proteins are continually being broken down into amino acids. This dynamic pool of amino acids is in equilibrium with tissue protein (see Figure 3-53).

Replenishment

Takes place through:

- De novo synthesis
- Dietary supply
- Protein degradation

Depletion

Occurs through:

- Protein synthesis
- Oxidation of excess amino acids

Any amino acid not immediately used must be converted to glycogen or fat stores, as protein cannot be stored.

ESSENTIAL AMINO ACIDS

Of the 20 amino acids in the body, 10 cannot be synthesized de novo in adequate amounts and must be consumed in the diet. These essential amino acids include:

- Phenylalanine (Phe)
- Valine (Val)
- Tryptophan (Trp)
- Threonine (Thr)
- Isoleucine (Ile)
- Methionine (Met)
- Histidine (His)
- Arginine (Arg)
- Leucine (Leu)
- Lysine (Lys)

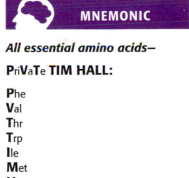

MNEMONIC

All essential amino acids—

PriVaTe TIM HALL:

Phe
Val
Thr
Trp
Ile
Met
His
Arg
Leu
Lys

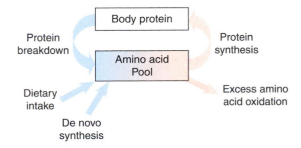

FIGURE 3-53.   **Amino acid pool.** Amino acids are taken in through the diet, recycled through the breakdown and synthesis of protein, and then removed by oxidation. Alternatively, amino acids can also be formed by de novo synthesis.

Histidine and arginine are essential only for periods when cell growth out-paces production such as during childhood.

NONESSENTIAL AMINO ACIDS

The remaining amino acids can be synthesized using the TCA cycle and other metabolic intermediates in reactions that are discussed below.

- Tyrosine (Tyr)
- Glycine (Gly)
- Alanine (Ala)
- Cysteine (Cys)
- Serine (Ser)
- Aspartate (Asp)
- Asparagine (Asn)
- Glutamate (Glu)
- Glutamine (Gln)
- Proline (Pro)

METABOLIC REACTIONS

Two simple reactions are the key to understanding amino acid metabolism: **transamination** and **oxidative deamination**.

Transamination

DEFINITION

Transfers an α-amino group to an α-keto acid group creating a new amino acid (see Figure 3-54).

- Transfer agent is an **aminotransferase/transaminase** (e.g., AST, ALT).
- Acceptor (usually α-ketoglutarate, can be pyruvate, oxaloacetate) becomes a new amino acid.
- Donor becomes a new α-keto acid.
- Reaction important for both synthesis and breakdown of amino acids.

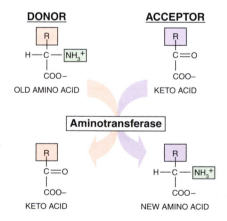

FIGURE 3-54. Transamination reaction. In this reaction, an α-amino group is transferred from the donor amino acid to the acceptor keto acid creating a new amino acid. In essence, the α-amino group is being transferred from one carbon skeleton to another.

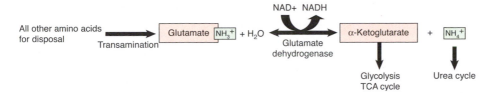

FIGURE 3-55. **Oxidative deamination reaction.** Glutamate is the only amino acid that undergoes rapid oxidative deamination. During this reaction, glutamate dehydrogenase catalyzes the removal of the α-amino group leaving an α-ketogluterate carbon skeleton. The carbon skeleton serves as a glycolytic or TCA cycle intermediate while the released ammonia enters the urea cycle.

SITE

Cytosol and mitochondria.

COFACTORS

All aminotransferases require the vitamin B₆ derivative **pyridoxal phosphate** (PLP).

Oxidative Deamination

DEFINITION

Removes an α-amino group, leaving a carbon skeleton (see Figure 3-55).

- Ammonia released enters urea cycle.
- Carbon skeletons used as glycolytic and TCA cycle intermediates.
- **Glutamate,** with the assistance of glutamate dehydrogenase, is the only amino acid that **undergoes rapid oxidative deamination.**

SITE

Mitochondria.

CONTROL

Reversible reaction driven by need for TCA intermediates.

- **Low energy (GDP, ADP) activates.**
- **High energy (GTP, ATP) inhibits.**

NONESSENTIAL AMINO ACID BIOSYNTHESIS

Nonessential amino acids can be synthesized in adequate amounts from essential amino acids and from intermediates of glycolysis and the TCA cycle.

Tyrosine

PRECURSOR

Phenylalanine.

SYNTHESIS

Irreversible hydroxylation catalyzed by **phenylalanine hydroxylase** and its required cofactor **tetrahydrobiopterin** (see Figure 3-56).

SIGNIFICANCE

Tyrosine is the precursor for catecholamines (e.g., dopamine, adrenaline, noradrenaline), melanin, and thryroxine. A genetic deficiency of phenylal-

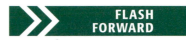

FLASH FORWARD

Aminotransferases are important liver enzymes used in diagnostic testing.

KEY FACT

Vitamin B₆ and niacin deficiencies affect the functioning of transaminases.

FLASH FORWARD

There are several major vitamin-derived cofactors that are essential for enzymatic reactions.

KEY FACT

Note: During breakdown, all amino acid α-amino groups are transferred to α-ketoglutarate since only glutamate undergoes rapid oxidative deamination.

FLASH BACK

Amino acid metabolism is intimately related to the urea and TCA cycles.

KEY FACT

Tetrahydrobiopterin is an electron carrier in redox reactions, such as tyrosine synthesis, and its deficiency is responsible for a minority of phenylketonuria cases.

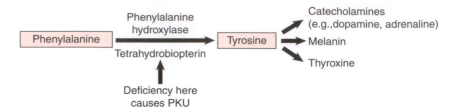

FIGURE 3-56. **Tyrosine synthesis.** Hydroxylation of phenylalanine by phenylalanine hydroxylase results in the formation of tyrosine. Tyrosine can then be used for the synthesis of other compounds. Deficiencies in either phenylalanine or its required cofactor tetrahydrobiopterin cause the disease phenylketonuria.

anine hydroxylase causes **phenylketonuria** (discussed below) which results in the build-up of phenylalanine and an inability to produce tyrosine.

Serine, Glycine, Cysteine

PRECURSORS

Glycolysis intermediates. Serine can act as precursor for glycine and cysteine. Cysteine synthesis from serine also requires the essential amino acid methionine.

SYNTHESIS

- **Serine:** Mainly a three-step process from glycolytic intermediates in the cytosol. Can also be synthesized in a reversible reaction by transfer of a hydroxymethyl group from glycine in the mitochondria (see Figure 3-57).
- **Glycine:** Mainly from CO_2, NH_4^+, and N_5N_{10}-methylene **tetrahyrdrofolate** in mitochondria. Can also be synthesized by the reverse of the serine synthesis reaction in the mitochondria (see Figure 3-60).
- **Cysteine:** Synthesis is a multistep process with four main steps (see Figure 3-58):
  1. Methionine activation.
  2. Homocysteine formation.
  3. Homocysteine and serine condensation to cystathionine.
  4. Cystathionine hydrolysis to cysteine and homoserine.

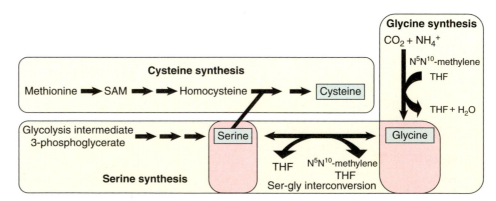

FIGURE 3-57. **Serine, glycine, cysteine synthesis.** Serine is mainly synthesized in a three-step process from the glycolytic intermediate 3-phosphoglycerate. Alternatively, serine can be formed from glycine by transfer of a hydromethyl carbon group. Glycine, in turn, can be synthesized from serine in a reversal of the previous reaction. However, it is mainly synthesized from CO_2, NH_4^+, and N_5N_{10}-methylene tetrahydrofolate. Cysteine synthesis requires methionine and serine. SAM, S-adenosyl methionine.

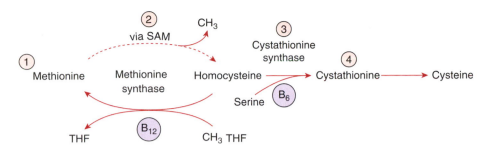

FIGURE 3-58. Cysteine synthesis. Synthesis of cysteine from serine occurs in the cytosol and requires the essential amino acid methionine. The key steps are (1) activation of methionine, (2) formation of homocysteine, (3) condensation of serine and homocysteine to from cystathionine, and (4) hydrolysis of cystathionine to form cysteine.

SIGNIFICANCE

- Glycine is notably a component of **collagen** and an inhibitory **neurotransmitter.** It is also used in the antioxidant glutathione (along with glutamate and cysteine), creatine, porphyrins, and purines.
- Cysteine synthesis interruption can lead to a buildup of homocysteine in the urine known as **homocystinuria** (discussed below).

Alanine

PRECURSOR

Pyruvate.

SYNTHESIS

One-step transamination of pyruvate (see Figure 3-59).

Aspartate, Asparagine

PRECURSOR

TCA cycle intermediate oxaloacetate.

SYNTHESIS

- Aspartate: One-step transamination of oxaloacetate (see Figure 3-60).
- Asparagine: Amide group transfer from glutamine (see Figure 3-60).

SIGNIFICANCE

- Aspartate serves as an amino donor in the **urea cycle** and in **purine and pyrimidine synthesis.**
- Asparagine provides a site of carbohydrate attachment for N-linked glycosylation.

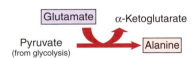

FIGURE 3-59. Alanine synthesis. Alanine is synthesized from the glycolytic intermediate pyruvate by a one-step transamination.

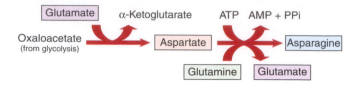

FIGURE 3-60. **Aspartate and asparagine synthesis.** Aspartate is formed in a one-step transamination from the TCA cycle intermediate oxaloacetate. Asparagine is then formed by amidation of aspartate.

Glutamate, Glutamine, Proline, Arginine

PRECURSOR

α-Ketoglutarate. Glutamate also serves as a precursor to glutamine, proline, and arginine.

SYNTHESIS (see Figure 3-61)

- **Glutamate:** Reductive amination of α-ketoglutarate. Also commonly from transamination of most other amino acids.
- **Glutamine:** Amidation (the addition of an amide group) of glutamate.
- **Proline:** Three-step synthesis from glutamate involving reduction, spontaneous cyclization, and another reduction.
- **Arginine:** Two-step synthesis from glutamate involving reduction and transamination to ornithine. Ornithine is then sent to the urea cycle where it is metabolized to arginine.

Although the details of these synthetic pathways can seem overwhelming, it is important to have a familiarity with the overall picture of nonessential amino acid synthesis and from where in the TCA cycle the precursors are obtained (see Figure 3-62).

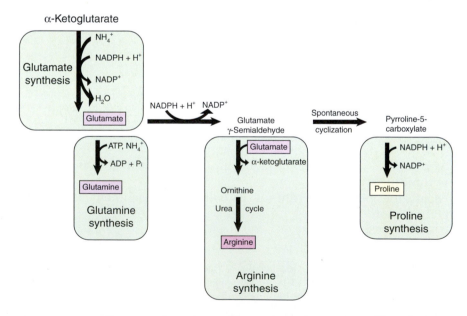

FIGURE 3-61. **Glutamate, glutamine, proline, and arginine synthesis.** These four amino acids are formed from α-ketoglutarate. (1) Glutamate is formed from a direct reductive amination. (2) Glutamine can then be formed from glutamate by amidation. At this branch point, either (3) proline can be formed in three steps or (4) ornithine can be formed in two and sent to the urea cycle, where it is metabolized to arginine.

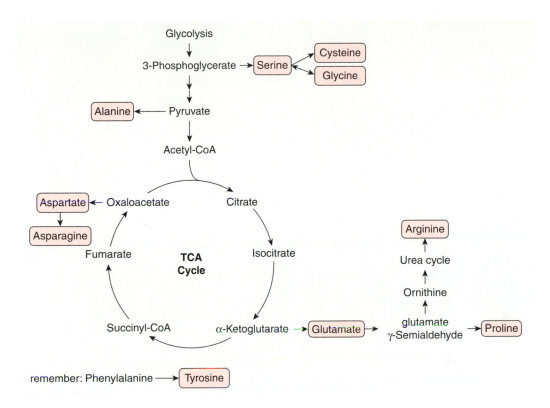

FIGURE 3-62. Biosynthesis of nonessential amino acids. This overview highlights the precursors and pathways used in nonessential amino acid synthesis.

Amino Acid Transport

Protein digestion begins in the stomach, where gastric juice and pepsin break proteins down to large peptides. Degradation continues in the small intestine to free amino acids, dipeptides, and tripeptides. These components are taken into epithelial cells via specific transporters and hydrolyzed into free amino acids (see Figure 3-63). Amino acid transport is an energy-requiring process, since the amino acid concentration in the cell is much higher than that outside of the cell. Luminal transport is Na^+ dependent, whereas contraluminal transport is Na^+ independent, much like glucose transport. There are four main transport systems based on their amino acid side chain specificity (see Table 3-22).

> **FLASH FORWARD**
>
> Amino acid transport is an important step in protein digestion.

Amino Acid Transport Deficiency

HARTNUP'S DISEASE

Rare autosomal recessive defect in the intestinal and renal transporters for **neutral amino acids.** The symptoms are due to a **loss of tryptophan,** which is a nicotinamide precursor. Thus, many aspects of the presentation **mimic niacin (vitamin B₃) deficiency** (pellagra).

PRESENTATION

Patients exhibit pellagra-like skin lesions and neurologic manifestations ranging from ataxia to frank delirium.

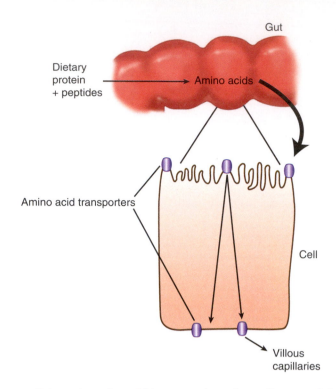

FIGURE 3-63. **Enterocyte amino acid transport.** An active, sodium-coupled transport carries dipeptides and tripeptides into the cell where they are broken down into individual amino acids by peptidases. There are also transporters for individual amino acids. At the basolateral membrane, amino acids diffuse into villous capillaries destined for the liver via portal circulation.

DIAGNOSIS

Diagnosis is made by detection of neutral aminoaciduria, which is not present in pellagra.

TREATMENT

Management is targeted at replacing niacin and providing a high-protein diet with nicotinamide supplements.

CYSTINURIA

Autosomal recessive defect in kidney tubular reabsorption of the **basic amino acids** resulting in high levels of their excretion. The low solubility of cysteine leads to precipitation and **kidney stone** formation.

TABLE 3-22. **Important Amino Acid Transport Systems**

AMINO ACID SPECIFICITY	AMINO ACIDS TRANSPORTED	DISEASES RESULTING FROM DEFECTIVE CARRIER SYSTEM
Small, aliphatic	Alanine, serine, threonine.	Nonspecific
Large, aliphatic, aromatic	Isoleucine, leucine, valine, tyrosine, tryptophan, phenylalanine.	Hartnup's disease
Basic	Arginine, lysine, cysteine, ornithine.	Cystinuria
Acidic	Glutamate, aspartate.	Nonspecific

PRESENTATION

Most of the symptoms are due to stone formation.

DIAGNOSIS

Quantitative urinary amino acid analysis confirms the diagnosis.

TREATMENT

Management strives to eliminate precipitation and stone formation by increasing urine volume (high daily fluid ingestion) and urinary alkalination.

ABSORPTIVE STATE METABOLISM

Once amino acids are absorbed, most are transaminated to **alanine, the main amino acid secreted by the gut,** and released into the portal vein destined for the liver (see Figure 3-64). In the liver, amino acids meet a use-it-or-lose-it fate. They can either be used for protein synthesis or transaminated to glutamate for rapid oxidative deamination and urea excretion. Excess amino acids must either be used directly for energy or converted to glycogen or fat stores. They **cannot be stored as protein**.

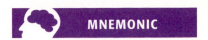

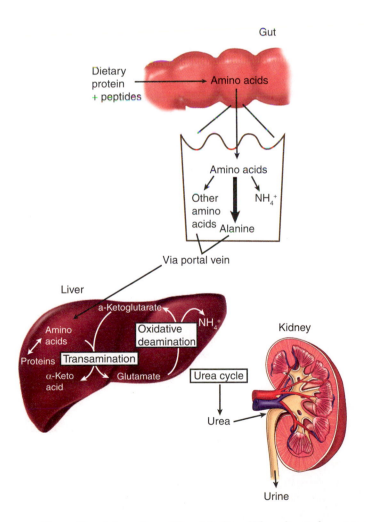

FIGURE 3-64. **Absorptive state amino acid metabolism.** When digested, protein is broken down into amino acids, most of which are converted to alanine and shuttled via the portal vein to the liver. The liver can use the amino acids for protein synthesis or lose the amino acids via entry to the urea cycle and excretion from the kidney.

AMINO ACID DERIVATIVES

Amino acids serve as precursors to synthesize many important compounds. Three simple reactions are the key to understanding amino acid derivatives: decarboxylation, hydroxylation, and methylation.

Decarboxylation: Removal of a carboxyl group (−COOH) from a compound.
Hydroxylation: Addition of a hydroxyl group (−OH) to a compound, thus oxidizing it.
Methylation: Addition of a methyl group (−CH3) to a compound.

Methionine Derivative

S-ADENOSYLMETHIONINE (SAM)

Main biosynthetic reaction methyl donor.

- **Synthesis location:** All living cells.
- **Synthesis reaction:** Methionine and ATP condensation.

Tyrosine Derivatives

THYROID HORMONES

Control the body's metabolic rate.

- **Synthesis location:** Thyroid follicle cells.
- **Synthesis reaction:** See Figure 3-65.
  - Tyrosine converted to the glycoprotein thyroglobulin.
  - Iodide oxidized to iodine (I_2) and incorporated into the tyrosine side chains of the thyroglobulin.
  - Tyrosine + one I_2 = monoiodinated tyrosine (MIT).
  - Tyrosine + two I_2 = diiodinated tyrosine (DIT).
  - DIT + DIT = thyroxine (T_4).
  - MIT + DIT = triiodothyroxine (T_3, active form).

MELANIN

Provides pigmentation, forms cap over keratinocytes for protection from UV rays.

- **Synthesis location:** Hair and skin melanocytes.
- **Synthesis reaction:** See Figure 3-66.
  - Tyrosine hydroxylation at two sites.
    - Catalyzed by **tyrosinase.**
    - Requires cofactors copper and ascorbate.
  - Reactive molecules variably polymerize to form different melanins.

CATECHOLAMINES

Control body's stress responses acting as neurotransmitters or hormones.

- **Synthesis location:** Central nervous system, adrenal medulla.
- **Synthesis reaction:** See Figure 3-67.
  - Tyrosine hydroxylation and decarboxylation to **dopamine.**
  - Dopamine hydroxylation to **norepinephrine.**
  - Norepinephrine methylation to **epinephrine** using the methyl donor SAM.
  - Metabolism occurs through the enzymes **catecholamine O-methyltransferase (COMT)** and **monoamine oxidase (MAO).**

KEY FACT

Much like the amino acid pool, there exists a dynamic one-carbon pool. These one-carbon units are used for molecular synthesis and elongation, but require activation by a carrier (usually SAM or folate) to enable their transfer.

MNEMONIC

SAM is the methyl donor man.

FLASH FORWARD

This would be good time to review the regulation of thyroid hormone synthesis.

KEY FACT

Tyrosinase, also known as tyrosine hydroxylase, deficiency is one cause of albinism.

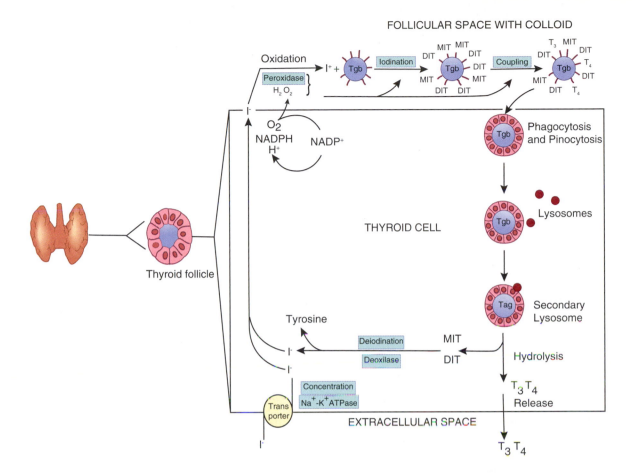

FIGURE 3-65. **Thyroid hormone synthesis.** Thyroglobulin (Tgb), which is rich in tyrosine, is transported to the lumen, where its tyrosine residues are iodinated. The various forms of thyroid hormones (T_3, T_4) produced can then be released in a regulated manner.

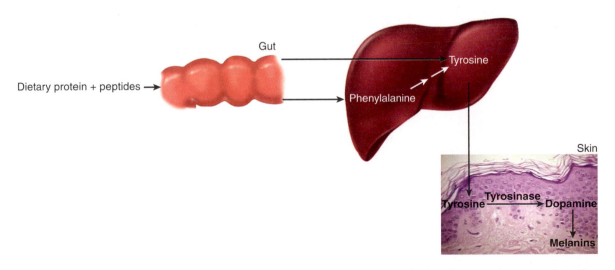

FIGURE 3-66. **Melanin synthesis.** Tyrosine can be converted by the enzyme tyrosine hydroxylase to a more active form that polymerizes to four different melanins. (Histology image courtesy of PEIR Diginal Library [http://peir.net].)

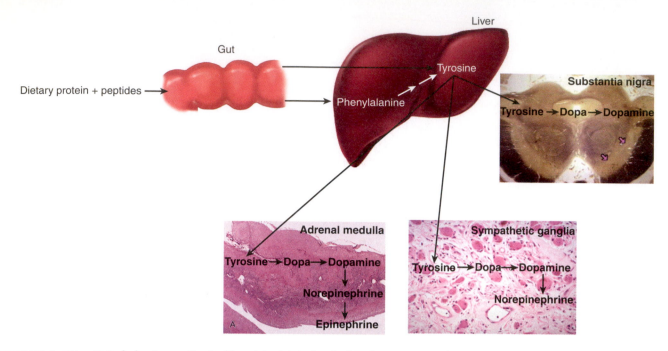

FIGURE 3-67.   Catecholamine synthesis. Phenylalanine is absorbed in the intestine and converted to tyrosine in the liver. Tyrosine can then be converted to dopamine in the substantia nigra or further processed to norepinephrine in sympathetic ganglion neurons or to epinephrine in the adrenal medulla. (Histology images courtesy of PEIR Digital Library [http://peir.net].)

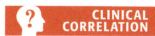
KEY FACT

The body derives energy from the many redox (oxidation-reduction) reactions that transfer electrons. NAD+ (mainly in mitochondria for oxidative, catabolic reactions) and NADP+ (mainly in cytosol for reductive, anabolic reactions) act to accept and donate these electrons.

CLINICAL CORRELATION

Serotonin levels can be diminished in patients with depression. For this reason, selective serotonin reuptake inhibitors (SSRIs) are widely used.

CLINICAL CORRELATION

Pharmacologically, melatonin has been used to treat circadian rhythm disorders such as jet lag.

Tryptophan Derivatives

NIACIN (VITAMIN B₃)

Forms essential redox reaction cofactors NAD+, NADP+.

Synthesis location: Liver.

Synthesis reaction:

- Tryptophan five-membered aromatic ring cleaved and rearranged to six-membered ring using its α-amino group.
- Reaction very slow and requires cofactors pyridoxine (vitamin B₆), riboflavin (vitamin B₂), and thiamine (vitamin B₁).

SEROTONIN

- **Synthesis location:** CNS serotonergic neurons, GI tract enterochromaffin cells.
- **Synthesis reaction:** Tryptophan aromatic ring hydroxylation and then decarboxylation (see Figure 3-68).

Serotonin is also present in high levels in platelets, but is taken up rather than synthesized.

MELATONIN

Controls circadian rhythm functions.

- **Synthesis location:** Pineal gland pinealocytes.
- **Synthesis reaction:** (See Figure 3-69).
  - Tryptophan conversion to serotonin (see above).
  - Serotonin acetylation and methylation.

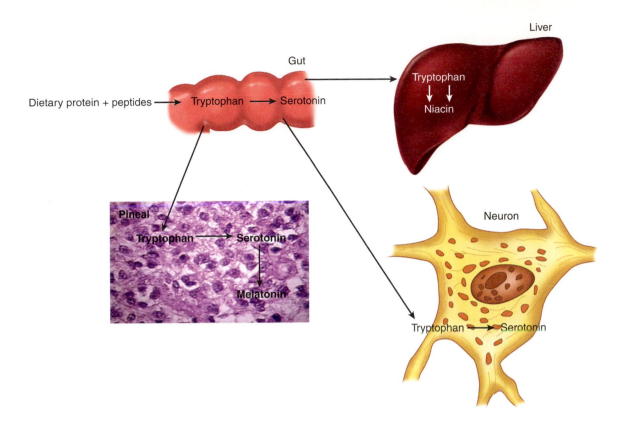

FIGURE 3-68. Serotonin and melatonin synthesis. Serotonin is derived from tryptophan via hydroxylation and decarboxylation of the aromatic ring. Melatonin can then be derived from serotonin via acetylation and methylation. (Histology image courtesy of PEIR Digital Library [http://peir.net].)

Histidine Derivative

HISTAMINE

Mediates inflammatory responses, acts as neurotransmitter, stimulates gastric acid secretion.

- **Synthesis location:** Connective tissue mast cells, GI tract enterochromaffin cells.
- **Synthesis reaction:** Histidine decarboxylation.

Glycine Derivative

HEME

Electron carrier in cytochromes and enzymes, O_2 carrier in hemoglobin and myoglobin.

- **Synthesis location:** Mitochondria and cytosol of bone marrow erythroid cells (for hemoglobin), liver hepatocytes (for cytochromes).
- **Synthesis reaction:** See Figure 3-69.
  - Eight-step reaction with first three and last three occurring in the mitochondria.
  - Δ-Aminolevulinic acid (ALA) synthesis—irreversible, rate-limiting step
    - Glycine and succinyl-CoA condensation.
    - Catalyzed by ALA synthase, requires PLP cofactor.
  - Porphobilinogen (PBG) formation—dehydration of two ALA molecules.

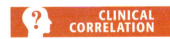

CLINICAL CORRELATION

Histidine can be metabolized to histamine, which is rapidly deactivated or stored in the granules of mast cells. These cells are degranulated when exposed to an allergen.

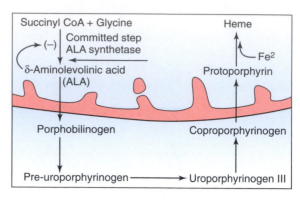

FIGURE 3-69. **Heme synthesis.** Glycine and succinyl-CoA combine to form protoporphyrin IX, which is used to form aminolevulinic acid (ALA). Two ALA molecules then condense to form porphobilinogen (PBG). Four molecules of PBG then condense to form pre-uroporphyrinogen. The remaining reactions alter side chains and the degree of porphyrin unsaturation.

- Uroporphyrinogen I (UROgen I) formation—condensation of four PBG molecules (inactive).
- Uroporphyrinogen III (UROgen III) formation—produces an active molecule.
- Coproporphyrinogen III formation, protoporphyrin IX formation, which alters side chains and porphyrin unsaturation degree.
- Heme formation—insertion of Fe^{2+}.

Arginine Derivatives

CREATINE

High-energy phosphate storage.

- **Synthesis location:** Liver, precursor formed in kidney.
- **Synthesis reaction:** See Figure 3-70.
  - Arginine and glycine formation of guanidoacetate in kidney.
  - Guanidoacetate methylation using SAM as methyl donor.

For storage, phosphate of ATP can be transferred to creatine forming creatine phosphate. Phosphate transfer can be reversed in energy depleted muscle generating creatine and ATP. Creatine and creatine phosphate spontaneously cyclize creating creatinine for excretion in urine.

UREA

Nontoxic disposable form of ammonia that is generated during amino acid turnover.

- **Synthesis location:** Liver.
- **Synthesis reaction:** Arginine cleavage to urea and ornithine in the urea cycle.
- Urea travels via the blood to the kidneys, where it is excreted in the urine.

NITRIC OXIDE

Positively regulates vessel dilation through smooth muscle relaxation.

- **Synthesis location:** Small-vessel endothelial cells.
- **Synthesis reaction:** Arginine oxidation.

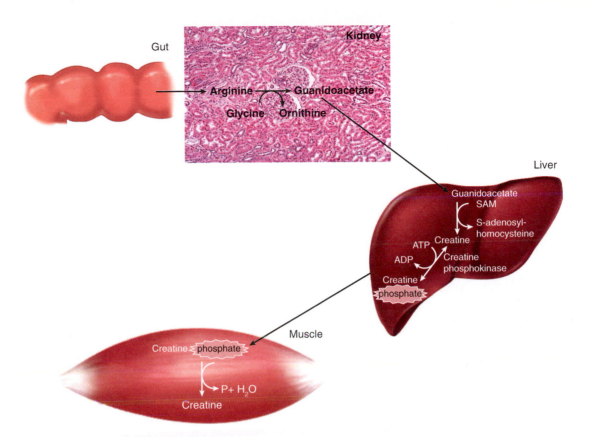

FIGURE 3-70. **Creatine synthesis.** Arginine reacts with glycine in the kidney to form the precursor guanidoacetate. Guanidoacetate is then methylated, using SAM, in the liver forming creatine. A high-energy phosphate group from ATP can then be transferred creating creatine phosphate. In muscle, when energy demand is high, the high-energy phosphate can be removed and creatine phosphate is converted back to creatine. (Histology image courtesy of PEIR Digital Library [http://peir.net].)

Glutamate Derivative

GABA

Acts as inhibitory neurotransmitter.

- **Synthesis location:** Central nervous system.
- **Synthesis reaction:** Glutamate decarboxylation.

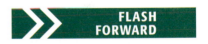

FLASH FORWARD

GABA analogs, such as gabapentin, were initially designed for use as anticonvulsants.

AMINO ACID BREAKDOWN

Excess amino acids and used amino acids must be degraded and eliminated from the body. This process can be thought of as consisting of two steps: disposal of the α-amino group and disposal of the carbon skeleton.

DISPOSAL OF THE α-AMINO GROUP

The α-amino group can be disposed of by two possible routes, both of which begin with transamination to create a common pool of glutamate (see Figure 3-71). In the first route, the glutamate formed in the cytosol undergoes oxidative deamination in the mitochondria and the amino group is sent to the urea cycle for disposal. In the second route, the glutamate is transaminated a second time with a transfer of the α-amino group to oxaloacetate to form aspartate. This occurs mainly in the liver and is catalyzed by aspartate transaminase (AST). The aspartate can then enter the urea cycle via condensation with citrulline and the amino group is again disposed.

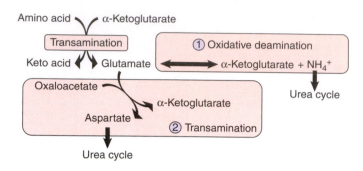

FIGURE 3-71. α-**Amino group disposal.** The first step in disposal is the transamination of amino acids to form a common pool of glutamate. This glutamate can undergo (1) oxidative deamination with the resulting amino group sent to the urea cycle or (2) a second transamination with aspartate being sent to the urea cycle.

ALANINE-GLUCOSE CYCLE

During amino acid catabolism the ammonium accumulated in skeletal muscle must be transported to the liver for disposal. However, ammonium is a toxic molecule (the reason we have the urea cycle), so alanine is used as a carrier in the circulation (see Figure 3-72). In muscle, a common pool of glutamate is again created via transamination. Glutamate is transaminated a second time, transferring the α-amino group to pyruvate, which forms alanine. This reaction is catalyzed by alanine aminotransferase (ALT). Alanine is released into the circulation, as occurs during amino acid absorption. The alanine is taken up by the liver and the reaction is reversed, adding the glutamate from the muscle to the common pool in the liver which is processed as described above.

DISPOSAL OF THE CARBON SKELETON

The remaining carbon skeleton can then be salvaged as TCA cycle and glycolytic intermediates. All 20 amino acids break down to seven common products: acetyl-CoA, acetoacetyl-CoA, pyruvate, oxaloacetate, fumarate, succinyl-CoA, and α-ketoglutarate (see Figure 3-73). Ketogenic amino acids are those that are broken down into the **ketone body formers acetyl-CoA and acetoacetyl-CoA.** Glucogenic amino acids are those that are broken down to **pyruvate or TCA intermediates** that can be channeled into gluconeogenesis. Only leucine and lysine are considered to be purely ketogenic. **Isoleucine, phenylalanine, tyrosine,** and **tryptophan are both ketogenic and glucogenic.** All other amino acids are purely glucogenic.

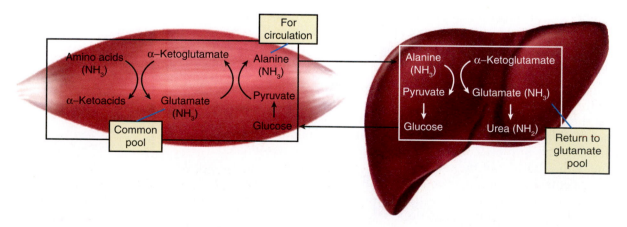

FIGURE 3-72. **Alanine-glucose cycle.** Alanine is used as a carrier to transport α-amino acid groups from the skeletal muscle to the liver for disposal via the urea cycle. This cycle allows carbon skeletons to be converted between protein and glucose.

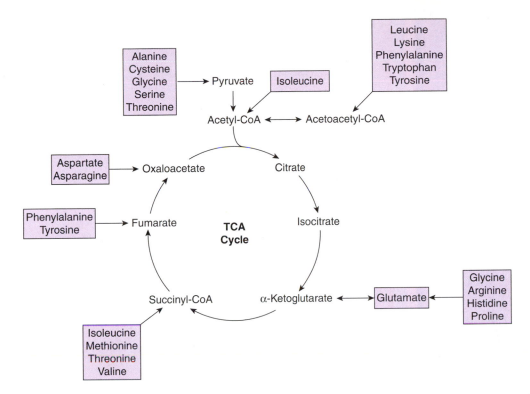

FIGURE 3-73. **Amino acid carbon skeleton recycling.** The 20 amino acids can be broken down to seven common carbon skeletons, which can be feed into the TCA cycle. Depending on the energy needs of the cell, these products can also be used to synthesize fat or glycogen.

AMINO ACID DEFICIENCIES

Phenylketonuria (PKU)

Autosomal recessive deficiency of **phenylalanine hydroxylase** or in some cases its cofactor tetrahydrobiopterin (see Figure 3-74). The lack of this enzyme causes a **buildup of phenylalanine** and an **inability to produce tyrosine.** Excess phenylalanine is converted into the phenylketones: phenylpyruvate, phenyllactate, and phenylacetate.

INCIDENCE

PKU is one of the most common amino acid deficiencies with an incidence of 1 in 13,500–19,000 live births.

PRESENTATION

If untreated, infants present at 6–12 months with CNS symptoms of developmental delay, seizures, and failure to thrive. Patients also exhibit characteristics of hypopigmentation such as fair hair, blue eyes, and pale skin.

DIAGNOSIS

All neonates are screened for raised blood levels of phenylalanine.

TREATMENT

Classically, management of the condition is accomplished by **restriction of dietary phenylalanine,** which is contained in aspartame (e.g., NutraSweet), and an increase in dietary tyrosine along with monitoring of blood phenylalanine levels. However, new treatments are in development.

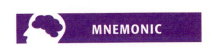

MNEMONIC

PKU: Disorder of **aromatic** amino acid metabolism—musty body **odor.**

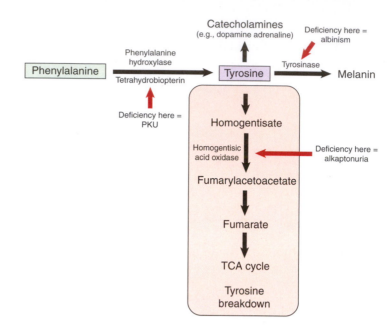

FIGURE 3-74. **Phenylalanine derivative amino acid deficiencies.** Blockades in the metabolism of phenylalanine lead to the enzyme deficiencies alkaptonuria, albinism, and phenylketonuria.

Alkaptonuria

Congenital deficiency of **homogentisic acid oxidase,** an enzyme used in the degradation of tyrosine (see Figure 3-75). This deficiency results in a buildup of homogentisate that polymerizes to a black-brown pigment. This pigment deposits in connective tissue, including cartilage.

PRESENTATION

Alkaptonuria is one of the few inborn errors of metabolism that does not present until **adulthood.** In this disease, joint damage and arthritis become apparent at presentation. However, it may be detected at an earlier age, since **urine and sweat may turn black** upon standing owing to the formation of alkapton.

DIAGNOSIS

This condition may be diagnosed by allowing the patient's urine to stand and monitoring for colorimetric change. The results can be confirmed quantitatively with a measurement of homogentisate in the urine.

TREATMENT

There is no specific treatment for alkaptonuria, and the clinical effects of dietary restriction are limited.

Albinism

Deficiency of the enzyme **tyrosinase,** which catalyzes conversion to melanin, or defective **tyrosine transporters** (see Figure 3-75). The disorder can also result from lack of migration of neural crest cells.

PRESENTATION

Neonates present with amelanosis (whitish hair, pale skin, gray-blue eyes), nystagmus, and photophobia (low pigment in iris and retina leads to failure to develop fixation reflex).

The **pentose phosphate pathway** functions to synthesize the nucleotide ribose for nucleic acid formation and to increase the amount of NADPH for fatty acid and cholesterol synthesis. Oxidative decarboxylation of pyruvate to acetyl-CoA is necessary for carbohydrate metabolism (the acetyl-CoA produced irreversibly enters the **TCA cycle**). Oxidative decarboxylation of α-ketoglutarate, found in the **TCA cycle** could not take place without TPP. Also, thiamine is used by **branched-chain α-keto acid dehydrogenase** to metabolize the three-branched chain amino acids: leucine, isoleucine, and valine (mitochondrial branched-chain α-keto acid dehydrogenase is structurally similar to pyruvate dehydrogenase).

In the United States, thiamine deficiency is most commonly due to chronic alcoholism. This is because patients with chronic alcoholism may have impaired intestinal absorption of thiamine, decreased dietary intake of thiamine, or poor thiamine metabolism. Absence of thiamine decreases the amount of acetyl-CoA available to enter the TCA cycle and increases the amount of pyruvate available for anaerobic oxidation. This leads to increased lactic acid production.

Clinically, signs of thiamine deficiency include:

- Muscle cramps
- Paresthesias
- Irritability
- Beriberi (wet or dry)

Beriberi is divided into wet and dry. Wet beriberi involves the cardiovascular system, whereas dry beriberi involves the nervous system (dry beriberi with Wernicke-Korsakoff syndrome).

Wet beriberi is characterized by neuropathy as well as heart failure, which may be high output, and includes a **triad** of **peripheral vasodilation, biventricular failure,** and **edema.** It is often brought on by physical exertion and increased carbohydrate intake.

Dry beriberi occurs with little physical exertion and decreased caloric intake and may affect peripheral nerves (motor and sensory neuropathy). **Wernicke-Korsakoff syndrome** occurs in chronic alcoholics with thiamine deficiency. **Wernicke's** encephalopathy consists of the triad: **ophthalmoplegia** (and nystagmus), **truncal ataxia,** and **confusion.** Untreated encephalopathy progresses to **Korsakoff's** syndrome. Korsakoff's syndrome consists of **impaired short-term memory** and **confabulation,** with otherwise grossly normal cognition.

Vitamin B₂—Riboflavin

Riboflavin, used as a cofactor in the oxidation and reduction of various substrates, is found in milk and other diary products. It serves as a precursor to the **coenzymes flavin mononucleotide (FMN)** and **flavin adenine dinucleotide (FAD).**

In the formation of both FMN and FAD, riboflavin reacts with ATP. In the formation of FMN, riboflavin reacts with a single ATP, yielding FMN and ADP as a by-product. In the formation of FAD, FMN reacts with a second ATP molecule, yielding FAD and pyrophosphate as a by-product.

Because of their ability to add/subtract two hydrogen atoms, FMN and FAD are favored in **fatty acid oxidation, amino acid oxidation,** and the **TCA**

KEY FACT

It is traditional to give thiamine before glucose in alcoholic patients to avoid precipitating Wernicke's encephalopathy (although thiamine is taken up by cells more slowly than glucose).

cycle. Riboflavin is also important for **erythrocyte integrity**, through erythrocyte glutathione reductase, and also for the conversion of **tryptophan to niacin.**

Deficiencies in riboflavin, leading to deficiencies in FMN and FAD, clinically cause glossitis, cheilosis, and corneal vascularization. It may also cause angular stomatitis, seborrhetic dermatitis, and weakness. Because erythrocyte glutathione reductase is dependent on riboflavin, patients may also have anemia secondary to red blood cell lysis.

Vitamin B₃—Niacin

Niacin, found in liver, milk, and unrefined grains, is another coenzyme used in oxidation and reduction reactions. Niacin appears in the diet as tryptophan, **nicotinamide adenine dinucleotide (NAD)** or its phosphorylated form, **nicotinamide adenine dinucleotide phosphate (NADP)**, both forms are hydrolyzed by intestinal enzymes to form nicotinamide. Intestinal flora convert NAD and NADP to nicotinic acid. The body is also capable of converting tryptophan to niacin.

Pharmacologically, nicotinic acid can be a treatment option to decrease total and LDL cholesterol (and has some effects to raise HDL). Its side effects include flushing, pruritus (both of which are treated with aspirin), hives, nausea, and vomiting.

Pellagra is the name of niacin deficiency. Patients can get pellagra from lack of dietary niacin, isoniazid use, Hartnup's disease, or malignant carcinoid syndrome. Pellagra is characterized by **diarrhea, dermatitis,** and **dementia** (see Figure 3-75). If untreated, pellagra can be fatal. Dietary replacement of both tryptophan and niacin is the treatment.

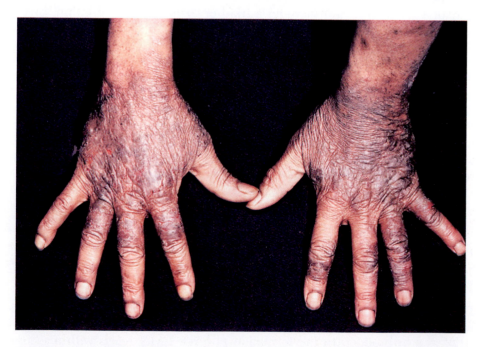

FIGURE 3-75.   Pellagra. Signs of pellagra include hyperpigmented, brittle, cracked, and scaly skin. (Reproduced, with permission, from Wolf K, Johnson RA, Suurmond D. Fitzpatrick's Color Atlas & Synopsis of Clinical Dermatology, 5th ed. New York: McGraw-Hill, 2005: 457.)

Hartnup's disease is a genetic defect in tryptophan membrane transport that causes intestinal malabsorption and poor renal resorption. Therefore, simple replacement therapy is insufficient. Similarly, in **malignant carcinoid syndrome**, tryptophan is used for excessive 5-hydroxytryptamine (5-HT) production and is less available for NAD synthesis, causing pellagra that is nonresponsive to therapy.

VITAMIN B$_5$—PANTOTHENIC ACID

Pantothenic acid is the major constituent of CoA, and it is found in most foods. It is a cofactor for acyl transfers (pantothen-A is in the CoA complex). These reactions take place in the TCA cycle, fatty acid oxidation, acetylations, and cholesterol synthesis. Deficiency of vitamin B$_5$ is rare in humans, but may result in paresthesias or dysesthesias, and gastrointestinal distress.

VITAMIN B$_6$—PYRIDOXINE

A pyridine derivative, pyridoxine, along with pyridoxal and pyridoxamine, serve as building blocks for **PLP**, which is the coenzyme involved in **amino acid metabolism** (e.g., conversion of serine to glycine). These molecules are found in wheat, egg yolk, and meats. The coenzyme is responsible for numerous reactions including transamination, deamination, decarboxylation, and condensation and creation of the liver enzymes **AST** and **ALT**.

Although clinical manifestations are rare, a deficiency of vitamin B$_6$ can result in **convulsion** as well as **hyperirritability**. Decreased concentrations of vitamin B$_6$ deficiency may occur after use of oral contraceptives, isoniazid, cycloserine, and penicillamine. Too much vitamin B$_6$ can cause sensory neuropathy that is unrelieved when toxicity is corrected.

VITAMIN B$_{12}$—COBALAMIN

Animal products (meat or dairy) are the only dietary source of vitamin B$_{12}$. Absorption of cobalamin starts in the stomach after ingestion. Vitamin B$_{12}$, bound to animal protein, is released by mechanical and chemical digestion. The parietal cells, located primarily at the gastric fundus, secrete both hydrochloric acid and **intrinsic factor** in response to the meal. As the cobalamin is released from the animal protein, it is bound by **R protein (haptocorrin)**, forming a stable complex in the low pH. **The R protein–cobalamin complex** and the secreted intrinsic factor move into the duodenum, where pancreatic enzymes degrade R protein. The R protein–cobalamin complex is broken down and allows intrinsic factor to bind B$_{12}$. **The intrinsic factor–cobalamin complex** formed in the duodenum moves toward the distal ileum and binds to the **intrinsic factor–cobalamin receptor** expressed on the enterocytes. Once bound, the entire unit is internalized by the enterocyte. Intrinsic factor is degraded in the enterocyte, freeing cobalamin. The available cobalamin is bound to plasma **transcobalamin II** (TCII) forming yet another complex. The TCII/cobalamin complex then migrates through the basolateral side of the enterocyte into circulation, stored in the liver, and made available for B$_{12}$-dependent enzymes.

B$_{12}$-dependent enzymes:

- Methylmalonyl-CoA mutase (converts proprionyl-CoA to methylmalonyl-CoA and then to succinyl-CoA)
- Leucine aminomutase
- Methionine synthase

Cobalamin is used as a cofactor for **methionine synthase** and **methylmalonyl-CoA synthase.** Methionine synthase catalyzes homocysteine to methionine via a one-carbon transfer from methyl-THF to create THF (see Figure 3-76). These one-carbon transfers are necessary for **de novo synthesis of purines** and work in tandem with folate. Deficiency in cobalamin causes a buildup of methyl-THF (unconjugated form), which eventually leaves the cell and can lead to a corresponding folate deficiency.

Vitamin B_{12} deficiency can be caused by a myriad of disorders. **Dietary deficiency** is rare, because the liver stores large quantities of vitamin B_{12}. **Pernicious anemia** is a common cause of megaloblastic anemia (MCV greater than 100 fL). It is typically caused by an autoimmune attack on gastric parietal cells, which leads to decreased production of intrinsic factor (accompanied by achlorhydria and atrophic gastritis). **Gastrectomy** (and similarly gastric bypass surgery) disrupts secretion of intrinsic factor by gastric parietal cells, leading to decreased absorption of vitamin B_{12}. **Infectious** causes include *Helicobacter pylori*, which causes chronic gastritis, *Diphyllobothrium latum*, in which the fish tapeworm competes for vitamin B_{12} absorption in the intestine, and blind loop syndrome, in which bacterial overgrowth also competes for vitamin B_{12} absorption in the intestine. **Structural abnormalities of the terminal ileum** (Crohn's disease, surgical resection) can cause decreased absorption of vitamin B_{12}. **Pancreatic insufficiency** leads to a decrease in enzymes necessary to break down the R protein–cobalamin complex, preventing cobalamin to bind with intrinsic factor. Finally, **deficiency of transcobalamin II** prevents cobalamin from entering systemic circulation.

Clinical signs of vitamin B_{12} deficiency include a neuropathy characterized by defective myelin formation and consequent subacute degeneration of the posterior and lateral spinal columns. This results in symmetric paresthesias and ataxia, loss of proprioception and vibration senses, and, in severe cases, spasticity, clonus, paraplegia, and fecal and urinary incontinence. The mechanism for this defect is uncertain, but it may be that lack of vitamin B_{12} causes

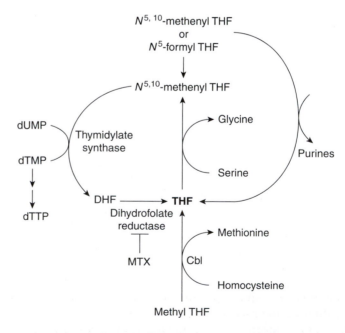

FIGURE 3-76. Tetrahydrofolate metabolism. (Modified, with permission, from Kasper DL, Braunwald E, Fauci AS, et al. *Harrison's Principles of Internal Medicine*, 16th ed. New York: McGraw-Hill, 2005: 602.)

decreased folate, which in turn decreases methionine levels and leads to impaired myelin production.

The most evident sign of vitamin B_{12} deficiency, however, is megaloblastic change of the red blood cells (seen on a peripheral blood smear) and mean cell volume (MCV). **Elevated MCV (> 110 fL)** and **hypersegmented neutrophils** (lobe count of 4 or greater) indicate deficiency. The megaloblastic changes due to vitamin B_{12} deficiency are indistinguishable from those due to folate deficiency; however, **only vitamin B_{12} deficiency causes neuropathy.**

FOLIC ACID

Present in fruits and vegetables, folic acid is required for erythropoiesis and one-carbon transfers. It is responsible for the conversion of homocysteine to methionine (where vitamin B_{12} is a cofactor), conversion of serine to glycine (where B_6 is a cofactor), and conversion of deoxyuridylate to thymidylate for DNA synthesis, and it is indirectly responsible for purine ring formation (through its derivatives) (see Figure 3-76).

Folate is maintained in the body via the **folate enterohepatic cycle.** Dietary folate (available as polyglutamates) undergoes hydrolysis and reduction from enzymes on mucosal cell membranes to form monoglutamate. **Dihydrofolate reductase** found in the duodenal mucosa methylates the folate and allows it to be absorbed by enterocytes in the jejunum. Folate then joins with plasma-binding proteins and travels systemically or to the liver, where it is converted and secreted in bile back to the duodenum to repeat the cycle.

Causes of folate deficiency include **inadequate dietary intake, malabsorptive diseases, liver dysfunction, medications,** and states of **increased folate consumption.** Inadequate dietary intake is seen in alcoholics or persons who consume only cooked or boiled (not raw) vegetables because folate is easily destroyed by heat. Malabsorptive diseases that affect the jejunum, celiac sprue, sprue, and biliary diseases alter the folate enterohepatic cycle. Hepatic dysfunction, seen in alcoholics and those with liver cirrhosis, also interfere with the enterohepatic cycle and may interfere with production of plasma-binding proteins. Medications such as methotrexate and trimethoprim inhibit dihydrofolate reducatase and decrease absorption of dietary folate. Other medications (phenytoin) can also interfere with absorption. Finally, pregnancy, hemolytic anemias, and other states that require a large amount of folate can simply deplete the available stores of folate and create a relative deficiency because of increased demand.

Clinical symptoms of folic acid deficiency consist of megaloblastic anemia (with mucosal changes). However, there are no neurologic sequelae from folic acid deficiency (in contrast to what occurs with vitamin B_{12} deficiency, which consists of a megaloblastic anemia and neurologic symptoms).

BIOTIN

Biotin is a water-soluble vitamin found in peanuts, cashews, almonds, and other foods. Intestinal flora also synthesize biotin. Raw egg whites contain **avidin,** which binds to biotin, forming a nonabsorbable complex. The biotin coenzyme **carries carboxylate** and is involved in carboxylation reactions important for carbohydrate and lipid metabolism. Biotin participates in several key reactions including conversion of **pyruvate to oxaloacetate** (by pyruvate carboxylase in the TCA cycle) and conversion of **propionyl-CoA to methylmalonyl-CoA** (by proprionyl-CoA carboxylase, in synthesis of odd-chain fatty acids).

KEY FACT

Folate deficiency leads to hyperhomocysteinemia (elevated levels of homocysteine), which leads to atherosclerosis.

VITAMIN C—ASCORBIC ACID

Vitamin C or ascorbic acid is found in citrus fruits. Dietary vitamin C is taken up in the ileum. It provides reducing equivalents for several enzymatic reactions, particularly those catalyzed by **copper- and iron-containing enzymes,** and is linked to increased iron absorption in the intestine. Vitamin C is necessary for proper hydroxylation of proline and lysine used in **collagen synthesis.** It also serves as an antioxidant and facilitates iron absorption by keeping iron in its reduced state. Many copper-containing or iron-containing hydroxylases require ascorbic acid to maintain normal metabolism. **Dopamine β-hydroxylase,** involved in the conversion of tyrosine to norepinephrine and epinephrine, requires ascorbate to reduce copper after it has been oxidized in the reaction. Likewise, **proline and lysine hydroxylase** are required for the post-translational modification of procollagen to form collagen, because hydroxylated residues are required for the formation of stable triple helices and for cross-linking of collagen molecules to form fibrils.

Scurvy results from vitamin C deficiency. Swollen gums, bruising, anemia, and poor wound healing are signs of scurvy and are due in part to impaired collagen formation (see Figure 3-77).

KEY FACT

Genetic disorders of collagen synthesis include osteogenesis imperfecta and Ehlers-Danlos syndrome.

Fat-Soluble Vitamins

VITAMIN A—RETINOIDS

Vitamin A (e.g., retinol, retinaldehyde, retinoic acid) is found in fish oils, meats, dairy products, and eggs. β-Carotene, a precursor of vitamin A that is metabolized by intestinal mucosal cells into retinaldehyde, is found in green vegetables. Vitamin A in the form of retinol is absorbed into the **intestinal mucosal cells** and is transported **to the liver via chylomicrons.** Vitamin A is delivered to the rest of the body via prealbumin and retinol-binding protein.

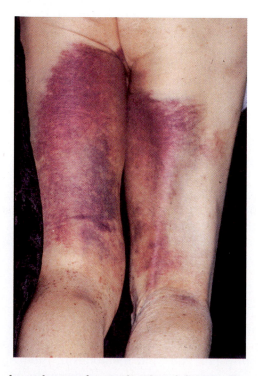

FIGURE 3-77. Ecchymosis secondary to vitamin C deficiency. (Reproduced, with permission, from Wolff K, Johnson RA, Suurmond D. *Fitzpatrick's Color Atlas and Synopsis of Clinical Dermatology,* 5th ed. New York: McGraw-Hill, 2005: 453.)

Vitamin A combines with opsin in the eye to form rhodopsin in the rod cells of the retina. A similar reaction produces iodopsin in cone cells. These proteins play a crucial role in sensing light in the retina and are essential for vision. Vitamin A also has a role in the differentiation and proliferation of epithelial cells in the respiratory tract, skin, cornea, conjunctiva, and other tissues.

Deficiency of vitamin A, therefore, causes vision problems, disorders of epithelial cell differentiation and proliferation, and impaired immune response. Symptoms may include headaches, skin changes, sore throat, and alopecia. Progression of visual symptoms for vitamin A deficiency are loss of green light sensitivity, poor adaptation to dim light, night blindness (loss of retinol in rod cells). **Xerophthalmia** (squamous epithelial thickening), **Bitot's spots** (squamous metaplasia), and **keratomalacia** (softening of the cornea) also occur in vitamin A deficiency. Metaplasia of respiratory epithelia is seen (often common in cystic fibrosis due to failure of fat-soluble vitamin absorption) as well as frequent respiratory infections (secondary to respiratory epithelial defects).

Because vitamin A is stored in the liver and is lipophilic, the body can store large amounts of the vitamin. Toxicity can occur acutely, chronically, or as a teratogenic effect. Acute toxicity can be caused from a large, single dose of vitamin A and results in nausea, vertigo, and blurry vision. Chronic toxicity can manifest as ataxia, alopecia, hyperlipidemia, or hepatotoxicity. In the first trimester of pregnancy, excess vitamin A can be very teratogenic and can lead to fetal loss.

VITAMIN D—CHOLECALCIFEROL

Vitamin D plays an important role in bone metabolism by regulating plasma calcium concentrations. Vitamin D is absorbed from dietary sources and is also synthesized in the skin. Vitamin D absorption is regulated by serum calcium concentrations.

In the presence of UV light, 7-dehydrocholesterol present in the skin is converted to previtamin D. Once previtamin D is formed, it can be converted to cholecalciferol, which enters the circulation. Before cholecalciferol can be effective in calcium homeostasis, it must be activated. Activation of cholecalciferol takes place in the liver and the kidney. The **liver** converts cholecalciferol to **25-hydroxy derivative**. The **kidney** converts the 25-hydroxy derivative into **1,25-hydroxy vitamin D (calcitriol)**, its active metabolite. The kidney also converts 25-hydroxy derivative into 24,25-hydroxyvitamin D, an inactive metabolite (see Figure 3-78). Vitamin D–binding globulin stores vitamin D and is also responsible for its systemic transport in the circulation.

Vitamin D maintains the plasma calcium concentration by increasing intestinal absorption of calcium, minimizing calcium excretion in the distal renal tubules, mobilizing bone mineral in bones. It also stimulates osteoblasts and improves calcification of bone matrix (and, hence, bone formation). In addition, vitamin D has various roles in the skin, immune cells (lymphocytes, monocyctes), thyroid, and parathyroid.

Vitamin D, when activated, behaves like a steroid hormone in that it binds to the nuclear receptor of cells of interest (intestinal cells, renal cells, and osteoblasts) and induces gene expression. It is regulated by a series of feedback mechanisms involving PTH (parathyroid hormone), calcium, and phosphate. Low levels of calcium stimulate PTH synthesis and secretion, which in turn

KEY FACT

The consumption of polar bear liver, which contains high levels of vitamin A, resulted in the discovery of vitamin A toxicity.

KEY FACT

Calci**TRI**ol works on the **TRI**ad of intestines, kidneys, and bone to maintain plasma calcium levels.

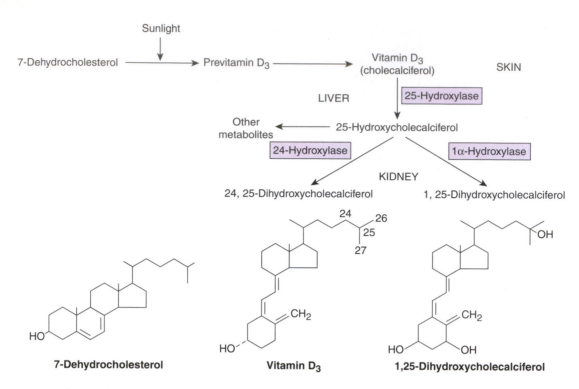

FIGURE 3-78. **Various pathways of vitamin D formation.** (Modified, with permission, from Ganong WF. *Review of Medical Physiology*, 22nd ed. New York: McGraw-Hill, 2005: 388.)

prompt the conversion of 25-hydroxy derivative to 1,25-dihydroxyvitamin D (calcitriol). In turn, calcitriol has a negative feedback effect on its own production as well as PTH production. In excess, calcitriol also promotes the conversion of 24,25-dihydroxyvitamin D. As previously described, calcitriol acts to regulate calcium homeostasis. In the presence of excess calcium from either bone or intestinal absorption, high levels of calcium act to decrease PTH production, and high levels of phosphate act to decrease conversion of 25-hydroxy derivative to 1,25-dihydroxyvitamin D by blocking the 1α-hydroxylase (see Figures 3-79 and 3-80).

Deficiency of vitamin D leads to **rickets** in children and **osteomalacia** in adults, the differences being open (in children) or closed (in adults) epiphyseal plates. Rickets results from not receiving enough calcium and phosphate going to the sites where bone mineralization is taking place.

Clinically, children with rickets show signs of hypocalcemia, bowing of the lower extremities, and poor dentition. The treatment for vitamin D–deficient rickets and osteomalacia is vitamin D therapy. In vitamin D–resistant rickets, vitamin D repletion does not treat the syndrome, and a genetic abnormality may be present.

- **Type I vitamin D–resistant rickets** occurs when there is a genetic mutation of 1α-hydroxylase. This can be treated with 1,25-dihydroxyvitamin D by passing the conversion of 25-hydroxy derivative in the kidney. If supplementation of 1,25-dihydroxyvitamin D does not treat the underlying problem, then the patient has **type II vitamin D–resistant rickets**.
- Type II vitamin D–resistant rickets. The 1,25-dihydroxyvitamin D receptor is mutated and therefore unresponsive to both vitamin D and calcitriol.
- **X-linked rickets** is entirely due to renal phosphate wasting. In this condition, 1,25-OHD levels are elevated.

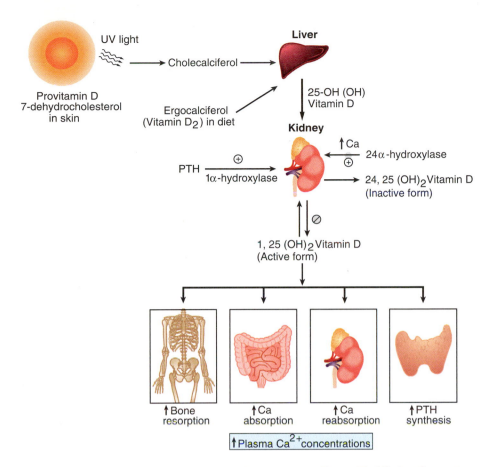

FIGURE 3-79. **Vitamin D target organs and consequent effects.** (Modified, with permission, from Molina PE. *Endocrine Physiology*, 2nd ed. New York: McGraw-Hill, 2006: 110.)

Excess vitamin D leads to hypercalcemia and all of the sequelae associated with it (e.g., kidney stones, dementia, constipation, abdominal pain, depression). Sarcoidosis can lead to excess vitamin D since pulmonary macrophages can produce calcitriol. Similarly, lymphoma can produce calcitriol.

VITAMIN E—α-TOCOPHEROL

Vitamin E is a lipid-soluble antioxidant found in sunflower oil, corn oil, soybeans, meats, fruits, and vegetables. It can be found in cell membranes and serves as an antioxidant like glutathione and vitamin C. It is used to react to the radicals formed by peroxidation of fatty acids. Like other fat-soluble vitamins, vitamin E is absorbed in the intestine and travels to the liver via chy-

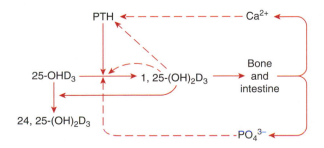

FIGURE 3-80. **Vitamin D regulation.** Solid lines indicate stimulation. Dashed lines indicate inhibitory. (Modified, with permission, from Ganong WF. *Review of Medical Physiology*, 22nd ed. New York: McGraw-Hill, 2005: 389.)

lomicrons to the liver. Fat malabsorption diseases (cystic fibrosis, liver disease) decrease the amount of vitamin E available. Deficiency of vitamin E is uncommon, but can cause hemolytic anemia, peripheral neuropathy, and ophthalmoplegia. In excess, vitamin E can interfere with vitamin K metabolism.

Vitamin K—Phylloquinone

Vitamin K is found in either vegetable or animal sources (phylloquinone) or through bacterial flora (menaquinone). It is used by the liver in clotting proteins for the carboxylation of glutamate residues. It forms γ-carboxyglutamate (**Gla**) in the in the postsynthetic modification of clotting proteins. Prothrombin and Factors VII, IX, and X, and the antithrombotic proteins C and S all use these residues (see Figure 3-81). They are essential because Gla acts as a chelator, trapping calcium ions. This allows the clotting proteins to bind to negatively charged phospholipids at the surface of platelets and to function at these membranes.

The reduced form of vitamin K is oxidized by γ-glutamyl carboxylase (and epoxidase) to form the γ-carboxyglutamate (Gla) in the postsynthetic modification. The oxidized form of vitamin K or **vitamin K epoxide** needs to be converted back to the reduced form to be used again. **Warfarin** blocks the use of the **2,3-epoxide reductase** in its reaction with **vitamin K epoxide and NADH** (see Figure 3-82). The resulting vitamin K epoxide is solubilized in

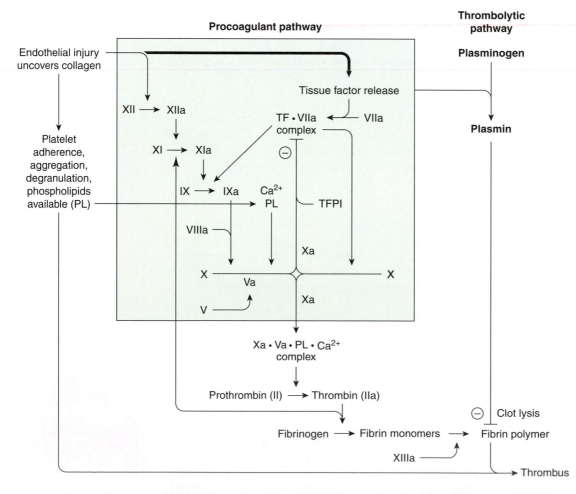

FIGURE 3-81. **Procoagulation and thrombolytic coagulation pathways.** (Modified, with permission, from McPhee SJ, Ganong WF. *Pathophysiology of Disease: An Introduction to Clinical Medicine*, 5th ed. New York: McGraw-Hill, 2006: 120.)

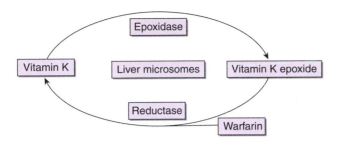

FIGURE 3-82. **Warfarin prevents conversion of vitamin K epoxide to vitamin K.** (Modified, with permission, from Kasper DL, Braunwald E, Fauci AS, et al. *Harrison's Principles of Internal Medicine*, 16th ed. New York: McGraw-Hill, 2005: 683.)

water and excreted from the body. The overall effect is anticoagulation, reducing the total amount of biologically active coagulation factors.

Vitamin K deficiency is rare in otherwise healthy adults. Symptoms of vitamin K deficiency are similar to those of warfarin toxicity in that both have an apparent lack of vitamin K, resulting in a decrease of clotting factor function. Signs and symptoms of vitamin K deficiency include gastrointestinal bleeding, intracranial bleeding, ecchymoses, epistaxis, and hematuria.

Fed versus Unfed State

ENDOCRINE PANCREAS

The pancreas contains both exocrine and endocrine functions. The **exocrine** function of the pancreas is performed by acinar cells, which form lobules and secrete **digestive enzymes** and bicarbonate-rich fluids into the duodenum. The **endocrine** function of the pancreas is responsible for **insulin, glucagon,** and **somatostatin** production and secretion.

Insulin is an anabolic polypeptide hormone (i.e., induces growth through intracellular processes) produced by the β-cells (75% of total mass of pancreatic endocrine cells) of the **islet of Langerhans**. The α-cells (20% of total mass of pancreatic endocrine cells) secrete glucagon. Finally, δ-cells (5% of total mass of pancreatic endocrine cells) secrete somatostatin. The β-cells are typically located centrally with α-cells and δ-cells located around them, allowing for **paracrine regulation.**

Insulin

Synthesis of insulin, like all hormones, starts in the nucleus. The insulin gene is transcribed to produce mRNA. The insulin mRNA is translated on RER-bound ribosomes which produce **preproinsulin.** This molecule enters the RER because it contains an N-terminal signal sequence. The signal sequence is cleaved off in the lumen of the RER to generate **proinsulin** (see Figure 3-83). Proinsulin contains the "C peptide" region, which links the insulin α- and β-chains and allows the protein to fold properly during its formation. Proinsulin is packaged in a vesicle and sent to the Golgi apparatus, where it is again cleaved, forming **insulin** and **C peptide.** Mature insulin consists of two polypeptide chains linked together by disulfide bonds. When β-cells are stimulated by increased blood glucose concentration, calcium enters the cells and triggers exocytosis of secretory granules containing both insulin and C peptide (see Figure 3-84).

CLINICAL CORRELATION

Rat poison is a type of "superwarfarin," and causes severe coagulopathy. Treatment for ingestions is with high doses of vitamin K.

KEY FACT

Multiple endocrine, neoplasia (MEN) type 1 or **Werner's syndrome** consists of parathyroid, pituitary, and enteropancreatic tumors. Among the pancreatic tumors are **insulinomas** (causing fasting hypoglycemia), **glucagonomas** (causing diabetes mellitus and migratory necrolytic erythema), and **somatostatinomas** (also causing diabetes mellitus, steatorrhea, and cholelithiasis).

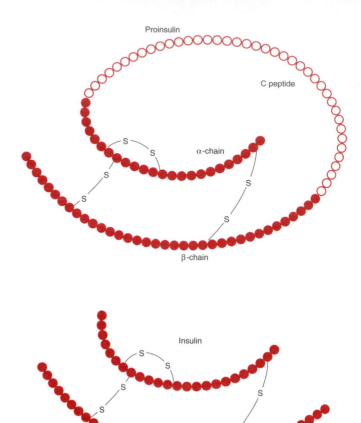

FIGURE 3-83. **Structure of proinsulin and insulin.** (Modified, with permission, from Molina PE, *Endocrine Physiology*, 2nd ed, New York: McGraw-Hill, 2006: 159.)

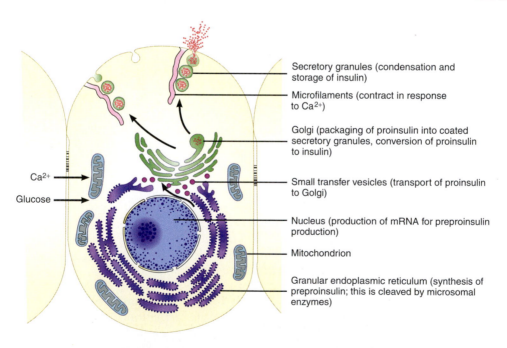

FIGURE 3-84. **Formation and secretion of insulin.** Structural components of the pancreatic B cell involved in glucose-induced insulin biosynthesis and release. Schematic representation of secretory granular alignment on microfilament "tracks" that contract in response to calcium.

Insulin secretion is **stimulated** by:

- **Glucose** (most important stimulus)
- Amino acids (arginine)
- Secretin (as well as other gastrointestinal hormones)
- Free fatty acids
- Ketone bodies
- Sulfonylurea drugs (inhibit ATP-sensitive K^+ channels)
- Cholecystokinin
- Acetylcholine
- Glucagon

Insulin secretion is **inhibited** by:

- Epinephrine
- Norepinephrine
- Cortisol
- Growth hormone

Insulin serves as an anabolic hormone used by the body to **maximize the storage of dietary glucose in the well-fed state**. Its actions serve to decrease serum glucose levels, and it targets tissues responsible for glucose storage and utilization. Its main targets are the liver, muscle, and adipose tissues (see Figure 3-85).

In the **liver**, insulin:

- Inhibits gluconeogenesis
- Inhibits breakdown of glycogen
- Promotes glycogen synthesis

In **muscle** cells, insulin:

- Promotes glycogen synthesis
- Increases glucose entry into cells (mediated by GLUT4 glucose transporters)
- Stimulates the entry of amino acids (desirable for protein synthesis)

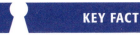

KEY FACT

Oral glucose has a greater effect on insulin secretion than does the same amount of intravenous glucose.

KEY FACT

In adipocytes, insulin regulates the entry and metabolism of glucose. Glucose, once it enters the fat cell, is converted to glycerol 3-phosphate, the substrate used for triacylglycerol synthesis.

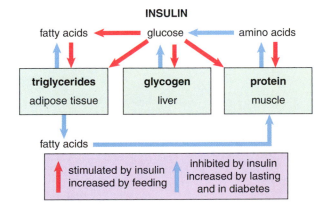

FIGURE 3-85. **Targets of insulin.** Pathways in blue indicate targets that are stimulated by insulin. Pathways in white indicate targets that are inhibited by insulin. The blue pathways are increased by feeding, whereas the white pathways are increased by fasting. (Modified, with permission, from Brunton LL, Lazo JS, Parker KL. *Goodman and Gilman's The Pharmacological Basis of Therapeutics*, 11th ed. New York: McGraw-Hill, 2006: 1621.)

KEY FACT

Cells that **do not** require insulin for the uptake of glucose:

- Hepatocyctes
- Erythrocytes
- Cells of the nervous system
- Intestinal mucosa
- Renal tubules
- Cornea

In **adipose** tissue, insulin:

- Increases glucose uptake/entry into cells (mediated by GLUT4 transporters)
- Increases triacylglycerol synthesis
- Decreases triacylglycerol degradation
- Inhibits activity of hormone-sensitive lipase
- Increases lipoprotein lipase activity

INSULIN SECRETION

Insulin secretion starts with glucose entering the β-islet cells through the **GLUT2 transporter.** Glucose is then phosphorylated by glucokinase and is trapped in the β-cells. The glucose molecule is used to form ATP, which inhibits the ATP-sensitive potassium channels that are used to pump potassium out of the cell. Retention of intracellular potassium causes the cell membrane to depolarize, which causes an influx of extracellular calcium through voltage-sensitive calcium channels. The rise in intracellular calcium triggers the release of vesicles containing insulin and C-peptide (see Figure 3-86).

MECHANISM OF ACTION OF INSULIN

Insulin binds to the insulin receptor, a tyrosine kinase (once insulin binds to the external part of the receptor, tyrosine residues on the internal part of the receptor become autophosphorylated). Once activated, the tyrosine kinase phosphorylates insulin receptor substrate (IRS) proteins. The newly activated IRS proteins in turn, activate cellular kinases and phosphatases that vary depending on the type of cell. After insulin binds to its receptor, both

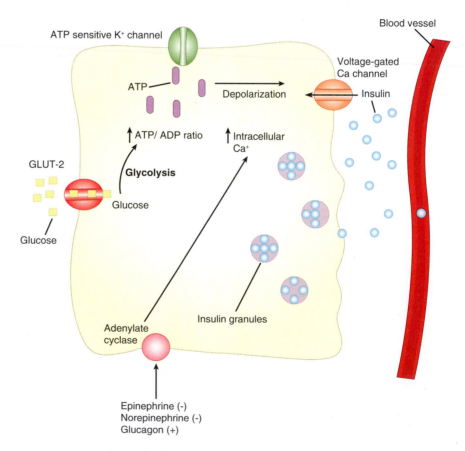

FIGURE 3-86. Pancreatic β cell insulin secretion.

are taken up into the cell. Although insulin is then degraded, its receptor may return to the cell membrane.

Seconds to minutes: Transports glucose into cells.
Minutes to hours: Induces changes in enzymatic activity.
Hours to days: Increases **glucokinase, phosphofructokinase** and **pyruvate kinase**.

Glucagon

Glucagon is a polypeptide hormone secreted by α **cells of the pancreatic islets**. Glucagon regulates the actions of insulin and **maintains serum glucose levels**. It does so by activation of hepatic glycogenolysis and gluconeogenesis.

Stimuli for glucagon release include:

- Hypoglycemia (primary stimulus)
- Amino acids
- Epinephrine

Release of glucagon is inhibited by:

- Insulin
- Hyperglycemia

Glucagon:

- Activates **phosphorylase** (causing **glycogen***lysis*)
- Increases uptake of amino acids by the liver, providing carbon skeletons for **gluconeogenesis**
- Has **no** effect on muscle glycogen stores
- Promotes ketone body formation from acetyl-CoA produced by hepatic oxidation

In all of these actions, glucagon acts via generation of cAMP. See Table 3-23 for a summary of the action of insulin and glucagon.

TABLE 3-23.   Summary of Action of Insulin and Glucagon

	LIVER	ADIPOSE TISSUE	MUSCLE
Increased by insulin	Fatty acid synthesis Glycogen synthesis Protein synthesis	**Glucose** uptake Fatty acid synthesis	**Glucose** uptake Glycogen synthesis Protein synthesis
Decreased by insulin	Ketogenesis Gluconeogenesis	Lipolysis	
Increased by **glucagon**	Glycogenolysis Gluconeogenesis Ketogenesis	Lipolysis	

(Reproduced, with permission, from Murray RK, Granner DK, Rodwell VW. *Harper's Illustrated Biochemistry*, 27th ed, New York: McGraw-Hill, 2000: 174.)

MNEMONIC

When it comes to glucagon's effects on glucose and glycogen storage, you can consider your glucose all gone from the liver:
Glucagon = **gluc-all-gone.**

KEY FACT

Amino acids cause the release of **both** insulin and glucagon. The release of glucagon opposes the action of secreted insulin on cellular intake of serum glucose.
Catecholamines released in the sympathetic nervous system "fight or flight" response allow for elevated serum glucose for use by muscles, organs, and other tissues.

KEY FACT

Epinephrine activates *muscle* phosphorylase. **Glucagon** activates *liver* phosphorylase.

Fatty Acid Metabolism

Lipogenesis occurs in the brain, liver, kidney, lung, and adipose tissue. The main substrate is acetyl-CoA, and the major product is palmitate. The first step in the formation of palmitate is the formation of malonyl-CoA. The substrate, acetyl-CoA, must be produced from citrate, which must be transported from the mitochondria (where it was created in the citric acid cycle), to the extramitochondrial cytosol. Acetyl-CoA serves as the substrate for the synthesis of long-chain fatty acids containing an even number of carbons, and forms carbons numbers 15 and 16 of the molecule palmitate. Propionyl-CoA, not acetyl-CoA, acts as the substrate for long-chain fatty acids containing an odd number of carbons.

Citrate is formed from the condensation of acetyl-CoA and oxaloacetate. The tricarboxylate transporter allows citrate to travel from the mitochondria to the extramitochondrial cytosol. Acetyl-CoA and oxaloacetate are then catalyzed by ATP-citrate lyase. Well-fed states increase ATP-citrate lyase activity. It is also the only enzyme used in both fatty acid synthesis and cholesterol synthesis.

Carboxylation of acetyl-CoA to malonyl-CoA by **acetyl-CoA carboxylase** (a multienzyme protein) takes place in two reactions (see Figure 3-87):

- Carboxylation of biotin using ATP.
- Transfer of the carboxyl to acetyl-CoA, forming malonyl-CoA.

The fatty acid synthase complex starts with acetyl-CoA joining **acetyl transacylase** and malonyl-CoA joining **malonyl transacylase** thus triggering the cycle (see Figure 3-93).

Acyl-CoA activates the newly formed palmitate so that it can be used by other processes, including:

- Chain elongation
- Desaturation
- Cholesteryl ester
- Acylglycerols

Fatty acid elongase uses malonyl-CoA and NADPH to attach two carbons to unsaturated fatty acyl-CoAs at carbon 10.

Fatty Acid Oxidation

Carnitine palmitoyltransferase-I converts long-chain acyl-CoA to acylcarnitine. This allows entry into the β-oxidation system of enzymes.

The chain is broken at the bond between the α and β carbons, and is appropriately titled β-oxidation (see Figure 3-88). The product (two-carbon units) is acetyl-CoA; palmitoyl-CoA therefore forms eight acetyl-CoA molecules. Fatty acids with an odd number of carbon atoms produce acetyl-CoA, until propionyl-CoA (3-carbon), which can be converted into succinyl-CoA.

The $FADH_2$ and NADH formed from β-oxidation is transported and used in the electron transport chain for the generation of ATP. The β-oxidation of one palmitate produces 106 molecules of ATP.

KEY FACT

Acetyl-CoA carboxylase requires: NADPH, ATP, Mn^{2+}, biotin, and carbonate.

KEY FACT

One gene encodes all of the enzymes in the fatty acid synthase complex.

KEY FACT

Stearyl-CoA is used in the brain during myelination for sphingolipids.

KEY FACT

Acyl-CoA synthetases are found:
- In ER
- In peroxisomes
- On the outer membrane of mitochondria

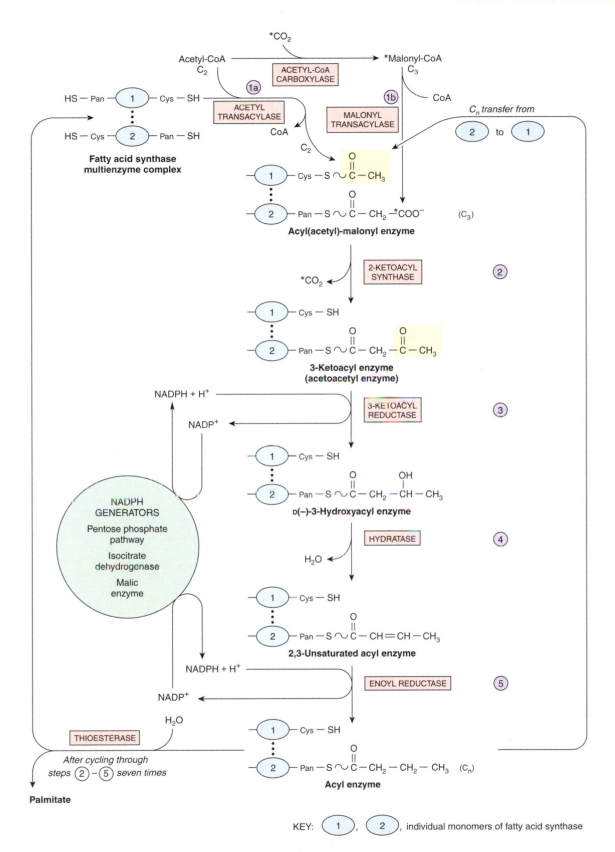

FIGURE 3-87. **Biosynthesis of long-chain fatty acids.** Details of how addition of a malonyl residue causes the acyl chain to grow by two carbon atoms. (Cys, cysteine residue; Pan, 4′-phosphopantetheine.) The blocks shown in dark color contain initially a C_2 unit derived from acetyl-CoA (as illustrated) and subsequently the C_n unit formed in reaction 5. (Modified, with permission, from Murray RK, Granner DK, Rodwell VW. *Harper's Illustrated Biochemistry*, 27th ed. New York: McGraw-Hill, 2006: 198.)

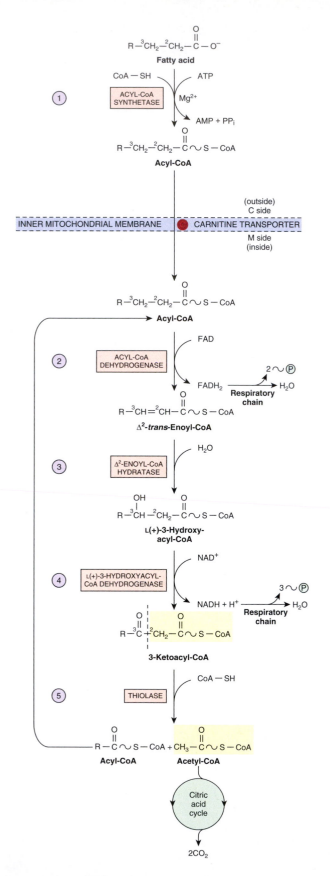

FIGURE 3-88. **Fatty acid oxidation.** β-Oxidation of fatty acids. Long-chain acyl-CoA is cycled through reactions 2–5, acetyl-CoA being split off, each cycle, by thiolase (reaction 5). When the acyl radical is only four carbon atoms in length, two acetyl-CoA molecules are formed in reaction 5. (Modified, with permission, from Murray RK, Granner DK, Rodwell VW. *Harper's Illustrated Biochemistry*, 27th ed. New York: McGraw-Hill, 2006: 189.)

KETONES

Structure and Classification

In a **prolonged fasting state** (including overnight fast) in which liver glucose stores are depleted, the body relies on two chief sources of energy to maintain blood glucose levels:

- Endogenous protein
- Triglycerides

These two fuels are broken down into their building blocks at their site of origin and are then released into the circulation for use by other organs. Thus, muscle (the chief protein repository) contributes free amino acids, whereas adipose tissue (triglyceride storage) supplies free fatty acids (FFA) and glycerol.

The liver utilizes glucogenic amino acids and glycerol for gluconeogenesis; however, the amount of glucose produced by the fasting body is not sufficient for the energy needs of the brain. FFA are a rich source of energy, but they bind to albumin and thus cannot cross the blood-brain barrier to feed the CNS. The body is unable to convert FFA into glucose (the brain's favorite food). Therefore, **the liver must convert fatty acids (and ketogenic amino acids) into ketone bodies, which can be utilized by the brain** (see Figure 3-89).

The two ketone bodies made by the liver are **acetoacetate** and **β-hydroxybutyrate.** The term "ketone body" ("ketone" for short) used here is historical. In fact, only acetoacetate contains ketone functional groups. However, both are organic **acids,** and their presence in blood is associated with lowering of blood pH.

Anabolism

Low insulin/glucagon ratio stimulates the ketogenic pathway:

- All the material for ketone body synthesis comes from acetyl-CoA, the breakdown product of most fatty acids and ketogenic amino acids (see Figure 3-90).
- Two molecules of acetyl-CoA unite with the help of β-ketothiolase, forming acetoacetyl-CoA.

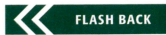

FLASH BACK

The last step of β-oxidation of odd-chain fatty acids produces a molecule of propionyl-CoA, which can contribute to gluconeogenesis. Thus, odd-chain fatty acids represent an exception to the rule that fatty acids cannot be converted to glucose.

KEY FACT

Ketone bodies are best thought of as "acid bodies."

FLASH FORWARD

Statins block HMG-CoA reductase, the committed step in cholesterol synthesis.

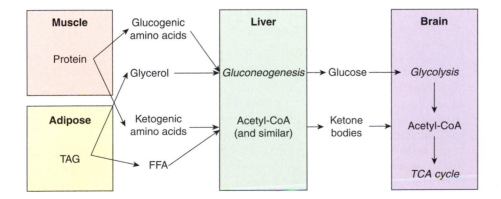

FIGURE 3-89. **Brain energy supply in the prolonged fasting state.**

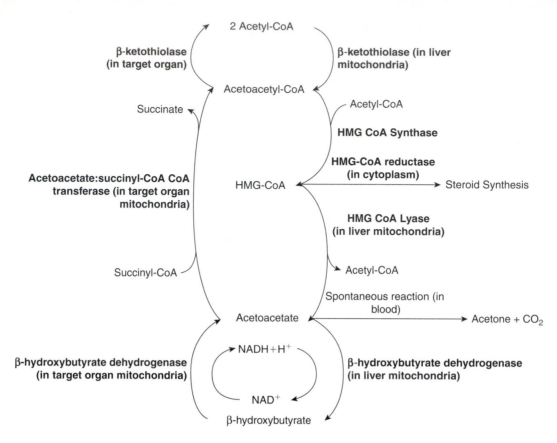

FIGURE 3-90. Ketone body synthesis.

- There is no hydrolase to split this molecule into acetoacetate and CoA, so a two-step detour must be taken:
  1. A synthase enzyme combines acetoacetate-CoA with another molecule of acetyl-CoA, forming β-hydroxy-β-methylglutaryl-CoA (HMG-CoA), and a subsequent cleavage by HMG-CoA lysase yields the ketone body acetoacetate.
  2. Reduction with NADH-dependent β-hydroxybutyrate dehydrogenase provides the second ketone body, β-hydroxybutyrate.

Notice that HMG-CoA is also a precursor for **sterol synthesis**. The difference is that all ketone body synthesis takes place in liver mitochondria, whereas sterols are produced in the cytosol. Formation of β-hydroxybutyrate requires NADH. Hence, the ratio of [β-hydroxybutyrate] / [acetoacetate] in the blood reflects the ratio of [NADH] / [NAD$^+$] in the mitochondria.

- Blood tests are the most reliable gauge of ketone levels because urine tests (using nitroprusside strips) only detect acetoacetate. Routine tests do not typically screen for β-hydroxybutyrate.
- Alcohol consumption leads to NADH accumulation, which drives the conversion of acetoacetate to β-hydroxybutyrate. Hence, ketone levels in alcoholics may be underestimated if nitroprusside strips are used.
- High ketone concentrations often manifest a fruity smelling breath; acetoacetate decomposes into acetone, which has a low vapor pressure and is therefore largely cleared by the lungs.

Catabolism

Although the brain **requires** ketone bodies for survival in low glucose states, virtually all tissues give preference to ketones over other fuels.

- Once β-hydroxybutyrate and acetoacetate reach the mitochondria of the target organ, the former is converted to the latter by β-hydroxybutyrate dehydrogenase (acting in the opposite direction than in the liver, see Figure 3-91).
- Acetoacetate: Succinyl-CoA transferase subsequently attaches coenzyme A to acetoacetate, making it a ready substrate for β-ketothiolase.
- Thus, each ketone body delivers two units of acetyl-CoA to the target organ; β-hydroxybutyrate also provides an NADH. Note that synthesis and subsequent degradation of one acetoacetate molecule results in net energy loss due to cleavage of one succinyl-CoA molecule.

Ketosis

Fasting ketosis refers to an increase in the concentration of ketone bodies when liver glycogen is diminished. An overnight fast or high-intensity exercise is enough to result in ketosis, which becomes more prominent if the subject is on a low-carbohydrate diet and thus has low liver glycogen stores. Ketosis alone is not a pathologic process, and a glass of juice (i.e., sugar) is the fastest remedy.

Alcoholic ketoacidosis presents in chronic alcoholics following episodes of binge drinking. The hypoglycemia resulting from depleted glycogen and lack of gluconeogenesis (blocked by high NADH/NAD$^+$) causes mobilization of fat stores and their conversion to ketones. The resulting acidosis is usually not life-threatening, but may result in further complications.

Diabetic ketoacidosis (DKA) is a life-threatening condition, which may occur in type 1 diabetics with poorly controlled blood glucose. With insufficient insulin available, glucagon and other stress hormones rise, despite high blood glucose concentration. As seen in Figure 3-91, the liver produces exceptional amounts of ketone bodies, thus causing a high anion gap metabolic acidosis. The resulting potassium shift from cells into blood causes **hyperkalemia**.

High blood glucose levels raise the blood osmolarity. Hyperosmolar diuresis can ensue, resulting in dehydration and loss of electrolytes, including potassium (see Figure 3-92).

Symptoms of DKA are those of untreated diabetes (polydipsia, polyuria, nocturia) and dehydration (dry, warm skin, sunken eyes). Patients often present with increased respiratory rate and tidal volumes (**Kussmaul** respirations). As with all metabolic acidoses, a high respiratory rate is the primary respiratory compensation.

Typical causes of DKA include not taking insulin (common in teenagers with DM), infection, and other physiologic stressors that raise cortisol and consequently blood sugar in type 1 diabetics. Treatment includes:

- Isotonic IV saline
- Insulin
- K$^+$ replacement (high blood [K$^+$], but low total body K$^+$)

DKA is rare in type 2 diabetics. The best (though not universally accepted) explanation is that some insulin is always present in type 2 DM, and thus glucagon levels never rise to the point of permitting accumulation of ketones.

CLINICAL CORRELATION

Diabetes mellitus type 1 is an autoimmune disease in which β-cells in the pancreas are attacked. There is virtually no insulin produced.

In type 2 DM, the pancreas often produces more insulin than is normal, but peripheral tissues are relatively resistant to insulin action.

KEY FACT

In DKA, potassium shift causes apparent hyperkalemia, but the hyperosmolar diuresis results in actual total body potassium depletion.

MNEMONIC

The common causes of high anion gap metabolic acidosis are **I** am **SLUMPED**:

Isopropyl alcohol
Salicylates
Lactate
Uremia
Methanol
Paraldehyde (paint sniffing)
Ethylene glycol (anti-freeze)
Diabetic ketoacidosis

KEY FACT

Intravenous fluids are the first-line treatment for many acute disorders and should be administered even before starting an "actual medication." However, be careful in anyone with a history of L sided heart failure.

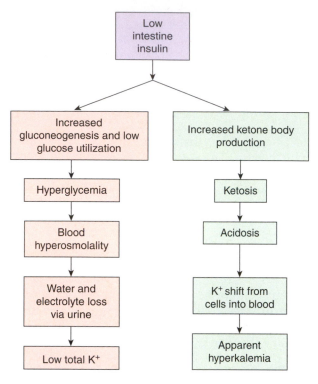

FIGURE 3-91.   Development and consequences of DKA.

LIPOPROTEINS

Function and Structure

Because fat is hydrophobic and does not dissolve in blood, lipids require carrier molecules to enter the circulation.

- **Albumin** can carry fat in the form of free fatty acids from adipose tissue. Fatty acids are "free" in that they are not covalently attached to glycerol, but they are noncovalently bound to albumin in blood; albumin is not considered a lipoprotein.
- Dietary fat from the intestine and fat from the liver associates with specialized amphiphilic (detergent-like) proteins, called **apolipoproteins**. Together with various lipids (cholesterol, cholesterol esters [CE], triglycerides [TG], and phospholipids [PL]), the apolipoproteins form **lipoproteins**.
- Lipoproteins are spherical. Like a cell, their shell is formed by PL, cholesterol, and protein, whereas the core is composed of the more hydrophobic lipids.

Most lipoproteins are named according to their density. From low- to high-density:

- **Chylomicrons < VLDL < IDL < LDL < HDL**

In general, higher density implies more protein, more cholesterol, more CE content, less TG, and smaller particle size. HDL is an exception in that its cholesterol content is only moderately high (see Table 3-24).

TABLE 3-24. Lipoproteins

LIPOPROTEIN	SCHEMA	DENSITY (G/ML)	DIAMETER (NM)	% CHOLESTEROL AND CE/% TG
Chylomicron	B-48	< 0.95	> 100	8/83
VLDL	B-100	1.00	60	22/50
IDL	B-100	1.01	30	29/31
LDL	B-100	1.04	20	45/9
HDL	A1 A1	1.14	10	30/8

IDL = intermediate-density lipoproteins; HDL = high-density lipoproteins; LDL = low-density lipoproteins; VLDL = very-low-density lipoproteins.

CHYLOMICRONS AND REMNANTS

- The dietary lipids (mostly TG, some cholesterol) in the cytoplasm of enterocytes enters the ER, where they co-assemble with a freshly translated, large apolipoprotein, called **ApoB-48,** and a smaller protein **ApoA-1.** The resulting lipoprotein is called **chylomicron.** "Chylo-," because these particles enter the lymphatic (chyle) vessels and the thoracic duct before actually reaching blood (see Figure 3-92A and B).
- When a chylomicron meets an HDL particle, they exchange ApoA-1 for **ApoC-2** (Figure 3-92C).
- ApoC-2 is a cofactor for lipoprotein lipase (**LPL**), so that when chylomicrons reach **muscle** and **adipose tissue,** LPL cleaves the TG content. The resulting fatty acids are taken up by muscle or adipose cells then either stored or β-oxidized. Note that LPL is on the apical membranes of the blood vessel **endothelium** (not on or in the adipose/muscle cells), so this enzyme digests the chylomicrons already in the blood (see Figure 3-92D).
- As TG, but not PL leave the lipoprotein, a relative buildup of PL results in large amount of surface shell and a small core. To avoid rupture of an

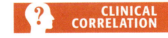

CLINICAL CORRELATION

Familial hypercholesterolemia results from dysfunctional LDL receptors. LDL cannot be removed, cholesterol levels spike, and patients suffer from premature atherosclerosis.

Chylomicron flow	Schema of main event	Description
Intestine	Apolipoproteins + Dietary lipids → Chylo [B-48] [A-1]	Chylomicrons are synthesized in enterocyte ER.
Lymph		
Blood	Chylo [B-48] / C-2 / A-1 / HDL	Chylomicrons exchange ApoA-1 for ApoC-2 with HDL.
Blood vessels in target organ	PLTP → PL ← HDL / Chylo [B-48] / CE → CETP / TG / LPL / C-2 / FFA + 2-acylglycerol / TG Adipocyte / Vessel Lumen	LPL, activated by ApoC-2, cleaves TG. The products are re-esterified in the target cell, e.g. an adipocyte. Meanwhile, PLTP and CETP mediate lipid exchange between HDL and the chylomicron.
Blood	Chylo [B-48] / C-2 / E / HDL	Depleted chylomicrons exchange ApoC-2 for ApoE and become "remnants."
Liver	CR [B-48] E / LDLR / E / LRP / Hepatocyte	Liver endocytoses chylomicron remnants (CR) in an ApoE-dependent and/or ApoB-dependent fashion.

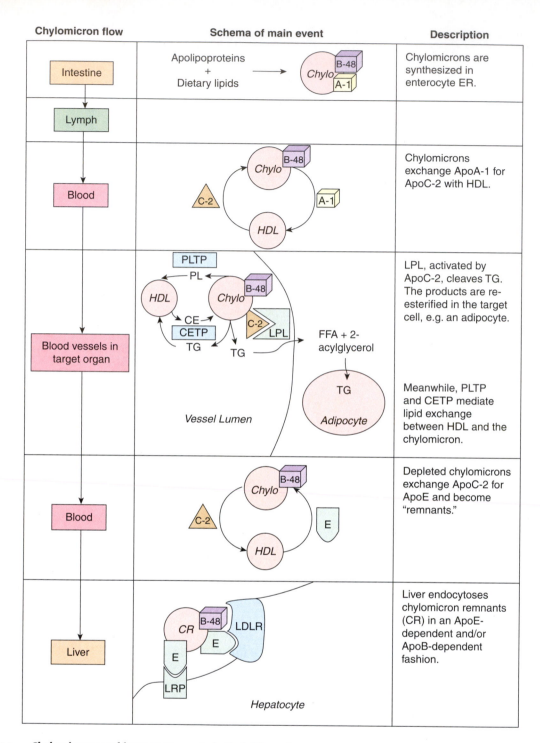

FIGURE 3-92. **Chylomicrons and important events in their life cycle.**

enzyme, phospholipid transfer protein (**PLTP**) moves PL from chylomicrons to HDL.

■ In addition, blood contains cholesterol ester transfer protein (**CETP**), which moves TG from chylomicrons to HDL, and CE in the opposite direction.

■ Once most TGs have been lost to LPL digestion, the chylomicron returns ApoC2 to an HDL particle, so that no further cleavage takes place. In exchange, HDL provides yet another apolipoprotein, called **ApoE**. The resulting shrunken, TG-depleted, CE-enriched, ApoE-labeled lipoprotein is known as the **chylomicron remnant** (Figure 3-92E).

- The remnants are ready to leave the circulation by entering the liver (Figure 3-93F). Hepatocytes have two receptors for chylomicrons. **The LDL receptor** requires both ApoE and ApoB-48 (or B-100) to bind. The **LRP** receptor is specific for ApoE-labeled chylomicrons. So even when LDL receptors are not functional, as in familial hypercholestrolemia, chylomicron remnants do not accumulate, because of sufficient LRP activity.

VLDL, IDL, AND LDL

Like the intestine, the liver packages all of its would-be secreted lipids into lipoproteins, called very-low-density lipoproteins (**VLDL**). VLDL is the hepatocyte's analog to the enterocyte's chylomicrons, with a few differences:

- The main VLDL apolipoprotein is the larger ApoB-100 (not ApoB-48).
- Although VLDL still contains more TG than cholesterol, it has a higher cholesterol content than do chylomicrons.
- The lipids packaged into VLDL are synthesized in the liver. This contrasts with the lipids in chylomicrons, which are from the diet.
- The VLDL remnants are called intermediate-density lipoproteins (**IDL**).
- Although IDL can be taken up by the liver, it often loses some of its ApoE, and shrinks even further, resulting in **LDL.**
- Liver's LDL receptors can still recognize LDL. However, LDL also tends to cross the endothelium into various tissues. In capillaries, this is not a problem, but in large arteries, LDL can get trapped and oxidized in the vessel intima. Oxidation of LDL renders it recognizable by macrophages as a pathogen (scavenger receptors), resulting in endocytosis and formation of foam cells. Thus begins **atherosclerosis.**

HDL

High-density lipoproteins (HDL) differ from the other lipoproteins in the following:

- HDL contains no large apolipoprotein (such as ApoB-48 or B-100). ApoA-1 is the most characteristic protein.
- HDL is not synthesized in the ER (exact site of synthesis unknown, probably at least part of its synthesis is in the plasma).

HDL, commonly referred to as the "good cholesterol," has multiple functions (see Figure 3-93):

- **Cholesterol collection:** Cells secrete cholesterol using a pump called **ABC1.** HDL then collects this peripheral cholesterol, using the plasma enzyme lecithin: cholesterol acyl transferase (**LCAT**).
- **LPL activation:** HDL supplies ApoC-2 to chylomicrons and VLDL in exchange for ApoA-1. Hence, the TGs in these large lipoproteins can be digested by LPL.
- **Lipoprotein size control:** Takes up excess phospholipids from other lipoproteins via phospholipid transfer protein.
- **Refills lipoproteins with CE:** HDL supplies CE to other lipoproteins in exchange for TG via CETP.
- **Provides the "exit" signal:** HDL supplies ApoE to depleted chylomicrons and VLDL in exchange for ApoC-2. Hence, the remnant lipoproteins (chylomicron remnants and IDL) can leave circulation.

Because liver endocytoses and degrades a portion of HDL particles, there is a net flow of cholesterol from peripheral tissues into the liver. This is referred to as the **"reverse cholesterol transport."** Notice that the enzyme CETP "short-circuits" this transport, by feeding the HDL cholesterol back into the tissue-

FLASH BACK

The primary DNA transcript (pre-mRNA) typically undergoes some modifications before exiting the nucleus as a finalized mRNA. The two main types of such **post-transcriptional processing** are **alternative splicing** (variable intron excision) and **nucleotide editing.** An example of the latter is seen with the intestinal ApoB pre-mRNA, which undergoes deamination at C6666 (resulting in U6666). This introduces a stop codon into the mRNA sequence so that only 48% of the full sequence gets translated—hence the name ApoB-48. No such editing occurs in the liver, which produces the full-length ApoB-100.

KEY FACT

HDL is the **"good cholesterol."** It collects peripheral cholesterol, including that of atherosclerotic plaque, and brings it back to the liver.

CLINICAL CORRELATION

In **Tangier disease,** there is no functional cholesterol pump (**ABC1**). HDL levels are therefore low, but cholesterol accumulates in the intracellular milieu.

CLINICAL CORRELATION

High LDL is correlated with increased CHD risk, whereas high HDL is correlated with a lower risk.

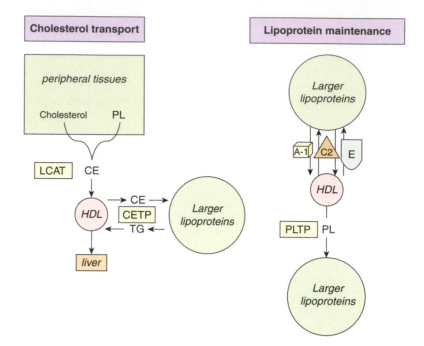

FIGURE 3-93. High-density lipoproteins (HDL). The functions of HDL can be split into two main categories: cholesterol transport and maintenance of other lipoproteins.

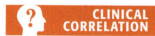
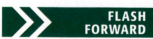
targeted lipoproteins. Consequently, drugs inhibiting CETP can be expected to lower peripheral cholesterol and are currently in clinical trials.

LIPASES

Lingual and gastric lipases only partially digest dietary TG. Their primary purpose is to emulsify the lipids for further digestion.

Pancreatic lipase, present in the small intestine, cleaves TG at positions 1 and 3, giving rise to FFA and 2-monoacylglycerol. These products then enter the enterocyte and re-esterify into a TG that can be exported in a chylomicron.

Lipoprotein lipase (LPL) mediates the same reaction as pancreatic lipase. However:

- LPL is present on vascular endothelium of adipose and muscle.
- It requires ApoC-2 as a cofactor.
- LPL activity decreases when insulin levels rise.
- The TG substrate comes from VLDL and chylomicrons.

Once again, the products of LPL digestion (FFA and 2-acylglycerol, which then become FFA and glycerol) enter the target cells. The myocytes use the FFA to fuel their β-oxidation, whereas adipocytes re-esterify them back to TG for storage. A minor point is that in this re-esterification the adipocyte uses its endogenously synthesized glycerol phosphate from adipocyte carbohydrate metabolism. The glycerol from the LPL cleavage actually travels back to the liver.

Hormone-sensitive lipase is an intracellular enzyme, mainly present in adipocytes.

- It is induced in response to stress hormones such as glucagon, adrenocorticotropic hormone (ACTH), epinephrine, and norepinephrine.

- These hormones raise intracellular cAMP concentrations, and hence PKA activity.
- PKA phosphorylates hormone-sensitive lipase, thus activating the cleavage of stored TG into FFA and glycerol. These then enter the bloodstream and, mostly attached to albumin, travel back to the liver.
- Insulin inhibits this activation by favoring dephosphorylation of the enzyme.

Hepatic TG lipase degrades TG from IDL and chylomicron remnants previously endocytosed by the liver.

Note that LPL and hormone-sensitive lipase both respond to insulin, though in opposite ways. However, their roles in diabetes are still being elucidated (see Tables 3-25 and 3-26).

Dyslipidemias

A standard lipid profile measures LDLc (LDL cholesterol), HDLc (HDL cholesterol), total cholesterol, and TG in blood. Any significant difference from normal values constitutes a **dyslipidemia**.

- High LDLc and low HDLc are well-established risk factors for atherosclerosis and coronary artery disease. High TG is probably less important.
- Very high LDLc may also cause cholesterol to be deposited in skin or tendons (xanthomas), eyelids (xanthelasma), and cornea (arcus senilis).

TABLE 3-25. Key Proteins Involved in Lipoprotein Turnover

PROTEIN	LOCATION	FUNCTION
ApoB-48	Chylomicrons	Structural, chylomicron transport from small intestine → lymph → blood to bind LDLR.
ApoB-100	VLDL, IDL, LDL	Structural, transports liver apoliprotein (VLDL) → peripheral LDLR.
ApoA-1	HDL	Cholesterol collection and activation of LCAT.
ApoC-2	VLDL, chylomicrons	Lipoprotein lipase cofactor, release FA/glycerol from chylomicrons, VLDL, LDL.
ApoE	IDL, chylomicron remnants	Binds to LDLR, helps lipoproteins exit blood into liver.
PLTP	Blood	Moves phospholipids from large lipoproteins to HDL.
CETP	Blood	Exchanges CE for TG between HDL and large lipoproteins.
LCAT	Blood	Allows HDL to collect cholesterol.
ABC1	Cellular membrane	Secretion of cholesterol by tissues.

CE = cholesterol esters; HDL = high-density lipoproteins; IDL = intermediate-density lipoproteins; LCAT = lecithin cholesterol acyl transferase; LDL = low-density lipoproteins; LDLR = low-density lipoprotein receptor; TG = triglycerides; VLDL = very-low-density lipoproteins.

TABLE 3-26. Important Lipases

Lingual, gastric lipases	Saliva, stomach	Fat emulsification.
Pancreatic lipase	Pancreatic juice	Fat absorption by intestine.
Lipoprotein lipase	Endothelium	Fat absorption by muscle and adipose.
Hormone-sensitive lipase	Adipocyte cytoplasm	Release of fat during fast.
Hepatic TG lipase	Hepatocyte cytoplasm	Remnant TG IDL digestion.

IDL = intermediate-density lipoproteins; TG = triglycerides.

In most dyslipidemias, LDLc, HDLc, and TG are altered simultaneously. Isolated changes in one lipid are less common and are usually indicative of familial dyslipidemias.

Primary causes of elevated blood lipids:

- Polygenic hypercholesterolemia (i.e., family history)
- Familial dyslipidemias (often present with isolated lipid elevations)
- Gender (male > female) and age (increase with age)

Secondary causes of elevated blood lipids:

- Saturated fat, *trans* fat, cholesterol, and carbohydrates in diet
- Lack of exercise (low HDLc)
- High body mass index (BMI)
- Metabolic syndrome and diabetes (low HDLc, high TG, LDLc usually normal)
- AIDS (high TG owing to HIV infection *and* to treatment)
- Smoking (low HDLc)
- Hypothyroidism (due to reduced LDL receptors)
- Nephrotic syndrome
- Anorexia nervosa and stress

Causes of decreased lipid levels are:

- Infections, malignancies, hematologic disorders
- Liver disease
- Hyperthyroidism
- Genetic disorders (Tangier's disease and abetalipoproteinemia)

Selected pathologic states are discussed below.

Diabetes (types 1 and 2) can cause hyperglycemia, which in turn causes:

- Increased VLDL synthesis, and impaired VLDL and chylomicron removal. Thus, TG accumulates in the plasma.
- Decreased turnover of lipoproteins causes HDLc levels to decrease.
- LDLc usually stays normal.
- First treat diabetes. If that fails to correct lipids, start lipid-lowering drugs.

See Table 3-27 for a summary of familial hyperlipidemias.

FLASH FORWARD

Smoking may cause a decrease in HDLc, which is a risk factor for coronary artery disease. However, smoking also causes damage to vessel walls, which is an **independent risk factor** for coronary artery disease.

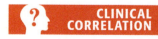

CLINICAL CORRELATION

Xanthomas are accumulations of lipid-laden macrophages in tissues. Erruptive xanthoma = high TG Tendinous xanthoma = high cholesterol Palmar xanthoma = dysbetalipoproteinemia

TABLE 3-27. **Characteristics of Familial Dyslipidemias**

FAMILIAL DYSLIPIDEMIA	LIPOPROTEINS ELEVATED	LIPIDS ELEVATED	PATHOPHYSIOLOGY	MAIN COMPLICATION
Type I: Hyperchylomicronemia	Chylomicrons	Cholesterol:+ TG:+++	ApoC-2 or LPL deficiency	Pancreatitis, no atherosclerosis
Type IIa: Hypercholesterolemia	LDL	Cholesterol:+++ TG: no change	LDL receptor deficiency	Atherosclerosis
Type IIb: Combined hyperlipidemia	VLDL, IDL	Cholesterol:+++ TG:+++	VLDL overproduction	Atherosclerosis
Type III: Dysbetalipoproteinemia	IDL, chylomicron remnants	Cholesterol:++ TG:++	ApoE deficiency	Atherosclerosis
Type IV: Hypertriglyceridemia	VLDL	Cholesterol: + TG:+++	VLDL overproduction	Atherosclerosis
Type V: Mixed hypertriglyceridemia	VLDL, chylomicrons	Cholesterol:+ TG:+++	VLDL overproduction	Pancreatitis, no atherosclerosis

FA = fatty acids; IDL = intermediate-density lipoproteins; LDL = low-density lipoproteins; LPL = lipoprotein lipase; TG = triglycerides; VLDL = very-low-density lipoproteins.

Familial hyperchylomicronemia (type I) is a rare disease.

- Lack of LPL or its cofactor, ApoC-2, prevents the breakdown of chylomicrons, and their TG content in particular. Hence, TG accumulates in blood.
- Since no treatment is available, patients must avoid fatty food for life.
- Acute pancreatitis and eruptive xanthomas are major complications, whereas atherosclerosis is usually **not** a problem.

Familial hypercholesterolemia (type IIa) is an autosomal dominant disease.

- Usually results from a defective LDL receptor (or ApoB-100). The cholesterol-laden LDL particles cannot be reclaimed by the liver (unlike chylomicron remnants, which are still recognized by the LRP receptor).
- Not only does LDL accumulate in the blood, but liver cholesterol synthesis is deprived of negative feedback, which further contributes to high cholesterol levels.
- **Homozygous** patients have extreme levels of blood LDL cholesterol (LDLc > 600 mg/dL) and suffer from severe premature atherosclerosis and coronary artery disease, which tends to be the cause of death before age 30 (without treatment).
- **Heterozygotes** have a slightly better prognosis, with LDLc of 200–400 mg/dL.
- Tendon xanthomas, particularly on Achilles tendon, are fairly pathognomonic.
- Treatment consists of:
  - Healthy diet
  - Cholesterol-lowering drugs (statins, niacin, cholestyramine but not fibrates)
  - LDL apheresis (a weekly plasmapheresis, used in homozygous patients)
  - Portocaval anastomosis (mechanism unknown)
  - Liver transplantation (the ultimate measure)

KEY FACT

LDL receptor mutations are either **null** (complete absence of the gene product) or affect receptor **trafficking** (either to or from the membrane). The actual affinity for LDL tends not to be affected.

FLASH FORWARD

There are five main classes of lipid-lowering drugs:
Resins and **ezetimibe:** Lower cholesterol
Fibrates: Lower TG
Niacin and **statins** (especially atorvastatin): Lower cholesterol *and* TG

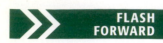

FLASH FORWARD

Think of **niacin** as the opposite of hyperlipidemia type IIb. This drug lowers TG and cholesterol by **inhibiting VLDL secretion.**

Familial combined hyperlipidemia (type IIb) is a fairly common autosomal dominant disease.

- Liver overproduces VLDL. Consequently, VLDL, LDL, or both accumulate in blood.
- As a result, TG, cholesterol, or both can be elevated.
- As with type Ia, patients can get atherosclerosis and coronary artery disease.
- Likewise, the treatment consists of diet, exercise, and lipid-lowering drugs, which may include fibrates to lower TG (unlike with type IIa, for which their application is of little usefulness).

Dysbetalipoproteinemia (type III) is an autosomal recessive disease.

- It is also known as **remnant removal disease** because lipoproteins lack functional ApoE and cannot "exit" the bloodstream.
- This is not sufficient to cause any pathology, but a concomitant condition (e.g., obesity) can cause dysbetalipoproteinemia to manifest itself.
- Both blood TG and cholesterol become high, since chylomicron remnants and VLDL remnants (i.e., IDL) accumulate.
- Patients present with palmar xanthomas (fairly pathognomonic) and atherosclerosis.
- Exercise, diet modification, and lipid-lowering drugs reduce the risk of atherosclerosis.

Familial hypertriglyceridemia (type IV) is a common autosomal dominant disorder.

- As in type IIb, there is an elevation in VLDL production, but TG accumulates in preference to cholesterol.
- There is some association with insulin resistance.
- Risk for IHD and atherosclerosis can be reduced with TG-lowering drugs, diet change, and exercise.

Familial mixed hypertriglyceridemia (type V) is an uncommon mixture of types I and IV familial dyslipidemias.

- VLDL and chylomicrons are elevated, probably as a result of overproduction. TG levels are high, whereas cholesterol concentration increases only moderately.
- Like type I, but unlike type IV, there is no major risk of atherosclerosis, so that pancreatitis and eruptive xanthomas remain the main complications.

Tangier disease is a rare autosomal recessive disorder.

- It is found in communities in Virginia.
- Tangier's disease is due to lack of ABC1 cholesterol transporter gene.
- Cholesterol accumulates inside cells.
- Blood HDL and cholesterol are low.
- The disease is characterized by atherosclerosis (compare with other dyslipidemias), hepatosplenomegaly, polyneuropathy (compare with metabolic storage diseases), and pathognomonic **orange tonsils**.
- No specific treatment. Enlarged organs are sometimes excised.

Abetalipoproteinemia is a rare autosomal recessive disease.

- Cells are unable to make functional ApoB-48 and ApoB-100, resulting in a deficiency of most lipoproteins.
- Lipids and lipid-soluble vitamins (especially **A** and **E**) are poorly absorbed **(steatorrhea).**

- CNS disease—vitamin deficiency causes progressive neurologic and optic degeneration.
- Hemolytic anemia—lipid imbalance causes RBC membranes to pucker (**acanthosis**).
- No treatment other than vigorous vitamin supplementation.

SPECIAL LIPIDS

Cholesterol

The highly lipophilic core of cholesterol contains several carbon rings and very few polar hydroxyl substituents; hence, it is poorly soluble in water. Cholesterol is found in:

- Plasma in the core of VLDL and LDL. It is mostly esterified to a fatty acid.
- In all plasma membranes, conferring rigidity (lipid rafts).
- In bile, where it is solubilized by phospholipids and bile salts.

Although all cells can synthesize cholesterol, some cells are able to further process it to:

- **Steroids** (adrenal cortex, ovary/testes, placenta)
- **Vitamin D** (skin, then liver and kidney)
- **Bile acids** (liver, then intestinal bacteria)

ANABOLISM

Cholesterol synthesis can be characterized by a few major enzymatic conversions (see Figure 3-94):

- Cholesterol synthesis begins with conversion of three molecules of **acetyl-CoA** into **HMG-CoA**. The reactions are the same as in ketone body synthesis except that they occur in the **cytoplasm.**
- **HMG-CoA reductase**, the **rate-limiting** enzyme in cholesterol synthesis, converts HMG-CoA to **mevalonic acid**. This enzyme is anchored to the ER and utilizes two molecules of NADPH per reduction.
- Mevalonic acid then gives rise to either isopentenyl pyrophosphate (IPP) or dimethylallyl pyrophosphate (DPP). IPP and DPP are known as **activated isoprene units.**
- IPP and DPP combine, forming geranyl pyrophosphate (GPP).

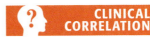

CLINICAL CORRELATION

Statins are HMG-CoA reductase blockers.

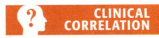

CLINICAL CORRELATION

Terbinafine inhibits the conversion of squalene to lanosterol (step 7) in fungi. It is a useful antifungal, especially for treating onychomycosis.
Imidazole and triazole antifungals (fluconazole, ketoconazole, etc.) inhibit conversion of lanosterol to ergosterol in fungi. They are important P-450 inhibitors.

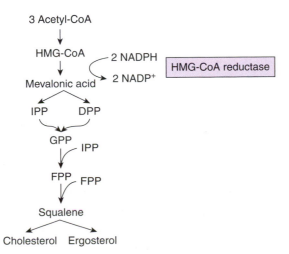

FIGURE 3-94. **Cholesterol synthesis.** DPP, dimethylallyl pyrophosphate; FPP, farnesyl pyrophosphate; GPP, geranyl pyrophosphate; IPP, isopentenyl pyrophosphate.

CLINICAL CORRELATION

The **triple screen** (an assay of blood α-fetoprotein, β-human chorionic gonadotropin, and estriol) detects congenital abnormalities in a second-trimester fetus.

Estriol can also be detected in urine during third-trimester gestation and indicates general well-being of the fetus. A low E3 level can indicate serious congenital diseases, including Down's syndrome.

CLINICAL CORRELATION

Congenital deficiency in any of the "numbered" enzymes in Figure 3-101 leads to serious disease. Missing enzymes 3, 11, 17, or (most commonly) 21 present as the various forms of **congenital adrenal hyperplasia** (CAH).

5α-reductase deficiency in genetic males results in ambiguous genitalia that virilize during puberty.

- GPP and IPP combine, forming farnesyl pyrophosphate (FPP).
- Two FPP molecules combine, forming **squalene**.
- Squalene then cyclizes, forming **lanosterol**.
- Finally, lanosterol is converted (via several steps) into cholesterol.

Plants and fungi convert lanosterol to **ergosterol**, a cholesterol analog.

CHOLESTEROL DERIVATIVES

Most cholesterol in the body actually exists in the form of **CE**. These are usually formed with a fatty acid.

Steroid hormones are derivatives of cholesterol (see Figure 3-95). The main adrenal cortical hormones are **dehydroepiandrosterone** and its sulfate (DHEA and DHEA-S, respectively), **cortisol**, and **aldosterone**. **Androstenedione** and **testosterone** are produced by theca and Leydig cells. In women, granulosa cells along with several extraovarian tissues use aromatase to convert these androgens to **estrogens**. Similarly, in men, Sertoli cells convert testosterone to **dihydrotestosterone** (DHT).

Additional steroid hormones, especially **estriol** (E3) are produced by the placenta, which uses fetal DHEA as its substrate.

Another cholesterol derivative, **7-dehydrocholesterol,** is converted to **cholecalciferol** (vitamin D_3) in skin upon UV light exposure. Subsequent hydroxylations in liver and kidney produce the biologically active 1,25-dihydroxy-cholecalciferol, known as **calcitriol** (see Figure 3-96). Note that irradiation of the plant lipid **ergosterol** produces vitamin D_2, which can undergo the same set of hydroxylations, but displays lower activity than vitamin D_3.

Liver also converts cholesterol into **bile salts** (see Figure 3-97). These detergents are secreted into the intestine (in bile) and render dietary fat more

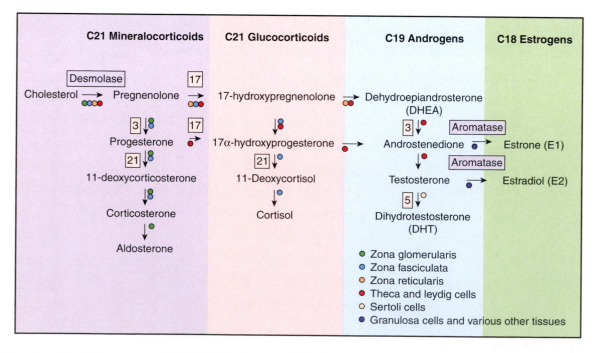

FIGURE 3-95. **Steroid hormone synthesis.** 3, 3β-hydroxysteroid dehydrogenase; 5, α-reductase; 11, 11β-hydroxylase; 17, 17β-hydroxylase; 21, 21β-hydroxylase.

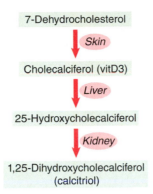

FIGURE 3-96. **Vitamin D metabolism.**

absorbable. Although the intestine reclaims most bile salts (enterohepatic circulation), some are excreted. Therefore, bile excretion is one of the body's ways of reducing cholesterol load.

- **Liver** forms the primary bile salts, **cholate** and **chenodeoxycholate**, in its smooth ER and mitochondria. The primary salts are secreted only after **conjugation** to **taurine** or **glycine**, which improves their solubility.
- After cecal and colonic **bacteria deconjugate** the primary salts, they proceed to modify them into secondary and tertiary bile salts. Cholate becomes **deoxycholate**, whereas chenodeoxycholate turns into **ursodeoxycholate** and the highly insoluble **lithocholate**.
- Most bile salts are reclaimed and **reconjugated** by the liver. In addition, sulfation of lithocholate also occurs in hepatocytes. The resulting **sulfolithocholate** is not reclaimed by the intestine, thus constituting an important "leak" in enterohepatic circulation.

Glycerophospholipids and Sphingolipids

STRUCTURE AND FUNCTION

Glycerophospholipids and sphingolipids can be thought of as substituted glycerol molecules. Fatty acids usually attach to two of the glycerol carbons, leaving the third carbon with a polar group. Therefore, most of these lipids are amphiphilic and consequently ideal constituents of lipid bilayers. See Figure 3-98 for a summary of their structures.

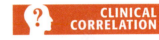

CLINICAL CORRELATION

Ursodeoxycholate (Ursodiol) is used in treatment of radiolucent gallstones. It not only solubilizes cholesterol, but also inhibits its production. However, cholecystectomy is usually the preferred treatment, so ursodiol is reserved mostly for poor surgical candidates.

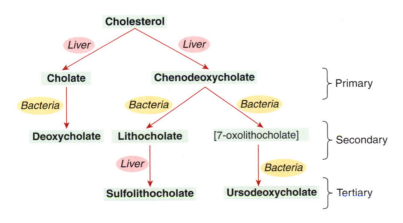

FIGURE 3-97. **Bile salts.**

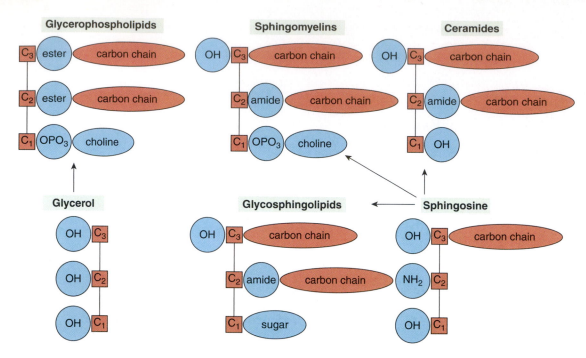

FIGURE 3-98. **Glycerophospholipids, sphingolipids, and their backbone molecules.** Choline is used here as an example of a polar head group component and can be replaced by several others, such as ethanolamine, inositol, and serine. Polar groups are blue and lipophilic groups are brown.

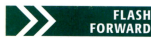

PIP$_2$ is an important membrane phospholipid, cleaved by **PLC** into **IP$_3$** and **DAG.** PLC responds to **G$_q$,** a G-protein subunit activated by: muscarinic, angiotensin, α_1-adrenergic, 5-HT$_{1C}$, 5-HT$_2$, TRH, and vasopressin V$_1$ receptors.

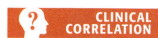

Lecithin and sphingomyelin are key components of **lung surfactant,** and their ratio (L:S) is a predictor of fetal viability. Premature infants born at < 37 weeks of gestation with a L:S < 2.2 have an increased risk for neonatal respiratory distress syndrome.

GLYCEROPHOSPHOLIPIDS

- C2 and C3 carry **esterified fatty acids.**
- C1 carries a **polar head group,** consisting of a phosphate coupled to a polar molecule such as choline, ethanolamine, serine, or inositol. The resulting phospholipids are named accordingly: phosphatidylcholine, phosphatidylethanolamine, and so on.
- The synthetic pathways vary depending on the phospholipid. Note that the phosphate group is often derived from cytidine triphosphate (**CTP**) (rather than ATP).

SPHINGOLIPIDS

- C3 carries a **carbon chain** (attached directly, not as an ester).
- The alcohol group on C2 is changed into an **amine.** In some sphingolipids, this amine condenses with a fatty acid, thus becoming an **amide.**
- A glycerol molecule with the above modifications (carbon chain on C3 and C2 alcohol changed to amine) is called **sphingosine.**
- C1 carries a polar head group, which varies widely among the different sphingolipids:
  - **Ceramides** use a plain alcohol group as their polar heads.
  - Just like glycerophospholipids, **sphingomyelins** use a phosphate coupled to another polar molecule, including choline, ethanolamine, and others.
  - **Glycosphingolipids** carry a sugar on their C1 and are subdivided into **cerebrosides** and **gangliosides.**

LYSOSOMAL STORAGE DISEASES

These diseases include **sphingolipidoses, mucopolysaccharoses, mucolipidoses,** and the **type II glycogen storage disease** (Pompe's disease). Their "taxonomy" is summarized in Figure 3-99.

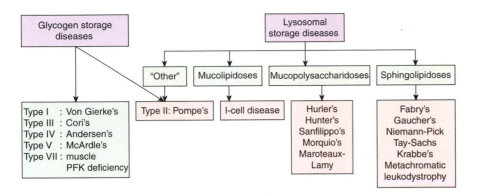

FIGURE 3-99.   The storage diseases. Pompe's disease can be classified as both a glycogen and a lysosomal storage disease.

Note that only the sphingolipidoses result from defects in lipid metabolism. We include other main lysosomal storage diseases in this chapter because of their clinical similarity; however, their etiology is not related to lipid metabolism.

SPHINGOLIPIDOSES

These are rare, autosomal recessive diseases (except Fabry's disease, which is X-linked recessive). They share the following characteristics:

- A missing enzyme leads to the accumulation of its substrates in lysosomes (see Figure 3-100).
- As with many autosomal recessive diseases, the incidence is higher in closed communities (such as Tay-Sachs disease among Ashkenazi Jews).
- Each disease has many subtypes, usually organized by age of onset. Gaucher's and Fabry's diseases often present in adulthood, whereas most other sphingolipidoses are diagnosed in early infancy.
- Variable expressivity is often present (especially Gaucher's disease). The early-onset diseases often include neurodegeneration.
- There is usually no effective treatment for the sphingolipidoses, and individuals who have early-onset of disease die early. Bone marrow transplantation can rarely rescue some patients, and enzyme replacement/gene therapy might prove useful.

Table 3-28 summarizes the sphingolipidoses.

FLASH BACK

The two layers of a plasma membrane bilayer have distinct phospholipid composition. The inner layer consists primarily of negatively charged phospholipids (e.g., phosphatidylserine), whereas the outer face contains phospholipids with no net charge (e.g., phosphatidylcholine). In cells undergoing **apoptosis**, this polarization is lost; the negatively charged phospholipids displayed on the exterior of the cell serve as a "kill me" signal for leukocytes.

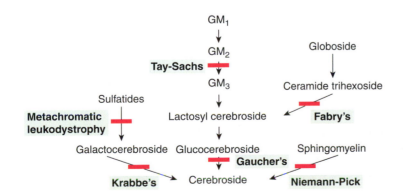

FIGURE 3-100.   Sphingolipidoses. Several sphingolipid catabolic pathways are shown. Steps affected by sphingolipidoses are designated with a red bar.

TABLE 3-28. Sphingolipidoses

DISEASE	DESCRIPTION	DEFICIENT ENZYME, ACCUMULATED SUBSTRATE, AND TREATMENT IF POSSIBLE
Fabry's disease	▪ **Peripheral neuropathy of hands/feet.** ▪ X-linked recessive; heterozygous females display mild phenotype. ▪ Angiokeratomas (small, raised purple spots on skin). ▪ Cardiovascular/renal disease and strokes. ▪ Cataracts. ▪ Usually survive till adulthood––die with kidney and heart failure.	▪ α-Galactosidase A missing. ▪ Ceramide trihexoside accumulates.
Gaucher's disease	▪ **Bone involvement: aseptic necrosis of femur, bone crises.** ▪ Several types, affect different ages. ▪ 1:1000 incidence among Ashkenazi Jews. ▪ Hepatosplenomegaly. ▪ Can present late in adulthood–– expressivity varies. ▪ Anemia, thrombocytopenia. ▪ Mental retardation in some types. ▪ Gaucher's cells (macrophages); "crinkled tissue paper cells" because of their large, foamy cytoplasm.	▪ δ-Glucocerebrosidase missing. ▪ Glucocerebroside accumulates. ▪ β-Glucocerebrosidase IV for treatment.
Niemann-Pick disease	▪ Types A and B; type A patients die by age 2–3; type B patients live longer. ▪ Progressive neurodegeneration, esp. in type A. ▪ Hepatosplenomegaly. ▪ Cherry-red spot (on macula). ▪ Foam macrophages in bone marrow.	▪ Sphingomyelinase missing. ▪ Sphingomyelin accumulates.
Tay-Sachs disease	▪ Multiple types, most common is infantile (death by 3 years). ▪ Ashkenazi Jews at increased risk. ▪ Progressibe neurodegeneration, developmental delay, microcephaly. ▪ Cherry-red spot. ▪ Lysozymes with onion skin.	▪ Hexosaminidase A missing. ▪ GM_2 ganglioside accumulates.
Christensen-Krabbe's disease	▪ Peripheral neuropathy. ▪ Developmental delay. ▪ Optic atrophy. ▪ Decerebrate posture. ▪ Death by 2 years. ▪ Globoid macrophages full of galactocerebroside, stain PAS+. ▪ Reported successful treatment with bone marrow transplantations.	▪ β-Galactosidase missing. ▪ Galactocerebroside and psychosine (which is the main toxin killing oligodendroglia) accumulate.
Metachromatic leukodystrophy	▪ Multiple types, but disease rarely presents before 6 months. ▪ Central and peripheral demyelination with ataxia, dementia.	▪ Arylsulfatase A missing. ▪ Cerebroside sulfate accumulates.

The syndromes associated with these diseases tend to be complex and variable, with no "typical presentation." We include hypothetical presentations only to differentiate between the different sphingolipidoses:

- **Fabry's:** A young man presents with a stroke. History reveals recurring pain in his hands and feet. Physical exam is significant for raised dark-red lesions all over his body and mitral valve prolapse.
- **Gaucher's:** A Jewish girl presents with chronic fatigue due to anemia. History reveals painful bone crises and pathologic fractures. Physical exam shows massively enlarged spleen and liver.
- **Niemann-Pick:** A 3-month-old infant presents with hepatosplenomegaly. Initially hypotonic, the infant later becomes spastic, rigid, and eventually unresponsive. He fails to meet developmental milestones and dies at age 2.
- **Tay-Sachs:** A 6-month-old infant becomes unresponsive and paralyzed and dies at age 3. Autopsy reveals microcephaly.
- **Christensen-Krabbe:** A 3-month-old infant will not feed and is irritable. He gradually becomes hypertonic, suffers from seizures, and assumes decerebrate posture. Eventually, he stops responding to all stimuli and dies.
- **Metachromatic leukodystrophy:** A 6-year-old girl's performance in school is declining. She becomes clumsy and unable to walk. She dies at age 16.

MUCOPOLYSACCHARIDOSES

Table 3-29 summarizes a subset of lysosomal storage diseases, called **mucopolysaccharidoses** (MPS). These result from lysosomal enzyme defects that

TABLE 3-29. **Some Major Mucopolysaccharidoses**

DISEASE	DESCRIPTION	DEFICIENT ENZYME AND ACCUMULATED SUBSTRATE
Hurler's syndrome	- Most common. - Onset age is 1 year, death by age 14. - Starts with developmental delay, and coarse facial features with enlarged forehead (gargoylism). - Corneal clouding, enlarged tongue, airway obstruction.	- Iduronidase missing. - Heparan sulfate and dermatan sulfate accumulate.
Hunter's syndrome	- X-linked recessive. - Like Hunter's, but milder, with longer survival. - No corneal clouding. - Type B has a very mild phenotype.	- Iduronate sulfatase missing. - Heparan sulfate and dermatan sulfate accumulate.
Sanfilippo's syndrome	- Developmental delay, with severe mental retardation. - Onset in preschool children, death in mid-teens. - Relatively little somatic change.	- Heparan-N-sulfatase (or others) missing. - Heparan sulfate accumulates.
Morquio's syndrome	- Diagnosis by age 2. - Skeletal deformities, corneal clouding. - No mental abnormalities. - Death due to atlantoaxial instability (minor trauma can cause injury to spinal cord).	- N-acetyl-alactosamine-6-sulfate sulfatase missing. - Keratan sulfate accumulates.
Maroteaux-Lamy syndrome	- Multisystemic disease, but spares the CNS.	- N-acetylhexosamine-4-sulfatase missing. - Dermatan sulfate accumulates.

lead to accumulation of GAGs, the principal glycopeptide components of ECM in connective tissue.

The four most important GAGs are heparan sulfate, dermatan sulfate, chondroitin sulfate, and keratan sulfate.

- In general, accumulation of GAGs causes **skeletal deformities** (usually leading to coarse facial features), **corneal clouding, cardiovascular disease** (especially valvulopathies), and **excessive hair.**
- Heparan sulfate accumulation is particularly deleterious to the nervous tissue, causing **cognitive defects.**
- Keratan sulfate accumulation damages mostly corneal and cartilaginous tissues, while sparing the brain.

Note the following:

- Morquio's and Maroteaux-Lamy syndromes are the only MPS listed that spare cognitive function.
- All the listed MPS are autosomal recessive except **Hunter's** syndrome.
- Multiple subtypes exist for each disease.

MUCOLIPIDOSES

I-cell disease is an autosomal recessive disease.

- Caused by defective phosphotransferase. This Golgi enzyme targets newly synthesized enzymes to the lysosome by "labeling" them with mannose-6-phosphate. With a defective targeting system, these enzymes never reach the lysosome, thus preventing the organelle from working properly.
- Similar presentation to Hurler's syndrome.
- Pathology significant for many membrane-bound inclusion bodies in fibroblasts.

OTHER LYSOSOMAL STORAGE DISEASES

Pompe's disease is an autosomal recessive disorder that can also be classified as a type II glycogen storage disease. It has several subtypes (here we discuss the infantile form).

- It is caused by defective lysosomal α-1,4-glucosidase, a glycogen-breakdown enzyme.
- Unlike most other glycogen storage diseases, Pompe's disease does not severely violate the cell's energy economy. This is because the main glycogenolytic pathway (e.g., phosphorylase) is intact to break down most of the glycogen. However, the accumulation of glycogen in the lysosomes causes pathology (the glycogen storage diseases associated with energy economy are most frequently defects in the synthesis or degradation of glycogen granules in liver and muscle cytosol).
- Death occurs by 8 months of age.
- Pompe's disease is characterized by cardiomegaly, hepatomegaly, macroglossia, hypotonia, and other systemic findings.
- As in most systemic diseases, several blood lab values tend to be abnormal. However, glucose, lipids, and ketones tend to be normal (in contrast to other glycogen storage diseases).

KEY FACT

Sanfilippo's disease is associated with severe mental retardation but little somatic symptoms. Morquio's and Maroteaux-Lamy syndromes are the opposite.

Eicosanoids

Eicosanoids are derivatives of polyunsaturated long-chain fatty acids, most notably **arachidonic acid.** Whereas steroid hormones play the role of systemic, long-term messengers, eicosanoids are involved in **local (autocrine or paracrine) signaling.**

They include:

- Prostaglandins
- Thromboxanes
- Leukotrienes

Arachidonic acid resides in membranes as part of phospholipids, and is released by the action of **phospholipase A$_2$ (PLA$_2$).**

Arachidonic acid is then modified by several different pathways:

- **Cyclooxygenase (COX)** 1 and 2 lead to the production of prostaglandin G$_2$ (PGG$_2$) and subsequently PGH$_2$, from which most other prostaglandins, prostacyclin (PGI$_2$), and thromboxane A$_2$ (TXA$_2$) are synthesized.
- **Lipoxygenase (LOX)** converts arachidonic acid into 5-hydroperoxyeicosatetraenoic acid (5-HPETE) and is later transformed into leukotrienes.

The main synthetic pathways of the arachidonic acid–derived eicosanoids are summarized in Figure 3-101. Note that not all eicosainoids are derived from arachidonic acid. For example, TXA$_3$, a thromboxane that prevents platelet aggregation, is a derivative of omega-3 fatty acids. For this reason, consuming fish oil (high in omega-3 fatty acids) is thought to reduce one's risk of coronary artery disease.

The important eicosanoids and their functions are summarized in Table 3-30. Synthetic analogs of several prostaglandins are employed in clinical medicine.

FLASH FORWARD

Corticosteroids block PLA$_2$ and interrupt COX synthesis.
NSAIDs, acetaminophen, and coxibs block COX-1, 2, or both.
Zileuton blocks lipoxygenase.
Zafirlukast and montelukast block leukotriene receptors.

CLINICAL CORRELATION

To keep the PDA open in a neonate, use PGE$_2$ (or PGI$_2$). To promote closure of a PDA, use a COX inhibitor, such as indomethacin.

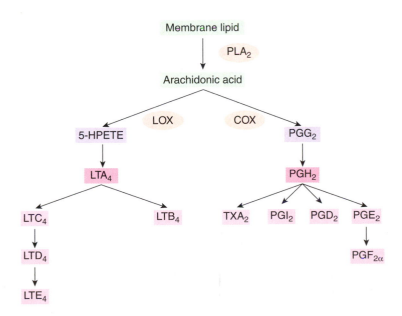

FIGURE 3-101. **Eicosanoid synthesis.**

TABLE 3-30. Eicosanoids and Their Function

EICOSANOID	FUNCTION
LTA_4	Very little (only a transient compound).
LTB_4	Neutrophile chemotactic factor.
LTC_4, LTD_4, LTE_4	Bronchoconstriction, vasoconstriction, smooth muscle contraction, and increased vascular permeability. Known as slow-reacting substance of anaphylaxis (SRS-A).
PGG_2, PGH_2	Very little (only transient compounds).
PGE_1	Smooth muscle relaxant, vasodilator. Keeps patent ductus arteriosus (PDA) open and beneficial in male erectile dysfunction (available as **alprostadil** for these purposes). Inhibits platelet aggregation. **Misoprostol** is a synthetic analog. Used in prevention of NSAID-induced peptic ulcers and (in combination with mifepristone) as an abortificant.
PGE_2	■ Similar to PGE_1. ■ Uterine contraction (**dinoprostone** can be used clinically to induce labor or abortion), bronchodilation. ■ Keeps PDA patent.
PGF_2	Like PGE_2 it causes uterine contractions and is used to induce labor or abortion. Increases outflow of aqueous humor (**latanoprost** is an analog available for treatment of open-angle glaucoma). Bronchoconstrictor.
PGI_2 (prostacycline)	Synthesized by vascular endothelium. Vasodilator and inhibitor of platelet aggregation. Bronchodilator and uterine relaxant. Keeps PDA open.
TXA_2	Synthesized by platelets. Opposite to prostacyclin (platelet aggregator, vasoconstrictor, bronchoconstrictor).

LT = leukotriene; PG = prostaglandin; TX = thromboxane.

HEME

Structure

Many proteins use **heme** as their prosthetic group (a tightly bound cofactor that is not peptide). Heme consists of a large, planar aromatic ring, called **protoporphyrin IX** and a **ferrous ion** (i.e., Fe in its +2 state).

Heme Proteins

Heme plays a vital role in O_2-binding proteins, such as **hemoglobin** and **myoglobin**. These proteins hold the heme in place using proximal histidine, which binds directly to the ferrous iron. O_2 binds to the ferrous ion opposite to proximal histidine, but is stabilized by another, "distal histidine" (see Figure 3-102).

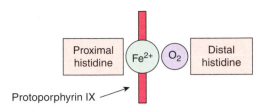

FIGURE 3-102.   Heme in hemoglobin (or myoglobin). In this figure, the flat aromatic ring of protoporphyrin IX ring is seen from the side.

Although best known as part of myoglobin and hemoglobin, heme's function is not limited to **O$_2$ storage/transport.** Heme resides in several enzymes, such as **peroxidase.** It also functions in mitochondrial electron transport as part of **cytochrome c** and in some detoxification reactions as part of the **cytochrome P-450** system.

Heme Synthesis

- Given the preceding list of heme-containing proteins, it is not surprising that most heme synthesis occurs in **erythroid** and **liver** cells.
- The building blocks of heme are **succinyl-CoA, glycine,** and ferrous ion (**Fe^{2+}**).
- Knowing that succinyl-CoA is a product of citric acid cycle, it is easy to remember that heme synthesis begins in the mitochondrion. Although the final reactions are also mitochondrial, some steps occur in the cytosol.
- Heme synthesis begins in the mitochondria → cytosol → mitochondria again.

The reactions occur as follows:

- **Succinyl-CoA** and **glycine** combine, forming δ-aminolevulinic acid (**ALA**). This is catalyzed by **PLP**-requiring (vitamin B6) **ALA synthase** and constitutes the first committed and rate-limiting step.
- ALA leaves the mitochondrion and is converted to **porphobilinogen** (**PBG**) by the cytosolic, zinc-containing **PBG synthase.**
- Four BPG molecules then condense, forming **uroporphyrinogen III,** catalyzed by uroporphyrinogen III cosynthase, along with porphobilinogen deaminase. The latter enzyme is also known as uroporphyrinogen I synthetase.
- This product is decarboxylated, yielding **coproporphyrinogen III,** which then returns to the mitochondrion.
- Here the action of coproporphyrinogen oxidase results in **protopophyrinogen IX.**
- Another oxidase yields protoporphyrin IX.
- Finally, addition of Fe^{2+} due to **ferrochelatase** yields heme.

Since ALA synthase catalyzes the first committed step, it is also the main site of regulation of heme synthesis in the liver. This enzyme is feedback-inhibited by:

- its own product (**ALA**).
- the final pathway product (**heme**).
- oxidized heme (**hematin,** which is heme carrying Fe^{3+} rather than Fe^{2+}).

In erythroid cells, this regulation is absent, so that all primordial RBCs produce heme without inhibition.

Porphyrias and Lead Poisoning

Porphyrias are diseases resulting from defects in heme synthesis.

- Since heme is generally made in the blood and liver, porphyrias tend to affect these two systems (although virtually every organ suffers damage). In children, porphyrias often present as encephalopathy.
- In addition, the various synthetic precursors of heme are large aromatic rings that absorb light; their accumulation in skin thus causes a photosensitivity rash in many porphyrias.
- The inheritable forms of each disease are generally autosomal dominant, except eythropoietic porphyria, which is recessive.
- The intermittent or sporadic nature of some porphyrias may complicate their diagnosis. In general, symptoms of porphyrias are triggered by events that increase heme synthesis and thus increase accumulation of heme synthetic precursors.
- Although not a true porphyria, we include lead poisoning, because it has major effects on heme synthesis.

ACUTE INTERMITTENT PORPHYRIA (AIP)

This congenital disease results from an **autosomal dominant** deficiency of **porphobilinogen deaminase** (also known as **uroporphyrinogen I synthetase**). The precursors that accumulate are ALA and PBG.

- Patients are often normal until adulthood, at which point they may begin experiencing attacks. Attacks usually subside after patients reach age 40. Most patients never experience symptoms.
- Patients are usually asymptomatic between attacks, which are precipitated by multiple factors, including **fasting** and ingestion of certain **drugs** (often inducers of the P-450 system).
- An attack may last several days and often consists of the following symptom triad:
    - **GI problems** (abdominal colic, nausea, constipation).
    - **Peripheral motor neuropathy** (can mimic Guillain-Barré).
    - **CNS symptoms** (psychosis, depression, seizures).
- Unlike most other porphyrias, there is **no skin rash.**
- Diagnosis is made by detection of increased **PBG in urine** (Watson-Schwartz test).
- Although the enzyme defect is not amenable, treatment of symptomatic attacks involves **carbohydrates** (in diet or as IV glucose) or **hematin** (to inhibit ALA synthase).
- If the disease is misdiagnosed, the various drugs that may have been used to address specific symptoms (e.g., barbiturates for psychosis) can severely exacerbate AIP.

PORPHYRIA CUTANEA TARDA (PCT)

This disease results from dysfunctional **uroporphyrinogen decarboxylase** and consequent uroporhyrinogen accumulation. It is the most common porphyria in the United States.

- Symptoms of PCT can be present in affected families and may manifest after exposure to some **substances** (estrogen, excess iron, and P-450 inducers such as alcohol), **dietary restriction,** and **contraction of viruses** (HepC, HIV) or hepatocellular **carcinoma.** The **most common cause is hepatitis C.**
- Symptoms usually appear in adulthood.
- Sun-exposed areas show **photosensitivity rash and blisters,** which leave pigmented scars upon healing.

- Although proper diagnosis is made by detecting elevated porphyrin levels in urine, tea-colored urine that turns **pink upon Woods' lamp illumination** is suggestive of PCT. PBG levels are normal.
- Treatment for PCT must address underlying or triggering condition (e.g., phlebotomy if patient has excess iron, chloroquine).

HEREDITARY COPROPORPHYRIA

This **autosomal dominant** defect in **coproporphyrinogen oxidase** can be thought of as AIP with the rash of PCT.

- In addition to ALA and PBG (as in AIP), there is accumulation of **coproporphyrin**.
- As in AIP, patients experience bouts of gastrointestinal, CNS, and peripheral neurological symptoms, which are usually triggered by medications.
- As in PCT, patients with hereditary coproporphyria develop a photosensitivity rash and blisters.
- Diagnosis is usually made by demonstrating elevated porphyrins in the stool (better than urine).
- Treatment similar to AIP.

ERYTHROPOIETIC PORPHYRIA

This rare and highly variable **autosomal recessive** disease results from defective **uroporphyrinogen III cosynthase**. It is also known as Gunther's disease.

- **Photosensitivity rash** (as in PCT) is present and can be very severe.
- In addition, **hemolytic anemia** and **port-wine urine** can be present.
- Diagnosis is made by detection of corresponding porphyrin pattern in urine (Watson-Schwartz test). CBC may reveal hemolytic anemia.
- The only successful prevention consists of total avoidance of sun exposure. Blood transfusions and possibly bone marrow transplantation constitute more extreme treatment measures.

LEAD POISONING

Lead poisoning occurs both in children (**GI exposure** via chewing on objects with lead-based paint or working in a battery factory) and adults (plumbers **inhale** lead dust). Although best known as heme synthesis inhibitor, lead poisons physiologic processes and can affect virtually every organ.

- Lead is chemically similar to calcium and zinc. This has two main consequences:
    - Lead is better absorbed when the above metals are lacking in the diet. For this reason, it is especially important for children's diet to be replete in calcium and zinc.
    - Lead inhibits zinc-dependent enzymes and deposits in bone (relpaces calcium), and may affect brain physiology (again, replacing calcium, which is important for neurotransmitter release).
- Lead **inhibits ferrochelatase** in the heme pathway so that protoporphyrin IX accumulates.
- Lead inhibits PBG synthase (because it relies on zinc), resulting in the accumulation of ALA. ALA chemically resembles γ-aminobutyric acid (GABA), which may explain the psychosis manifested in acute lead poisoning.
- Chronically, lead accumulates in kidneys, causing interstitial nephritis and eventually renal failure.

MNEMONIC

Porphyria cutanea **tarda** (PCT) is "**tardy**" compared with acute intermittent porphyria (AIP). (The enzyme defective in AIP precedes the enzyme defective in PCT in the synthetic pathway.)

FLASH FORWARD

When RNA precipitates in RBCs, it appears as blue dots in the cytosol (on a stained blood smear). Although this **basophilic stippling** can be seen in several other anemias (e.g., the thalassemias), it remains very specific to lead poisoning.

? CLINICAL CORRELATION

Dimercaprol requires intramuscular injection, which is often painful. Succimer is a water-soluble form of dimercaprol that can be given by mouth. This makes it the preferred drug, particularly when treating children (unless lead poisoning is very severe).

FLASH BACK

Most chelating drugs are not selective for the metal they chelate. In addition to toxins other than lead (e.g., mercury, arsenic), they may also remove useful physiologic ions (e.g., zinc), resulting in deficiency.

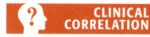

? CLINICAL CORRELATION

Causes of sideroblastic anemias include alcohol abuse, lead poisoning, myelodysplastic syndrome, and others. In all cases, the developing RBC is unable to insert iron into hemoglobin. Free iron accumulates in mitochondria, causing them to stain as blue dots around the nucleus. Remember that these **ringed sideroblasts** are seen only on bone marrow smears, in contrast to **basophilic stippling,** which appears on a regular peripheral blood smears and represents ribosomal RNA.

Clinically, lead poisoning can be subdivided into three categories:

1. In utero exposure even at very low concentrations has primarily neurologic consequences. It is an independent risk factor for spontaneous abortion.
2. Days or weeks after acute lead exposure, patients may develop the symptomatic triad of **abdominal colic, CNS symptoms (with cerebral edema),** and **sideroblastic anemia.** CNS symptoms can range from nonspecific cognitive problems and headache to frank **encephalopathy** with seizures.
3. **Chronic lead poisoning** can present with the same symptoms, but is less clear-cut. In addition, patients can also present with **renal insufficiency, gout,** and (in children) **growth retardation.** Peripheral motor neuropathy may be present with characteristic **wrist drop.** Heart disease and **hypertension** can also occur.

Diagnosis of lead poisoning is established directly by measuring elevated lead levels in blood. Bone X-ray fluorescence can demonstrate chronic lead exposure (X-ray shows "lead lines" on epiphyseal bones).

Blood tests show **sideroblastic anemia** (microcytic, hypochromic RBCs), and **basophilic stippling** of RBCs. Erythrocyte protoporphyrin IX is increased.

Severe symptoms (e.g., encephalopathy) should be treated with **EDTA calcium disodium, dimercaprol,** and **succimer.** Mild symptoms and prophylaxis may only require succimer.

Heme Catabolism

PATHWAY (see Figure 3-103)

- When RBCs age, they are collected by the spleen, where their heme is released and degraded to **biliverdin** and subsequently **indirect bilirubin,** a linearized molecule devoid of iron.
- Indirect bilirubin is poorly water-soluble, but it attaches to albumin and is transported liver, where it is conjugated to glucuronic acid molecules. The resulting **direct bilirubin** is water soluble.
- Conjugated bilirubin then enters the intestine via bile.

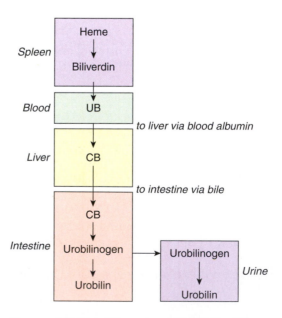

FIGURE 3-103. **Heme catabolism.** CB, conjugated bilirubin; UB, unconjugated bilirubin.

- Colonic bacteria deconjugate bilirubin and convert it to urobilinogen, which subsequently turns into **urobilin.** Urobilin contributes to the characteristic color of stool.
- Small portion of urobilinogen is reabsorbed, enters the blood, and is filtered into urine. The resulting urobilin also lends its color to urine.
- Note that in jaundice, it is bilirubin (not urobilin), that causes yellow skin discoloration.

CAUSES OF ELEVATED BILIRUBIN

Elevated **indirect (unconjugated) bilirubin** is caused by defects of heme catabolism prior to and including conjugation:

- Overabundance of heme: mainly due to hemolytic anemia.
- Defects in bilirubin conjugation in the liver (Gilbert's syndrome, Crigler-Najjar syndrome, and neonatal hyperbilirubinemia).

Direct (conjugated) bilirubin elevation results from dysfunctional steps down the excretion pathway:

- Defects of bilirubin secretion from the liver (Dubin-Johnson and Rotor syndromes).
- Obstruction of the biliary pathway (variety of hepatic and biliary disorders, including hepatitis, cirrhosis, or choledocholithiasis).

Hemoglobin

STRUCTURE

Hemoglobin is the chief O_2-binding protein in RBCs. In adults, it exists as a **tetramer,** mostly consisting of two α and two β subunits ($\alpha_2\beta_2$). Each subunit contains one heme molecule, each of which may bind one O_2 atom.

With no O_2 bound, the tetramer remains in a taut (T) conformation, notable for its low O_2 affinity. Once an O_2 molecule binds to one of the subunits, the entire tetramer twists into a relaxed (R) conformation, which is more willing to accommodate second, third, and fourth O_2 molecules. In other words, the more O_2 is around, the more likely the transition from T to R, and the higher the O_2 affinity of hemoglobin.

- This is an example of **cooperative binding,** in which affinity of a protein increases as more ligand is bound.
- Cooperative binding is a subtype of **allostery,** a more general concept, in which binding of one molecule to a protein somehow affects the binding of another molecule (may or may not be identical with the former).

Cooperative binding results in a sigmoidal hemoglobin binding curve (see Figure 3-104). At low partial pressures of O_2 (Po_2), such as in peripheral tissues, the affinity of hemoglobin for O_2 is low. This allows hemoglobin to release its cargo O_2 to supply tissues. Conversely, at high Po_2 (as in the lungs), O_2 binding is enhanced.

Compare this with **myoglobin,** the O_2-binding protein in muscles. The amino acid sequence of myoglobin is similar to that of a hemoglobin subunit, except it does not form tetramers. As a result, the monomeric protein does not show allosteric binding, and its binding curve is therefore hyperbolic.

CLINICAL CORRELATION

Carbon monoxide (CO) is released as heme is converted to biliverdin; this is the only biological reaction that produces CO, which is therefore a highly specific marker for the amount of heme catabolism.

KEY FACT

Indirect bilirubin = unconjugated bilirubin (water-insoluble).
Direct bilirubin = conjugated bilirubin (water-soluble).

FLASH FORWARD

Approximately 95% of the bile acids secreted into bile undergo **enterohepatic circulation.** They are reabsorbed from the intestine and re-enter the liver. Bile pigments are recirculated less efficiently and may be resecreted into urine.

CLINICAL CORRELATION

Cholelithiasis (gallstones) is the most common cause of **cholecystitis,** inflammation of gallbladder along with obstruction of cystic duct. Since the common bile duct remains patent, cholecystitis does not usually cause jaundice. However, once the calculus moves from the cystic duct into the common bile duct (i.e., **choledocholithiasis**), bile regurgitates into liver. This elevates direct bilirubin in the blood and causes jaundice.

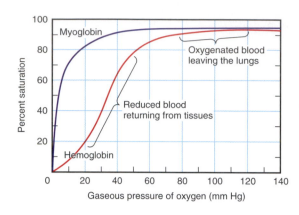

FIGURE 3-104. **Hemoglobin binding curve.** Myoglobin curve is included for comparison. (Modified, with permission, from Scriver CR, et al. *The Molecular and Metabolic Basis of Inherited Disease*, 7th ed. New York: McGraw-Hill, 1995.)

FLASH FORWARD

One of the major complications in thalassemias is iron overload. Hence, pharmacologic treatment includes iron chelation with **desferroxamine.** Sickle cell disease patients can be managed with **hydroxyurea,** which moderately augments HbF levels.

CLINICAL CORRELATION

Since hemoglobin becomes glycated in proportion to blood glucose concentration and HbA_{1c} has a long half-life, its levels reflect how well blood sugars have been managed for the previous **6–8 weeks.** In the treatment of diabetes mellitus, the goal is to keep $HbA_{1c} < 7\%$.

HEMOGLOBIN ISOTYPES

Two gene clusters encode hemoglobin subunits: A and B (see Figure 3-105). Ideally, two chains from cluster A and two chains from cluster B form the hemoglobin tetramer. For example, the major adult hemoglobin isotype (called HbA_1) comes in the form $\alpha_2\beta_2$, where α chains come from cluster A and β chains come from cluster B.

Tables 3-31 and 3-32 describe some normal and pathologic hemoglobin isotypes, respectively.

ALLOSTERIC EFFECTORS

Several molecules may bind to hemoglobin (at a site distinct from O_2), either increasing or decreasing the stability of the R conformation. This results in changes in the net affinity of hemoglobin for O_2, visualized as horizontal shifts in the sigmoidal binding curve. Molecules that stabilize the R conformation increase O_2 affinity and therefore cause a **left shift.** As a result, the partial pressure at which 50% hemoglobin capacity is saturated (P_{50}) **decreases.** Conversely, stabilization of the T conformation results in lower affinity, **right shift** of the binding curve, and **higher P_{50}** (see Figure 3-106).

Allosteric effectors producing a **left shift** in the O_2-binding curve include:

- Low partial pressure of CO_2 (Pco_2)
- Low temperature
- Alkaline environment (low H^+ concentration, high pH)

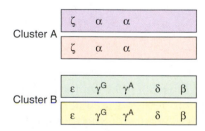

FIGURE 3-105. **Hemoglobin genes.** Clusters are shown in duplicates to emphasize the availability of two copies of each gene in a diploid cell. Only the most relevant genes are included.

TABLE 3-31. Normal Hemoglobin (Hb) Isotypes

COMPOSITION	NAME	COMMENTS
$\alpha_2\beta_2$	HbA$_1$	Comprises vast majority of adult hemoglobin.
$\alpha_2\delta_2$	HbA$_2$	Minor component of adult hemoglobin. Unknown function. Becomes more important in β-chain deficiencies (e.g., β-thalassemia).
$\alpha_2\gamma_2$	HbF	The major hemoglobin in the fetus. Low in adult, unless pathology present. Low affinity for 2,3-BPG. In effect, HbF has a lower P_{50} than adult HbA$_1$, i.e., higher affinity for O_2. This allows O_2 to travel from maternal blood (umbilical veins) to fetal blood.
$\zeta_2\varepsilon_2$	Hb Gower-1	Embryonic hemoglobin.
$\zeta_2\gamma_2$	Hb Portland	Embryonic hemoglobin.

TABLE 3-32. Blood Dyscrasias and Abnormal Hemoglobin Isotypes

	DISEASE	GENOTYPE	HEMOGLOBIN EXPRESSED
α-Thalassemia	Hydrops fetalis	All four α genes deleted.	HbH (δ_4) and Hb Barts (γ_4). Death in utero.
	HbH disease	Three α genes deleted.	HbH and Hb Barts, some HbA$_2$. Death by age 8.
	Thalassemia trait	Two α genes deleted.	HbA$_2$ and Hb Barts early in life. Mild phenotype.
	Carrier	One α gene deleted.	Normal HbA$_1$ content. Silent phenotype.
β-Thalassemia	Thalassemia major	Both β genes affected by a severe mutation (so that no or little β produced).	HbF and HbA$_2$ are the main isotypes available. HbA$_1$ reduced or absent.
	Thalassemia intermedia	Both β genes affected by a mild mutation.	As in thalassemia major, but more HbA$_1$.
	Thalassemia trait	Only one β gene affected by a mutation (mild or severe).	Normal HbA$_1$, but increased HbA$_2$.
Sickle cell anemia		Both β genes have a mutation at position 6 (glutamate $\rightarrow$ valine).	HbSS present, no HbA$_1$. HbF increased.
Sickle cell anemia carrier		One β gene with the above mutation.	HBSS present along with HbA$_1$.
Diabetes		Normal hemoglobin genes.	Normal hemoglobin pattern in addition to HbA$_{1c}$, a glycated form of HbA$_1$.

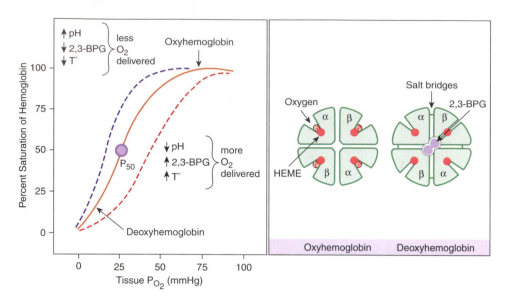

FIGURE 3-106. **Hemoglobin allostery.** (Modified, with permission, from Kasper DL, Braunwald E, Fauci FS, et al. *Harrison's Internal Medicine*, 16th ed. New York: McGraw-Hill, 2005: 593.)

2,3-BPG (made via a biochemical shunt in an RBC's glycolytic pathway) stabilizes the T conformation of adult hemoglobin. It has dual physiologic function:

- It becomes abundant in the face of O_2 shortage (e.g., in patients with chronic obstructive pulmonary disease, but also in normal subjects living at high altitude). This leads to more effective O_2 release in peripheral tissues.
- It affects fetal hemoglobin (HbF) less than maternal HbA_1. Hence, HbF has effectively higher O_2 affinity, thus aiding fetal blood oxygenation.

An infant fed formula made with nitrate-contaminated water is particularly prone to developing methemoglobinemia (known as the **blue baby syndrome**). The abundant gastrointestinal flora in a newborn can convert the nitrate contaminant into nitrite, a very potent oxidant.

- Low 2,3-bisphosphoglycerate (2,3-BPG)
- Carbon monoxide poisoning
- Fetal hemoglobin (HbF; note that HbF is a hemoglobin variant, not an allosteric effector, its binding curve is left-shifted compared with the adult variant)

Allosteric effectors producing a **right shift** in the O_2-binding curve include:

- High P_{CO_2}
- High temperature
- Acidic environment (high [H^+], low pH)
- High 2,3-BPG

METHEMOGLOBINEMIA

In methemoglobinemia, an unusually high percentage of hemoglobin contains iron in the ferric (Fe^{3+}) rather than ferrous (Fe^{2+}) state, thus preventing O_2 from binding. Normally, the methemoglobin reductase system is responsible for restoration of the ferrous state.

- In the uncommon, congenital forms of methemoglobinemia, methemoglobin reductase is faulty or there is a defect in hemoglobin itself that makes the reductase less effective.
- More commonly, methemoglobinemia is **acquired** by exposure to strong oxidants that overwhelm the reductase system. Such oxidants include **nitrates, nitrates** (typically from fertilizer-contaminated water, wells, and so on), **aniline** dyes, **naphthalene** (in mothballs), **local anesthetics** (lidocaine), **vasodilators** (nitric oxide, nitroprusside), **antimalarials** (chloroquine, primaquine), **sulfonamides, dapsone,** and others.
- Laboratory tests usually show normal Pao_2, but decreased Sao_2. Direct tests for methemoglobin detection are available.
- Cyanosis is usually the chief sign. Blood is dark and "chocolate-colored" and does not turn bright red on exposure to O_2.
- Treatment consists of removal of the offending toxin by using **methylene blue,** and sometimes **ascorbic acid.**
- Because methylene blue utilizes G6PD, it is ineffective (and may even cause hemolysis) in patients with concurrent G6PD deficiency.

Carbon Monoxide Poisoning

Carbon monoxide is a colorless, odorless gas. Intoxication occurs either directly by inhalation of fumes from incompletely combusted fuel (car exhaust, heaters) or by inhalation of certain organic solvents (methylene chloride, a paint-stripper), which are metabolized to CO in the liver.

- CO binds to heme in hemoglobin with much higher affinity than does O_2. As a result:
  - CO diminishes the O_2 carrying capacity of hemoglobin by competing for the binding sites.
  - CO shifts the O_2-binding curve of hemoglobin to the left. In other words, binding of a CO molecule to one hemoglobin subunit increases the affinity of the other three subunits for O_2. Although this results in better O_2 uptake in the lungs, it also prevents O_2 unloading in the tissues.
- Symptoms of CO poisoning are usually very **nonspecific**. Cherry-red discoloration of skin is specific but not sensitive (pale skin is more common).
- As with methemoglobinemia, arterial blood gas tests show normal Pao_2 but diminished hemoglobin saturation. Direct CO detection tests are available. Note that smokers often present with values indicative of mild CO poisoning as a result of the CO in inhaled cigarette smoke.
- Treatment consists of 100% O_2 supplementation. Patients with severe cases may require hyperbaric O_2.

Carbon Dioxide

Although hemoglobin is primarily known for its O_2 carrying capacity, it is also an important transporter for CO_2. There are two main mechanisms by which this occurs (see Figure 3-107):

- **Isohydric transport** accounts for 80% of CO_2 movement. As CO_2 diffuses into an RBC, the enzyme **carbonic anhydrase** combines it with water, yielding carbonic acid (H_2CO_3). As the word "acid" implies, H_2CO_3 tends to lose a proton, leaving behind the bicarbonate ion (HCO_3^-). The proton can bind to several **histidine** residues on hemoglobin, while bicarbonate leaves the RBC in exchange for chloride ion (the chloride shift). Note that in isohydric transport the CO_2 is not directly carried by hemoglobin.

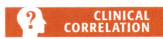

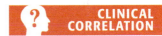
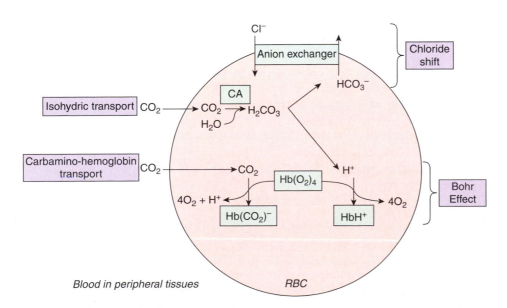

FIGURE 3-107. O_2/CO_2 exchange in peripheral tissues. CA, carbonic anhydrase; Hb, hemoglobin.

- In **carbamino-hemoglobin transport,** which carries up to 20% of CO_2, the CO_2 molecule reacts directly with amino groups on hemoglobin. This reaction produces one free proton.

The reactions involved here are reversible, so the opposite processes take place in the lungs, where CO_2 is unloaded.

Recall that CO_2 and H^+ are allosteric effectors of hemoglobin, both causing an increase in P_{50} and thus lower affinity for and increased release of O_2. In other words, the presence of CO_2 and protons is a signal for the hemoglobin molecule that it has reached the periphery and that its time to release its O_2 cargo. This is called the **Bohr effect.** Conversely, as blood returns to the lungs it faces high Po_2, which prompts the release of protons and CO_2. This is the **Haldane effect.**

Laboratory Tests and Techniques

Hospital laboratories often use basic techniques of molecular biology and biochemistry to analyze clinical samples from patients. Although these tests are often developed and used in basic science research, they aid in diagnosis and help guide clinical decision making.

DNA-BASED LAB TESTS

DNA Gel Electrophoresis

PRINCIPLE

Because DNA carries an **overall negative charge** (due to its phosphate backbone), it migrates toward the positive cathode in an electric field. When loaded into an agarose gel, the internal structure of the gel provides a physical barrier for the movement of DNA. The **rate of movement is directly proportional to the size of the DNA fragment,** making it possible to separate and visualize DNA fragments of different sizes from a clinical sample. Visualization is typically carried out by using a fluorescent dye, ethidium bromide, which intercalates between the DNA bases, making it possible to detect DNA fragments within the gel using UV light.

USE

DNA electrophoresis is a fundamental technique used mainly in conjunction with other techniques to analyze samples. The ability to separate DNA fragments based on their size is critical in polymerase chain reaction (PCR), DNA sequencing, DNA restriction digestion, and Southern blotting, all of which provide important information about the genetic makeup of clinical samples.

DNA Sequencing

PRINCIPLE

A single-stranded DNA fragment from a clinical sample is used as a template in the presence of DNA polymerase, a short primer, four standard deoxynucleotide bases (A, T, G, C), and a small amount of radiolabeled or fluorescently labeled dideoxynucleotide base. Although these bases are otherwise identical to the standard A, T, G, and C nucleotides, they terminate the growth of the DNA chain when they are incorporated into a growing DNA molecule because they lack a second O_2 atom (**dideoxy**nucleotide), thus making it impossible for the chain to accept and chemically react with the base that would follow. During chain synthesis, at a certain point in the growing DNA chain, one of the dideoxynucleotide bases gets incorporated. This causes that particular growing DNA molecule to stop elongating. Statistically, this random incorporation of the dideoxynucleotides produces a sample with DNA fragments of different sizes, corresponding to each of the positions of a particular nucleotide in the DNA chain. Repeating this process for each of the four bases and separating the resulting fragments using DNA gel electrophoresis makes it possible to determine the sequence of bases in the DNA sample fragment because the relative positions of the fragments on the DNA gel reveal the order of the bases in the DNA molecule (see Figure 3-108).

USE

DNA sequencing is used to confirm or exclude known sequence variants (genotyping) or to fully characterize a defined DNA region. It is most commonly used to detect specific mutations in diagnosis of genetic diseases.

CLINICAL EXAMPLES

In patients with a clinical diagnosis of **osteogenesis imperfecta,** a blood sample can be analyzed for mutations in *COL1A1* or *COL1A2* genes. Similarly, DNA of patients with **Ehlers-Danlos syndrome (EDL)** would be analyzed for mutations in *COL3A1*. Genotyping is also used to diagnose **cystic fibrosis, β-thalassemia, muscular dystrophies,** and **sickle cell anemia.**

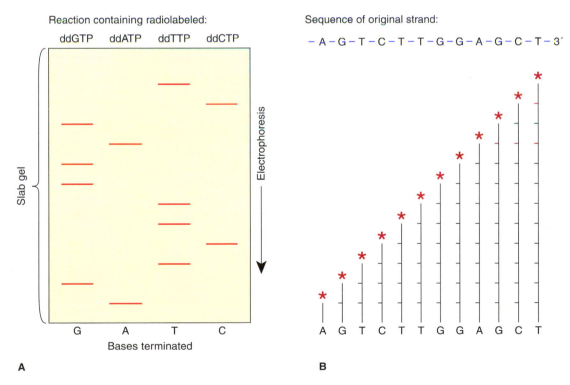

FIGURE 3-108.   DNA sequencing. (A) DNA fragments formed in each of the four reactions containing one of the four nucleotides are run on a DNA gel and separated by size. (B) Radiolabel (asterisk) allows for the visualization of the DNA fragments containing dideoxynucleotides, which makes it possible to deduce the order of individual bases. (Modified, with permission, from Murray RK, Granner DK, Rodwell VW. *Harper's Illustrated Biochemistry*, 27th ed. New York: McGraw-Hill, 2006: 411.)

Polymerase Chain Reaction

PRINCIPLE

Polymerase chain reaction (PCR) is an important method for amplifying DNA, making it possible to increase the amount of DNA available for analysis from a clinical sample. The original double-stranded DNA serves as a template. This reaction also requires a thermally stable DNA polymerase, primers flanking the region that needs to be amplified, and nucleotides. The mixture then undergoes the following procedure in an automated cycle (see Figure 3-109). Of note, the polymerase usually used is Taq polymerase, which was first isolated from *Thermus aquaticus,* a bacterium found in **hot springs.**

- **Denaturing:** Heating to approximately 95°C separates the double-stranded DNA.
- **Annealing:** Cooling to approximately 45°C causes the primers to attach to single strands of DNA in complementary regions.
- **Elongation:** Heating to approximately 72°C causes Taq polymerase to synthesize a complementary DNA strand, starting at the primer.

This cycle is usually repeated approximately 30 times, resulting in an exponential increase in the number of synthesized copies of the original DNA fragment. The DNA is then available for further analysis.

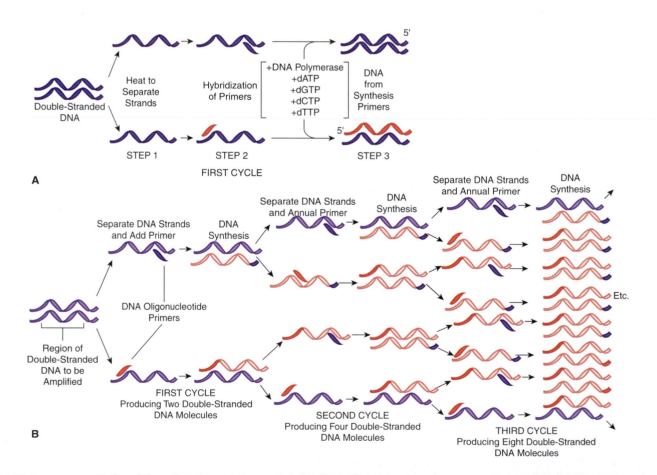

FIGURE 3-109.   Cycles of the polymerase chain reaction. (A) In the first cycle, the primers anneal to the complementary sequences on the DNA in the sample, and the polymerase extends the strands in either the 3′ or the 5′ direction. (B) In each of the subsequent cycles, the newly synthesized strands are separated from the template, the primers re-anneal, and the steps are repeated. The result is an exponential rise in the number of DNA fragments synthesized between the positions of the two original primers. Typically, about 30 cycles are conducted.

USE

PCR is used to genotype-specific mutations, detect hereditary diseases, diagnose viral diseases, genetic fingerprinting, and paternity testing. It is now also used in clinical microbiology to identify pathogenic microorganisms.

CLINICAL EXAMPLES

PCR is used in early detection of hepatitis B virus (**HBV**), HCV, HIV, varicella-zoster virus (**VZV**), herpes simplex virus (**HSV**), cytomegalovirus (**CMV**), Epstein-Barr virus (**EBV**), **parvovirus** B19, and **influenza** viruses—often following initial antibody-based approaches. PCR detects the actual presence of the virus by amplifying viral DNA, even in the absence of the host's antibody response. **Group A streptoccoci,** *Legionella* **spp,** *Bordetella pertussis,* and vancomycin-resistant enterococcus (**VRE**) are examples of bacterial infections often identified using PCR. PCR is most widely used for identification of microbial pathogens, but it is also used for detection of tumor factors, profiling of cytokines, expression of various genes, and as an integral part of many approaches used in human genetic testing.

DNA Restriction Digest

PRINCIPLE

DNA restriction digest refers to a technique in which a **DNA sample is cut into pieces using restriction enzymes** (also known as restriction endonucleases). Each restriction enzyme cleaves double-stranded DNA within a certain base sequence (recognition sequence), and does so consistently (see Figure 3-110). Therefore, a specific DNA sample that is fragmented using a known combination of restriction enzymes always results in a reproducible and unique pattern of DNA fragments. These fragments can then be visualized using DNA gel electrophoresis.

USE

DNA restriction is often used as a part of **restriction fragment length polymorphism (RFLP) analysis.** This method relies on the fact that random mutations sometimes introduce or eliminate a restriction site. It is one of the methods used for DNA fingerprinting, in which different patterns of polymorphisms (variations in a population's DNA) in individuals are used as a basis for identification. More commonly, it is used in **single nucleotide polymorphism (SNP) analysis,** in which changes in single nucleotides within a restriction enzyme recognition sequence are present in certain alleles, and are correlated with genetic diseases. It is important to note that these are not disease-causing mutations; they are normal variations occurring within a population (alleles) that are **correlated** with certain genetic diseases.

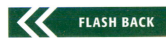

◀◀   FLASH BACK

In DNA gel electrophoresis, the **rate of movement is directly proportional to the size of the DNA fragment,** making it possible to separate and visualize DNA fragments of different sizes from a sample.

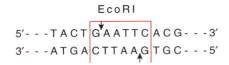

FIGURE 3-110.   Typical endonuclease recognition site. This is an example of a specific sequence recognized by the EcoRI restriction endonuclease. EcoRI always recognizes this specific site and cleaves the DNA chain at the positions marked by the arrows.

Fluorescence In Situ Hybridization (FISH)

PRINCIPLE

In the cytogenetic technique known as fluorescence in situ hybridization (FISH), a **fluorescently labeled DNA probe** is used to determine not just the **presence or absence of a particular DNA sequence in a sample,** but also to **visualize its actual location on the chromosome** (see Figure 3-111).

- Single-stranded DNA that has been tagged with a fluorophore, antibody epitope, or biotin is added to a preparation of nuclear DNA, either in intact nuclei (interphase FISH) or chromosomes arranged on a slide (fiber FISH).
- After binding to the complementary sequence in the sample, the excess unbound probe is washed away.
- The sample is then imaged using fluorescence microscopy.

USE

FISH is used to map specific DNA sequences such as genes or rearrangements to a particular position on a chromosome. It plays a particular role in detect-

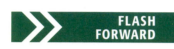

FLASH FORWARD

Cri du chat—partial deletion of the **short arm of chromosome 5** → characteristic **cry similar to the mewing of kittens.** Patients exhibit failure to thrive and severe cognitive and motor delays, but typically are able to communicate socially. Often present are microcephaly and coarsening of facial features.

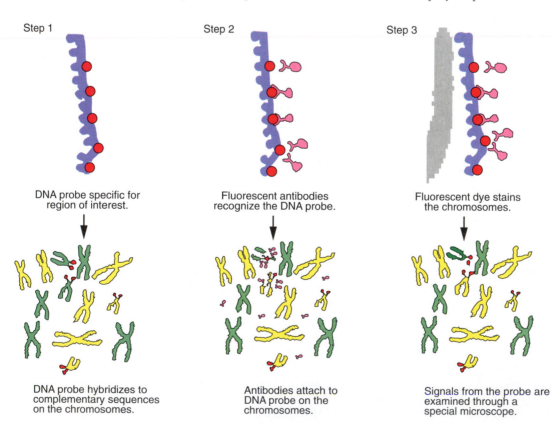

Step 1

DNA probe specific for region of interest.

DNA probe hybridizes to complementary sequences on the chromosomes.

Step 2

Fluorescent antibodies recognize the DNA probe.

Antibodies attach to DNA probe on the chromosomes.

Step 3

Fluorescent dye stains the chromosomes.

Signals from the probe are examined through a special microscope.

FIGURE 3-111. Fluorescence in situ hybridization. Step 1, A DNA probe complementary to the gene of interest is added to the chromosomal preparation. Step 2, A fluorescent antibody against the epitope that was used to tag the DNA probe is added, and it binds to the DNA probe. Step 3, Chromosomes are counterstained with a fluorescent dye of a color different from that of the antibody. This enables clear visualization of the regions of interest under a fluorescent microscope.

ing chromosomal abnormalities such as inversions or translocations. When using labeled primers for the 16S rRNA region of specific bacteria as probes, it can also determine the presence of microorganisms in clinical samples.

CLINICAL EXAMPLES

FISH is often used for detection of **aneuploidies** (e.g., trisomy 21, 18, 13), including **sex chromosome number abnormalities** (e.g., Klinefelter's, Turner's, and triple X syndromes). It can be used on tissue samples, as well as amniotic fluid. It is also used in the diagnosis of certain **cancers,** such as the Philadelphia chromosome (i.e., BCR-ABL t(9,22) translocation) in CML. Furthermore, it can be used for detection of **microdeletions,** such as 5p- in cri du chat, and 15q11.2–q13 in Prader-Willi and Angelman syndromes.

Southern Blotting

PRINCIPLE

Southern blotting refers to a technique whereby a **DNA sample is separated according to fragment size** using gel electrophoresis and is then transferred on to a nitrocellulose or nylon membrane, where it is fixed in place. Much like FISH, a single-stranded DNA probe, usually labeled with a radioactive isotope, is allowed to incubate with the membrane containing the sample. This **radioactive DNA probe binds to complementary sequences** in the DNA sample. After the nonbound probe has been washed away, X-ray film is placed on top of the membrane. The radioactivity from the bound probe exposes the X-ray film in the exact position of the radiolabeled probe. This indicates the presence, and the position of the sequence of interest, within a particular DNA fragment from the original sample (see Figure 3-112).

FLASH FORWARD

Angelman syndrome (AS)—loss of **maternal 15q11** (both copies of paternal origin) → mental retardation, seizures, **inappropriate outbursts of laughter.**

Prader-Willi syndrome (PWS)—loss of **paternal 15q11** (both copies of maternal origin) → mental retardation, obesity, hypotonia, weak cry.

AS and PWS are examples of **genomic imprinting,** in which the expression of a particular allele and the associated phenotype are exclusively determined by which parent contributed it.

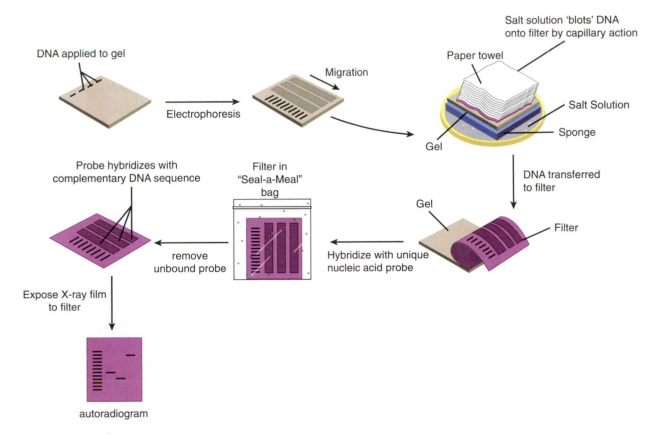

FIGURE 3-112. **Southern blotting.** DNA is separated according to size, transferred on to a nitrocellulose filter, and hybridized with radiolabeled probes specific for the sequence of interest. Exposure of the X-ray film reveals the position and size of the DNA fragments that contain the sequence of interest.

USE

Southern blotting is used in diagnosis of genetic disorders, especially those involving nucleotide expansions. It is also used in detection of viral and bacterial pathogens, as well as for certain forensic applications.

CLINICAL EXAMPLES

Southern blots are often used to detect trinucleotide expansion in **fragile X syndrome, Friedreich's ataxia,** and **myotonic dystrophy,** as well as **methylation or deletion of the SNRPN locus in the Prader-Willi/Angelman syndromes.** Southern blotting has also been used to directly detect malaria parasites (*Plasmodium* spp.) in the blood of patients.

PROTEIN-BASED LAB TESTS

Protein Gel Electrophoresis

PRINCIPLE

Sodium dodecyl sulfate-polyacrylamide gel electrophoresis or SDS-PAGE, as it is almost exclusively known, is a fundamental technique for **separating proteins based on size.** It is the protein counterpart to DNA agarose gel electrophoresis. Proteins are denatured using SDS detergent and then loaded on to a polyacrylamide gel. The buffer used in this technique gives the denatured proteins an **overall negative charge.** Therefore, when placed into an electric field, the proteins move through the gel matrix toward the positive electrode. Because the internal gel structure serves as a barrier for the movement of proteins, their migration toward the positive electrode is directly proportional to the size of the protein, with the **smallest proteins migrating farthest** (closest to the positive electrode). A standard mix of proteins of known sizes (ladder) is also run on the gel for comparison (see Figure 3-113).

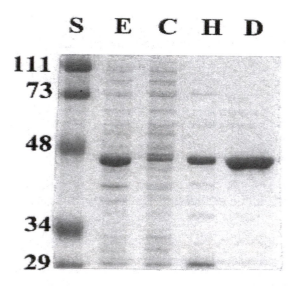

FIGURE 3-113. **Example of an SDS-PAGE (sodium dodecyl sulfate-polyacrylamide gel electrophoresis) gel.** The appearance of an actual protein electrophoresis gel, in which the protein was stained using Coomassie blue dye. Lane S contains protein standards of known molecular weights for comparison (numbers represent the size in kDa). Other lanes contain samples with different amounts of a particular protein (around 45 kDa in size). (Reproduced, with permission, from Murray RK, Granner DK, Rodwell VW. *Harper's Illustrated Biochemistry*, 27th ed. New York: McGraw-Hill, 2006: 25.)

Use

Much like DNA gel electrophoresis, SDS-PAGE is a basic technique used in conjunction with other methods to analyze clinical samples. One of the most common uses is as part of Western blot analysis for detection of pathogens.

Western Blot

Principle

In Western blotting (or protein immunoblotting), a **protein** sample is denatured using the SDS detergent and run on a polyacrylamide gel to separate the proteins present according to their size (see SDS-PAGE in preceding text). The second step involves using an **electrical field perpendicular to the gel to transfer the proteins from the gel on to a nitrocellulose membrane**. To prevent nonspecific antibody binding to the membrane, it is **blocked** by incubating in a solution of bovine serum albumin (BSA) or nonfat dry milk. The membrane is then incubated with a **primary antibody** specific for the protein of interest. After washing off the excess unbound primary antibody, a **secondary antibody** is added. This secondary antibody is conjugated to an enzyme; it is also specific for the primary antibody that was used in the previous step. Subsequent addition of a **substrate** for the enzyme causes a colorimetric reaction in the bands containing the protein of interest (see Figure 3-114).

Use

Western blotting is used to detect the presence of a protein in a clinical sample, indicating an infection with a specific agent. This may refer to both antigens native to the pathogen (e.g., in the case of **bovine spongiform encephalopathy** or **BSE**) or to the actual host antibodies that have developed in response to the infection (e.g., **HIV** and **Lyme disease** [*Borrelia burgdorferi*]). Note that Western blots can also be used for relative quantification of the amount of protein present.

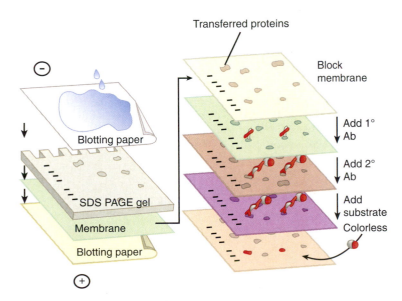

FIGURE 3-114. **Western blotting.** After they are separated by size using SDS-PAGE (sodium dodecyl sulfate-polyacrylamide gel electrophoresis), the proteins are transferred on to a membrane with the aid of an electric field. The membrane is then blocked and incubated with the primary and the secondary antibodies. Using a substrate, a color signal is produced showing the fragments that contain the protein of interest.

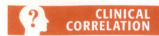

CLINICAL CORRELATION

In HIV testing, when an initial positive result is obtained using ELISA, a Western blot is always done to confirm the results and reduce the number of false-positives.

- **Known HIV viral antigens** are run on an SDS-PAGE gel, transferred to a membrane, and then incubated with the patient's serum.
- The test is considered positive if the patient's serum contains HIV antibodies against at least two of the following antigens: **p24, gp41, gp120/160.**
- It is generally accepted that only the absence of all bands is considered a negative result. If only a single band is present, the test is considered intermediate and needs to be repeated (almost all turn positive).

CLINICAL EXAMPLES

Western blotting is a confirmatory test performed when the results of an ELISA (see below) test are positive for HIV antibodies.

Enzyme-Linked Immunosorbent Assay (ELISA)

PRINCIPLE

ELISA is an immunologic technique widely used for the detection of antigens and antibodies in clinical samples. There are two types of assay:

- **Indirect ELISA**
  - A known amount of an **antigen is fixed to a surface.**
  - A clinical sample (usually the patient's serum) is then added on to the surface.
  - If the sample contains antibodies against the antigen, the **antibodies bind the antigen** and remain attached to the surface.
  - The surface is washed to remove any unbound (nonspecific) antibody.
  - A **secondary, enzyme-linked antibody**, specific for the Fc portion of the human IgG, is then added to the reaction.
  - This **secondary antibody binds the primary antibodies** present from the patient's serum.
  - A substrate is then added, which results in a **colorimetric reaction catalyzed by the enzyme linked to the secondary antibody.**
  - The color change can be quantified using a spectrophotometer and related to the amount of the antibody present in the clinical sample.
- **Direct, or "sandwich," ELISA** (see Figure 3-115)
  - The **antibody** specific for the antigen of interest is first **fixed to a surface** (1).
  - A sample potentially containing the antigen of interest is added to the reaction.
  - If the **antigen** is present in the sample, it **will bind to the fixed antibodies,** while the rest is washed away (2).
  - A **second "layer" of the antibody** is then added, "sandwiching" the bound antigen (3).
  - As in the indirect ELISA, an **enzyme-linked secondary antibody** and the substrate are then added, and the **colorimetric reaction** is read in a spectrophotometer (4 and 5).

ELISA is used for the detection of antibodies against many pathogens, as a means of establishing present or past infection with the pathogen. It is also sometimes used by the food industry to detect the presence of certain common allergens.

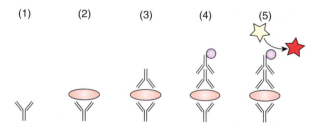

FIGURE 3-115. ELISA. See text for a step-by-step explanation.

ELISA is the most *sensitive* screening test for HIV in individuals at risk for infection. A positive result is followed up by the more *specific* Western blot assay. ELISA is also used to screen for other viral pathogens, such as the West Nile virus.

Immunohistochemistry

PRINCIPLE

Similar to ELISA and Western blotting, immunohistochemistry (IHC) is a general technique that relies on visual detection of proteins in a sample using antibodies. The main difference is that IHC usually refers to the detection of antigens in **tissue samples.** Some authors refer to a variant of this technique under the term immunocytochemistry, which differs from immunohistochemistry in that immunocytochemistry uses cells grown in laboratory culture.

In both techniques, an antibody raised against the protein of interest is incubated with the tissue sample; the tissue is subsequently washed to remove unbound primary antibody. If the antigen is present in the tissue, bound antibodies stay attached. A secondary, enzyme-conjugated or fluorophore-conjugated antibody against the primary antibody is added to the reaction. Finally, the addition of the substrate causes a color change in the locations that contain the antigen of interest. These can be directly observed using a microscope. In the case of a fluorophore-labeled antibody, a fluorescent microscope would be used for visualization, eliminating the need for the substrate-enzyme reaction (see Figure 3-116).

USE

In a clinical setting, immunohistochemistry is commonly used in histopathology, often to detect a specific cancer antigen in a tissue sample, thus confirming the tumor type. Tissue can come from diagnostic biopsies or tumor samples following resection.

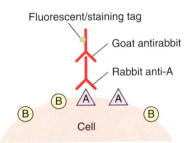

FIGURE 3-116. **Immunohistochemical detection.** An antibody specific to the protein of interest is incubated with a clinical sample and allowed to bind to it. Then a secondary antibody is used to provide a visual signal, which identifies and localizes the protein of interest if it is present in the sample.

CLINICAL EXAMPLES

Immunohistochemical techniques are used to detect the presence of markers such as the **carcinoembryonic antigen (CEA)** in adenocarcinomas, **CD15** and **CD30** in Hodgkin's disease, **α-fetoprotein** in yolk sac tumors and hepatocellular carcinoma, **CD117** in gastrointestinal stromal tumors (GIST), and **prostate-specific antigen (PSA)** in prostate cancer.

Radioimmunoassay

PRINCIPLE

Radioimmunoassay (RIA) is a technique used to measure small amounts of antigen in clinical samples. The protein of interest is first **labeled with a radioactive isotope** and allowed to bind to the antibody against that protein until the point of saturation. The clinical sample is then added to the mix, **causing any antigen in the sample to displace the radioactively labeled one from the antibodies.** This free radiolabeled antigen is then measured in the solution, making it possible to calculate the amount of the antigen in the original sample.

USE

RIA is used most commonly to measure various hormone levels in patients. It is also sometimes used to measure the amounts of vitamins, enzymes, and drugs in clinical samples.

CLINICAL EXAMPLES

RIA is routinely used to measure the levels of **TSH, T_3,** and **T_4** as part of a thyroid disease workup, as well as **insulin** levels in patients with suspected diabetes mellitus or insulinomas.

RNA-BASED LAB TESTS

Northern Blotting

PRINCIPLE

Northern blotting is similar to Southern and Western blotting, except that the substance being analyzed is **RNA,** rather than DNA or protein. In Northern blotting, a sample of RNA is run on an agarose gel and is then transferred to a nitrocellulose membrane. A radiolabeled RNA or single-stranded DNA is used as a probe. Finally, an X-ray film is exposed to the membrane, revealing the location of the RNA sequences of interest (see Figure 3-117).

USE

Northern blotting is usually used in special laboratory studies to detect the levels of expression of a certain gene in clinical samples, as indicated by the amount of mRNA present.

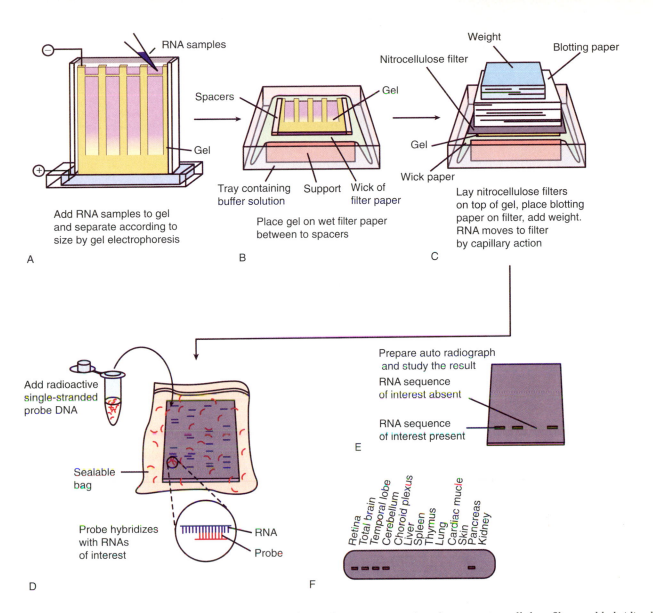

FIGURE 3-117. Northern blotting. (A–E) RNA is separated according to size, transferred on to a nitrocellulose filter, and hybridized with radiolabeled probes specific for the sequence of interest. Exposure of the X-ray film reveals the position and size of the RNA fragments that contain the sequence of interest. (F) The presence or absence of a particular RNA fragment can be determined and compared in several clinical samples, such as from different patients or different organs from the same patient.

Genetics

HARDY-WEINBERG GENETICS

Humans carry two copies of each gene (one inherited from each parent). These copies, known as alleles, each can be dominant or recessive. **Hardy-Weinberg genetics** are used to describe the frequency of these alleles in large populations.

The percentage of each of the two alleles (p and q) in the population must total 100%.

$$p + q = 1.00$$

EXAMPLE

In a sample population, there are only two eye colors: brown and blue. If 90% of the alleles in the population are for brown eyes (p=.90), then the other 10% must be for blue eyes (q=.10).

To determine the number of people with each combination of alleles:

$$p^2 + 2pq + q^2 = 1.00$$

where p^2 and q^2 are the fractions of the population homozygous for p and q, respectively, and 2pq is the fraction heterozygous for p and q.

Using the above example of eye color, if p = 0.90 and q = 0.10, then:

$p^2 = .90^2 = .81$	81% homozygous for brown eyes
$2pq = 2 \times .90 \times .10 = .18$	18% heterozygous for eye color
$q^2 = .10^2 = .01$	1% homozygous for blue eyes

Disease inheritance depends on the number of copies of the mutant gene required to produce the condition and on which chromosome the gene is located.

Non–Sex Chromosome Diseases

Autosomal dominant and **autosomal recessive** diseases are caused by genes carried on chromosomes other than the X and Y sex chromosomes.

- **Autosomal dominant** diseases require the presence of only one mutant gene (or allele). These individuals are termed heterozygotes. Affected persons may be of both sexes and appear in most generations (see Figure 3-118).
- **Autosomal recessive** diseases require the presence of two mutant genes (homozygous). Affected persons are of both sexes, but autosomal recessive diseases appear sporadically and infrequently throughout a family tree (see Figure 3-119).

Sex Chromosome Diseases

- **X-linked recessive** diseases affect males because they carry one X chromosome that is always inherited from the mother. Because they have only one allele for each gene on the X-chromosome, the recessive mutant gene is always expressed (there can be no second, dominant allele to disguise the recessive allele) (see Figure 3-120).
- **X-linked dominant** diseases affect both sexes. An affected male has only one X chromosome and thus always passes the disease to daughters. Affected mothers have a 50% chance of passing on the disease to offspring of either sex (see Figure 3-121).

MITOCHONDRIAL DISEASES

Mitochondria carry their own DNA, which is inherited from the mother. Because the mother passes all mutations to her offspring, the inheritance pattern is essentially a dominant one (all offspring of an affected mother are affected) (see Figure 3-122).

These modes of inheritance are summarized in Table 3-33.

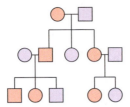

FIGURE 3-118.   **Autosomal dominant inheritance.**

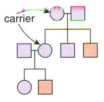

FIGURE 3-119.   **Autosomal recessive inheritance.**

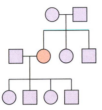

FIGURE 3-120.   **X-linked recessive inheritance.**

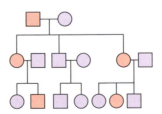

FIGURE 3-121.   **X-linked dominant inheritance.**

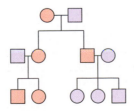

FIGURE 3-122.   **Mitochondrial inheritance.**

TABLE 3-33. Modes of Inheritance

Mode	Chromosome Carried On	Sex Affected	Generations Affected	Parent Who Transmits	Types of Disease	Hints When Looking at Pedigree Tree
Autosomal dominant	Non-X, non-Y chromosomes	Both equally	Multiple serial generations.	Parent who is also affected.	Often structural and not fatal at early age.	Most generations affected.
Autosomal recessive	Non-X, non-Y chromosomes	Both equally	Usually multiple offspring of one generation.	Both parents are carriers.	Most metabolic diseases and cystic fibrosis.	Often sporadically appears in one generation.
X-linked recessive	X chromosome	Males	Variable depending on presence of male offspring.	Mother.	Fragile X, muscular dystrophy, hemophilias, Lesch-Nyman.	Mostly males.
X-linked dominant	X chromosome	Females > males	Multiple serial generations.	Both parents can give gene to a female, only mother gives to male offspring.	Hypophosphatemic rickets.	All female children of affected male are affected.
Mitochondrial	None (carried in mitochondrial DNA)	Both equally	Multiple serial generations.	Mother.	Leber's optic neuropathy, MELAS, many myopathies.	All offspring of affected mother.

MELAS = mitochondrial encephalomyopathy with lactic acidosis and stroke-like episodes.

Inheritance Properties

- **Incomplete penetrance** occurs when a person with a mutant genotype does not show signs of the **disease** (phenotype).
- **Variable expression** occurs when the severity and nature of the disease phenotype varies between individuals with the same mutant **genotype.**

TRISOMIES

Trisomies occur when three homologous chromosomes combine in a zygote.

Nondisjunction

Either the sperm or the egg may carry the extra chromosome, as shown in Figure 3-123.

Chromosomal Translocation

Trisomy can also occur when a piece of one chromosome attaches to another and "hitches a ride" during meiosis. As a result, two homologous chromosomes can be sorted to the same zygote, as shown in Figure 3-124.

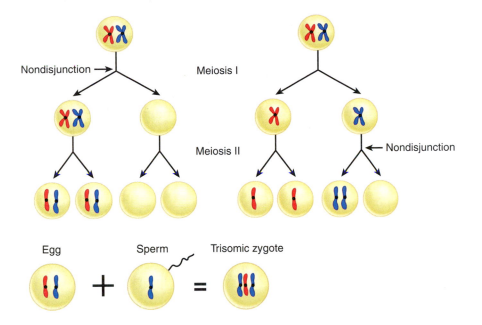

FIGURE 3-123.   Nondisjunction during meiosis I and meiosis II.

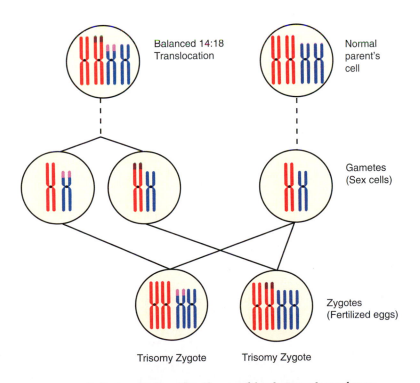

FIGURE 3-124.   Robertsonian translocation resulting in Down's syndrome.

Common Trisomies

All trisomies are characterized by mental retardation, abnormal facies, and often heart disease. Few trisomies routinely survive to birth.

Trisomy 21 (Down's syndrome) is the most common trisomy and the most common cause of mental retardation. Mothers may express **low α-ferroprotein and high β-hCG** during pregnancy and ultrasound may show **nuchal translucency**. Patients are characterized by:

- Epicanthal folds
- Simian crease
- Atrial septal defect (ASD) or other congenital heart disease
- Acute lymphocytic leukemia (ALL)
- Duodenal atresia
- Celiac disease

Trisomy 18 (Edward's syndrome) is often fatal by < 1 year of age. Patients are characterized by:

- Micrognathia
- Overlapping, clenched fingers
- Rocker-bottom feet
- Big occiput

Trisomy 13 (Patau's syndrome) is often fatal by < 1 year of age. Patients are characterized by:

- Micropthalmia
- Polydactyly
- Cleft lip/palate

MNEMONIC

Drink at 21, **E**lection age is 18, **P**uberty at 13.
Downs=Trisomy 21
Edwards=Trisomy 18
Patau's=Trisomy 13

Trisomy 8 is rare, but can also result in live births.
Trisomy 16 is a very common cause of miscarriage.

IMPRINT DISORDERS

Imprinting occurs when identical genes are expressed differently, depending on which parent they are inherited from.

Prader-Willi and Angelman's syndrome create two different phenotypes based on whether the paternal or the maternal portion of the same segment on chromosome 15 is deleted in the fetus.

Prader-Willi Syndrome

Occurs when a portion of the **paternal** chromosome 15 is deleted in the fetus:

- Neonatal hypotonia and failure to thrive
- Later childhood hyperphagia and obesity
- Mild mental retardation
- Aggressive/psychotic behavior
- Short stature, with small hands, feet, and gonads

Angelman's Syndrome

Occurs when a portion of the **maternal** chromosome 15 is deleted in the fetus:

- Inappropriate laughter (also known as happy puppet syndrome)
- Jerky, flexed movements
- Microcephaly
- Minimal speech
- Severe mental retardation and seizures
- Sleep disturbance

NOTES

Embryology

STAGES OF PRENATAL DEVELOPMENT

Human prenatal development is a complex process that allows a single cell to develop into an organism. The right cues must occur at the right time and in the right place to guide cellular proliferation, migration, and differentiation. Development occurs in three main stages (see Figure 4-1).

Germinal Stage (Weeks 0–2)

- Zygote formation
- Cell division
- Zygote attachment to the uterine wall

Embryonic Stage (Weeks 3–8)

- Organ formation
- Teratogen sensitivity

Fetal Stage (Week 9–Birth)

- Rapid fetal growth
- Sex organ formation
- Organ systems function

EMBRYOLOGY DECODER RING

There are several key terms that define the language of embryology and are instrumental to understanding the field (see Table 4-1).

GAMETOGENESIS

Meiosis

Prior to fertilization, the gametes that are going to fuse must undergo meiosis (see Figure 4-2). During meiosis, the genetic information in diploid germ cells is ultimately halved ($2n \rightarrow n$). The genetic material is **initially doubled (4n)** prior to the first meiotic division. Meiosis produces **two diploid (2n) daughter cells.** Each daughter cell then undergoes a second meiosis that is not preceded by a doubling. This results in the production of **four haploid (n) daughter cells.** These haploid cells then fuse to produce a genetically unique offspring.

> **KEY FACT**
>
> **Down's syndrome (trisomy 21)** is usually caused by a **nondisjunction** (failure of separation) during meiosis of the female gametes.

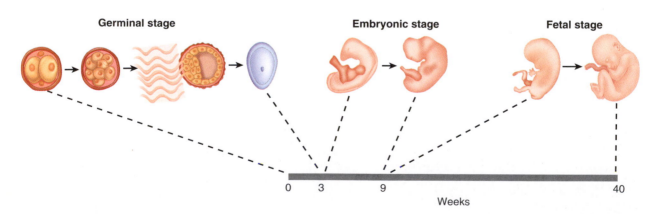

Germinal stage   Embryonic stage   Fetal stage

0   3   9   40

Weeks

FIGURE 4-1.   Human prenatal development time line. The germinal period (weeks 1 and 2) includes zygote formation and implantation. The embryonic period (weeks 3–8) includes organ formation. The fetal period (week 9 until birth) includes rapid growth and organ function.

TABLE 4-1. **Embryology Vocabulary**

TERM	DEFINITION
Atresia	Blind pouch
Blast	Precursor cell
Caudal	Hind part, tail, posterior.
Cephalic	Upper part, head
Coelom	Cavity
Cranial	Skull, head part, anterior
Dorsal	Back or top side
Ecto-	Outer
Endo-	Inner
Epi-	Above
Extraembryonic	Outside the embryonic body
Fistula	Abnormal connection
Gastrulation	Formation of the three germ layers.
Hypo-	Below
Intraembryonic	Inside the embryonic body
Meso-	Middle
Mesenchyme	Any loosely organized tissue of fibroblast-like cells and extracellular matrix, regardless of the origin of the cells.
Neurulation	Formation of the neural tube.
Splanchnic	Belonging to the internal organs as opposed to its framework.
Somatic	Belonging to the framework of the body rather than the internal organs.
Ventral	Front or bottom side

Spermatogenesis

Just before **puberty,** the primordial sperm cells (2n) differentiate into **spermatogonia (2n)** (see Figure 4-3) in the seminiferous tubules.

- **Type A spermatogonia**
  - Stem cell population lining the basal compartment.
  - Produce progenitor type B spermatogonia.

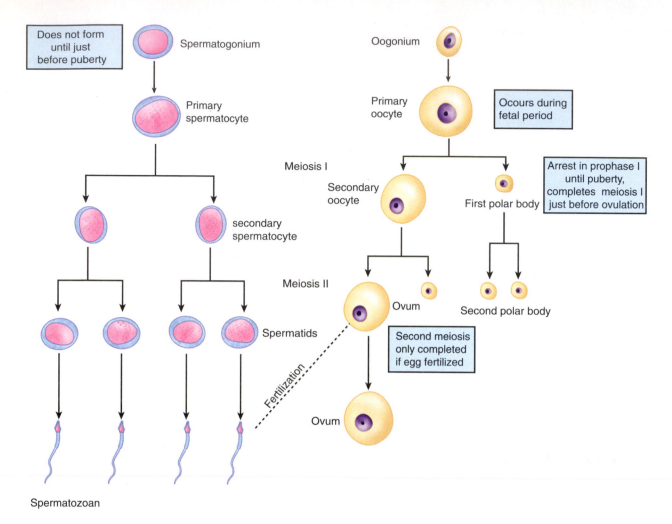

FIGURE 4-2. **Meiosis of male and female germ cells.** Gametogenesis begins with a doubling of the genetic information by mitosis. Subsequent meiosis results in halving of the DNA. This process takes place on a different timescale for male and female gametes.

- **Type B spermatogonia:** Mature as they move toward the testicular lumen.
  - Mitosis → **primary spermatocytes (4n).**
  - Meiosis after prolonged prophase → **secondary spermatocytes (2n).**
  - Rapid second meiosis → **spermatids (n).**

The spermatids undergo several morphologic changes to form spermatozoa, including (see Figure 4-4):

- **Cytoplasm reduction:** Discarded and phagocytosed by Sertoli cells.
- **Nuclear condensation.**
- **Flagellum formation:** Mitochondria pack tightly.
- **Acrosome formation:** Cap containing enzymes for penetration of the oocyte zona pellucida.

Components of a mature spermatozoon (see Figure 4-4):

- **Head:** Nucleus covered by an acrosome and a cell membrane.
- **Neck:** Two centrioles + tightly packed mitochondria.
- **Tail:** A central pair of microtubles (**axoneme**) surrounded by nine doublets ($9 \times 2 + 2$).
  - Proximal: Axoneme + inner layer dense fibers + outer layer mitochondria.

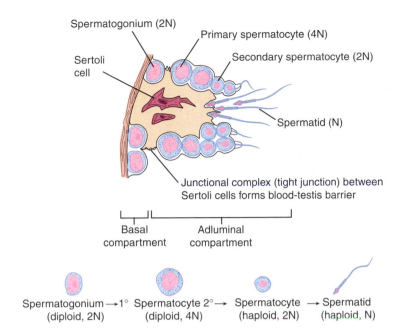

FIGURE 4-3. **Spermatogenesis.** Spermatogonia are produced from primordial germ cells just before puberty. Type A cells reside in the basal compartment and act as a stem cell population. As type B cells travel toward the testicular lumen, they continue to mature to the haploid spermatid state.

- Distal: Axoneme + dense fibers + outer fibrous sheath.
- Terminal: Only axoneme.

Sertoli cells release spermatozoa into the lumen of the **seminiferous tubules**, which are connected to the rete testis. The **rete testis** is in turn connected to efferent ductules, which empty into the epididymis. In the **epididymis**, spermatozoa mature further and become motile.

Oogenesis

In contrast to spermatogenesis, primordial eggs differentiate into **oogonia (2n) during the fetal period** (see Figure 4-5). By the end of the first trimester, after several mitotic divisions, the oogonia differentiate into **primary oocytes.** The primary oocytes replicate their DNA and **enter meiosis I (4n)**, but **arrest in prophase I until puberty**. After entry into meiosis I, further mitosis does

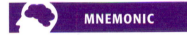

MNEMONIC

The neck, or **M**iddle part, of the sperm contains **M**itochondria.

KEY FACT

Oogonia form during fetal development (arresting in prophase I until puberty) and there is not continual replenishment by a resident stem cell.

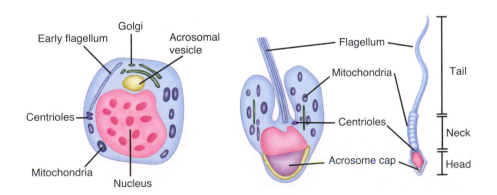

FIGURE 4-4. **Spermatid maturation.** A fresh spermatid cell must undergo several morphologic changes on its way to becoming a mature sperm cell. These changes include cytoplasmic reduction, nuclear condensation, flagellum formation, and acrosome formation.

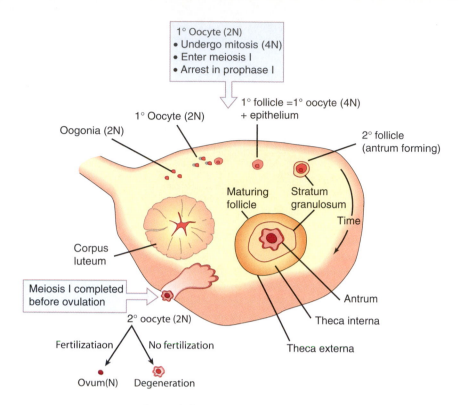

FIGURE 4-5. **Oogenesis.** Primordial germ cells differentiate into oogonia during the fetal stage. This maturation is arrested at the primary oocyte stage until puberty, although the surrounding follicle does continue to develop. Meiosis I is completed, creating a secondary oocyte just before ovulation.

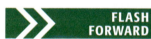

FLASH FORWARD

Spermatogenesis and oogenesis are regulated by several crucial hormonal signals originating from both the endocrine and reproductive systems.

not occur, and unlike in males, there is no stem cell system. Each primary oocyte becomes enveloped in a single layer of epithelial cells, which together form the **primordial follicle.** The follicle can develop through stages, while the primary oocyte remains dormant. After puberty, **a few primordial follicles begin to mature during each ovarian cycle,** but only one will ultimately be released. Prior to release, meiosis I is completed. This forms a secondary oocyte (2n), which then begins meiosis II, but arrests in metaphase. If the secondary oocyte is fertilized within 12–36 hours, it can escape degradation and complete meiosis II, forming the **ovum (n).**

EARLY LANDMARKS

Day 0: Fertilization

For the male and female gametes to fuse, they must first find their way to each other. Once introduced to the cervix, the **spermatids traverse the hostile environment of the female genital tract to meet the secondary oocyte** in the fallopian tube at the infundibulum. During this journey, a maturation process called **capacitation** results in hyperactivity and activation of the sperm's acrosomal coat. When the sperm encounter the pellucid zone of the oocyte, the **acrosomal reaction** releases enzymes that degrade the zone. Once a single sperm reaches the oocyte:

- Sperm and oocyte membranes fuse.
- Oocyte cortex granules release enzymes that render the zona pellucida impenetrable (polyspermy block).
- The second meiosis of the oocyte is completed.

- Maternal and paternal pronuclei come together and nuclear membranes between them dissolve.
- A zygote is formed.

Week 1: Cleavage and Implantation

CLEAVAGE

As the zygote travels through the fallopian tube, it is cleaved into progressively smaller daughter cells (see Figure 4-6).

- **Morula:** 16- to 32-cell stages; resides at the os.
- **Compaction:** Tight junction formation that leads to flattening and separation of the inner and outer blastomeres; a pole is formed.
- **Blastocoele:** Fluid pumped into the intercellular spaces of the morula.

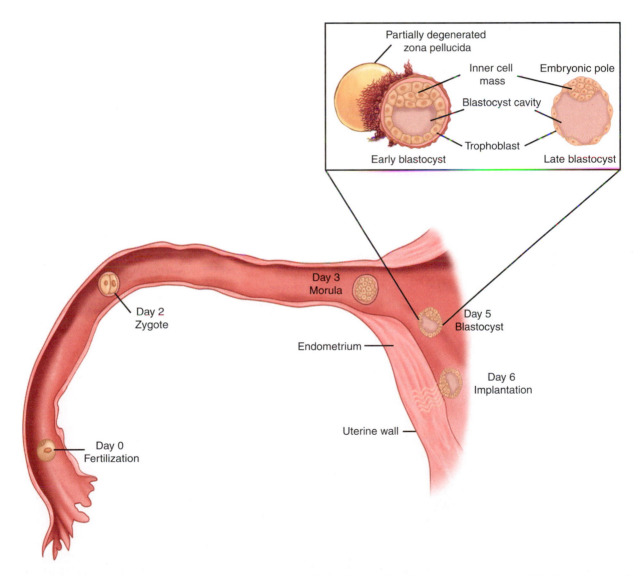

FIGURE 4-6. **Fertilization to implantation.** The oocyte is usually fertilized in the fallopian tube at the infundibulum. As it travels to the uterus, it goes through several maturational stages. While in the blastocyst stage, it "hatches" from the zona pellucida and implants in the uterine wall.

- **Blastocyst**
    - Free of the zona pellucida (hatching, "first birth").
    - Inner cell mass (**embryoblast**, embryonic stem cells).
    - Outer cell mass (**trophoblast**).

IMPLANTATION

The zygote attaches to and invades the endometrium using the trophoblast cells over the embryoblast pole.

Week 2: "Week of Twos"

At this stage, the embryo resembles a sandwich cookie without icing suspended between two cavities (see Figure 4-7).

TWO GERM LAYERS

The embryoblast organizes into two layers resembling a sandwich with only two slices of bread.

- **Epiblast:** Dorsal layer composed of high columnar cells.
- **Hypoblast:** Ventral layer composed of low cuboidal cells.

TWO CAVITIES

- **Amniotic cavity:** Dorsal to the epiblast, lined by proliferative edges of the epiblast.
- **Yolk sac:** Ventral to the hypoblast, lined by proliferative edges of the hypoblast.

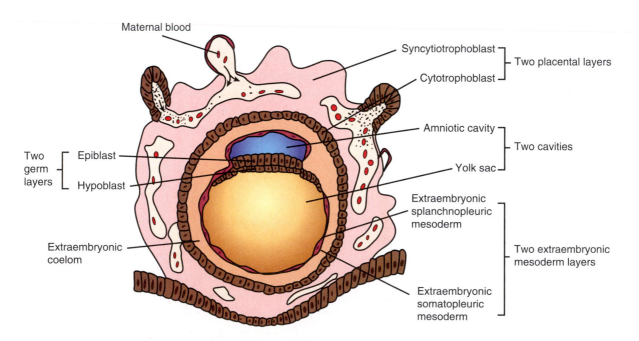

FIGURE 4-7. Second week of embryologic development. During the second week of embryologic development, there are two germ layers (epiblast and hypoblast), two cavities (amniotic cavity and yolk sac), two placental layers (syncytiotrophoblast and cytotrophoblast), and two extraembryonic mesoderm layers (splanchnopleuric and somatopleuric).

TWO PLACENTAL LAYERS

The trophoblast organizes into two layers.

- **Cytotrophoblast:** Inner proliferative layer that provides additional trophoblast cells.

- **Syncytiotrophoblast:** Thick outer layer without cell boundaries that invades the endometrium as the chorionic villi.

TWO EXTRAEMBRYONIC MESODERM LAYERS

Extraembryonic mesoderm, a **loose connective tissue layer,** forms between the cytotrophoblast and two cavities. During the second week, fluid-filled spaces appear, pushing aside the mesenchyme to **form a coelom,** or cavity (see Figure 4-8). This **splits the mesoderm** into two layers that will remain connected at the connecting stalk. The connecting stalk will later contribute to the umbilical cord.

- **Splanchnopleuric:** Inner layer lining the yolk sac.
- **Somatopleuric:** Concentric layer lining the inner surface of the cytotrophoblast.

UTEROPLACENTAL CIRCULATION

The syncytiotrophoblast erodes the maternal vessels, forming **lacunae**—intervillous spaces—that bring nutrients closer to the embryo.

DECIDUAL REACTION

The cells of the decidua, the functional layer of the endometrium, enlarge. They accumulate lipid and glycogen to provide nourishment to the embryo until the placenta is vascularized.

Week 3: "Week of Threes"

THREE GERM LAYERS

During the process of **gastrulation,** mesoderm fills in the middle of the bilaminar sandwich (see Figure 4-9). Gastrulation begins with the formation of a

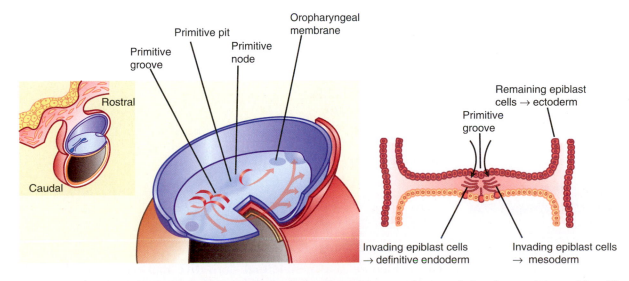

FIGURE 4-8. Gastrulation. During gastrulation, epiblast cells detach, proliferate, and migrate below the remaining epiblast. The migrating cells displace the hypoblast, forming the endoderm, and fill in the space between the epiblast and hypoblast, forming the mesoderm. The remaining epiblast cells form the ectoderm.

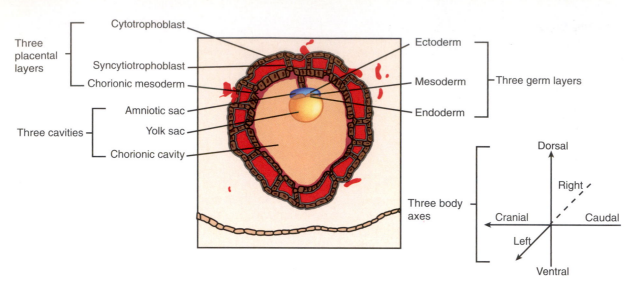

FIGURE 4-9. **Third week of embryologic development.** During week 3 of embryologic development, there are three germ layers (ectoderm, mesoderm, endoderm), three cavities (amniotic sac, yolk sac, chorionic cavity), three placental layers (cytotrophoblast, syncytiotrophoblast, chorionic mesoderm), and three body axes (craniocaudal, dorsoventral, right-left).

groove and pit at the caudal end of the epiblast called the **primitive streak.** The pit and elevated cells around the cranial end comprise the **primitive node.** Cells proliferate from the streak and node, detach, and migrate beneath the remaining epiblast.

- **Ectoderm:** Remaining epiblast.
- **Mesoderm:** New layer formed between old layers.
- **Endoderm:** Original hypoblast displaced by the definitive endoderm.

THREE CAVITIES

In addition to the yolk sac and amniotic cavity, the chorionic cavity is defined by complete separation of the mesoderm layers.

- **Chorionic:** Former extraembryonic coelom
- **Yolk sac**
- **Amniotic**

THREE PLACENTAL VILLI LAYERS

In addition to the two existing layers, the chorionic (extraembryonic) mesoderm invades the core.

- **Syncytiotrophoblast**
- **Cytotrophoblast**
- **Chorionic mesoderm**

THREE BODY AXES

- **Craniocaudal** (anteroposterior)
- **Dorsoventral**
- **Right-left**

NOTOCHORD AND NEURAL PLATE

The notochord is a **mesodermal derivative** that establishes the midline. It sends signals for **induction of the neural tube, somites,** and **other surrounding structures.**

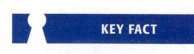
KEY FACT

To visualize the process of notochord formation, picture a finger pressing into an inflated balloon while staying close to the surface.

- **Notochordal process:** Formed during gastrulation, when future notochord cells migrate through the primitive node.
- **Notochordal plate:** Formed when the chordal process fuses with underlying endoderm.
- **Neurenteric canal:** Formed when the floor of the chordal process and the fused endoderm degenerate, creating a temporary passage between the yolk sac and amniotic cavity.
- **Definitive notochord:** Formed when notochordal cells detach from the endoderm and reside in the middle of the mesoderm.
- **Neural plate:** Formed when the notochord induces a thickening of the ectoderm above it; this will eventually form the neural tube.

ALLANTOIS

The allantois, which is mostly vestigial in humans, begins as a diverticulum of the yolk sac at the posterior wall (see Figure 4-10).

Weeks 3–8

During this time of intense organ formation, the embryo is very fragile and susceptible to harmful teratogens.

ECTODERM

During week 3, the process of **neurulation** continues. The neural plate invaginates, forming the **neural groove** at the midline and **two neural folds** laterally (see Figure 4-11). The plate rolls up like a tube, with the edges of these neural folds, the **neural crests,** fusing together at the midline. This **neural tube** formation begins in the neck region, at the fourth somite, and proceeds in both cephalic and caudal directions, with the cephalic being completed first. The cephalic end dilates, forming the forebrain, midbrain, and hindbrain, while the rest of the neural tube forms the spinal cord.

As the neural folds elevate and join at the midline, cells at the neural crests differentiate, forming **neural crest cells** (see Figure 4-11). When they reach their final destinations, they differentiate into numerous cell types, including spinal ganglia, melanocytes, and support cells of the nervous system. **Gut tube** formation is concurrently occurring ventrally, forming a **tube beneath a tube** held together by mesodermal glue.

KEY FACT

To visualize the process of neural tube formation, imagine a zipper starting in the middle and being pulled in both directions.

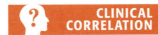

CLINICAL CORRELATION

If the neural tube does not close completely, a variety of congenital **neural tube defects** can occur. A cranial defect results in **anencephaly,** while a defect along the spinal cord results in **spina bifida.**

CLINICAL CORRELATION

Neural crest cells migrate to become precursors of colonic ganglion cells. If this migration is incomplete, segments of the bowel cannot relax and a functional obstruction occurs. This disorder is known as **Hirschsprung's disease.**

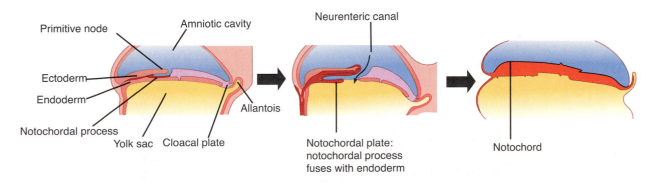

FIGURE 4-10. Notochord development. The notochord begins as an invagination of the mesoderm known as the notochordal process. This process then fuses with the endoderm, forming the notochordal plate. A portion of this plate degenerates, creating the neurenteric canal. Finally, a subset of the notochordal cells detaches from the endoderm, forming the definitive notochord.

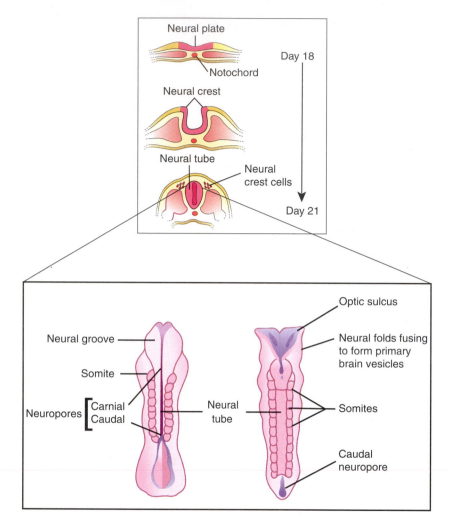

FIGURE 4-11. **Neural tube development.** The notochord induces a thickening of the ectoderm above it, known as the neural plate. This plate then rolls up to form the neural tube. The closing of the neural tube begins at the fourth somite and proceeds in both directions. A group of cells, the neural crest cells, migrate away from the tube and eventually form a variety of cell types, including spinal ganglia, melanocytes, and nervous system support cells.

MESODERM

While the neural and gut tubes are forming, the mesoderm proliferates and rearranges itself into **three distinct regions:** Paraxial, intermediate, and lateral.

The **paraxial mesoderm** forms paired, segmentally arranged columns on either side of the neural tube. These segments, called somites, will divide into **sclerotomes, dermatomes,** and **myotomes** that give rise to bone/cartilage, dermis/subcutaneous, and skeletal muscles, respectively (see Figures 4-11 and 4-12).

The **intermediate mesoderm** forms between the paraxial mesoderm and lateral mesoderm. Cranially, it arranges into segments of cell clusters that represent the future **nephrotomes** (see Figure 4-12). In the lumbosacral region,

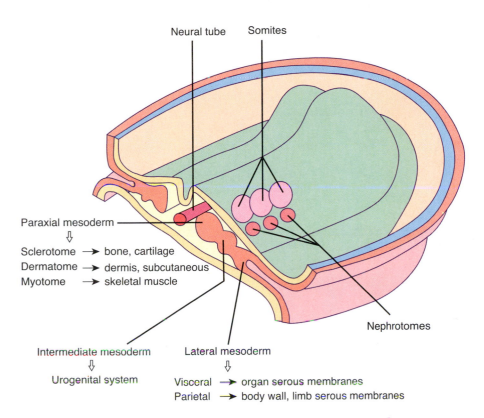

Neural tube   Somites

Paraxial mesoderm

Sclerotome → bone, cartilage
Dermatome → dermis, subcutaneous
Myotome → skeletal muscle

Nephrotomes

Intermediate mesoderm
⇩
Urogenital system

Lateral mesoderm
⇩
Visceral → organ serous membranes
Parietal → body wall, limb serous membranes

FIGURE 4-12. Mesoderm segmentation. The mesoderm separates into three segments. Paraxial mesoderm lies alongside the neural tube and gives rise to sclerotomes, dermatomes, and myotomes. Intermediate mesoderm lies lateral to the paraxial mesoderm and forms the urogenital system. Lateral mesoderm lies lateral to the intermediate mesoderm and forms the serous membrane lining of organ systems, limbs, and the body wall.

an unsegmented mass of tissue known as the **nephrogenic cord** forms. These structures and their duct system contribute to the urogenital system.

The **lateral mesoderm** lies on the lateral edge of the embryo and is further divided by the intraembryonic coelom or cavity into **somatic or parietal** (wall), and **splanchnic or visceral** (organ). Vacuoles begin to form in the lateral mesoderm and ultimately fuse, creating a U-shaped cavity, the **intraembryonic coelom** (see Figure 4-13). The outer parietal or somatic mesoderm layer forms the serous membrane lining of the body wall, anterior abdominal wall, and limbs. The inner visceral or splanchnic mesoderm layer forms the serous membrane lining of the gut, pericardial, pleural, and peritoneal cavities.

ENDODERM

The endoderm forms the primitive **gut tube**—the future respiratory and digestive systems—via cephalocaudal and lateral folds of the embryonic disk. The folding is similar to pulling the strings on a cinched sac and leaves the embryonic disk in the traditional "fetal position." This folding is driven by rapid longitudinal growth of the central nervous system, creating caudal and cephalic bending known as the **head and tail folds.** The head fold brings the cardiogenic region cephalic to the brain. As the sac is cinched and folds in, part of the yolk sac is pinched off and becomes the **foregut** and **midgut,** while the allantois contributes to the **hindgut** (see Figure 4-14).

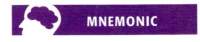

MNEMONIC

Mesoderm segment locations—

Paraxial mesoderm: Lies **next to (para)** the neural tube (axis).
Intermediate mesoderm: Lies **between (intermediate)** the other mesoderm segments.
Lateral mesoderm: Lies **lateral** to the other mesoderm segments.

KEY FACT

Gut tube + neural tube = tube on top of a tube held together with mesodermal glue.

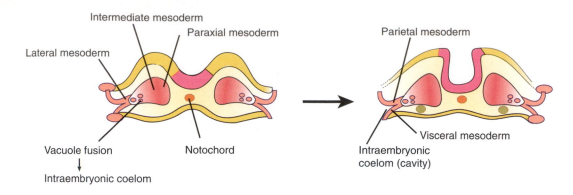

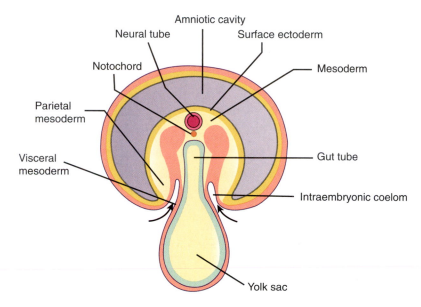

FIGURE 4-13. **Separation of the lateral mesoderm.** The lateral mesoderm is further divided by the formation of the intraembryonic coelom into parietal and visceral mesoderm. The outer parietal mesoderm forms the serous membrane lining of the body wall and limbs. The inner visceral mesoderm remains invested around the gut tube and forms the serous membrane lining of the gut and the pericardial, pleural, and peritoneal cavities.

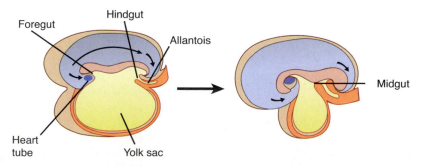

FIGURE 4-14. **Endodermal gastrulation.** The gut tube is formed by "cinching" the embryo with a combination of cephalocaudal and lateral folds. The yolk sac contributes to the formation of the foregut and midgut, while the allantois contributes to the hindgut.

Other Landmarks

WEEK 4

- Body system appears in rudimentary form.
- Heart beats.
- Upper and lower limb buds form.

WEEK 5

- Muscle and cartilage formation begins.
- Cardiac septa form and atrioventricular cushions fuse.
- Craniofacial development begins.

WEEK 10

- Genitalia have male or female characteristics.

FETAL MEMBRANES AND PLACENTA

The placenta supplies nutrients to and removes waste from the embryo via interaction with the maternal circulation.

Placenta

The **chorion** constitutes the **fetal contribution to the placenta** and includes the somatic extraembryonic mesoderm, cytotrophoblast, and syncytiotrophoblast. The **syncytiotrophoblast** invades and erodes maternal tissue and vessels, forming tissue lacunae, which fill with maternal blood. **Placental villi,** the exchange units, begin to form in stages.

- **Primary villi:** Syncytiotrophoblast covering + cytotrophoblast core.
- **Secondary villi:** Primary villi + invasion of the extraembryonic mesoderm at the core.
- **Tertiary villi:** Secondary villi + vessel formation in the extraembryonic mesoderm core.

On the maternal side, a **cytotrophoblastic shell** develops as the cytotrophoblast grows through the villi and connects with the cytotrophoblast of the adjacent villi (see Figure 4-15). On the embryonic side, the extraembryonic mesoderm remains connected at its base, known as the **chorionic plate.** Extension of the villi from the chorionic plate to the cytotrophoblastic shell anchors the

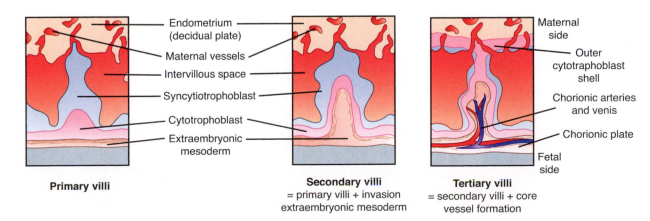

Primary villi

Endometrium (decidual plate)
Maternal vessels
Intervillous space
Syncytiotrophoblast
Cytotrophoblast
Extraembryonic mesoderm

Secondary villi
= primary villi + invasion extraembryonic mesoderm

Tertiary villi
= secondary villi + core vessel formation

Maternal side
Outer cytotraphoblast shell
Chorionic arteries and venis
Chorionic plate
Fetal side

FIGURE 4-15. **Placental villi development.** The placental villi form in stages. Primary villi consist of a cytotrophoblast core with a syncytiotrophoblast covering. Secondary villi form when the core of the primary villi is invaded by extraembryonic mesoderm. Tertiary villi form when the core of secondary villi develops vasculature.

FLASH FORWARD

In addition to facilitating nutrient exchange and physically anchoring the fetus to the endometrium, the placenta also releases several important hormones.

CLINICAL CORRELATION

In **placenta previa,** the placenta implants in the lower part of the uterus, covering the cervix and effectively blocking entrance to the vagina. As such, cesarean section is the preferred mode of delivery.

CLINICAL CORRELATION

Mothers who lack the Rh antigen (Rh⁻) on the surface of their blood cells can develop an **Rh antibody** during pregnancy with a child who has the antigen (Rh⁺). Any subsequent Rh⁺ children are attacked by this maternal antibody, and **anemia, congestive heart failure,** and **even fetal death may occur.** Initial antibody development can be prevented with the delivery of **Rh immunoglobulin.**

placenta to the uterus. The epithelial lining of the endometrium that participates in this anchoring is known as the **decidua.** As the heart develops, circulation is established in the placenta. The cytotrophoblast layer of the villi degenerates, thinning the wall and facilitating diffusion.

Similar to the polarization of the fetus, the placenta also becomes polarized, resulting in portions of the chorion and decidua becoming distinct (see Figure 4-16).

- **Chorion frondosum:** Villi on the embryonic side grow and differentiate.
- **Chorion laeve:** Villi on the nonembryonic side degenerate, leaving this part of the chorion smooth.
- **Decidua basalis:** Over the embryonic pole, the chorion frondosum adheres tightly, forming an anchoring decidual plate.
- **Decidua capsularis:** The decidual layer covering the embryonic side.
- **Decidua parietalis:** The decidua covering the remaining uterus.

As the fetus grows, the decidua capsularis contacts the decidua parietalis on the opposite uterine wall and degenerates. The underlying chorion laeve can then fuse directly with the decidua parietalis. As amniotic fluid fills the amniotic cavity, the amnion contacts the chorion laeve and also fuses, leaving one large amniotic cavity.

In the fourth month, the decidual plate begins to separate groups of villi into compartments called **cotyledons** by forming septa or walls (see Figure 4-17). The septa grow toward but do not contact the chorionic plate, allowing maternal blood from the spiral arteries to flow between compartments. Maternal blood is subsequently drained by endometrial veins. Deoxygenated fetal blood is brought to the chorionic villi by two umbilical arteries, and oxygenated blood is returned by the umbilical vein. There is **no mixing of the maternal and fetal blood,** just an exchange of nutrients, antibodies, etc. The placenta is also responsible for producing hormones, such as progesterone, estrogen, and human chorionic gonadotropin.

Yolk Sac

The yolk sac functions as a **transfer agent for nutrients** from the trophoblast to the embryo (2–3 weeks), as a **source of primordial germ cells,** and as a **source of blood cells and vessels** that connect to the vitelline arteries and veins. The dorsal part of the yolk sac connects to the primitive gut and forms

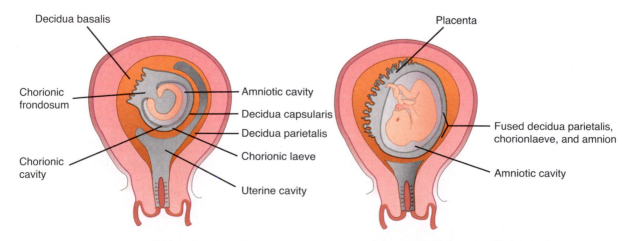

FIGURE 4-16.   Placenta polarization and cavity development. As the embryo grows, the placenta becomes polarized, with different segments of the chorion and decidua developing different characteristics. These layers eventually degenerate and fuse, leaving one large amniotic cavity.

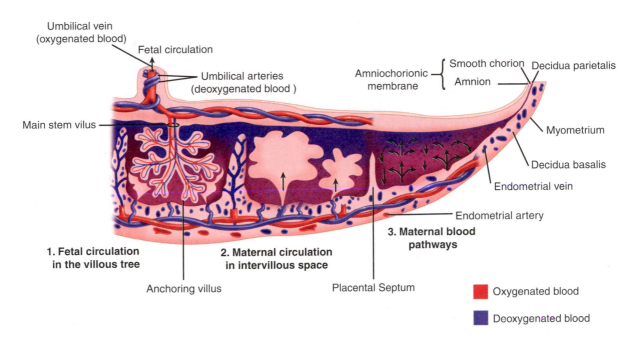

Umbilical vein (oxygenated blood)

Fetal circulation

Umbilical arteries (deoxygenated blood)

Main stem vilus

Amniochorionic membrane { Smooth chorion   Decidua parietalis

Amnion

Myometrium

Decidua basalis

Endometrial vein

Endometrial artery

3. Maternal blood pathways

1. Fetal circulation in the villous tree

2. Maternal circulation in the intervillous space

Anchoring villus   Placental Septum

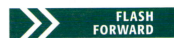

Oxygenated blood

Deoxygenated blood

FIGURE 4-17. Placental flow. As the placenta matures, it separates the villi into communicating compartments. As oxygenated maternal blood enters these compartments, via spiral arteries, it has access to all of the compartments. The now deoxygenated maternal blood is returned to the circulation via endometrial veins. Deoxygenated fetal blood enters the placenta via two umbilical arteries, and oxygenated blood is returned via the umbilical vein.

the epithelial linings and glands of the respiratory and digestive systems and the bladder, urethra, and lower vaginal canal in the female. The yolk sac is connected to the midgut via the **vitelline duct,** which, along with the yolk sac, forms part of the umbilical cord (see Figure 4-18).

Allantois

The allantois is used in some animals for removal of nitrogenous waste. However, humans have a well-developed chorionic placenta that removes waste through the maternal circulation, thus the allantois is mostly vestigial. It does, however, **provide vessels for the establishment of the definitive placenta and forms the umbilical blood vessels.** Beginning as an outpouching from

FLASH FORWARD

Meckel's diverticulum is a congenital outpouching in the small intestine, and is a remnant of the **vitelline duct.** It is a common malformation present in approximately 2% of the population.

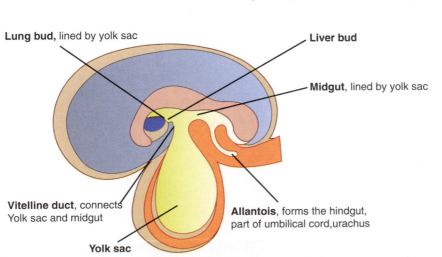

Lung bud, lined by yolk sac

Liver bud

Midgut, lined by yolk sac

Vitelline duct, connects Yolk sac and midgut

Allantois, forms the hindgut, part of umbilical cord, urachus

Yolk sac

FIGURE 4-18.   Yolk sac and allantois. The yolk sac connects to the primitive gut via the vitelline duct and forms the epithelial linings of the respiratory and digestive systems. The allantois contributes to the hindgut, part of the umbilical cord, and the urachus.

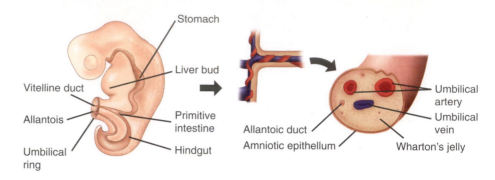

FIGURE 4-19. Umbilical cord development. The umbilical cord is created as the embryo is folded and cinched into the fetal position.

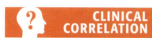

the yolk sac, it **forms the hindgut** (see Figure 4-18). It also becomes incorporated into the umbilical cord and persists from the urinary bladder to the umbilicus as the **urachus.** After birth, the urachus becomes a fibrous cord known as the **median umbilical ligament.**

Amnion

The amnion is a **thin nonvascular membrane** derived from the epiblast. It **lines the fluid-filled amniotic cavity** that cushions the embryo. The fluid filling of the cavity is initially derived from the maternal blood, but is later derived from fetal urine. The fluid is rapidly turned over as the fetus swallows it and passes it via the placenta to the maternal blood for waste removal. In the fifth month, the fluid is swallowed and returned via the gastrointestinal tract.

Umbilical Cord

The umbilical cord connects the embryonic circulation to the placenta. As the amniotic cavity is filled, the body stalk and yolk sac become incorporated into the umbilical cord. Initially, the umbilical cord is composed of:

- Vitelline vessels
- Umbilical vessels
- Allantois
- Chorionic cavity remnants
- Body stalk mesenchyme (Wharton's jelly)
- Intestinal loops (physiologic hernia)

Wharton's jelly is a gelatinous substance that contains no nerves and is a rich source for stem cells. As the umbilical cord develops, the vitelline vessels, allantois, yolk sac, and chorionic cavity remnants degrade and the intestinal loops are pulled back into the abdominal cavity. The cord ultimately consists of (see Figure 4-19):

- Umbilical vessels: Two arteries (return deoxygenated blood) and one vein (supplies oxygenated blood)
- Wharton's jelly
- Allantoic duct: Removes nitrogenous waste

EMBRYOLOGIC DERIVATIVES

Germ Layer Derivatives

The three embryonic germ layers form distinct subsets of adult tissue (see Table 4-2).

TABLE 4-2. **Germ Layer Derivatives**

GERM LAYER	DERIVATIVE
Ectoderm	
Surface ectoderm	■ Adenohypophysis (anterior pituitary)
	■ Sensory epithelium: Nose, ear, eye
	■ Lens of eye
	■ Epidermis, hair, nails
Neuroectoderm	■ Neurohypophysis (posterior pituitary)
	■ CNS neurons
	■ Oligodendrocytes
	■ Astrocytes
	■ Ependymal cells (glia)
	■ Pineal gland
Neural crest	■ Autonomic nervous system
	■ Dorsal root ganglia
	■ Cranial nerves
	■ Melanocytes
	■ Chromaffin cells of adrenal medulla
	■ Enterochromaffin cells
	■ Pia and arachnoid
	■ Celiac ganglion, autonomic ganglia
	■ Schwann cells
	■ Odontoblasts
	■ Parafollicular (C) cells of thyroid
	■ Laryngeal cartilage
	■ Bones of face, jaw, and ossicles of ear
Mesoderm	
Paraxial	■ Bones of skull
	■ Muscles
	■ Vertebrae
	■ Dura mater
	■ Connective tissue
	■ Bone
Intermediate	Urogenital system
Lateral	Serous membranes around organs
Splanchnic/visceral	■ Serous membranes
Somatic/parietal	■ Body wall
	■ Limbs
Endoderm	■ Gut tube epithelium
	■ Gut tube derivatives (lungs, liver, pancreas, thymus, parathyroid, thyroid follicular cells, gallbladder).

CNS = central nervous system.

TABLE 4-3. **Fetal-Postnatal Derivatives**

FETAL STRUCTURE	POSTNATAL DERIVATIVE
Umbilical vein	Ligamentum teres hepatic
Umbilical arteries	Medial umbilical ligament
Ductus arteriosus	Ligamentum arteriosum
Ductus venosus	Ligamentum venosum
Foramen ovale	Fossa ovalis
Alla**N**tois-urachus	Media**N** umbilical ligament
Notochord	Nucleus pulposus of the intervertebral disk
Inferior epigastric artery, vein	Lateral umbilical ligament

Fetal-Postnatal Derivatives

Some embryonic structures persist in the adult mostly as anatomical markers (see Table 4-3).

Aortic Arch Derivatives

At the beginning of the fifth week, a **series of paired arteries and veins** supply the head, body, yolk sac, and developing placenta. The head and body are specifically supplied by a pair of aortic and carotid arteries that form on either side of the pharynx as an extension of the **aortic sac** (see Figure 4-20 and Table 4-4). The *aortic* arches appear in cranial to caudal order, and each travels through the center of a *pharyngeal* arch. During the fifth week, **the vessels fuse, sprout,** and **regress** to form the adult vascular system.

Pharyngeal (Branchial) Apparatus

Lower head and neck development begins with the appearance of the pharyngeal apparatus. This apparatus is composed of **clefts, arches,** and **pouches.**

KEY FACT

The **urachus** is part of the **allantoic duct** between the bladder and the umbilicus.

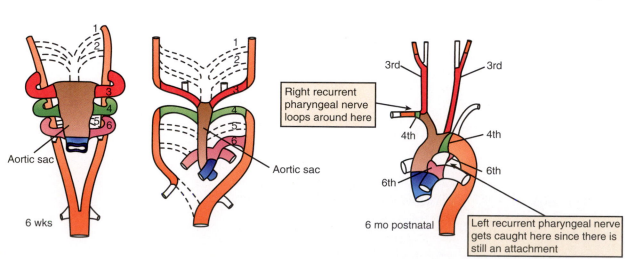

Right recurrent pharyngeal nerve loops around here

Left recurrent pharyngeal nerve gets caught here since there is still an attachment

Aortic sac

6 wks

Aortic sac

6 mo postnatal

3rd   3rd
4th   4th
6th   6th

FIGURE 4-20. Aortic arch development. To develop the adult vascular system, the rudimentary paired arteries and veins fuse, sprout, and regress.

TABLE 4-4. **Aortic Arch Derivatives**

ARCH	FATE	MNEMONIC
First	Part of **MAX**illary.	First arch is **MAX**imal.
Second	**S**tapedial artery, hyoid artery.	**S**econd = **s**tapedial.
Third	Common **C**arotid artery, proximal part of the internal carotid artery.	**C** is the third letter of the alphabet.
Fourth	Left = aortic arch; Right = proximal part of the right subclavian artery.	Fourth arch (four limbs) = systemic.
Fifth	*(Fails to form).*	
Sixth	Proximal part of pulmonary arteries; left only = ductus arteriosus.	Sixth arch = pulmonary and the pulmonary-to-systemic shunt (ductus arteriosus).

The clefts are an external lining derived from ectoderm. The arches are a mesenchyme derived from mesoderm and neural crest cells. The pouches are an internal lining derived from endoderm (see Figure 4-21).

Pharyngeal Arches

The mesenchymal core of the pharyngeal arches form the **bone and musculature of the face and neck** (see Figure 4-22). The cranial nerves (CNs) present in the core of each arch innervate the structures that are derived from that arch (see Table 4-5).

Pharyngeal Clefts and Pouches

The linings of the pharyngeal arches give rise to **epithelial linings, glandular structures**, and **cavities** (see Figure 4-23 and Table 4-6).

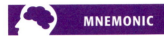

MNEMONIC

Pharyngeal apparatus—

CAP covers outside from inside:

Clefts = ectoderm
Arches = mesoderm
Pouches = endoderm

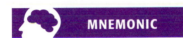

MNEMONIC

Pharyngeal arch 3 derivatives—

Think of pharynx:
Stylo**pharyngeus** is innervated by the glosso**pharyngeal** nerve.

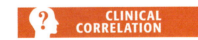

CLINICAL CORRELATION

DiGeorge's syndrome is a congenital immunodeficiency resulting from aberrant development of the third and fourth pharyngeal pouches. The syndrome is marked by **T-cell deficiency** (thymic aplasia) and **hypocalcemia** (failure of parathyroid development).

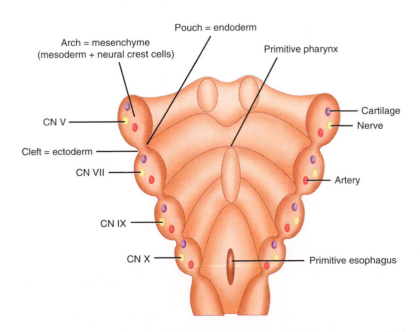

FIGURE 4-21. **The pharyngeal apparatus.** The pharyngeal apparatus consists of the outer pharyngeal clefts, the core pharyngeal arches, and the inner pharyngeal pouches.

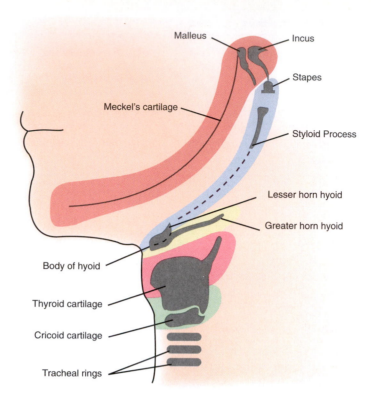

FIGURE 4-22. **The pharyngeal arch bone derivatives.** The pharyngeal arches contribute to the bone and musculature of the face.

TONGUE DEVELOPMENT

The **anterior two thirds** of the tongue is derived from the **first pharyngeal arch** (see Figure 4-24). Accordingly, its sensation is derived from V3 and its taste from CN VII. The **posterior one third** of the tongue is derived from the **third and fourth pharyngeal arches.** Accordingly, its sensation is derived from CN IX and the extreme posterior from CN X. All motor innervation for the tongue is derived from CN XII.

TERATOGENS

A teratogen is any agent that can cause birth defects following fetal exposure during a critical period of development. Teratogens include infectious agents, drugs, nutritional factors, chemicals, and ionizing radiation (see Table 4-7). There are three different periods during embryologic development during which a fetus may be exposed to a teratogen:

"All or None" Period (Weeks 1–3)

In early embryogenesis, the fetus will either die due to cellular injury induced by the teratogen or will survive unaffected if enough undifferentiated embryonic cells remain to replace the damaged or destroyed cells.

Embryonic Period (Weeks 3–8)

The fetus is most susceptible to teratogens at this time because organ systems and body regions are being established during this period. Teratogen exposure during this period generally results in **organ malformation.** Each organ system develops at different times and at different rates; therefore, each organ system will have different periods of susceptibility to various insults.

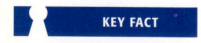

KEY FACT

Weeks 3–8 generate (organs).

TABLE 4-5. Derivatives of the Pharyngeal Arches

ARCH	CARTILAGE	MUSCLE	NERVE
1	**Meckel's** ■ **M**andible ■ **M**alleus ■ Incus ■ Spheno**M**andibular ligament	■ **M**uscles of **M**astication ■ Te**M**poralis ■ **M**asseter ■ Lateral pterygoid ■ **M**edial pterygoid ■ **M**ylohyoid ■ Anterior belly digastric ■ Tensor tympani ■ Tensor veli palatini	CN V$_3$
2	**Reichert's** ■ **S**tapes ■ **S**tyloid process ■ Lesser horn of the hyoid ■ **S**tylohyoid ligament	■ Muscles of facial expression ■ **S**tapedius ■ **S**tylohyoid ■ Posterior belly digastric	CN VII
3	Greater horn of the hyoid	Stylopharyngeus	CN IX
4–6	■ Thyroid ■ Cricoid ■ Arytenoids ■ Corniculate ■ Cuneiform	From fourth arch ■ Most pharyngeal constrictors ■ Cricothyroid ■ Levator veli palatini From sixth arch ■ All intrinsic muscles of the larynx **(except cricothyroid)**	Fourth = CN X Sixth = CN X (recurrent laryngeal branch)

CN = cranial nerve.

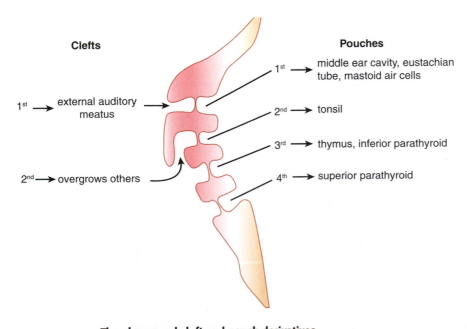

Clefts

1st → external auditory meatus

2nd → overgrows others

Pouches

1st → middle ear cavity, eustachian tube, mastoid air cells

2nd → tonsil

3rd → thymus, inferior parathyroid

4th → superior parathyroid

FIGURE 4-23. The pharyngeal cleft and pouch derivatives.

TABLE 4-6. Pharyngeal Cleft and Pouch Derivatives

ARCH	CLEFT DERIVATIVES	POUCH DERIVATIVES
1	External auditory meatus	▪ Middle ear cavity ▪ Eustachian tube ▪ Mastoid air cells
2		Epithelial lining of the palatine tonsil.
3	Temporary cervical sinuses obliterated by proliferation of the second arch mesenchyme.	▪ Dorsal wings → inferior parathyroids ▪ Ventral wings → thymus
4		Superior parathyroids

Fetal Period (Weeks 9–38)

The fetus has a decreased susceptibility to teratogens at this time because all organs have already been formed. Teratogen exposure during this period generally results in **organ malfunction** or growth disturbances.

Fetal infections can also cause congenital malformations.

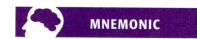

TWINNING

Dizygotic (Fraternal) Twins

Dizygotic twins are formed when **two different sperm** fertilize **two different secondary oocytes** (see Figure 4-25). This produces two separate zygotes, which form two separate blastocysts. These unique blastocysts implant into the endometrium of the uterus independently and eventually form **two distinct placentas**, **chorions**, and **amniotic sacs.** The end result is two siblings that are genetically distinct, just like siblings born at two different times.

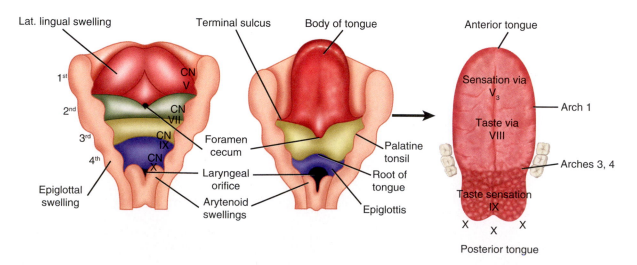

FIGURE 4-24. **Tongue development.** As the tongue develops from the pharyngeal arches, its taste and sensation are derived from the cranial nerves innervating the corresponding arches.

TABLE 4-7. Examples of Teratogens

TERATOGEN	EFFECTS ON FETUS
Alcohol	Birth defects and mental retardation (leading cause), fetal alcohol syndrome.
ACE inhibitors	Renal damage.
Cocaine	Abnormal fetal development and fetal addiction.
DES	Vaginal clear cell adenocarcinoma (occurs later in life).
Iodide	Congenital goiter or hypothyroidism.
13-*cis*-retinoic acid	Extremely high risk of birth defects.
Thalidomide	Limb defects ("flipper" limbs), cardiovascular defects, ear defects.
Tobacco	Preterm labor, placental problems, ADHD.
Warfarin	Multiple anomalies.
X-rays	Multiple anomalies.

ACE = angiotensin-converting enzyme; ADHD = attention deficit/hyperactivity disorder; DES = diethylstilbestrol.

Monozygotic

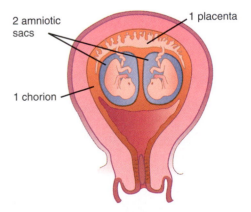

1 zygote splits evenly to develop 2 amniotic sacs with a single common chorion and placenta.

Dizygotic (fraternal) or monozygotic

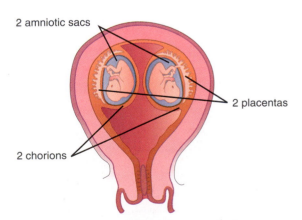

Dizygotes develop individual placentas, chorions, and amniotic sacs.

Monozygotes develop 2 placentas (separate/fused), chorions, and amniotic sacs.

FIGURE 4-25. Twinning.

Monozygotic (Identical) Twins

Monozygotic twins are formed when **one sperm** fertilizes **one secondary oocyte**. This produces one zygote, which forms one blastocyst. Instead of the single blastocyst forming a single fetus, however, the inner cell mass splits into two, resulting in the formation of two genetically identical siblings. Monozygotic twins most commonly develop a **single placenta and chorion** and two separate amniotic sacs (65% of the time), but may also develop two separate placentas, chorions, and amniotic sacs (35% of the time).

Conjoined (Siamese) Twins

Conjoined twins are considered monozygotic twins in whom the inner cell mass never fully separated. The two embryos are genetically identical and remain fused by a tissue bridge of variable proportions at birth.

In Vitro Fertilization (IVF)

IVF of oocytes and the subsequent transfer of cleaving embryos into the uterus is an assisted reproductive technology that includes several steps:

- Gonadotropins are given to the female to stimulate growth and maturity of the ovarian follicles.
- Maturing oocytes are monitored via ultrasound, and oocytes are collected from the ovary via needle aspiration.
- Sperm is collected via masturbation.
- In vitro culture of capacitated sperm and secondary oocytes is performed in a specialized medium to allow fertilization to occur.
- Once fertilization occurs, the zygote (an oocyte that has been fertilized) undergoes two to three rounds of cell division to become a 4- to 8-cell totipotent blastocyst.
- The cleaved embryo or blastocyst is then implanted into the uterus. (Typically, three or more blastocysts are implanted to increase the chances of success.)
- The remaining blastocysts are frozen for safekeeping for future use if needed or desired.

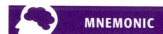

MNEMONIC

Young **L**iver **S**ynthesizes **T**he **B**lood:

Yolk sac (3–8 weeks)
Liver (6–30 weeks)
Spleen and **T**hymus (9–28 weeks)
Bone marrow (28 weeks onward)

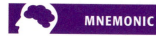

MNEMONIC

Fetal **F**ights (with the mother for O$_2$).

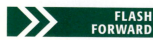

FLASH FORWARD

Thalassemia syndromes are disorders characterized by defects in either the α-globin (α-thalassemia) or β-globin (β-thalassemia) chain of hemoglobin.

FETAL ERYTHROPOIESIS

Erythropoiesis begins in the **third week of development**, when blood islands appear in the **mesoderm** around the wall of the yolk sac. Within the center of the blood islands are hemangioblasts, the pluripotent hematopoietic stem cells that will form all future blood cells. Although the first blood cells arise in the yolk sac, this site of blood formation is only temporary. By the fifth week, intraembryonic hematopoiesis begins to take place in different organs in a sequential manner:

1. Yolk sac (3–8 weeks)
2. Liver (6–30 weeks)
3. Spleen and thymus (9–28 weeks)
4. Bone marrow (28 weeks onward)

Hemoglobin

Three types of hemoglobin are synthesized during fetal erythropoiesis, corresponding to the organ involved in production (see Table 4-8). Fetal hemoglobin ($\alpha_2\gamma_2$) is the primary form during gestation because it has a higher affin-

TABLE 4-8. Timing of Various Hemoglobin Expressions During Fetal Erythropoiesis

PERIOD	HEMOGLOBIN TYPE
Yolk sac (3–8 wk)	Embryonic hemoglobin = $\delta_2\varepsilon_2$
Liver period (6–30 wk)	Fetal hemoglobin = $\alpha_2\gamma_2$
Bone marrow period (28 wk onward)	Adult hemoglobin = $\alpha_2\beta_2$

ity for O_2 than the adult form ($\alpha_2\beta_2$) and is therefore able to "steal" O_2 from maternal blood for fetal use. The switch between the fetal and adult forms occurs gradually, beginning at 30 weeks' gestation, and ultimately results in the fetal form being entirely replaced by the adult form.

NOTES

Microbiology

Bacteriology

BACTERIAL STRUCTURES

Prokaryotic organisms exhibit several structural components (see Figure 5-1).

Cytoplasmic Structures

Differ between eukaryotes and prokaryotes (see Table 5-1). Bacteria carry the following intracellular components:

KEY FACT

Because bacterial ribosomes and RNA polymerases differ from humans', they are ideal targets for antibiotics.

- **Bacterial chromosome:** Circular, double-stranded, and contained within the nucleoid.
- **Plasmids:** Smaller extrachromosomal DNA, often containing important genes, such as those that confer resistance to antibiotics.
- **Bacterial ribosome:** Consists of 30S and 50S subunits that form a 70S ribosome. Coupled in bacterial transcription and translation.

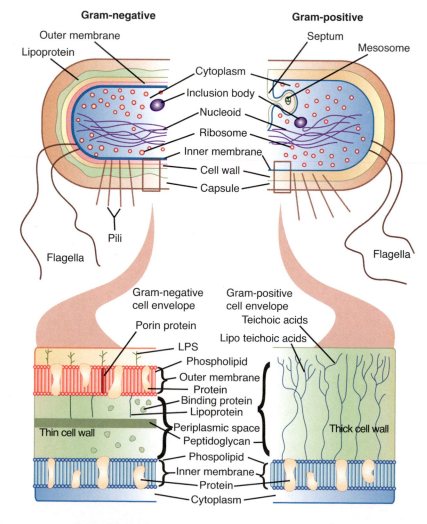

FIGURE 5-1. **Bacterial structures.**

TABLE 5-1. Eukaryotic versus Prokaryotic Cytoplasmic Structures

CYTOPLASMIC STRUCTURES	EUKARYOTE	PROKARYOTE
Nucleus	Nuclear membrane present	Nuclear membrane absent
Chromosomes	Linear, diploid DNA	Circular, haploid DNA
Ribosome	80S (60S + 40S)	70S (50S + 30S)
Cell membrane	Contains sterols	No sterols[a]
Mitochondria	Present	Absent
Golgi bodies	Present	Absent
Endoplasmic reticulum	Present	Absent
Respiration	Via mitochondria	Via cell membrane

[a]Mycoplasmas are an exception; as they incorporate sterols.

Bacterial Cell Walls

Composed of layers of **peptidoglycan** that surround the cytoplasmic membranes of bacteria, with the exception of **mycoplasma**, which has **no cell walls** (see Figure 5-1). The most important functions of the cell wall include:

- Resistance to osmotic stress.
- Necessary for cell division; serves as a primer for its own synthesis.
- Defines the shape of the bacteria; **coccus**, **bacillus** (Coccobacillus, Vibrio), **spirillum** (spirochete).
- Provides some protection from innate immune responses in humans.

Peptidoglycan synthesis occurs in several steps:

- **Glucosamine** is converted into N-acetylmuramic acid (MurNAc) and activated by UTP (uridine triphosphate) to UDP (uridine diphosphate)-MurNAc.
- A UDP-MurNAc-pentapeptide **precursor** is assembled.
- The UDP-MurNAc pentapeptide is attached to **bactoprenol** in the cytoplasmic membrane.
- **N-acetylglucosamine (GlcNAc)** is added to make a disaccharide.
- The bactoprenol translocates the disaccharide: **Peptide precursor** to the outside of the cell.
- The GlcNac-MurNac disaccharide is attached to a peptidoglycan chain by a **transglycosylase**.
- The pyrophosphobactoprenol is converted back to a phosphobactoprenol and recycled.
- Peptide chains from adjacent glycan chains are cross-linked to each other by **transpeptidation**.

External Bacterial Structures

There are several external bacterial structures of interest (see Figure 5-1):

- **Bacterial capsules** are usually composed of **glycocalyx**, with the **exception** of Bacillus anthracis (polypeptide capsule).
  - Important virulence factor. Capsules help to resist opsonization and phagocytosis.

KEY FACT

Mycoplasmas do not have cell walls.

KEY FACT

Some penicillin-binding proteins (PBPs) are **transpeptidases**; these are targeted by penicillin and other β-lactam antibiotics.

KEY FACT

Encapsulated bacteria:
Streptococcus pneumoniae, Haemophilus influenzae, Neisseria meningitidis, and Klebsiella pneumoniae.

Fimbriae adhering to other bacteria = F (sex) pili; transfer bacterial chromosomes to each other. Fimbriae adhering to **the host cell** (adhesion) = bacterial virulence factor.

- **Biofilms** are bacterial communities that can protect bacteria from antibiotics and host immune defenses.
- **Flagella** are **coiled protein subunits (flagellin)** anchored in bacterial membranes. They provide bacterial motility and express **antigenic (H antigen)** and **strain determinants** useful for serotyping bacteria.
- **Fimbriae** are hair-like structures on the outside of bacteria, composed of repeating subunits of the protein **pilin**. Fimbriae often promote **adherence** to other bacteria or to host cells.

Bacterial cell walls differ between gram-positive and gram-negative bacteria (see Figure 5-1 and Tables 5-2 and 5-3):

- **Gram-positive bacteria:** Thick cell wall, composed of many layers of **peptidoglycan.** The linkage between one layer of peptidoglycan and another (via the third and fourth amino acids of glucosamine pentapeptide) is further extended by a pentaglycine bridge, whereas gram-negative bacteria link their pentapeptide changes directly. Without peptidogylcan, the bacteria would lyse due to the differential in osmotic pressure across the cytoplasmic membrane. Gram-positive bacteria are also associated with **teichoic** and **lipoteichoic acids,** useful in distinguishing bacterial serotypes, promoting bacterial interactions with human cell receptors, and initiating host immune responses.
- **Gram-negative bacteria:** Consist of both a **peptidoglycan layer,** making up only 5%–10% of the cell wall, and **an outer membrane.**
  - **Periplasmic space**—area between the cytoplasmic membrane and the outer membrane. Contains **enzymes** necessary for metabolism and vir-

TABLE 5-2. **Gram-Positive and Gram-Negative Bacterial Membrane Structures**

GRAM-POSITIVE		GRAM-NEGATIVE	
STRUCTURE	**CHEMICAL CONSTITUENTS**	**STRUCTURE**	**CHEMICAL CONSTITUENTS**
Peptidoglycan	Chains of GlcNAc and MurNAc peptide bridges cross-linked by pentaglycine chains.	Peptidoglycan	Thinner version of that found in gram-positive bacteria with direct peptide bridging and no pentaglycine chains.
Teichoic acid	Glycerol phosphate or polyribitol phosphate cross-linked to peptidoglycan.	Periplasmic space	Enzymes involved in transport, degradation, and synthesis.
Lipoteichoic acid	Lipid-linked teichoic acid.	Outer membrane	Fatty acids and phospholipids.
Proteins	Porins, transport proteins.	Proteins	Porins, lipoprotein, transport proteins.
Plasma membrane	Phospholipids, proteins, and enzymes involved in generation of energy, membrane potential and transport.	Lipopolysaccharide (LPS)	Core polysaccharide, O antigen, lipid A.
Capsule	Disaccharides, trisaccharides, and polypeptides.	Plasma membrane	Same as gram-positive bacteria.
Pili	Pilin, adhesions.	Capsule	Polysaccharides and polypeptides.
Flagellum	Flagellin, motor proteins.	Pili	Pilin, adhesions.
		Flagellum	Flagellin, motor proteins.

TABLE 5-3. Summary of Gram-Positive and Gram-Negative Bacteria

MEMBRANE CHARACTERISTIC	GRAM-POSITIVE	GRAM-NEGATIVE
Outer membrane	–	+
Cell wall	Thick	Thin
Lipopolysaccharide (endotoxin)	–	+
Teichoic acid	Often present	–
Sporulation	Some strains	–
Capsule	Sometimes present	Sometimes present
Lysozyme	Sensitive	Resistant

ulence factors, such as proteases, phosphatases, lipases, nucleases, collagenases, hyaluronidases, and β-lactamases.

- There is **no** teichoic or lipoteichoic acid in gram-negative bacteria.
- Gram-negative bacteria contain **lipopolysaccharide (LPS-endotoxin)**, used for serotyping gram-negative bacteria. LPS is a potent activator of immune cells, and stimulates release of **interleukin-1 (IL-1), IL-6,** and **tumor necrosis factor (TNF)**, major pyrogenic substances.

KEY FACT

Neisseria contains a shorter version of LPS called lipo-oligosaccharide (LOS).

BACTERIAL GROWTH AND METABOLISM

Bacterial Growth and Death

The **minimum requirements** for bacterial growth are a source of carbon and nitrogen, an energy source, water, and various ions. When these conditions are met, bacteria must also obtain or synthesize the **amino acids, carbohydrates,** and **lipids** necessary for building proteins, structures, and membranes. A cascade of regulatory events then initiates **DNA synthesis**, which then runs to completion.

Bacterial growth occurs in **four phases** (see Figure 5-2):

- **Lag phase:** Gathering of necessary growth requirements, no divisions occur during this phase.
- **Log phase (or exponential phase):** Growth and cell division begins. The doubling time varies among different strains and conditions.
- **Stationary phase:** Depicts the point at which bacteria run out of metabolites, and toxic (metabolic) products start building up. This causes cessation of bacterial growth.
- **Decline phase:** Death of bacterial cells after stationary phase.

Bacterial growth is assessed in three ways: Viable cell counts, optical density, and metabolic products.

- **Viable cell counts** (colony-forming units—CFU/mL).
- **Optical density** (spectrophotometry).
- **Indirect measurement** of bacterial numbers by detection of metabolic by-products (CO_2).

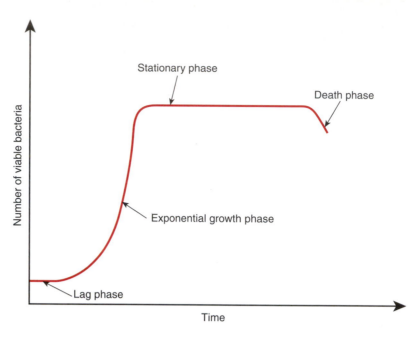

FIGURE 5-2. **Bacterial growth curve.** Depicted are lag phase, exponential growth phase, and stationary phase.

Bacterial growth is **controlled** by subjecting bacterial populations to heat, antimicrobial chemicals, and antibiotics (please see discussion below).

Key mechanisms of bacterial growth control include (see Table 5-4):

- Alteration of membrane permeability.
- Denaturation of proteins.
- Interference with DNA replication—alkylating agents.
- Oxidation.

Bacterial Metabolism

Major **essential elements** necessary for bacterial metabolism include carbon, hydrogen, nitrogen, sulfur, phosphorus, potassium, magnesium, calcium, iron, sodium, chloride, and O_2.

Bacterial needs for O_2 can be divided into four groups:

- **Obligate (or strict) anaerobes:** Cannot grow in the presence of O_2.
- **Facultative anaerobes:** Can grow either in the presence or absence of O_2.
- **Obligate (or strict) aerobes:** Require molecular O_2.
- **Microaerophilic:** Require very low levels of O_2 for growth.

A **carbon source** is required by all bacteria. Genre can be differentiated based on the type of carbon they use (i.e., **lactose**, **glucose**, and **galactose**).

Bacteria can produce energy either via aerobic respiration, anaerobic respiration, or fermentation.

- **Aerobic respiration:** Completely converts glucose into CO_2 and H_2O and forms adenosine triphosphate (ATP) through **substrate level** and **oxidative phosphorylation.**
- **Anaerobic respiration:** ATP is also formed through substrate level phosphorylation; however, another higher energy molecular such as SO_4^{2-} and NO_3^- are used as the terminal electron acceptors rather than O_2. Anaero-

KEY FACT

Not all bacteria require O_2 for survival and replication.

KEY FACT

Some bacteria are incapable of generating their own ATP and must dwell inside host cells that can. These **obligate intracellular pathogens** include *Rickettsia* and *Chlamydia*.

TABLE 5-4. **Methods of Controlling Bacterial Growth**

METHOD	ACTIVITY LEVEL, MECHANISM	SPECTRUM
Heat		
Steam autoclave	Sterilizing, membrane-active, protein denaturant.	All bacterial growth phases, viruses, fungi.
Boiling	Highly effective, membrane-active, protein denaturant.	Most growth phases, some spores, viruses, fungi.
Pasteurization	Intermediate, membrane-active, protein denaturant.	Vegetative cells.
Dry heat	High, membrane-active, protein denaturant.	All bacterial growth phases, viruses, fungi.
Chemical		
Ethylene oxide gas	Sterilizing, alkylating agent.	All bacterial growth phases, viruses, fungi.
Alcohol	Intermediate, membrane-active, protein denaturant.	Vegetative cells, some viruses, fungi.
Hydrogen peroxide	High, membrane-active, oxidizing agent.	Vegetative cells, viruses, fungi.
Chlorine	High, oxidizing agent.	Vegetative cells, viruses, fungi.
Iodine compounds	Intermediate, iodination, oxidation.	Vegetative cells, viruses, fungi.
Phenolics, phenol, hexochlorophene, chlorhexidine	Intermediate, membrane-active.	Vegetative cells, some viruses, fungi.
Glutaraldehyde	High, alkylating agent.	Vegetative cells, viruses.
Formaldehyde	High, alkylating agent.	Bacteria, viruses, fungi.
Quaternary ammonium compounds	Low, membrane-active, cations.	Bacteria, viruses, fungi.
Radiation		
Ultraviolet	Sterilizing.	Bacteria, viruses, fungi.
Ionizing	Sterilizing.	Bacteria, viruses, fungi.
Physical		
Filtration	High, size exclusion.	Bacteria, fungi, some viruses.

bic respiration produces slightly less ATP than aerobic respiration, but is more efficient than the fermentation.

■ **Fermentation:** In the absence of O_2 and following substrate level phosphorylation, certain bacteria are able to ferment pyruvic acid. The **end products** of this process are two- and three-carbon compounds. These organic molecules in lieu of O_2 as **electron acceptors** to **recycle NADH to NAD.**

The end products of fermentation can also be used to distinguish particular bacteria.

Bacterial Genetics

The bacterial **genome** consists of the single **haploid chromosome** of the bacteria in addition to extrachromosomal genetic elements (**plasmids** and **bacteriophages**). These elements may be independent of the bacterial chromosome and, in most cases, can be transmitted from one cell to another.

Exchange of genetic material between bacterial cells can occur via three mechanisms:

- **Conjugation** (see Figure 5-3): **One-way transfer of DNA** from a donor cell to a recipient cell through the sex (**F**) pilus. Conjugation typically occurs between members of the same species or related species.
  - The **donor bacterium** must carry the **F plasmid** (**F+, male**) and the other must not (**F−, female**). The F plasmid carries all the genes necessary for its own transfer.
  - Integration of the F plasmid into chromosomal DNA results in the **Hfr** (high-frequency recombination) **state.** This allows the donor to transfer whole pieces of the chromosome into the recipient bacteria.

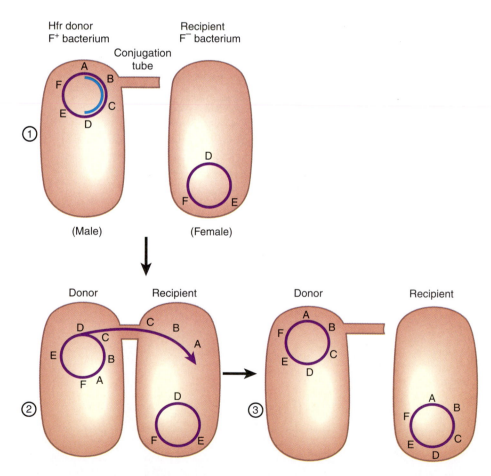

FIGURE 5-3. **Bacterial conjugation.** The transfer of genetic material from a donor bacterium to a recipient bacterium through contact is conjugation.

- If the F plasmid sequence is excised from the host chromosome, it may take some genes from the chromosome with it. This plasmid is called the F′ (F prime). Like F+, the prime plasmid can be transferred to an F- recipient and transfer the host gene along with it.
- **Conjugative R** = antibiotic resistance.
- **Transformation:** Bacteria take up **fragments of naked DNA** and **incorporate** them into their genomes if there is enough homology with the recipient chromosome for **homologous recombination** to occur. Certain species of bacteria such as *H. influenzae, S. pneumoniae, Bacillus* species, and *Neisseria* species are capable of taking up exogenous DNA.
- **Transduction:** Genetic transfer mediated by bacterial viruses, **bacteriophages.** The bacteriophages pick up fragments of DNA from a previous host bacterium and deliver it to newly infected cells. The new DNA may incorporate into the bacterial genomes with the phages. This is a very efficient way for bacteria to pass genetic information such as antibiotic resistance.

Bacterial Defenses—Pathogenic Factors

Bacteria have multiple levels of defense or **virulence factors** that allow them to protect themselves from the human immune system and/or promote disease. A few of these factors include capsules (explained above), spores, toxins, proteases, hemolysins, coagulase, and catalase (see Table 5-5).

TABLE 5-5. **Defensive Virulence Factors**

DEFENSE MECHANISMS	SPECIES OF BACTERIA
Spores	*Clostridium tetani* or *botulinum, Bacillus anthracis*
IgA proteases	*Streptococcus pneumoniae, Neisseria meningitidis, Neisseria gonorrhoeae, Haemophilus influenzae*
Cellular invasion	*Rickettsia* and *Chlamydia, Salmonella, Shigella, Brucella, Mycobacterium, Listeria, Francisella, Legionella, Yersinia*
Hemolysis	*Streptococcus pneumoniae, Staphylococcus pyogenes, Streptococcus agalactiae, Staphylococcus aureus, Listeria monocytogenes, Enterococcus*
Catalase	*Staphylococcus, Micrococcus, Listeria*
Coagulase	*Staphylococcus aureus*
Toxins	*Staphylococcus pyogenes, Staphylococcus aureus, Clostridium diphtheriae, Pseudomonas aeruginosa, Shigella dysenteriae, Escherichia coli, Vibrio cholerae, Bordetella pertussis, Clostridium difficile, Clostridium perfringens, Clostridium tetani, Clostridium botulinum*

SPORE

Dehydrated, multishelled structure that allows bacteria to survive when nutrients are limited. The spores are composed of:

- Inner membrane
- Two peptidoglycan layers
- Outer protein coat

The complete copy of the bacterium's chromosome, as well as the essential proteins and ribosomes necessary for germination, are confined within the spore. A spore can survive for decades, protecting bacterial DNA from heat, radiation, enzymes, and chemical agents (e.g., most disinfectants).

PIGMENT PRODUCTION

Pigment is often useful in the identification of particular bacteria. Three important pigment-producing bacteria are *Staphylococcus aureus, Pseudomonas aeruginosa,* and *Serratia marcescens*.

IgA PROTEASES

Cleave immunoglobulin A (IgA) found on mucosal surfaces and functions as a first line of defense against pathogens. Cleavage prevents opsonization, thus allowing bacteria to enter unnoticed by the host's immune system.

CELLULAR INVASION

Some bacteria are able to live and replicate intracellularly to avoid the host's immune system. There are **obligate** and **facultative** intracellular bacteria.

HEMOLYSIS

The breakdown of red blood cells in culture by hemolytic enzymes. Hemolysis is useful in categorizing types of streptococci. **Three types** of hemolysis are identified (see Figure 5-4):

- α-**Hemolysis** results in greenish darkening of the blood agar. Keep in mind that the green color change of the agar is actually caused by peroxide produced by the bacteria, not hemolysin, and therefore α-hemolysis is often referred to as **partial hemolysis.**
- β-**Hemolysis** complete clearing of the blood agar (complete hemolysis by hemolysin).
- γ-**Hemolysis** designates no hemolysis (there is no change to the blood agar).

CATALASES

These are enzymes that catabolize hydrogen peroxide into water and O_2. The presence or absence of catalase can be used to categorize gram-positive cocci.

COAGULASE

Used to **distinguish** S. *aureus* (the most common species of staphylococci found in humans that produces the enzyme coagulase) from other forms of staphylococci.

TOXINS

Three major types of toxins exist: endotoxin, exotoxin, and enterotoxin.

- **Endotoxin**, or **LPS**, is found in the outer cell membrane of gram-negative bacteria and can cause fever and shock.

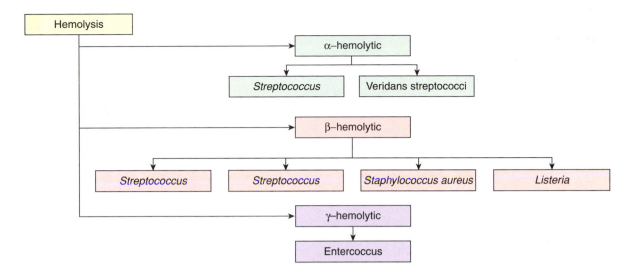

FIGURE 5-4. **Types of hemolysis.** Note that many other organisms besides enterococci are nonhemolytic, whereas enterococci can also be β, α, or γ.

- **Exotoxins** are **polypeptides** secreted by bacteria that cause harm to the host by altering cellular structure or function. Exotoxins are very potent and a very low minimum dose may be lethal to the host.
- **Enterotoxins** are toxins that act on the gut.

Toxins have **seven major mechanisms of action** (see Table 5-6):

1. **Facilitate spread through tissues:** Enzymes break down the extracellular matrix or degrade cellular debris in necrotic tissue.
2. **Damage membranes:** Cytolysins, pore-forming toxins cause death of the host cell.
3. **Stimulate production of excessive amounts of cytokines: Superantigens** bind to a site distinct from the antigen-binding site on the T-cell receptor, stimulating excess synthesis of cytokines including IL-2 and INF-γ.
4. **Inhibit protein synthesis:**
   - **Diphtheria toxin** and **P. aeruginosa** exotoxin A are ADP ribosyltransferases, which ribosylate and inactivate eukaryotic elongation factor 2 (EF-2), resulting in the cessation of protein synthesis.
   - **Shiga toxins** of **Shigella dysenteriae** and **Escherichia coli** are highly specific RNA N-glycosidases that remove one particular residue from the 28S RNA, thereby inactivating the ribosomes and halting protein synthesis.
5. **Activate second messenger pathways:** Exert hormone-like effects on the target cell, thus altering cell function without killing the cell.
   - **Heat-labile enterotoxins** Vibrio cholerae and E. coli are ADP ribosyltransferases that activate cell membrane–associated adenylate cyclase, thus activating **stimulatory (Gs) proteins**.
   - **Pertussis toxin (A and B components)** is an ADP ribosyltransferase that activates cell membrane–associated adenylate cyclase by ADP ribosylating the **inhibitory (Gi) protein** of the cyclase complex. Pertussis toxin can increase intracellular cAMP in many different target tissues, causing tissue-specific effects.
   - **Heat-stable enterotoxin I of E. coli** activates cell membrane–associated guanylate cyclase. Increased intracellular cGMP in enterocytes causes secretory diarrhea.

KEY FACT

In plasma, coagulase binds to serum factor and coverts fibrinogen to fibrin, forming a clot.

KEY FACT

Enzymes that facilitate spread through tissues: Hyaluronidase, DNAse, collegenase, elastase, streptokinase.

KEY FACT

Superantigens: Scarlet fever toxin of Streptococcus pyogenes, toxic shock syndrome toxin (TSST) of S. aureus, and Staphylococcus enterotoxins.

KEY FACT

Toxins that inhibit protein synthesis: Diphtheria toxin, exotoxin A of P. aeruginosa, Shiga toxins of S. dysenteriae, and E. coli.

TABLE 5-6. Bacterial Toxicity in Brief

Microorganism	Toxin Type	Mechanism	Molecular Result	Clinical Result
Corynebacterium diphtheriae	Diphtheria toxin.	Inactivates EF-2 via ADP–ribosyltransferases.	Inhibits protein synthesis.	Upper respiratory tract infection. Sore throat. Low fever.
Pseudomonas aeruginosa	Exotoxin A.	Inactivates EF-2 via ADP–ribosyltransferases.	Inhibits protein synthesis.	Urinary tract infection.
Escherichia coli	*Heat-labile* (LT) enterotoxin (ETEC).	Activates adenylate cyclase via ADP ribosylation of *Gs*.	Activates second-messenger pathway $\uparrow$ cAMP.	Secretory diarrhea.
	Heat-stable (ST) enterotoxin (ETEC).	Activates guanylate cyclase.	Activates second-messenger pathway $\uparrow$ cGMP.	Secretory diarrhea.
	Shiga toxins, e.g., EHEC strain *O157:H7.*	Inactivates ribosome via RNA N-glycosidase.	Inhibits protein synthesis.	Abdominal pain, fever. Bloody, mucoid, WBCs in stools. Reiter's symptoms. Toxin binds to Gb3 receptor on glomerular epithelial cells. Swelling and fibrin deposits in glomerulus.
Shigella dysenteriae	Shiga toxin.	Inactivate ribosome via RNA N-glycosidase.	Inhibits protein synthesis.	
Vibrio cholerae	Cholera toxin. Heat-labile (LT) enterotoxin.	Activates adenylate cyclase via ADP ribosylation of *Gs*.	Activates second-messenger pathway $\uparrow$ cAMP. CL(−) out Na (+) in	*Hypersecretory diarrhea* with great loss of fluid and electrolytes.
Bordetella pertussis	Pertussis toxin.	Activates adenylate cyclase via ADP ribosylation of *Gi*.	Activates second-messenger pathway $\uparrow$ cAMP.	$\uparrow$ Secretion in upper respiratory tract. Other tissue effects.
Clostridium tetani	Tetanus toxin.	Blocks release of glycine and GABA from inhibitory neurons.	Zinc-dependent proteases cleave VAMP.	Uncontrolled muscle spasms. *Spastic paralysis.*
Clostridium botulinum	Botulinum toxin (A, B, E).	Blocks release of acetylcholine at neuromuscular junctions.	Zinc-dependent proteases cleave VAMP.	*Flaccid paralysis.*
Bacillus anthracis	Anthrax toxin factor.	Calmodulin-dependent calcium activation.	Activates second-messenger pathway $\uparrow$ cAMP.	Edema, lethal.

- **Anthrax edema factor** is an adenylate cyclase toxin similar to that of *Bordetella pertussis*. Toxins enter target cells, increase intracellular cAMP, and produce cAMP-dependent effects. Their enzymatic activity is activated by **calmodulin**-dependent **calcium activation** in target cells.

6. **Inhibit release of neurotransmitters:** Botulinum and tetanus toxins.
   - **Botulinum toxin** causes **flaccid paralysis** by inhibiting the release of **acetylcholine** at myoneural junctions.
   - **Tetanus toxin** inhibits the release of neurotransmitters **(glycine and GABA)** from inhibitory interneurons in the spinal cord, resulting in stimulation of muscular contraction and tetany **(spastic paralysis).**

7. **Modify the cytoskeleton** of the target cell by glucosylating RhoA (a small GTP-binding protein), causing disaggregation of actin filaments. This results in the formation of pseudomembranes in the colon (e.g., *C. difficile* cytotoxin B).

MICROBIOLOGIC STAINS

The microscopic examination and subsequent identification of microorganisms are greatly aided by the use of stains, which generate artificial contrast so the organism can be visualized. Bacteriologic specimens are always submitted to one or more **differential stains**, which aid in identification by permitting visualization of certain cellular substructures. Further biochemical tests are used to definitively characterize the organism.

Staining Methods

Bacteria can be seen microscopically via:

- **Direct examination:** Performed by suspending bacteria in liquid (sometimes called a **wet mount**). This is useful for detecting motility, for distinguishing larger organisms such as yeasts and parasites from bacteria, and for visualizing *Treponema pallidum*, using darkfield microscopy.
- **Acid-fast stains** include **Ziehl-Neelsen**, **Kinyoun**, and **auramine-rhodamine**. They are used to stain the bacteria only if pretreated with acid-alkali solutions because the bacteria resist decolorization. Acid fast staining is particularly useful in identifying **mycobacteria**. However, other acid-fast organisms include *Nocardia, Rhodococcus, Tsukamurella, Gordonia, Cryptosporidium, Isospora, Sarcocystis,* and *Cyclospora*.
- **Fluorescent stains** include Acridine orange, auramine-rhodamine, calcofluor, and direct/indirect fluorescent antibody staining.
  - **The Acridine orange** stains DNA so that bacteria or fungi fluoresce a reddish orange at an acidic pH.
  - **Calcofluor staining** is used on fungi.

Fluorescent antibody staining is based on the recognition of pathogens by staining with fluorescently labeled antibodies specific for the pathogens.

Gram's Stain

The best-known and most widely used differential stain for bacteria (see Table 5-7; depicting respective staining patterns of different bacterial species) because it permits identification of the bacteria based on the chemical and physical properties of their cell walls. This method is fast and reliable when fast diagnosis is needed. It is usually performed on bodily fluids (e.g., cerebrospinal fluid [CSF] for meningitis or synovial fluid for septic arthritis).

CLINICAL CORRELATION

Increased cAMP in enterocytes causes secretory diarrhea.

CLINICAL CORRELATION

Tissue-specific effects of pertussis toxin: Islet cell activation (↑ hypoglycemia), increased histamine sensitivity, inhibition of immune effector cells.

KEY FACT

Toxins that activate second-messenger systems: Edema factor of *B. anthracis*, adenylate cyclase toxin and pertussis toxins of *B. pertussis*, heat-stable enterotoxin and heat-labile toxin of *E. coli*, heat labile toxin of *V. cholerae*.

KEY FACT

Botulinum toxin ↑ **flaccid paralysis**
Tetanus toxin ↑ **spastic paralysis**

KEY FACT

Toxins that modify the cytoskeleton: Cytotoxic necrotizing factor of uropathogenic *E. coli*, toxin of *C. difficile*.

KEY FACT

The waxy coat of mycobacteria resists acid, thus making them **acid-fast**. They stain red with the acid-fast stain.

TABLE 5-7. Gram-Staining Patterns of Various Bacterial Species

STAIN	GRAM-POSITIVE	GRAM-NEGATIVE
Bacteria	Staphylococcus, Streptococcus, Clostridium, Listeria, Bacillus, Corynebacterium	Neisseria, Haemophilus influenzae, Pasteurella, Brucella, Bordetella pertussis, Klebsiella, Escherichia coli, Enterobacter, Citrobacter, Serratia, Shigella, Salmonella, Proteus, Pseudomonas

KEY FACT

Following Gram's stain, some bacteria yield a **gram-variable** pattern; that is, a mix of pink and purple cells can be seen.

KEY FACT

Bacteria that **are not visualized on Gram's stain** are:
- *Treponema*
- *Rickettsia*
- *Mycobacteria*
- *Mycoplasma*
- *Legionella*
- *Chlamydia*

MNEMONIC

Gram-**p**ositive bacteria are **purple**; gram-**n**egative bacteria are **not**.

FLASH FORWARD

β-**Lactam** antibiotics target the enzymes—penicillin-binding proteins (PBPs)—responsible for cross-linking amino acids in peptidoglycan molecules. Eukaryotes (like us) possess neither peptidoglycan nor PBPs and thus are intrinsically "resistant" to these antibiotics.

In a Gram's stain preparation, gram-positive bacteria appear dark blue to **purple**, and gram-negative bacteria are **red.**

The procedure includes:

- Application of a sample to a glass slide and fixation under a flame.
- Application of the primary stain—crystal violet (CV).
- Application of iodine to bind and "set" the dye.
- Washing away of unbound CV from gram-negative organisms during decolorization.
- Counterstaining of gram-negative organisms with the red dye safranin.

The mechanism of staining is based on the following properties/interactions:

- CV penetrates the cell wall and membrane of both gram-positive and gram-negative cells.
- **Iodine** interacts with CV and forms complexes of CV and iodine within the inner and outer layers of the bacterial cells.
- **Decolorizer** disintegrates the lipids of the cell membranes, thus gram-negative cells lose their outer membrane, exposing the peptidoglycan layer, whereas gram-positive cells dehydrate following treatment with ethanol.
  - Decolorization washes out the CV–iodine complexes and outer membrane from gram-negative cells.
  - CV–iodine complexes remain "trapped" within the gram-positive cells owing to the multilayered composition of their peptidoglycan.
- Following decolorization:
  - **Gram-positive** bacteria remain (stain) **purple.**
  - **Gram-negative** bacteria **lose** their **purple** color.
- Application of the **counterstain** (either positively charged safranin or basic fuchsin) stains decolorized **gram-negative** bacteria **pink or red,** respectively.

GRAM-POSITIVE CELL WALL

The cell wall of gram-positive organisms consists principally of **peptidoglycan,** which form multiple layers of a thick mesh outside the plasma membrane, and captures the Gram's stain (hence gram-positive organisms are blue/purple—see Figure 5-5). **Teichoic acids** are exclusively found in gram-positive organisms, and are covalently linked to the peptidoglycan molecules and can act as virulence factors. The laboratory algorithm for biochemically identifying gram-positive organisms is shown in Figure 5-6.

GRAM-NEGATIVE CELL WALL

Compared with the cell wall of gram-positive bacteria, gram-negative cell wall has a much thinner layer of peptidoglycan immediately outside the plasma membrane. Crystal violet is easily washed out of this thin mesh by the decolorizer (hence the red color on Gram's stain).

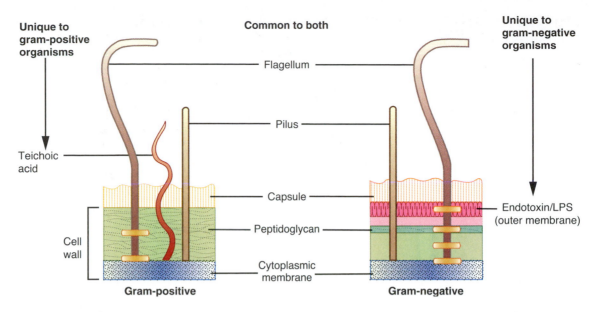

Unique to gram-positive organisms

Common to both

Unique to gram-negative organisms

Flagellum

Pilus

Teichoic acid

Capsule

Endotoxin/LPS (outer membrane)

Peptidoglycan

Cell wall

Cytoplasmic membrane

Gram-positive

Gram-negative

FIGURE 5-5. **Gram-positive and gram-negative cell wall structures.** The thick peptidoglycan mesh of the gram-positive cell wall effectively traps the crystal violet stain. LPS, lippopolysaccharide. (Modified, with permission, from Levinson W, Jawetz E. *Medical Microbiology and Immunology: Examination and Board Review.* 9th ed. New York: McGraw-Hill, 2006: 7.)

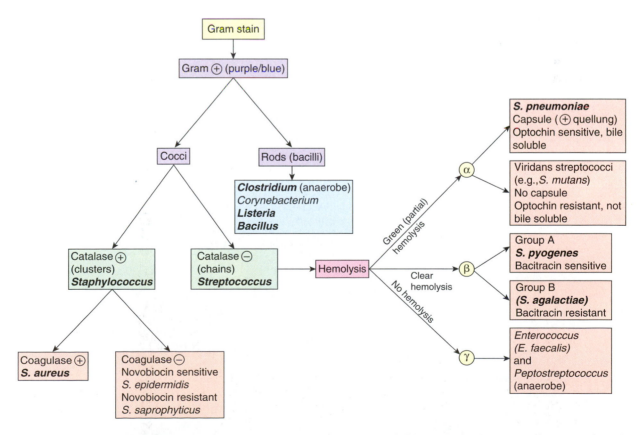

FIGURE 5-6. **Gram-positive laboratory algorithm.** Important pathogens are in bold type. Enterococcus is either α- or γ-hemolytic.

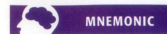

MNEMONIC

Gram-**ne**gative bacteria are the only ones containing **en**dotoxin.

External to the peptidoglycan layer is the **outer membrane,** a porous structure unique to gram-negative bacteria that contains phospholipids, embedded proteins, and most significantly LPS, a phospholipid molecule largely responsible for the virulence of gram-negative organisms.

LPS is often referred to as **endotoxin** (as opposed to an *exotoxin*) because it is an integral part of the bacteria. The space between the plasma membrane and the outer membrane is referred to as the **periplasmic space,** which contains various membrane-associated proteins as well as the thin peptidoglycan layer.

Cell wall structures related to motility, including **pili** and **flagella,** are common to both gram-positive and gram-negative cell walls. The laboratory algorithm for biochemically identifying gram-negative organisms is shown in Figure 5-7.

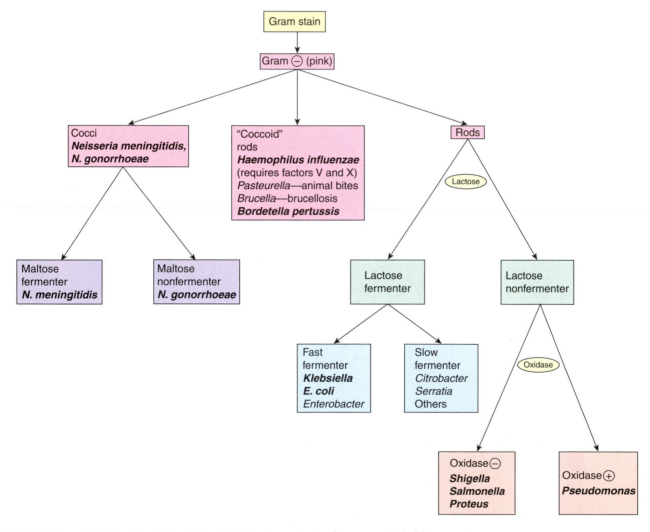

FIGURE 5-7. **Gram-negative laboratory algorithm.** Important pathogens are in bold type.

GRAM-INDETERMINATE ORGANISMS

Several medically important microorganisms are for a variety of reasons impossible to visualize on gram's stain preparation. Other techniques are necessary to visualize and/or identify these organisms in the laboratory.

MYCOBACTERIA. These intracellular organisms have a cell wall composed largely of mycolic acids, which are lipid-rich and prevent crystal violet from penetrating the cell wall. Mycobacteria can be visualized using an **acid-fast** (carbol fuschin) stain.

MYCOPLASMA. Truly gram-indeterminate organisms, these microbes possess **no cell wall.** Conventional laboratory stains do not work, so culture and serologic tests are used to make the diagnosis.

SPIROCHETES. The thin, corkscrew-shaped organisms in the genera *Treponema*, *Borrelia*, and *Leptospira* are too thin to be visualized via Gram's stain. Hence, darkfield microscopy, indirect immunofluorescence, serologic assays, and specialized tests (such as those for *T. palladium*) are used. Note that *Borrelia* microbes, fatter than the other two, can generally be seen on peripheral blood smears—the preferred mechanism for the laboratory identification of relapsing fever.

INTRACELLULAR MICROORGANISMS. *Rickettsia* spp. (including *Coxiella*), *Ehrlichia* spp., and *Chlamydia* spp. are all small, obligate intracellular parasites that live in the cytosol of infected cells. They stain poorly with Gram's stain, but share membrane characteristics with gram-negative organisms. Microscopy is generally not useful in the diagnosis of diseases caused by these organisms. *Listeria monocytogenes,* a gram-positive rod that is primarily intracellular, also does not take up crystal violet and is usually visualized on clinical specimens via a silver stain.

The limitations of Gram's staining (due to differences in composition of various microorganisms) are bypassed by using other staining methods (see Table 5-8).

Other Microbiologic Stains and Microscopic Techniques

For most common bacteria, Gram's stain is sufficient to make an accurate diagnosis. However, in certain cases, such as the identification of nonstainable organisms, fungi, and parasites, other techniques must be used (see Tables 5-9 and 5-10).

MNEMONIC

Gram-indeterminate organisms—

Some **E**rrant **R**ascals **M**ay **M**icroscopically **L**ack **C**olor:
Spirochetes
Ehrlichia
Rickettsia
Mycobacterium
Mycoplasma
Listeria
Chlamydia

FLASH FORWARD

Don't forget the important nonmicrobiologic tissue–based stains: **Congo red** for **amyloid**; **Sudan black** for **fat droplets**; **periodic acid–Schiff** for **glycogen**, and **trichrome** for **tissue collagen**.

BACTERIAL CULTURE

Growing bacteria on agar plates can provide additional diagnostic information for the identification of clinically relevant microorganisms. Bacteria often have a characteristic colony appearance when growing on conventional media. For example, bacteria with polysaccharide capsules generally have "wet" or **mucoid**-appearing colonies. Some bacteria also produce visibly pigmented colonies on agar:

- *Pseudomonas aeruginosa* produces a fluorescing blue-green pigment.
- *S. aureus* produces a **gold** pigment (think of **Au**reus, the abbreviation for gold on the periodic table).
- *Serratia marcescens* produces a red pigment.

TABLE 5-8. Gram Stain Limitations

BACTERIA	PREFERRED STAINING METHOD
Treponema	Darkfield microscopy and fluorescent antibody staining.
Rickettsia	Immunofluorescent and immunoperoxidase staining.
Mycobacterium	Acid-fast.
Mycoplasma	Do not stain.
Legionella pneumophila	Silver stain.
Chlamydia	Immunofluorescent staining.

Generally, bacteria from clinical specimens are grown on agar-based, permissive, nonselective medium, with an additional nutrient source (either hydrolyzed soy protein or sheep's blood). Isolated colonies from these agar plates can then be aseptically selected and used for further laboratory diagnosis via molecular, biochemical or serologic techniques, microscopy, or further culture.

TABLE 5-9. Microscopy Techniques and Stains Used in Microbiology

	ORGANISMS	RATIONALE
Darkfield microscopy	Spirochetes.	Thin organisms are more easily identified by this technique.
KOH (potassium hydroxide) preparation	Fungi.	*Fungal cell walls* are stable in strong alkali solution, unlike bacteria.
India ink	*Cryptococcus* in CSF specimens.	Cryptococcal *polysaccharide capsule* scatters ink, rendering it bright against dark background.
Wright/Giemsa	*Borrelia recurrentis* Blood parasites (*Plasmodium spp.,* *Trypanosoma spp.* and *Babesia microti*). *Chlamydia* and *Rickettsia.*	A routine stain for peripheral blood.
Silver (methenamine silver)	Fungi. *Listeria monocytogenes.* *Pneumocystis jiroveci.*	Tissue stain for *fungus*; is also used to detect certain poorly Gram's-staining organisms. Technically difficult.
Acid-fast (Ziehl-Neelsen or carbol-fuschin)	*Mycobacterium.* *Nocardia.* Some protozoa.	*High lipid content* of cell wall prevents stain from being washed out by acid alcohol decolorizer.
Iron hematoxylin and trichrome	Protozoa.	
Fecal wet mount (ova and parasites)	Protozoa, helminth eggs.	

TABLE 5-10. **Specialized Media for Microbial Growth**

ORGANISM	MEDIUM
All bacteria	Blood agar
Gram-negatives, lactose fermenters	MacConkey's agar
Gram-negatives, lactose fermenters	EMB (eosin-methylene blue) agar
Haemophilus influenzae	Chocolate agar
Neisseria	Thayer-Martin (VCN) agar
Bordetella pertussis	Bordet-Gengou medium
Corynebacterium diphtheriae	Tellurite agar
Group D streptococci	Bile esculin agar

- **Selective media** are supplemented with antibiotics or other substances that **prevent the growth** of certain contaminating bacteria.
- **Differential media** contain **indicators** that provide further biochemical information about the microorganisms.

Blood Agar

- Many clinical specimens are swabbed on to the common differential medium sheep's blood agar (5%).
- Allows discrimination between *Streptococcus* species based on the **hemolysis** pattern of the blood.
    - Complete (clear) lysis of the red cells allows text to be read through the agar plate; this is known as β-**hemolysis.**
    - Incomplete hemolysis yields a distinct green cast to the otherwise red agar and is termed α-**hemolysis.**
    - No color change is labeled γ-**hemolysis.**

MacConkey's Agar

- Selective and differential medium.
- Inhibits the growth of gram-positive bacteria.
- Also differentiates whether a microorganism can use lactose as a nutrient source.
- Lactose utilizers form red colonies.
- Used to distinguish among different enteric bacteria.

Eosin–Methylene Blue (EMB) Agar

- Like MacConkey's, EMB agar inhibits gram-positive bacterial growth and allows assay of lactose as a sugar source.
- Lactose utilizers form dark-green, metallic-appearing colonies.

Chocolate Agar

- *Haemophilus* spp. are pathogens that are highly fastidious in their growth requirements and require enriched medium to survive in vitro.
- **X factor** (hemin) and **V factor** (nicotinamide adenine dinucleotide or NAD) are required.

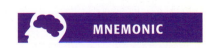

MNEMONIC

Say **HI** (*H. influenzae*) to the townsfolk on your way to the **five and dime** (**V** and **X**) to buy some **chocolate.**

- ■ Present in sheep's blood agar, but gentle heating (or "chocolatizing") is required to remove V factor inhibitors.

Thayer-Martin (VCN) Agar

Like *Haemophilus*, *Neisseria* spp. are highly fastidious microbes and require X and V factors for growth in the laboratory. Thayer-Martin (VCN) agar is a selective medium made of **chocolate agar supplemented with vancomycin, colistin,** and **nystatin.** It is used for the isolation of *N. gonorrhoeae* from mucosal surfaces. The three powerful antimicrobial agents strongly suppress growth of other commensal organisms present in vaginal, rectal, and pharyngeal specimens.

Bordet-Gengou Medium

B. pertussis is a highly fastidious respiratory pathogen that is very difficult to grow under typical laboratory conditions. Specimen collection must be performed with a calcium alginate swab (because ordinary sterile cotton is toxic to the microbe), and freshly prepared special medium (charcoal and horse blood required for growth).

Tellurite Agars

Various selective and differential media (potassium tellurite agar, cysteine-tellurite agar) are used to isolate *Corynebacterium diphtheriae* from the respiratory tracts of affected individuals. Positive colonies are characteristically black on these agar plates.

Bile Esculin Agar

This selective medium is used to differentiate group D streptococci (including *Enterococcus* spp.) from other streptococci, which are unable to grow in the presence of bile salts.

GRAM-POSITIVE COCCI

MNEMONIC

Stre**P**to**C**occi are seen in **p**airs and **C**hains.
STAPHylococci are in clusters, like the **staff** of the hospital.

KEY FACT

Streptococci are found in pairs and chains, and are catalase-negative. Staphylococci are found in clusters and are catalase-positive.

Microbes from the genera *Streptococcus* and *Staphylococcus* make up the bulk of medically relevant gram-positive cocci and are responsible for diseases affecting diverse organ systems. Streptococci and staphylococci can be easily differentiated based on microscopic morphology; staphylococci appear in clusters (often referred to as "bunches of grapes"), whereas streptococci are always seen in pairs (or **diplococci**) and chains. In addition, the **catalase** test easily discerns between the two genera; staphylococci are catalase-positive, and streptococci are catalase-negative.

Streptococcus and *Enterococcus*

The catalase-negative, gram-positive cocci (*Streptococcus* and the closely related *Enterococcus*, from now on referred to together as streptococci for simplicity) are a diverse group of coccoid organisms. Many medically important streptococci were first classified serologically by their **Lancefield group antigen,** a polymorphic immunogen located on the C carbohydrate component of the cell wall. Today, only three medically-important groups of streptococci are known by their Lancefield antigens. Streptococci can be differentiated among each other on the basis of hemolysis patterns on blood agar.

STREPTOCOCCUS PYOGENES (LANCEFIELD GROUP A)

CHARACTERISTICS

- **Pyogenic** or pus-producing organism.
- Responsible for a diverse collection of diseases.
- By microscopy, classically a 1- to 2-μm spherical coccus found in chains (see Figure 5-8).
- Easily discerned while growing on blood agar based on its wide zones of β-hemolysis.
- Like all streptococci, it is catalase-positive and sensitive to the antibiotic bacitracin.
- Colonizes the upper respiratory mucosa (especially the oropharynx). Asymptomatic carriage in healthy individuals is common.
- Spread by respiratory droplets, so crowded conditions (such as day-care facilities) facilitate person-to-person transmission.

PATHOGENESIS

S. pyogenes has a number of virulence factors that are important in causing a variety of diseases.

- **M protein** is a part of the cell wall that inhibits complement activation and thus prevents opsonization.
- Specific antibodies produced by the immune system are directed against the M protein.
- **Streptolysins S** and **O** are enzymes capable of causing hematopoietic cell death and are responsible for the characteristic β-hemolytic pattern in vivo.
- Streptolysin O is also a target for host cell antibodies and can be detected in blood (as an **ASO titer**).
- **Pyrogenic exotoxins** are superantigens capable of causing the characteristic rash of scarlet fever as well as the multiple organ system failure seen in streptococcal toxic shock syndrome.
- **Streptokinases** mediate the rapid spread of infection through infected tissues.

CLINICAL SYMPTOMS

Clinical sequelae of *S. pyogenes* infection can be easily divided into diseases caused by toxic effects of the bacteria themselves (often termed **suppura-**

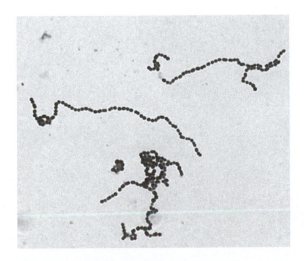

FIGURE 5-8. ***Streptococcus pyogenes* in long chains.** (Reproduced, with permission, from Brooks GF, Butel JS, Morse SA. *Jawetz, Melnick, & Adelberg's Medical Microbiology*, 23rd ed. New York: McGraw-Hill, 2004: 235.)

tive infections) and diseases caused by inappropriate activation of the host immune system.

- Local invasion or toxin released by the microbe:
  - Pharyngitis
  - Skin and soft tissue infection
  - Toxic shock syndrome (discussed under *S. aureus* infections)
- Cross-reacting antibodies produced by an infected host:
  - Rheumatic fever
  - Poststreptococcal glomerulonephritis

STREPTOCOCCAL PHARYNGITIS

CLINICAL SYMPTOMS

Strep throat is a common cause of sore throat among children and young adults. It is characterized by pain on swallowing, high fever, regional lymphadenopathy, and, most notably, erythema and frank white exudate on the palatine tonsils. Distinguishing viral from streptococcal sore throat can be difficult, and throat culture or a "rapid Strep test" is usually required.

A complication of streptococcal pharyngitis, caused by strains containing a lysogenized pyrogenic exotoxin, is **scarlet fever.** Following the sore throat, a sandpaper-like rash appears on the chest and spreads centrifugally (outward), sparing the palms, soles, and face. Complications from untreated pharyngitis include retropharyngeal and parapharyngeal abscesses, as well as immunologic complications (described below).

SKIN AND SOFT TISSUE INFECTIONS

CLINICAL SYMPTOMS

Several distinct syndromes are caused by *Streptococcus* infection of epidermal, dermal, or fascial components.

- **Impetigo** is a common childhood colonization of the upper epidermis characterized by perioral vesicular/blistered lesions that eventually develop a honey-colored crust (see Figure 5-9).
- **Erysipelas** and **cellulitis** are both acute infections of the skin characterized by erythema, edema, warmth, and systemic symptoms; cellulitis also involves deeper subcutaneous/dermal tissues. Both can be caused by other organisms as well (mainly *S. aureus* in immunocompetent individuals).
- **Necrotizing fasciitis** (or "flesh-eating bacteria") is a rapidly progressive infection of deep subcutaneous tissues. Symptoms include purple-blue **bullae** on the overlying skin following a cellulitis-like picture; overt gangrene, systemic symptoms, and multiorgan failure soon follow.

RHEUMATIC FEVER

PATHOGENESIS

Rheumatic fever is caused by cross-reaction of antibodies raised against the *Streptococcus* bacteria with antigens in the heart, causing an initial **pancarditis.** Further cardiac damage in the form of valvular disease may occur many years later.

CLINICAL SYMPTOMS

In addition to symptoms of valvular cardiac disease, joint, epidermal, and neurologic involvement is common.

KEY FACT

Centrifugal rashes spread outward from the chest to the extremities; centripetal rashes spread inward from the hands and feet to the body.

KEY FACT

Rheumatic fever follows untreated streptococcal pharyngitis, **not** strep skin or soft tissue infection!

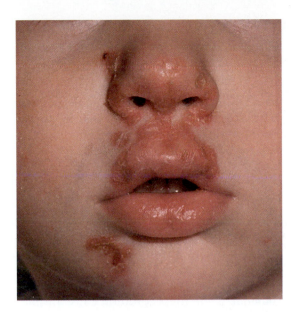

FIGURE 5-9. **Impetigo.** (Reproduced, with permission, from Wolff K, Johnson RA, Suurmond D. *Fitzpatrick's Color Atlas & Synopsis of Clinical Dermatology*, 5th ed. New York: McGraw-Hill, 2005: 589.)

TREATMENT

Rheumatic fever can recur after subsequent streptococcal infections, so patients are placed on lifelong prophylactic antibiotics.

POSTSTREPTOCOCCAL GLOMERULONEPHRITIS

PATHOGENESIS

Unlike rheumatic fever, renal sequelae of streptococcal infection can occur following either pharyngitis or skin/soft tissue infection. **Immune complexes** (antigen-antibody complexes) arising from streptococcal infection are deposited in the basement membrane of the glomerulus.

CLINICAL SYMPTOMS

The immune complex deposition causes typical glomerulonephritic symptoms of hematuria, hypertension, gross proteinuria, and tissue edema all secondary to glomerular inflammation. Prognosis is generally good in the pediatric population.

TREATMENT

In the case of poststreptococcal glomerulonephritis, treatment is generally supportive; immunosuppressive therapy to eliminate the immune complex deposition has been shown to have no impact on the disease course. *S. pyogenes* is highly sensitive to penicillin and other β-lactam agents, as well as macrolide antibiotics. Skin/soft tissue infections are usually treated with an antistaphylococcal penicillin (such as oxacillin) to cover for *S. aureus* as well. Prevention of rheumatic fever is effectively accomplished by the early diagnosis and treatment of streptococcal pharyngitis with antibiotics, thus preventing the synthesis of the responsible antistreptococcal antibodies.

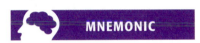

MNEMONIC

The **J♥NES** cr**ITERIA** are used to formally diagnose rheumatic fever.

Required criterion—documented evidence of recent group A streptococcal infection.

Major criteria:
Joint pains (migratory arthritis)
♥ (carditis)
Nodules (subcutaneous)
Erythema marginatum (spreading circular rash with red edges)
Sydenham's chorea

Minor criteria:
Inflammatory cells (leukocytosis)
Temperature (fever)
ESR (erythrocyte sedimentation rate) or CRP (C-reactive protein) elevated
Rheumatic fever (history of rheumatic disease)
Increased PR interval
Arthralgias
Two major criteria, or one major and two minor criteria are required for diagnosis.

STREPTOCOCCUS AGALACTIAE (LANCEFIELD GROUP B STREPTOCOCCUS)

S. agalactiae, a common cause of neonatal infection, is indistinguishable from *S. pyogenes* by microscopy and is also characterized by β-hemolysis on blood agar.

- Unlike *S. pyogenes*, it is resistant to the antibiotic bacitracin.
- Approximately 10%–30% of pregnant women are asymptomatically colonized with this organism. Transmission can occur transplacentally in utero or during delivery of the fetus.

CLINICAL SYMPTOMS

S. agalactiae infections fall broadly into two classes. It is a relatively common cause of **urinary tract infection** in pregnant women, for which the prognosis is excellent. Other group B streptococcal (GBS) infections of adults are uncommon and generally occur in immunocompromised individuals.

Given the high rate of asymptomatic carriage in pregnant females, it is no surprise that *S. agalactiae* is the most common cause of **neonatal septicemia** (sepsis) and meningitis. GBS can also cause **pneumonia in neonates.**

TREATMENT

Like *S. pyogenes*, GBS is also **penicillin-sensitive,** although higher concentrations are required for treatment. To prevent neonatal disease, current recommendations call for **screening** of pregnant women at 35–37 weeks' gestational age for GBS colonization via vaginal swab and culture. Women with positive cultures and those at high risk for intrapartum infection are given prophylactic penicillin G (or ampicillin) shortly before delivery.

VIRIDANS STREPTOCOCCI

CHARACTERISTICS

The viridans group of *Streptococcus* consists of several **nongroupable** (i.e., not classified according to the Lancefield classification) streptococci that produce α-hemolysis on blood agar. Important members of this group include:

- *S. mutans*, which is responsible for dental caries (cavities).
- *S. sanguis*, which causes subacute bacterial endocarditis (SBE).
- *S. intermedius* group, which can be found in abscesses.
- *S. bovis*, which is associated with malignancies of the GI tract.

S. viridans group are resistant to **optochin**, which allows discrimination from *S. pneumoniae*, which is optochin-sensitive.

CLINICAL SYMPTOMS

Several members of the viridans streptococci group are normal oropharyngeal flora; *S. mutans* is well known to cause dental caries. Several other members of the group are associated with SBE, an indolent infection affecting previously damaged (i.e., secondary to rheumatic fever or congenital bicuspid aortic valve) cardiac valves. Transient bacteremia is caused by dental procedures, and bacteria settle on the aforementioned valves. Associated symptoms include fevers, night sweats, fatigue, and new-onset murmurs. Resolution of this serious infection generally requires long-term use of parenteral antibiotics (typically ampicillin and an aminoglycoside).

KEY FACT

Antibiotic therapy for newborns with suspected meningitis is empiric; treatment should cover group B streptococcal infections, *Listeria*, and *E. coli*, the three most common bacterial CNS pathogens in this age group. **Ampicillin** (to cover *Listeria* and GBS) and **gentamicin** or cefotaxime are usually the agents of choice.

ENTEROCOCCUS AND OTHER GROUP D STREPTOCOCCI

CHARACTERISTICS

The genus *Enterococcus*, members of which possess the group D Lancefield antigen, are distinguished from non-enterococcal group D streptococci by their growth under harsh conditions, namely 6.5% sodium chloride and 40% bile salts. Hemolysis patterns on blood agar are variable. Two species of enterococci, *E. faecalis* and *E. faecium*, are clinically relevant.

- Responsible for disease in immunocompromised and hospitalized patients. Patients on extended courses of broad-spectrum antibiotics are also at risk.
- Urinary tract infections in catheterized patients, postsurgical peritonitis, and SBE are the most common clinical entities caused by these microorganisms.

Of note, *S. bovis* is an uncommon cause of endocarditis. It is associated with gastrointestinal malignancy for an unknown reason; all patients with documented *S. bovis* infections should be worked up completely for GI malignancies.

KEY FACT

Enterococci are responsible for up to 10% of all infections in hospitalized patients.

TREATMENT

In the past, therapy for enterococcal infections, like many serious bloodborne gram-positive coccal infections, has been the synergistic combination of ampicillin and an aminoglycoside. In the 1990s, rising resistance to these agents has prompted the use of vancomycin to treat resistant strains. Unfortunately, resistance to vancomycin is rising (up to 20% of *E. faecium* isolates), and novel antibiotic therapy has been required to treat these **vancomycin-resistant enterococci** (VRE) infections.

- **Linezolid** and **Synercid** (dalfopristin/quinupristin) are two new antimicrobial agents with activity against VRE; unfortunately they are bacteriostatic and have significant side effects.
- Urinary sterilizers such as nitrofurantoin are another option for the treatment of VRE urinary tract infections.

STREPTOCOCCUS PNEUMONIAE

CHARACTERISTICS

The nontypable *S. pneumoniae*, commonly known as **pneumococcus**, is one of the most clinically important gram-positive cocci due to its status as the **most common cause of bacterial pneumonia in adults**. Microscopically, pneumococci are commonly seen as "**lancet-shaped**" organisms in pairs or **diplococci**. Most pathogenic strains are encapsulated with a polysaccharide capsule (which serves as a virulence factor), and thus colonies appear mucoid (jelly-like) on blood agar. Hemolysis patterns on blood agar are variable, but usually α-hemolysis is seen.

Given the importance of this organism, it is fortunate that laboratory identification of the pneumococcus is facilitated by several individualized assays.

- The **Quellung** reaction can identify pneumococci in a clinically derived sample such as sputum; the polysaccharide capsule is microscopically visualized by the addition of anticapsular antibodies, which cause the capsule to swell.
- Colonies of *S. pneumoniae* are differentiated from other α-hemolytic streptococci (e.g., viridans streptococci) on agar plates by using optichin susceptibility and by adding bile to the culture medium.

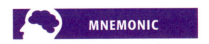

MNEMONIC

The **Quellung** reaction causes **swelling** of the polysaccharide capsule.

PATHOGENESIS

Virulence of pneumococcus is in large part mediated by the presence of a polysaccharide capsule, which serves to inhibit the microorganisms' phagocytosis by first-line immune cells such as macrophages and neutrophils.

A pyogenic immune response is ensured because of the ability of pneumococcal teichoic acid and peptidoglycan to activate the alternative complement pathway, thereby recruiting vast numbers of neutrophils.

Transmission of S. *pneumoniae* is respiratory, and prolonged, asymptomatic carriage is common. The capsule is highly immunogenic, and 84 serotypes have been identified in capsular antigens. Disease is caused by oropharyngeal infection with a noncolonizing serotype. The microorganism then spreads from the oropharynx via respiratory mucosa to the paranasal sinuses, the lower respiratory tract, or the meninges.

CLINICAL SYMPTOMS

- Pneumococcus is the most common cause of bacterial **pneumonia** in adults. A lobar pattern is seen on X-ray and high fevers with shaking chills are common. Frank blood and diplococci are found in an induced sputum sample.
- S. *pneumoniae* is also the number one cause of **meningitis** in adults.
- Pneumococcal **sinusitis** in adults and **otitis media** in children are commonly seen **owing** to facilitated transmission on mucosal surfaces.
- Pneumococcus can also cause **sepsis**, often preceded by meningitis. Individuals with **asplenia** (including functional asplenia seen in sickle cell disease) are also at increased risk for pneumococcal bacteremia and sepsis.

TREATMENT

Penicillin was once the mainstay of treatment for pneumococcal infection. However, rapidly increasing resistance has forced the use of alternate therapies in certain areas with intermediate or high rates of resistance. High-dose **amoxicillin** and/or **vancomycin** are used in these cases.

A 7-valent conjugated pneumococcal vaccine is recommended for all infants under the age of 2 years. Adults at high risk—including immunocompromised, asplenic, and elderly individuals as well as some transplant recipients—should receive a 23-valent polysaccharide vaccine to protect against pneumonia and invasive disease.

Staphylococcus

Staphylococci make up the other major medically relevant group of gram-positive cocci. Like streptococci, they are common colonizers of body surfaces and commonly cause skin and soft tissue substructure infections. Fortunately, they are easily differentiated from streptococci based on microscopy and the laboratory test for the **catalase** enzyme (using hydrogen peroxide as a substrate) (see Table 5-11). Staphylococci always assume the form of purple clusters (often called a "bunch of grapes") when gram-stained.

Three common and medically relevant species of *Staphylococcus* include S. *aureus*, S. *epidermidis*, and S. *saprophyticus*.

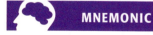

TABLE 5-11. Staphylococcus Compared With Streptococcus

	STAPHYLOCOCCUS	**STREPTOCOCCUS**
Microscopy	Clusters.	Pairs and chains
Catalase test	Positive.	Negative
Penicillin-sensitive	Never (except *Staphylococcus saprophyticus*).	Commonly

STAPHYLOCOCCUS AUREUS

CHARACTERISTICS

Because of its propensity for colonization and high degree of virulence, S. *aureus* is a major cause of both community-acquired and nosocomial morbidity and mortality. Like other staphylococci, its microscopic appearance looks like purple clusters (see Figure 5-10). Large β-hemolytic mucoid colonies that produce a **gold pigment** are seen when the organism is grown on blood agar.

S. *aureus* is unique among the staphylococci in that it contains the enzyme **coagulase.** Other species of *Staphylococcus* do not have this enzyme and are thus often referred to in laboratory reports as "coagulase-negative *Staphylococcus.*"

S. *aureus* is a part of the normal flora of human skin, and transient colonization of moist skin folds and the nasopharyngeal cavity is common. It also survives for long periods of time on dry surfaces. Transmission is either via shedding of microbes or contaminated **fomites,** inanimate objects that serve as vectors for microbial transmission. The rate of hospital-acquired multidrug-resistant S. *aureus* infections is almost certainly due to transmission via fomites such as bed linens.

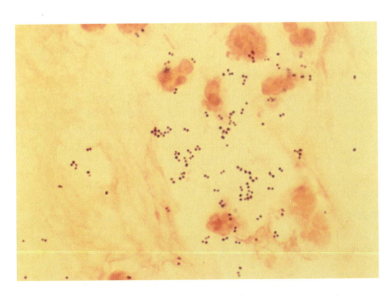

FIGURE 5-10. *Staphylococcus aureus.* Clusters of gram-positive cocci.

PATHOGENICITY

Like *S. pyogenes*, *S. aureus* features a number of different virulence factors that can be divided into several groups. Not all strains carry all virulence factors.

Immune modulators:

- **Protein A:** Specifically binds the Fc component of immunoglobulin, preventing immune-mediated destruction via **opsonization.**
- **Coagulase:** An enzyme that builts an insoluble fibrin capsule that surrounds the microorganism, thus preventing immune cell access.
- **Hemolysins** (also known as cytotoxins) α, β, γ, and δ—directly toxic to hematopoietic cells.
- **Leukocidin:** A toxin specific for white blood cells.
- **Catalase:** Prevents toxic action of neutrophil-derived hydrogen peroxide.
- **Penicillinase:** A secreted form of β-lactamase, can inactivate penicillin and derivatives.

Factors permitting penetration through tissues:

- **Hyaluronidase:** Hydrolyzes hyaluronic acid present in connective tissue.
- **Fibrinolysin** (also known as **staphylokinase**)—dissolves fibrin clots.
- **Lipases** allow for the survival and spread of *S. aureus* in fat-containing areas of the body, especially sebaceous glands.

Secreted toxins:

- **Exfolatin:** Result in the exfoliation of the middle skin layer, causing staphylococcal scalded skin syndrome.
- **Enterotoxins** (heat-stable): Cause vomiting and diarrhea.
- **Toxic shock syndrome toxin (TSST-1):** A **superantigen** that cross-links the MHC class II molecules on antigen-presenting cells, causing a massive nonspecific T-cell response, leading to toxic shock syndrome.

KEY FACT

Superantigens are substances that can cause a massive, **nonspecific** overstimulation of the immune system by chemically cross-linking the MHC class II molecules on antigen-presenting cells.

CLINICAL SYMPTOMS

S. aureus is capable of invading almost any organ. Signs and symptoms obviously differ, but because of the myriad virulence factors symptoms can be severe no matter what the organ. Both toxin-mediated (sterile) and invasive diseases are common (see Table 5-12).

STAPHYLOCOCCAL SCALDED SKIN SYNDROME

A relatively common disease of infants that presents with perioral exfoliation of the middle layer of the epidermis followed by the diffuse formation of blisters containing sterile fluid (see Figure 5-11). Unless there is bacterial super-infection, the disease resolves within approximately one week without further sequelae; morbidity and mortality rates are low.

GASTROENTERITIS

CHARACTERISTICS

Caused by *S. aureus*, gastroenteritis is common and notable for its rapid onset (within 4–6 hours of ingestion of the tainted foodstuffs).

PATHOGENESIS

Unusually rapid onset owing to the presence of **preformed heat-stable entero-toxin** in ingested food.

TABLE 5-12. Spectrum of Staphylococcal Disease

EXOTOXIN-MEDIATED	INVASIVE
Staphylococcal scalded skin syndrome (SSSS)	Skin/soft-tissue infections
Food poisoning	Endocarditis
Toxic shock syndrome	Pneumonia/empyema
	Osteomyelitis
	Septic arthritis

CLINICAL SYMPTOMS

Illness is often characterized by a rapid, abrupt onset of copious vomiting and nonbloody diarrhea. The illness generally runs a short (less than 24 hours) and uncomplicated course. Common culprit food items are room-temperature "salads" made with mayonnaise, such as **potato and tuna salad**, processed meats, custard, and nondairy creamer. The source is usually a human food preparer with a skin infection or asymptomatic nasal carriage.

TREATMENT

Supportive only; antibiotics do not significantly shorten the course of the diarrhea.

> **KEY FACT**
>
> *S. aureus* preformed enterotoxin is the only cause of food poisoning whose onset occurs acutely (within 4 hours).

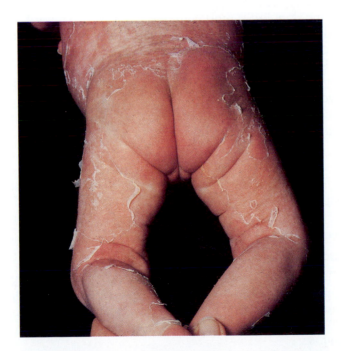

FIGURE 5-11. Staphylococcal scalded skin syndrome. The exfoliative dermatitis is widespread but not severe. (Reproduced, with permission, from Wolff K, Johnson RA, Suurmond D, *Fitzpatrick's Color Atlas & Synopsis of Clinical Dermatology*, 5th ed, New York: McGraw-Hill, 2005: 623.)

TOXIC SHOCK SYNDROME

CHARACTERISTICS

Occurs primarily in menstruating women using superabsorbent tampons left in place for long periods of time, but can also occur in wounds with draining fluid collections.

PATHOGENESIS

S. *aureus* microbes multiply in the nutrient-rich menstrual/wound fluid and secrete TSST-1, which causes a systemic inflammatory response due to the nonspecific activation of T cells.

CLINICAL SYMPTOMS

Abrupt onset of fever and hypotension, and multiple organ dysfunction are seen; a **desquamating rash of the palms and soles** is typical as well.

TREATMENT

Antibiotics have limited effectiveness, and supportive care is the rule.

SKIN AND SOFT-TISSUE INFECTIONS

CHARACTERISTICS

Like group A *Streptococcus*, S. *aureus* can also cause various **skin and soft-tissue infections,** such as cellulitis and impetigo. Skin substructure infections are more commonly caused by S. *aureus* and are listed below.

- **Folliculitis** is an infection of the base of the hair follicle. Patients present with a small, raised, erythematous bump. This infection can occur anywhere on the skin, but is most common in areas with abundant hair.
- A **furuncle** is a conglomeration of several adjacent inflamed follicles. It presents as a large, painful nodule that requires drainage.
- **Carbuncles** are furuncles that are coalesced and often extend into the dermis. They can cause systemic symptoms such as fever as well as staphylococcal bacteremia.
- Staphylococcal **wound infections** are common and are generally seen when a "dirty wound" containing foreign matter is present.

TREATMENT

Appropriate antibiotic therapy can be administered either systemically or locally via topical creams or ointments.

INFECTIVE ENDOCARDITIS (IE)

CHARACTERISTICS

IE of undamaged (native) valves is commonly caused by S. *aureus* migrating from infected surgical wounds or contaminated intravenous catheters. It is a serious disease with high (over 50%) mortality, especially when untreated.

CLINICAL SYMPTOMS

Unlike SBE, IE is characterized by a **rapid onset** of high fever with rigors, myalgias, and possibly a loud murmur. Large infective vegetations are seen on the affected valves (see Figure 5-12) and can embolize to the pulmonary or cerebral parenchyma.

KEY FACT

Most cases of IE occur on **left-sided** valves and have a poor prognosis due to brain emboli; IV drug users get **right-sided** IE, which has a much better prognosis.

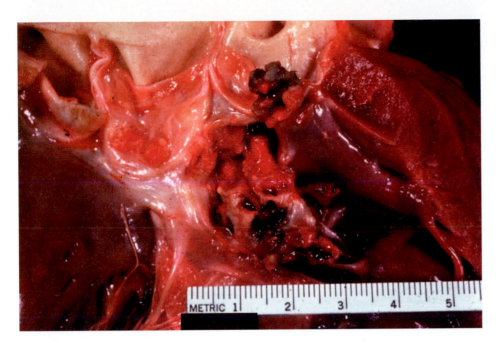

FIGURE 5-12.   **Infective endocarditis.** Note the large, friable-appearing vegetations on the mitral and aortic valves. (Image courtesy of PEIR Digital Library [http://www.peir.net].)

PNEUMONIA

CHARACTERISTICS

Staphylococcal **pneumonia** is rare in the community but a relatively more common cause of nosocomial pneumonia, especially in the elderly following viral (influenza) pneumonia.

CLINICAL SYMPTOMS

Characterized by the rapid onset of fever/chills and a nonspecific radiographic pattern. **Cavitations** in the lung tissue are seen on gross dissection. Infected parapneumonic effusions (known as **empyema**) are common as well. Certain strains can cause an even more severe variant known as **necrotizing** pneumonia, characterized by massive hemoptysis and septic shock.

OSTEOMYELITIS

CHARACTERISTICS

A deep-seated infection of the bone most often seen in preadolescent boys.

PATHOGENESIS

Seeded hematogenously from distant sites (usually cutaneous staphylococcal infections) or from contiguous, overlying skin infections (e.g., diabetic foot ulcers).

CLINICAL SYMPTOMS

Localized pain and fever are presenting symptoms, and further hematogenous spread is common. Bone scans are used to screen for distant disease.

TREATMENT

Several weeks to months of appropriate antibiotic therapy usually effects a complete cure.

FLASH FORWARD

Osteomyelitis is an important infection, especially in adolescents and immunocompromised individuals. **S. aureus** is the most common causative organism, but **Salmonella** osteomyelitis is common in patients with sickle cell disease.

SEPTIC ARTHRITIS

CHARACTERISTICS

S. *aureus* is the most common organism implicated in **septic arthritis** seen in pediatric and elderly age groups (N. *gonorrhoeae* is the most common cause among sexually active individuals).

PATHOGENESIS

Disease can be caused by local introduction of the organism by synovial puncture via needle or via hematogenous spread from distant foci of infection.

CLINICAL SYMPTOMS

Classic symptoms include an erythematous, swollen joint with decreased range of motion; the key laboratory finding upon **arthrocentesis** (joint aspiration) is an elevated neutrophil count.

TREATMENT

Drainage and prompt antibiotics generally produce an effective cure, especially in children.

Since most S. *aureus* isolates carry a penicillinase enzyme, first- and second-generation penicillins are not used for antibiotic therapy.

Methicillin-sensitive *Staphylococcus aureus* (MSSA) make up approximately 70% of S. *aureus* strains and are appropriately treated with semisynthetic penicillins such as nafcillin, oxacillin, and dicloxacillin, which are not broken down by penicillinase. First-generation cephalosporins are also highly efficacious. Note that methicillin is no longer used clinically because of concerns about nephrotoxicity.

Unfortunately, multidrug-resistant strains of S. *aureus* have developed in the past half century. These strains, termed **methicillin-resistant *Staphylococcus aureus*** or **MRSA**, contain an altered PBP, rendering them resistant to the semisynthetic penicillins. Previously, these strains were found only in settings where broad-spectrum antibiotics were commonly used. However, community-acquired MRSA is seen increasingly, especially as skin and skin substructure infections. **Vancomycin** is the cornerstone of MRSA therapy and is the correct answer to any exam question as such. However, clindamycin and trimethoprim-sulfamethoxazole (TMP-SMX) are effective in some nonserious infections as well.

COAGULASE-NEGATIVE STAPHYLOCOCCUS

CHARACTERISTICS

Staphylococcus epidermidis and S. *saprophyticus* are commonly isolated *Staphylococcus* species, but are much less clinically significant than S. *aureus*. Both appear as gram-positive cocci in small clusters and are catalase-positive, but do not contain the coagulase enzyme. Of note, S. *epidermidis* is sensitive to the antibiotic **novobiocin**, whereas S. *saprophyticus* is resistant.

CLINICAL SYMPTOMS

S. *epidermidis* is a constituent of the normal bacterial skin flora. In healthy, noninstrumented individuals, this species is not a major cause of disease. However, it can cause major infections of **mechanical prostheses** (e.g., prosthetic joints, mechanical heart valves) as well as **indwelling catheters** (intravenous, Foley) because of the organism's unique polysaccharide capsule. These dis-

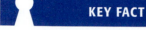

KEY FACT

S. *epidermidis* is one of the most frequently isolated organisms from blood cultures in hospitals. This is usually due to contamination of the venipuncture needle rather than true S. *epidermidis* bacteremia.

eases are usually characterized by an indolent course with systemic symptoms developing slowly, if at all.

S. saprophyticus is the second most common cause of community-acquired urinary tract infections in sexually active women (behind *E. coli*). Symptoms are typical and include dysuria, pyuria, and bacteruria.

TREATMENT

Over 50% of *S. epidermidis* isolates are methicillin-resistant and thus require vancomycin or alternative treatment. *S. saprophyticus* responds to typical empiric treatment for urinary tract infections with TMP-SMX, fluoroquinolones, and others.

GRAM-POSITIVE RODS

Gram-positive rods fall into two general categories: The spore-forming or **sporulating** rods, and the non–spore-forming rods. The anaerobic *Clostridium* spp. and the aerobic *Bacillus* spp. form **endospores** under conditions of metabolic stress, and these spores are seen under phase (wet-mount) microscopy, enabling easy differentiation. *L. monocytogenes*, *C. diphtheriae*, and the actinomycetes (*Actinomyces* spp. and *Nocardia* spp.) make up the heterogeneous group that is nonsporulating gram-positive rods.

Sporulating Gram-Positive Rods

The medically important gram-positive rods in this category are universally soil microbes. The endospore that they produce is actually thought to be an evolutionary adaptation to the dehydration these organisms can experience in exposed environments. Pathogenically, these microorganisms cause disease by secreting powerful exotoxins. Invasive disease is not characteristic and, since the toxins are usually preformed, antibiotics are of limited efficacy in treatment of disease.

CLOSTRIDIUM BOTULINUM

CHARACTERISTICS

C. botulinum is a gram-positive, sporulating rod that is anaerobic, thus growing only in specially designed anaerobic environments. It produces a highly virulent exotoxin leading to **flaccid muscular paralysis**.

PATHOGENESIS

The botulism exotoxin is a **heat-labile A-B neurotoxin** that inhibits the release of acetylcholine at neuromuscular junctions, leading to flaccid paralysis. There are seven serotypes, A–G; however, the serotypes that most commonly cause disease are **A**, **B**, and **E**. People never develop natural immunity to botulism toxin because of its extreme toxicity; even amounts too small to initiate an immune response can be fatal if untreated. Botulism toxin is a potential biologic weapon and is listed as a CDC Category A **bioterrorism agent.**

CLINICAL SYMPTOMS

There are three clinical presentations of botulism toxicity.

- **Food-borne botulism** is the only form that results from ingestion of preformed toxins.

- Patients complain of blurred or double vision, difficulty speaking or swallowing, droopy eyes or muscle weakness, and gastrointestinal symptoms. The paralytic effects progress in a descending fashion.
- This disease often occurs 1–2 days after eating homemade canned or preserved foods. Improperly processed food offers the anaerobic environment that spores need to germinate and synthesize botulism toxin.
- Once ingested, the exotoxin is absorbed through the gut and travels in the blood to nerve synapses.
- Patients need to be treated immediately because the toxin may compromise respiratory muscles. Treatment includes antitoxin and respiratory support.
- **Infant botulism** results when babies ingest spores found in household dust or (the classic scenario) **honey**.
  - The spores germinate in the gut and produce the exotoxin, which is absorbed into the blood.
  - Symptoms include constipation, limp body, loss of head control, dysphagia, weak feeding, and weak crying. This disease is sometimes referred to as **floppy baby syndrome** because of the severe loss of muscle tone and control.
  - Treatment includes respiratory support and human-derived polyvalent antitoxin (serotypes A, B, and E). A human-derived antitoxin rather than the equine-derived antitoxin is given to prevent any risk of type III hypersensitivity reaction.
  - Prognosis is good, even without the use of humanized antitoxin.
- **Wound botulism** occurs from traumatic implantation and germination of spores at the wound site.
  - Botulism toxin is produced in vivo and disseminated throughout the body. Symptoms are the same as food-borne botulism, without gastrointestinal symptoms.
  - Patients are treated with respiratory support, equine-derived polyvalent antitoxin, and antibiotics to eradicate the bacteria.

TREATMENT

Antitoxin is the cornerstone of treatment for all varieties of botulism. Antitoxin is a fraction of serum (usually equine) obtained from an animal that has been inoculated with the antigen in question. This serum contains polyclonal antibodies that can neutralize the botulism toxin. Antibiotics and supportive care are also important in selected situations.

CLOSTRIDIUM TETANI

CHARACTERISTICS

Like other *Clostridium* species, this anaerobic gram-positive rod produces spores that are generally found in the soil. These spores are inoculated into puncture wounds, which provide an ideal environment for germination.

PATHOGENESIS

The bacteria produce **tetanus toxin**, also known as tetanospasmin, a neurotoxin that binds peripheral nerve terminals and travels intra-axonally from the site of entry to the central nervous system. Like botulism toxin, tetanus toxin does not induce an immune response because of its sheer potency. It binds ganglioside receptors at the presynaptic inhibitory nerve ending, selectively cleaves synaptobrevin, a protein component of the synaptic vesicle, and **prevents the release of the inhibitory neurotransmitters** (GABA and glycine). Without inhibitory signals, excitatory neurons are unopposed, causing sustained muscle contraction or **tetany.**

KEY FACT

Never feed babies honey! Their immature gastrointestinal tracts do not have the normal flora that prevent spores from germinating.

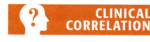

CLINICAL CORRELATION

Antitoxin of any variety given to a human can produce **serum sickness** because of the foreign protein antigens present in animal-derived sera.

CLINICAL SYMPTOMS

Patients with tetanus present with severe, unopposed muscle contractions. Often, this is most evident in the muscles of the jaw, producing the characteristic grin of **trismus** or lockjaw.

TREATMENT

The major modality for control and prevention of tetanus is the **tetanus toxoid** vaccine. This is a formalin-inactivated toxin that is first injected as part of the **DTaP** vaccine (diphtheria-tetanus-acellular pertussis). Since immunity is fleeting, booster shots are given every 10 years.

Treatment of active tetanus infection is accomplished with antibiotics (usually metronidazole), antitetanus immune globulin, an immediate tetanus booster, extensive débridement, and muscle relaxants. Rapid response is critical to prevent death secondary to respiratory complications.

CLOSTRIDIUM PERFRINGENS

CHARACTERISTICS

This anaerobic, spore-forming soil bacterium is well known for causing **gas gangrene**, a debilitating and often fatal infection of muscle tissue.

PATHOGENESIS

Traumatic implantation of the spores into muscle tissue (i.e., by a puncture wound) causes germination and the release of the α **toxin**, a lecithinase that can necrotize tissue and destroy blood and vascular cells. Other toxins are released as well, some of which are capable of catalyzing a **fermentation reaction**, causing the release of intraparenchymal **gas.**

CLINICAL SYMPTOMS

The most serious infection caused by *C. perfringens* is the aforementioned gas gangrene, also known as **clostridial myonecrosis**. This infection is characterized by **tissue crepitus** (the palpable/audible presence of subcuticular air or gas) and rapid, widespread necrosis of muscular tissue with rapidly ensuing death. Other soft tissue infections with significantly less severe presentations, and gastroenteritis, are also possible sequelae.

TREATMENT

Treatment of gas gangrene involves débridement, high-dose penicillin, and hyperbaric O_2 (to provide a toxic atmosphere for the anaerobic *clostridia*). Mortality is unfortunately still high in the most severe infections.

CLOSTRIDIUM DIFFICILE

CHARACTERISTICS

C. difficile is another anaerobic, spore-forming organism that causes **antibiotic-associated colitis** (the severe variant is known as **pseudomembranous colitis**), which is common among hospitalized patients, especially those on broad-spectrum antibiotics.

PATHOGENESIS

C. difficile is a normal component of the intestinal flora of some people (and is easily spread to others via its hardy spores). Because of its relative antibiotic resistance, it has the tendency to proliferate in the colon during treatment with broad-spectrum antibiotics, thus outcompeting the susceptible normal enteric flora. At this point, the organism produces **enterotoxin** and **cytotoxin**, which cause the characteristic secretory diarrhea.

CLINICAL SYMPTOMS

Clinically, patients present with an acute episode of watery diarrhea and abdominal cramping. In severe cases, a **pseudomembrane** composed of sloughed inflammatory cells, fibrin, and mucus is seen overlying intact colonic mucosa (see Figure 5-13).

TREATMENT

Appropriate treatment is discontinuation of broad-spectrum antibiotics and treatment with **oral metronidazole** (preferred) or **oral vancomycin**.

BACILLUS ANTHRACIS

CHARACTERISTICS

This spore-forming facultative anaerobe is the causative agent of **anthrax.** The microbe has received much press in recent years because of its potential as a bioweapon. It is a relatively large, sporulating, nonmotile gram-positive rod that primarily infects herbivores or lives in the soil as a resilient spore. Transmission to humans is usually via traumatic implantation or inhalation of spores from infected animals or, more recently, via inhalation of intentionally placed spores.

PATHOGENESIS

Three virulence factors are largely responsible for most of the clinical manifestations of *B. anthracis.* The organism possesses a unique, immunogenic **capsule** composed of a polypeptide that prevents phagocytosis. **Protective antigen** allows entry of other toxins into cells, and **edema factor** activates adenylate cyclase, causing osmotic cell swelling. The ominous-sounding **lethal**

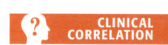

CLINICAL CORRELATION

Despite claims to the contrary, *C. difficile* colitis cannot be diagnosed based on the smell of the offending stool alone.

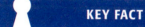

KEY FACT

The only organism with a polypeptide capsule is *B. anthracis.* All other known capsules are composed of polysaccharides.

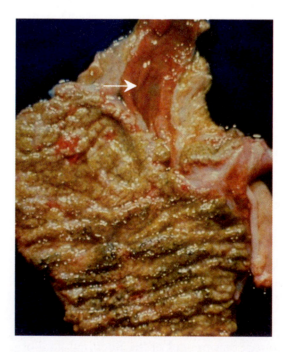

FIGURE 5-13. **Pseudomembranous colitis.** Note the confluent greenish pseudomembrane covering the colon, with relative sparing of the terminal ileum (arrow). (Reproduced, with permission, from Kasper DL, Braunwald E, Fauci AS, et al, *Harrison's Principles of Internal Medicine*, 16th ed, New York: McGraw-Hill, 2005: 760.)

factor is a cytotoxic protein that causes inflammation, macrophage activation, and cell death.

CLINICAL SYMPTOMS

There are three categories of clinical anthrax, which correspond completely with the route of contact with the pathogen or its spores.

- **Cutaneous anthrax** occurs when humans have direct epidermal contact with *B. anthracis* spores. A characteristic papule progresses to vesiculation/ulceration and subsequently to black eschar and central necrosis, all at the original site of inoculation (see Figure 5-14). The lesion itself is painless but painful regional lymphadenopathy and systemic disease can develop. The mortality is approximately 10%.
- **Pulmonary (inhalational) anthrax** occurs when spores are inhaled, either from animals (**woolsorter's disease**) or from **weaponized** preparations. Nonspecific symptoms such as fever, headache, cough, malaise, and chest pain are the usual initial manifestations. Untreated, this disease leads to **massively enlarged mediastinal lymph nodes**, pulmonary hemorrhage, meningeal symptoms, and often (50%) death.
- **Gastrointestinal anthrax** is caused by ingestion of live spores; it is highly lethal but rare.

TREATMENT

Immediate antibiotic treatment as soon as the diagnosis is suspected is the key to preventing fatality. Ciprofloxacin is the agent of choice, although several alternatives are available. Prevention is focused on **animal vaccination;** a human vaccine is available but has major side effects and is routinely given only to at-risk populations.

BACILLUS CEREUS

CHARACTERISTICS

B. cereus is another motile, spore-forming gram-negative rod, but its virulence is much lower than that of *B. anthracis*.

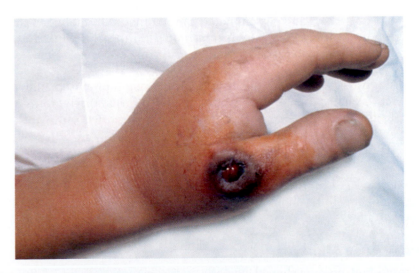

FIGURE 5-14. **Cutaneous anthrax on the thumb of a child.** (Reproduced, with permission, from Wolff K, Johnson RA, Suurmond D, *Fitzpatrick's Color Atlas & Synopsis of Clinical Dermatology*, 5th ed, New York: McGraw-Hill, 2005: 631.)

PATHOGENESIS

The spores are ubiquitously found in nature and are typically ingested in food sources. **Reheated fried rice** is a common source, since microwaving typically does not kill the spores.

CLINICAL SYMPTOMS

Two forms of gastrointestinal disease are possible: An **emetic** form manifesting as rapid-onset vomiting and diarrhea, and a **diarrheal** form characterized by a watery, secretory diarrhea.

TREATMENT

Both forms typically resolve without sequelae, and antibiotic treatment is not indicated.

Nonsporulating Gram-Positive Rods

LISTERIA MONOCYTOGENES

Listeria is an uncommon human pathogen responsible for important diseases affecting neonates. It is a short gram-positive rod that exhibits **tumbling motility** at room temperature and is easily grown on agar, **even at cold temperatures.** Like many opportunistic pathogens, it is ubiquitous in nature and can be found in animals, soil, and even as asymptomatic colonizers of the human gastrointestinal tract. When a source is identified, it is often a refrigerated, contaminated food product such as soft cheese, cabbage, or milk.

PATHOGENESIS

Infection is often precipitated by ingestion and subsequent transmucosal uptake by cells of the gastrointestinal tract. *L. monocytogenes* is also a facultative intracellular organism, enabling it to evade clearance by phagocytosis.

CLINICAL SYMPTOMS

Neonatal listeriosis can take on two forms. **Early-onset disease** (also known as **granulomatosis infantiseptica**) occurs as a result of transplacental transmission and is characterized by late miscarriage or birth complicated by sepsis, multiorgan abscesses, and disseminated granulomas. Mortality is extremely high. **Late-onset disease** typically is transmitted during childbirth and manifests as meningitis or meningoencephalitis occurring 2–3 weeks later.

Adult listeriosis (in pregnant, elderly, or immunocompromised individuals) can present as bacteremia, sepsis, or meningitis. Signs and symptoms are not unique to this organism, so other causes need to be ruled out. Mortality is rare.

TREATMENT

L. monocytogenes is intrinsically resistant to cephalosporins, and the mainstays of treatment are intravenous penicillin or ampicillin, often combined with gentamicin for synergy.

CORYNEBACTERIUM DIPHTHERIAE

This important comma-shaped bacteria is the causative agent of the once-prevalent childhood pharyngitis **diphtheria.** They are small, pleomorphic irregular-staining gram-positive rods that are observed to contain **metachromatic (red or blue) granules** when stained with methylene blue (see Figure 5-15). They can grow on most media, but **tellurite-containing medium**

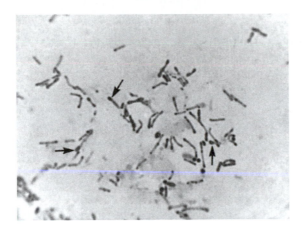

FIGURE 5-15. *Corynebacterium diphtheriae.* This specimen was stained with methylene blue; metachromatic granules are designated with arrows. (Reproduced, with permission, from Brooks GF, Butel JS, Morse SA, *Jawetz, Melnick, & Adelberg's Medical Microbiology*, 23rd ed, New York: McGraw-Hill, 2004: 214.)

is often used to selectively isolate the organism from pharyngeal swab specimens.

Because of an extensive childhood vaccination campaign, *C. diphtheriae* has become rare in the developed world, but cases are still relatively common in impoverished urban areas in the Third World. Transmission is via respiratory droplets from unvaccinated individuals or asymptomatic vaccinated carriers.

PATHOGENESIS

The virulence of *C. diphtheriae* is almost entirely due to the **diphtheria toxin**, an exotoxin that is encoded on a lysogenic bacteriophage virus called β-phage. Not all bacteria express the toxin, since expression relies on infection with the bacteriophage. The toxin itself is a classic A-B toxin; component B allows entry of the A subunit into the cells. The A subunit in this case is an ADP-ribosyltransferase enzyme that **inactivates elongation factor EF-2** via ADP-ribosylation, thereby inhibiting protein synthesis.

CLINICAL SYMPTOMS

Diphtheria generally manifests as an **exudative pharyngitis** causing dysphagia (pain on swallowing), fever, and malaise following an incubation period of less than 1 week. As the disease progresses, a thick **pseudomembrane** (made up of fibrin, dead cells, bacteria, and leukocytes) forms on the posterior oropharynx and tonsils. This membrane is gray and tightly adherent and **cannot be scraped off** without causing bleeding of the underlying tissue. After another week, this membrane spontaneously dislodges, although complications can arise from airway compromise from the membrane. Other features of the disease include cervical lymphadenopathy and edema, resulting in the characteristic **bull-neck** appearance. Cardiac and lower respiratory complications are rare but potentially fatal.

Diagnosis of diphtheria is usually clinical, but clinical specimens are generally tested for pathogenicity using the **Elek test**, an in vitro assay that tests for the production of exotoxin.

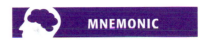
MNEMONIC

ABCDEFG:

ADP-ribosylation
Beta-phage
Corynebacterium
Diphtheriae
Elongation **F**actor EF-2
Granules (metachromatic)

TREATMENT

The cornerstone of treatment of active diphtheria is the early administration of **diphtheria antitoxin** to neutralize extant exotoxin, and appropriate antibiotic therapy (penicillin or erythromycin).

PREVENTION

Prevention has been largely successful in the United States, owing to routine childhood immunization with nontoxic **diphtheria toxoid** as part of the DTaP vaccine series.

ACTINOMYCETES

The actinomycetes are a group of gram-positive rods that typically live in soil and have unique, fungus-like microscopic morphology with branching and hyphal forms. There are a staggering number of these organisms, many of which cause rare opportunistic or pulmonary infections. Two actinomycetes are particularly important and are discussed here.

NOCARDIA SPECIES

CHARACTERISTICS

Nocardia is a strictly aerobic actinomycete that is distinguished from many others because it is partially **acid-fast** on carbol-fuschsin stain (unlike Actinomyces).

CLINICAL SYMPTOMS

This organism causes indolent bronchopulmonary infections, especially in individuals with **decreased T-cell immunity.** Cavitary pulmonary lesions as well as hematogenous spread to the skin and CNS are common. Primary cutaneous lesions such as **mycetomas**, cellulitis, and subcutaneous abscesses can develop as well.

TREATMENT

Treatment is with sulfonamides or TMP-SMX.

ACTINOMYCES ISRAELII

CHARACTERISTICS

Unlike its partner *Nocardia, A. israelii* is an anaerobic actinomycete that is not acid-fast. It is a constituent of the normal mouth flora of some humans.

CLINICAL SYMPTOMS

Typically causes slowly developing oral and facial abscesses with an underlying yellow color due to the presence of so-called **sulfur granules.** These granules are actually massive collections of *Actinomyces* organisms. Sinus tract drainage of these abscesses to the skin surface is common. Other potential sites for actinomycosis are the brain, chest cavity and abdominopelvic region. Mycetomas are also possible.

TREATMENT

Via surgical incision and drainage coupled with penicillin or ampicillin.

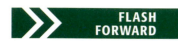

FLASH FORWARD

The causative agent of **Whipple's disease, *Tropheryma whipplei*,** is also an actinomycete.

KEY FACT

Actinomycotic mycetomas are chronic, destructive cutaneous lesions caused by actinomycetes that generally feature sinus tracts communicating with the epidermal surface, painless edema, and subcutaneous abscesses.

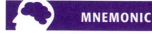

MNEMONIC

*Treatment of actinomycete infections is a **SNAP:***

Sulfa for **N**ocardia
Actinomyces needs **P**enicillin

GRAM-NEGATIVE COCCI

Neisseria

The only two medically important gram-negative cocci are N. *meningitidis* or **meningococcus**, which causes meningitis and sepsis; and N. *gonorrhoeae* or **gonococcus**, which causes gonorrhea, disseminated gonococcal disease, and ophthalmia neonatorum. All *Neisseria* are small aerobic gram-negative czocci typically seen on microscopy as coffee-bean-like **diplococci** or in clumps (see Figure 5-16). Both are oxidase-positive (in contrast to the oxidase-negative Enterobacteriaceae). N. *meningitidis* can be differentiated from N. *gonorrhoeae* by two distinguishing features:

- A polysaccharide capsule that inhibits phagocytosis.
- Metabolizes both glucose and maltose (N. *gonorrhoeae* only metabolizes glucose).

Eikenella and *Kingella* are uncommon opportunistic pathogens and rarely are implicated in SBE.

PATHOGENESIS

Except for the aforementioned meningococcal capsule, N. *meningitidis* and N. *gonorrhoeae* share the same virulence factors:

- **Pili** mediate mucosal surface attachment. The pili of N. *gonorrhoeae* undergo rapid antigenic variation, so there is a corresponding **lack of long-term immunity** to gonococcal infection.
- **Por** proteins form outer membrane pores that allow passage of nutrients and waste materials and, in some cases, prevent complement-dependent killing of the bacteria.
- **Opa** proteins are involved in surface adhesion.
- **LOS** (lipo-oligosaccharide) is a variant of gram-negative endotoxin (LPS) that does not possess the O-polysaccharide moiety present in LPS but still possesses endotoxin-like cytotoxic capabilities.

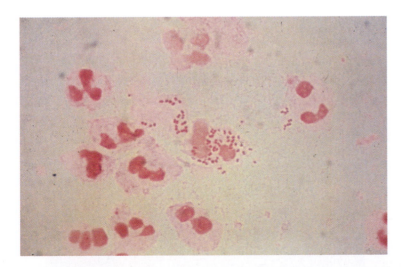

FIGURE 5-16. *Neisseria gonorrhoeae* **as seen on preparation from urethral discharge.** Microorganisms are arranged in side-by-side pairs and small clumps. (Reproduced, with permission, from Wolff K, Johnson RA, Suurmond D, *Fitzpatrick's Color Atlas & Synopsis of Clinical Dermatology*, 5th ed, New York: McGraw-Hill, 2005: 906.)

- **IgA proteases** cleave the immunoglobulin IgA into its inactive constituents thus foiling mucosal adaptive immunity.
- **Siderophores** allow collection of iron from human iron-binding proteins (transferrin).

NEISSERIA MENINGITIDIS

CHARACTERISTICS

Meningococcus is the organism responsible for most cases of bacterial meningitis in adolescents and certain at-risk populations (military trainees, dormitory residents). In addition, it can cause debilitating sepsis known as **meningococcemia**. The microorganism is transmitted by respiratory droplets and can be a normal constituent of the oropharyngeal flora.

PATHOGENESIS

As stated, this important pathogen possesses an antiphagocytic polysaccharide capsule, which is the basis of its subclassification into several serogroups. Serogroups A, B, C, Y, and W-135 are responsible for most infections. This capsule is immunogenic and is used to synthesize the meningococcal vaccine.

CLINICAL SYMPTOMS

Once resident in the nasopharynx, N. *meningitidis* can cause local symptoms, such as painful swallowing and fever. More important, it can easily spread to other subepithelial locations and cause significant disease.

Meningococcemia is life-threatening meningococcal sepsis results in severe multiorgan disease characterized pathologically by small vessel thrombosis and overwhelming consumptive coagulopathy. As a result, a characteristic **petechial** or **purpuric rash** is often seen on the trunk and lower extremities (see Figures 5-17). Fulminant menincococcemia can result in septic shock and bilateral **hemorrhagic destruction of the adrenal glands**; this symptom complex is known as **Waterhouse-Friderichsen syndrome**.

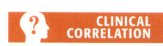

CLINICAL CORRELATION

Complement-mediated cytolysis is required for the immune system to clear a meningococcus infection. Repeated meningococcal infections in a child should prompt a search for hereditary terminal (C5–C9) complement deficiency.

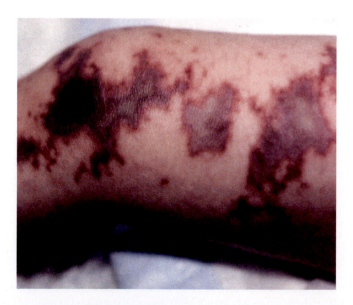

FIGURE 5-17. **Purpura fulminans due to acute meningococcemia.** (Reproduced, with permission, from Wolff K, Johnson RA, Suurmond D, *Fitzpatrick's Color Atlas & Synopsis of Clinical Dermatology*, 5th ed, New York: McGraw-Hill, 2005: 643.)

Meningococcal meningitis is the sequela of meningococcal invasion of the meninges of the central nervous system. Typical symptoms include an abrupt onset of fever, chills, stiff neck, headache, and vomiting. Meningeal signs are often present as well. Mortality rate is approximately 10% in appropriately treated patients, and complications such as long-term neurologic damage are rare.

Meningococcus is an uncommon cause of pneumonia and is usually observed with signs and symptoms of pharyngitis.

TREATMENT

N. *meningitidis* is almost universally sensitive to penicillin, which, owing to the severity of the disease, is usually given parenterally in cases of severe meningococcal infection. **Rifampin** can be used for chemoprophylaxis of close contacts of affected individuals. Currently, the American Academy of Pediatrics recommends vaccinating all adolescents at age 11–12 with the meningococcal conjugate vaccine, which covers four of the five most common disease–causing serogroups (capsule polysaccharide from serogroup B is not sufficiently immunogenic to synthesize a vaccine).

NEISSERIA GONORRHOEAE

CHARACTERISTICS

Like N. *meningitidis*, N. *gonorrhoeae* is an aerobic gram-negative coccus that is responsible for serious infections in humans. It possesses the same virulence factors as N. *meningitidis* except that it lacks a polysaccharide capsule. It is responsible for the sexually transmitted infection **gonorrhea** as well as a disseminated variant. Passage through an infected vaginal canal during parturition can result in purulent gonococcal infection of the eye, termed **ophthalmia neonatorum**. Transmission is otherwise via unprotected sexual contact.

Attempts to isolate gonococcus from clinical samples (e.g., urethral swabs) are usually performed on **Thayer-Martin medium**, which is supplemented with antibiotics to prevent overgrowth of normal genital flora.

CLINICAL SYMPTOMS

- Uncomplicated genital gonorrhea is generally found as acute, purulent **urethritis** in males (see Figure 5-18) and either as acute **cervicitis** or an asymptomatic finding in females. Most infected men present with acute onset of dysuria and discharge. Infected women may experience abdominal pain, vaginal discharge, and dysuria; often the infection is asymptomatic.
- **Gonococcal pharyngitis** is an uncommon cause of sore throat, inevitably caused by orogenital contact.
- A significant complication of untreated disease in females is ascending genital tract infection, termed **pelvic inflammatory disease (PID)**, in which the infection spreads to the uterus, salpinges, and ovaries. Symptoms are protean and include abdominal pain, cervical motion tenderness, dysuria, fever, nausea, and vomiting. Serious sequelae of PID include **tubo-ovarian abscess, infertility,** and increased probability of **ectopic pregnancy.**
- **Disseminated gonococcal infection** via hematogenous spread is also possible following local gonococcal infection. This is often manifested as acute, painful, asymmetric migratory polyarthralgia, frequently seen in a clinical triad with **tenosynovitis** (inflammation of the tendon capsule, often on the dorsum of the hand) and a painless, nonpruritic **rash**. Acute suppurative **septic arthritis** with swollen, painful knees, wrists, and ankles is also seen in disseminated infection.

KEY FACT

Meningeal signs include **nuchal rigidity** and **Kernig's** and **Brudzinski's signs**. All are signs of **meningeal irritation** (though with fairly low sensitivity) and their presence should prompt a meningitis workup.

KEY FACT

Gonorrhea is the second most common sexually transmitted infection in the United States, following only *Chlamydia trachomatis*.

KEY FACT

Pelvic inflammatory disease is usually polymicrobial; however, gonococcus and/or *C. trachomatis* are commonly involved.

MNEMONIC

The diagnosis of disseminated gonococcal infection is an ART:

Arthralgia
Rash
Tenosynovitis

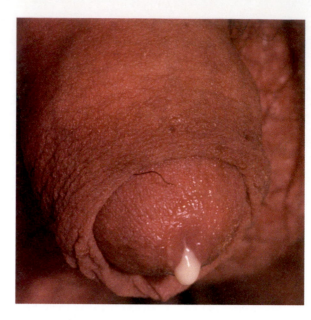

FIGURE 5-18. **Urethral discharge secondary to gonorrhea.** Frank purulent discharge is a common feature, especially in infected males. (Reproduced, with permission, from Wolff K, Johnson RA, Suurmond D. *Fitzpatrick's Color Atlas & Synopsis of Clinical Dermatology*, 5th ed. New York: McGraw-Hill, 2005: 907.)

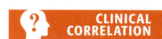

CLINICAL CORRELATION

Empiric antibiotic therapy for genital gonorrhea should always include coverage for coinfection with **C. trachomatis.** For this reason, **azithyromycin** or **doxycycline** is usually added to standard single-dose intramuscular **ceftriaxone** for gonorrhea.

- **Gonococcal ophthalmia neonatorum** presents as an acute purulent conjunctivitis several days after birth. All newborns routinely receive intraocular antibiotics as prophylaxis against ocular gonococcal and chlamydial infections.

TREATMENT

Resistance rates to penicillin and tetracycline are high, and resistance to the previous first-line therapy of fluoroquinolones is on the rise. Therefore, first-line therapy is usually a **third-generation cephalosporin,** such as intramuscular ceftriaxone. Prior infections do not confer immunity, so efforts at disease prevention are currently focused on barrier methods of contraception.

GRAM-NEGATIVE RODS

Because of the plethora of medically important gram-negative rods, many medical students find that keeping them straight is a difficult proposition. In this book, the microorganisms are grouped according to the major site of disease to allow for easier learning by categorization (see Table 5-13).

Gram-Negative Rods Causing Respiratory/Mucosal Infections

These organisms all appear as small, gram-negative "coccoid" rods when viewed under the microscope and are sometimes described as "coccobacillary" for this reason. The zoonotic bacteria *Brucella* spp. and *Pasteurella multocida* can also fall into this group, although for convenience they are described in the Zoonoses section.

HAEMOPHILUS INFLUENZAE

CHARACTERISTICS

Certainly the most clinically important member of the above-defined respiratory group is *H. influenzae*. Formerly a major cause of severe childhood respiratory disease, the highly virulent *H. influenzae* serotype **b** (Hib) has now

KEY FACT

H. influenzae does **not cause influenza,** although it is an important cause of post-influenza pneumonia.

TABLE 5-13. Gram-Negative Rods

Respiratory/Mucosal Pathogens	Enteric Pathogens	Zoonotic Pathogens
Haemophilus influenzae	Enterobacteriaceae family	Yersinia pestis
Haemophilus ducreyi	Vibrio spp.	Francisella tularensis
Gardnerella vaginalis	Pseudomonas aeruginosa	Brucella spp.
Bordetella pertussis	Bacteroides fragilis	Pasteurella multocida
Legionella pneumophila		Bartonella henselae

been largely relegated to the annals of pediatric history owing to remarkable success in vaccination.

- *H. influenzae* culture requires the addition of factors V and X, which are found in hydrolyzed blood ("chocolate") agar.
- They appear as small, gram-negative, nonmotile coccobacillary organisms.
- Both encapsulated and nonencapsulated (nontypable) strains exist.
- Encapsulated strains have been characterized as **serotypes a through f.**
- In the prevaccination era, **serotype b** (also known as **Hib**) was responsible for over 95% of invasive pediatric disease.
- Most *H. influenzae* disease is now caused by serotypes c, f, and nontypable strains (which can only cause local disease).

Nontypable *H. influenzae* contribute to normal bacterial flora of the nasopharyngeal mucosa from an early age, and endogenous infection from these sites is responsible for most localized disease (otitis media, sinusitis, pneumonia). Transmission is by respiratory droplets.

Children younger than three years old are uniquely susceptible to infection with encapsulated serotypes of *H. influenzae* because specific adaptive immune response to polysaccharide antigens is deficient in young children. Infants younger than six months have relative protection due to maternal antibodies passed transplacentally and via breast milk. Immunocompromised, nonvaccinated, and asplenic patients are also at risk.

PATHOGENESIS

Like all gram-negative organisms, *H. influenzae* possesses endotoxin, which is responsible for many of its deleterious effects. Other virulence factors include pili and nonpilus adhesins, which mediate attachment, and the antiphagocytic polysaccharide capsule if present.

CLINICAL SYMPTOMS

H. influenzae is responsible for a number of respiratory diseases with varying degrees of severity.

- **Epiglottitis** is perhaps the most memorable of the clinical entities caused by *H. influenzae*. It is uncommon now because it is **caused only by Hib.** Affected children are 2–4 years old and present sitting bolt upright with copious drooling, stridor, sore throat, fever, and dyspnea. Rapid airway obstruction leading to death can occur, and **laryngoscopy in the operating room** is required for definitive diagnosis.

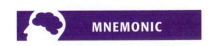

MNEMONIC

*Ha**EMOP**h**I**lu**S** influenzae* causes:

Epiglottitis
Meningitis
Otitis media
Pneumonia
eye –"**I**"– infections
Sinusitis

- **Meningitis** also only results from infection with serotype b. Formerly, it was the major causative organism of meningitis in infants six months to three years old. Since children at this age do not commonly present with the typical meningitic symptom of stiff neck, the diagnosis is suspected based on nonspecific signs such as fever, poor feeding, vomiting, and irritability. Mortality is low, but residual neurologic deficits are common.

- Upper and lower respiratory tract disease (**otitis media** in children, and **pneumonia**, **conjunctivitis**, and **sinusitis** in anyone) are common manifestations of endogenous *H. influenzae* infection caused by colonization with nontypable strains. The organism is among the top two causative agents of otitis media and sinusitis (*S. pneumoniae* is the other); pneumonia usually occurs only in previously damaged lungs (smokers and patients recovering from influenza viral pneumonia, for example).

TREATMENT

Minor respiratory tract infections generally respond to treatment with ampicillin or amoxicillin, although resistance rates are increasing (currently approximately 30%). Other options are azithromycin or a "respiratory" cephalosporin. Meningitis requires prompt therapy with CNS-penetrant third-generation cephalosporins (ceftriaxone or cefotaxime).

Chemoprophylaxis of susceptible close contacts is required and rifampin is the drug of choice. More important, immunization of all children with the univalent conjugate vaccine against the *H. influenzae* serotype b polysaccharide capsule is recommended—three doses are generally given before six months of age.

HAEMOPHILUS DUCREYI

CHARACTERISTICS

The causative organism of **chancroid**, a sexually transmitted infection.

CLINICAL SYMPTOMS

Patients have a tender perineal nodule that eventually ulcerates (see Figure 5-19) and is associated with inguinal lymphadenopathy. The differential diagnosis of this condition is important (see Table 5-14).

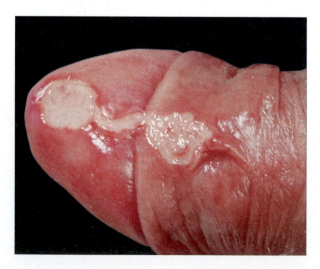

FIGURE 5-19. An enlarging chancroid with gray exudate. (Reproduced, with permission, from Wolff K, Goldsmith LA, Katz SI, et al. *Fitzpatrick's Dermatology in General Medicine*, 7th ed. New York: McGraw-Hill, 2008: Figure 202-2.)

TABLE 5-14. Differential Diagnosis of Genital Ulceration

	CHANCROID	SYPHILIS	GENITAL HERPES	LYMPHOGRANULOMA VENEREUM
Number of ulcers	Single.	Single, rolled edges.	Multiple, vesicular.	Single.
Ulcer painful?	Painful.	Painless.	Painful.	Painless.
Regional lymphadenopathy	Unilateral, painful, suppurative.	Bilateral, painless, nonsuppurative.	None, but systemic symptoms present.	Painless, suppurative; appear after ulcer disappears.

TREATMENT

Treatment is with erythromycin. The major complication is increased rate of transmission of other sexually transmitted diseases through the open sore.

GARDNERELLA VAGINALIS

CHARACTERISTICS

G. *vaginalis* is a coccobacillary gram-negative organism that has been isolated from the vaginal mucosa of both asymptomatic females as those with **bacterial vaginosis (BV)**.

CLINICAL SYMPTOMS

BV is a polymicrobial colonization of the vagina with G. *vaginalis* in addition to a number of anaerobic bacteria. Clinically, it is characterized by intense pruritus, dysuria, and a characteristic fishy odor of the copious, frothy secretions. **Clue cells**, which are vaginal epithelial cells covered with coccobacillary bacteria, are seen on wet mount of the discharge (see Figure 5-20).

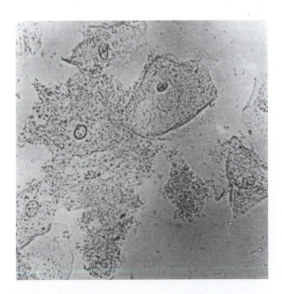

FIGURE 5-20. Clue cells of bacterial vaginosis. Note the stippled appearance of the epithelial cells, which is pathognomonic for *Gardnerella vaginalis* infestation. Reproduced, with permission, from Kuhn GJ, Vulvovaginitis. In Tintinalli JE, Kelen GD, et al. Stapczynski JS, eds., *Tintinalli's Emergency Medicine: A Comprehensive Study Guide*, 6th ed New York: McGraw-Hill, 2004: 691.)

TREATMENT

Treatment is with metronidazole to cover both G. *vaginalis* and anaerobes.

BORDETELLA PERTUSSIS

CHARACTERISTICS

Like H. *influenzae* serotype b, B. *pertussis* is a former major cause of pediatric respiratory morbidity and mortality that has been largely controlled by an effective vaccination program. It is responsible for **whooping cough.**

- B. *pertussis* is an extremely small, coccobacillary, gram-negative rod.
- It is highly sensitive to drying, so care must be taken when collecting and transporting patient samples.
- The microbe has fastidious nutritional requirements, so specialized media (Bordet-Gengou or Regan-Lowe agars) are required for growth.
- Only 50% of all clinically diagnosed patients have positive cultures.

B. *pertussis* is highly infective via the nasopharyngeal/respiratory route and infects only humans. Although it is traditionally considered a pediatric disease, whooping cough is now seen in older individuals as well, a phenomenon thought to be secondary to decreased protective effects of childhood vaccination.

PATHOGENESIS

B. *pertussis* has a number of virulence factors that contribute to its toxicity. **Filamentous hemagglutinin** and **pertactin** are proteins that mediate specific adhesion to ciliated respiratory epithelial cells. **Tracheal cytotoxin** destroys respiratory epithelium directly and may be responsible for the characteristic violent cough. **Pertussis toxin** is a two-part (A-B) exotoxin in which the B component binds the respiratory epithelial cell, allowing entry of the A component. The A component then constitutively inactivates the inhibitory G protein $G_{\alpha i}$, causing increased cyclic adenosine monophosphate (cAMP) levels and therefore increased respiratory secretions. The **adenylate cyclase toxin** also increases cAMP levels to the same effect.

CLINICAL SYMPTOMS

Pertussis, or whooping cough, is characterized by four stages with relatively distinct clinical features.

- The asymptomatic **incubation** period is 7–10 days.
- The **catarrhal stage** lasts about 10 days. This stage is characterized by typical upper respiratory infection symptoms such as sneezing, low fever, and rhinorrhea. Despite its nonspecific symptoms, this stage harbors the period of maximum infectivity.
- The **paroxysmal stage** then lasts for two weeks to one month and characterized by the "whoops" of whooping cough. Patients have periodic paroxysms consisting of repetitive nonproductive coughing followed by an inspiratory "whoop"; this then continues to cycle and is often terminated only by post-tussive emesis or exhaustion. Hypoxemia and cyanosis are also seen.
- Finally, the **convalescent stage** lasts for approximately one month and is characterized by the gradual reduction in intensity and frequency of paroxysms.

TREATMENT

Macrolide antibiotic therapy is effective only when given during the incubation or catarrhal stages of the disease. Other treatment is generally supportive in nature and is focused on maintenance of a patent airway. Household contacts of patients with pertussis undergo chemoprophylaxis with 14 days of erythromycin.

The acellular pertussis vaccine—which has replaced the complication-prone whole cell pertussis vaccine—is a key component of the diphtheria-tetanus-acellular pertussis combination vaccine (DTaP) recommended for all infants. Five total doses are given. TdaP (tetanus-acellular pertussis) was recently approved as a booster vaccine to reimmunize adolescent and adult individuals who have probable waning immunity from their childhood DTaP series.

LEGIONELLA PNEUMOPHILA

CHARACTERISTICS

L. pneumophila, the causative organism of **Legionnaires' disease**, was discovered in 1976 after an outbreak of severe lower respiratory disease at a convention in Philadelphia. During the workup of this epidemic, this novel organism was discovered to preferentially inhabit natural and artificial bodies of water. Transmission is usually via the inhalation of infectious aerosols. In the case of the Legionnaires' convention, the microbe was found in the air-conditioning system.

L. pneumophila is a highly motile, pleomorphic, gram-negative rod that is poorly visualized on Gram's staining; therefore, silver or fluorescent antibody staining is generally used. Culture is possible on **buffered charcoal yeast extract agar** supplemented with cysteine, but diagnosis is usually made using urine serology.

PATHOGENESIS

The Legionella organism is a facultative intracellular microbe, meaning that it multiplies inside the phagosomes of alveolar macrophages following phagocytosis, specifically inhibiting lysosome fusion so that it is not destroyed.

CLINICAL SYMPTOMS

The mild form of legionellosis is an influenza-like illness called **Pontiac fever.** It is characterized by epidemic outbreaks with a high attack rate, as well as a clinical syndrome of fever, chills, and myalgias with resolution in about 1 week without treatment. Legionnaires' disease itself is a severe community-acquired pneumonia that generally affects elderly persons with underlying lung disease. Clinically presentation includes a nonproductive cough, high fevers, and headache, with a rapid deterioration often leading to death if antibiotic therapy is not promptly started.

TREATMENT

The mainstay of treatment is erythromycin; penicillins are not effective because of the presence of β-lactamase. Following diagnosis, an effort to discover and eradicate the source of infection should be undertaken.

Enteric Gram-Negative Rods

Enteric pathogens are microbes that commonly infect the lumen of the lower alimentary canal. This site is relatively accessible to bacteria, as evidenced by the vast number of commensal organisms (such as E. coli) that happily coexist with the human host. Pathogenic microbes that cause enteric pathology can produce syndromes along two clinical spectra: Diarrheal disease and systemic disease.

There are four taxonomic families of enteric organisms important in medicine:

- **Enterobacteriaceae:** a large, diverse family made up of typical enteric organisms.
- **Vibrionaceae:** containing the causative agents of cholera and some others.
- **Pseudomonadaceae:** *P. aeruginosa*, commonly seen in hospitalized patients.
- **Bacteroidaceae:** *Bacteroides fragilis*, an anaerobe that can cause visceral infections.

ENTEROBACTERIACEAE

CHARACTERISTICS

This family of enteric gram-negative rods is huge, but they fortunately share many common characteristics. Microscopically, they all appear as medium-sized nonsporulating gram-negative rods; when cultured, they have relatively relaxed nutrient requirements and grow handily on most basic media. The **lactose fermentation test** (often accomplished on the selective and differential EMB or MacConkey's agars) and the ability to **produce hydrogen sulfide (H_2S) gas** are two biochemical tests that help technologists characterize and differentiate members of the Enterobacteriaceae family.

PATHOGENESIS

Common virulence factors include the **O**, **K**, and **H** antigens, which differ between genera and species and are used to serologically classify clinical isolates. The heat-stable **O antigen** is the outermost polysaccharide layer of the LPS (endotoxin) component of the cell wall. The heat-labile **K antigen** refers to the polysaccharide capsule if present, and the heat-labile **H antigen** is a flagellar protein that may be present.

SHIGELLA SPECIES

CHARACTERISTICS

The four species that make up the genus *Shigella* are highly virulent enteric bacteria responsible for many cases of gastrointestinal disease, especially in pediatric populations with relaxed standards of hygiene (e.g., day-care centers). It is a **nonmotile**, gram-negative rod that, when cultured, does **not ferment lactose** but is able to **produce H_2S gas.**

Humans are the only host of *Shigella*; unlike many other Enterobacteriaceae there is **no animal reservoir.** Transmission is from person to person via the fecal-oral route, and as few as 10 organisms may cause symptomatic infection!

PATHOGENESIS

Shigella causes an invasive gastroenteritis by specifically attaching to and invading immune cells located in Peyer's patches. Much of *Shigella's* virulence can be ascribed to the presence of the highly virulent exotoxin called **Shiga toxin.** This is a typical A-B toxin wherein the B subunit binds to enterocytes, allowing the A unit to penetrate the cells and cause cell death.

CLINICAL SYMPTOMS

The invasive diarrhea caused by *Shigella* spp. is called **shigellosis** and is characterized by **bloody stools** with frank pus, fever, and abdominal pain occurring 1–3 days after ingestion of the organism. The diarrhea is often initially watery. *S. dysenteriae* specifically produces the Shiga toxin and can cause a

MNEMONIC

COFFEe:

Capsulated
O antigen
Flagellar antigen
Ferment glucose
Enterobacteriaceae

MNEMONIC

*OKH antigens: **O**utside **K**apsule **H**ello.*

Outside
Kapsule
H is a flagellum waving **"hello"**

MNEMONIC

The four **F**'s of *Shigella* transmission: **F**ood, **F**ingers, **F**lies, and **F**eces.

more severe form of the disease termed **bacterial dysentery;** this species is also occasionally associated with the **hemolytic-uremic syndrome** (discussed in greater detail in the *E. coli* text).

TREATMENT

Empiric antibiotic therapy with a fluoroquinolone or TMP-SMX can shorten the course of disease. Other treatment is supportive in nature.

SALMONELLA SPECIES

CHARACTERISTICS

The enteric pathogen *Salmonella* is another common cause of invasive diarrhea, although unlike infection with *Shigella*, the disease is normally acquired by eating contaminated food products. *Salmonella* spp. is a **motile,** gram-negative rod that, like *Shigella*, **produces H$_2$S gas,** but does **not ferment lactose.** Several species exist, but the most important distinction is between *Salmonella typhi* (the causative agent of typhoid fever) and everything else (*S. enteritidis*, others that cause gastrointestinal disease).

Transmission of *Salmonella* is usually via ingestion of contaminated chicken, egg, or dairy products. *S. typhi* is propagated by the fecal-oral route, often from infected, asymptomatic carriers that harbor the organism in their gallbladders.

PATHOGENESIS

Like *Shigella*, the main route of initial *Salmonella* invasion is via the M cells of the Peyer's patches of the intestine, which then may result in hematogenous spread. The organism is remarkably tolerant to stomach and lysosomal acid. *S. typhi* is able to reside in macrophage vesicles, allowing it to be carried to extraintestinal sites to cause typhoid fever. The organism possesses a polysaccharide capsule known as the **Vi antigen.**

CLINICAL SYMPTOMS

Four different clinical syndromes can result from *Salmonella* infection: Gastroenteritis, bacteremia/sepsis, typhoid fever, and an asymptomatic carrier state.

- *Salmonella* **gastroenteritis** is the most common form of *Salmonella* infection. It presents as an invasive diarrhea characterized by nausea, frequent stools ranging from watery to slightly bloody with mucus, and abdominal pain. Notably, antibiotic therapy does not shorten the course of the disease.
- *Salmonella* **sepsis** is uncommon and has a higher incidence in immunocompromised, pediatric, and elderly patients. Asplenic individuals (i.e., those with sickle cell) have difficulty clearing the organism because of the polysaccharide capsule, so hematogenous spread to various end organs (bone, joints, heart) is possible in these cases.
- **Typhoid fever** (also known as enteric fever) results from *S. typhi* invasion into enterocytes and subsequent intracellular residence in circulating macrophages. It is characterized by the onset of fever, headache, and abdominal pain, mimicking appendicitis, approximately 1–3 weeks after exposure. Signs include splenomegaly and a transient rash (termed **rose spots**) on the abdomen (see Figure 5-21).
- **Asymptomatic carriers** of *S. typhi* constitutively excrete the organism in stool due to colonization of the gallbladder but are completely asymptomatic. This represents the source and reservoir of *S. typhi* infections.

KEY FACT

Typhoid Mary was an asymptomatic carrier of *S. typhi* in early 20th century New York. Via her job as a cook, she infected several people who later died of typhoid fever. She was incarcerated by the state against her will as a public health measure.

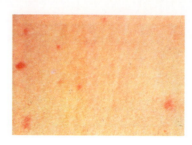

FIGURE 5-21. **Rose spots of typhoid fever.** These pathognomonic spots appear transiently on light-skinned individuals. (Reproduced, with permission, from Kasper DL, Braunwald E, Fauci AS, et al. *Harrison's Principles of Internal Medicine*, 16th ed. New York: McGraw-Hill, 2005: 899.)

TREATMENT

Ciprofloxacin or ceftriaxone, among other agents, are appropriate treatments for disseminated disease or typhoid fever. Treatment of asymptomatic carriers is strongly suggested as a public health measure and may require surgical excision of the gallbladder. A vaccine for *S. typhi* is available but is only routinely given to individuals traveling to endemic areas.

ESCHERICHIA COLI

E. coli is definitely the most important of the enteric bacteria. It can be associated with many diseases affecting different organ systems.

- *E. coli* is a motile, gram-negative, medium-sized rod.
- It is a **lactose fermenter,** thus appearing purple on MacConkey's agar, and does **not** produce H_2S gas.
- It is the most common aerobic gram-negative rod in the digestive tract.

CLINICAL SYMPTOMS

Diseases caused by *E. coli* are numerous and varied. The spectrum ranges from relatively trivial infections such as bacterial cystitis and traveler's diarrhea to neonatal meningitis and gram-negative sepsis.

- *E. coli* **infectious diarrhea** is a major cause of infant mortality worldwide, usually due to dehydration. Several variants of diarrheal illness caused by *E. coli* have been characterized in humans. They differ from each other based on affected populations, clinical presentation, pathogenic factors, and severity (see Table 5-15).
- The **hemolytic-uremic syndrome (HUS)** is one of the most feared complications of enterohemorrhagic *E. coli* (EHEC) infection in children. Approximately 5%–10% of infected children younger than 10 years go on to have the clinical triad of renal failure, hemolytic anemia, and thrombocytopenia in addition to bloody diarrhea.
- *E. coli* is by far the number one cause of urinary tract infections. Strains of *E. coli* possess pili-bound adhesion factors allowing them to attach to the urethral wall and ascend the urinary tract, causing **bacterial cystitis.** This is characterized by dysuria, hematuria, and increased urinary frequency. A common complication of cystitis is **pyelonephritis** or ascending infection of the kidney parenchyma, in which fever, flank pain, and vomiting are common.
- *E. coli* is the second most common cause of **neonatal meningitis.**
- Gram-negative sepsis is usually nosocomially acquired and caused by *E. coli*. It primarily affects debilitated, hospitalized patients, especially following instrumentation or intra-abdominal infection. Septic shock is the most

TABLE 5-15. Diarrhea Caused by *E. coli*

VARIANT	EPIDEMIOLOGY	PRESENTATION	PATHOGENESIS	SEVERITY
Enterotoxigenic *E. coli* (ETEC)—traveler's diarrhea. Found in contaminated water.	Affects infants in developing countries, travelers.	Copious, watery, nonbloody diarrhea up to 20 L/day, abdominal cramping.	Cholera-like heat-labile toxin **LT-I** and heat-stable toxin **STa** stimulate secretion of Cl⁻ and HCO_3^- ions into intestinal lumen; water follows osmotic load.	Can be fatal in infants if not rehydrated.
Enteropathogenic *E. coli* (EPEC).	Affects infants in developing countries.	Watery diarrhea.	Microcolony formation on the surface of intestinal epithelium with subsequent loss of microvilli → decreased absorption.	Mild to moderate disease.
Enteroinvasive *E. coli* (EIEC).	Rare in developed countries, uncommon worldwide.	Bloody diarrhea with pus, fever, abdominal pain.	Shares virulence factors with *Shigella* (not Shiga toxin) and can invade enterocytes directly, causing an inflammatory reaction and colitis.	Usually mild; can progress to dysentery.
Enterohemorrhagic *E. coli* (EHEC), including strain O157:H7. Found in ground beef.	Most common strains causing disease in developed world; O157:H7 most common in U.S.	Hemorrhagic colitis— abdominal pain, bloody diarrhea, no fever; can cause hemolytic-uremic syndrome (HUS).	Expresses Shiga toxin, inhibiting protein synthesis and causing enterocyte death.	Usually resolves without treatment; HUS can be fatal.

common cause of death in this group, presumably caused by the endotoxin component of the cell wall.

TREATMENT

Antibiotics are not necessarily indicated in most diarrheal infections. Antibiotic choice is dictated by susceptibility testing in the case of disseminated or serious disease. Urinary tract infections are usually treated empirically with TMP-SMX, fluoroquinolones, or urinary sterilants.

CAMPYLOBACTER JEJUNI

CHARACTERISTICS

This organism is not actually a member of the Enterobacteriaceae family, but is included here because it also causes severe invasive **diarrhea.**

- *C. jejuni* is a small, curved (comma-shaped), motile gram-negative rod.
- Culture conditions require special nutrients contained in **Campy agar** as well as a **microaerophilic** atmosphere (5% O_2).
- Acquisition of the organism is from contaminated foodstuffs and water; **undercooked chicken,** and **unpasteurized milk** are common sources.
- Although usually not stressed by microbiology textbooks, *Campylobacter* is the single most common cause of invasive diarrhea.
- Over two million incident cases of *C. jejuni* occur in the United States each year.

PATHOGENESIS

As indicated by its species name, *C. jejuni* causes an invasive diarrhea with tissue invasion largely in the distal small bowel. Pathologic specimens show ulceration, crypt abscesses, and acute inflammation. Unfortunately, neither the virulence factors causing *Campylobacter*'s tropism to this area nor the toxins involved in invasion have been well characterized.

CLINICAL SYMPTOMS

Like other invasive infectious diarrheas, *C. jejuni* enteritis is characterized by bloody diarrhea, fever, malaise, and abdominal pain. The disease is self-limited. Complications are rare and include sepsis and spontaneous abortion.

TREATMENT

Routine regional enteritis of *C. jejuni* infection usually responds to fluid replacement and does not require antibiotic therapy. More serious infections require erythromycin, tetracyclines, or fluoroquinolones.

HELICOBACTER PYLORI

CHARACTERISTICS

The recently discovered bacterium *H. pylori* has been found to be a highly important cause of gastroduodenal pathology.

- *H. pylori* is a corkscrew-shaped, highly motile, gram-negative rod that grows best under microaerophilic conditions.
- It is uniquely found in biopsy specimens of **duodenal ulcers** and **chronic gastritis,** but without evidence of tissue invasion.
- It possesses a **urease** enzyme capable of splitting urea into alkaline ammonia, which allows it to survive in the highly acidic gastric microenvironment.
- Diagnosis is usually made either by examination of endoscopic biopsies or a highly specific **urease breath test**.
- **Triple therapy** (either bismuth-metronidazole-tetracycline/amoxicillin or metronidazole-omeprazole-clarithromycin) eradicates the organism and prevents ulcer/gastritis recurrence.
- **Vaccine development** is currently underway.

KLEBSIELLA PNEUMONIAE

CHARACTERISTICS

Klebsiella is an **encapsulated**, **lactose-fermenting** member of the Enterobacteriaceae family that causes community-acquired pneumonia.

CLINICAL SYMPTOMS

Alcoholics and others with conditions causing aspiration of oral secretions are particularly at risk for this condition, which is characterized by frankly bloody, **currant-jelly** sputum. The pneumonia is lobar, severe, and often necrotizing and cavitating. It can also cause gram-negative sepsis.

PROTEUS MIRABILIS

CHARACTERISTICS

This organism is uniquely characterized by its extreme motility and its ability to chemically split urea into two molecules of ammonia via its **urease** enzyme.

CLINICAL CORRELATION

Prior **C. jejuni infection** has been shown to be associated with the development of **Guillain-Barré syndrome** and **reactive arthritis** resulting from the cross-reactivity of antibodies directed against the bacteria.

KEY FACT

H. pylori infection is associated with increased risk of gastric adenocarcinoma and gastric lymphoma.

CLINICAL SYMPTOMS

P. mirabilis is a common cause of urinary tract infections; in these cases, urinalysis confirms the bacterial diagnosis owing to the **alkaline pH of the urine.**

YERSINIA ENTEROCOLITICA

CHARACTERISTICS

This bacterium is actually a fully zoonotic pathogen, infecting mostly farm animals and pets. It is transmitted by the ingestion of contaminated water or milk.

CLINICAL SYMPTOMS

Y. enterocolitica causes an invasive gastroenteritis associated with fever, abdominal pain, and diarrhea (sometimes bloody). It can also spread to the mesenteric lymph nodes and produce symptoms of abdominal pain that closely mimic acute appendicitis.

CITROBACTER, ENTEROBACTER, MORGANELLA, SERRATIA, EDWARDSIELLA, PROVIDENCIA

CHARACTERISTICS

Certain other Enterobacteriaceae rarely infect immunocompetent patients and are included here for completeness only. *Enterobacter* infections are known for resistance to multiple antibiotics. *S. marcescens* culture produces characteristic bright-red colonies on agar.

VIBRIONACEAE

CHARACTERISTICS

Vibrio spp. are curved, motile, gram-negative rods with a single polar flagellum. Three medically relevant members of the *Vibrio* genus exist. The well-known *V. cholerae* produces the profuse watery diarrhea of cholera. *V. parahaemolyticus* and *V. vulnificus* are both acquired by eating contaminated shellfish and cause self-limiting gastroenteritides and wound infections, respectively.

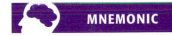

MNEMONIC

Vibrio spp. have **vibrating** motility.

VIBRIO CHOLERAE

CHARACTERISTICS

V. cholerae is a major cause of infant mortality worldwide due to the effects of its exotoxin. It is a comma-shaped gram-negative rod that has no particular specific culture requirements (see Figure 5-22). Many serogroups are found in nature; the **O1 and O139 serogroups** are specifically associated with epidemic full-blown cholera.

V. cholerae is generally found in developing or impoverished countries in standing or brackish water contaminated by human feces. The organism can easily multiply and contaminate drinking water, causing epidemics and pandemics. The **el tor** biotype of serogroup O1 was responsible for the most recent worldwide pandemic in the latter half of the previous century. Person-to-person transmission is rare, and inhabitants of endemic areas often are immune.

PATHOGENESIS

The **cholera toxin,** also known as choleragen, is an A-B exotoxin that is secreted upon binding of the cholera bacteria to the enterocytes. Once the A subunit gains entry to the cell, it causes constitutive activation of the G protein $G_{\alpha s}$, resulting in the buildup of cAMP in a manner similar to the action

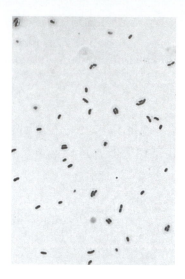

FIGURE 5-22. ***Vibrio cholerae* in broth culture.** These organisms appear black because this is a phase-contrast micrograph; on Gram's stain they would appear red. (Reproduced, with permission, from Brooks GF, Butel JS, Morse SA. *Jawetz, Melnick, & Adelberg's Medical Microbiology*, 23rd ed. New York: McGraw-Hill, 2004: 271.)

of pertussis toxin. Because of this cAMP accumulation, sodium and chloride ions are actively extruded into the colon lumen and reabsorption is inhibited.

CLINICAL SYMPTOMS

Affected individuals are rapidly afflicted with so-called **rice-water stools** named for their appearance. Massive fluid catharsis due to osmotic pull of the secreted sodium chloride occurs, with isotonic fluid losses potentially up to 20 liters per day. Massive electrolyte imbalances (hypokalemia, metabolic acidosis) and hypovolemic shock can occur and lead to death if affected persons are untreated.

TREATMENT

The cornerstone of therapy for cholera is fluid replacement; the use of inexpensive **oral rehydration therapy** in developing countries has saved countless lives. Antibiotic therapy with doxycycline or TMP-SMX in children can shorten the course of the disease.

PSEUDOMONACEAE

CHARACTERISTICS

P. aeruginosa and related organisms constitute a group of microbes that serve mainly as **opportunistic pathogens** of humans; that is, they mainly infect patients with specific defects in their immune or antimicrobial defenses. These large, **strictly aerobic,** gram-negative rods do **not ferment lactose** and are differentiated from the nonfermentative Enterobacteriaceae (*Shigella, Salmonella*, and others) by the fact that they contain the enzyme oxidase and are thus **oxidase-positive.** *P. aeruginosa* is by far the most common and important of these organisms; the others that make up this group are listed only for completeness: *Burkholderia* spp., *Stenotrophomonas maltophila*, and *Acinetobacter* spp.

PSEUDOMONAS AERUGINOSA

CHARACTERISTICS

Pseudomonas is an oxidase-positive, gram-negative rod that can be immediately identified in a microbiology lab because of its characteristic odor and color. Cultures of this organism (as well as infected surface wounds) have a bluish-green tint due to the production of the **water-soluble** pigments **pyocyanin** and **fluorescein.** In addition, the bacteria produces a sweet (some people liken it to grapes) odor.

The epidemiology of *Pseudomonas* is relatively uncomplicated. It is naturally a soil contaminant and is commonly found in moist environments, especially within hospitals. The organism is uniquely **resistant** to many antibiotics and disinfectants, and direct transmission from contaminated surfaces is the rule.

PATHOGENESIS

This organism features a number of virulence factors that are key to its unique patterns of toxicity. It does not possess significant invasive ability in healthy hosts, but easily infects hospitalized, immunocompromised patients.

- **Exotoxin A** serves as an inhibitor to elongation factor EF-2, effectively disrupting protein synthesis in mammalian cells.
- **Endotoxin** (LPS) is a major player in pseudomonal sepsis.
- Some strains have an antiphagocytic polysaccharide **capsule.**
- Connective tissue hydrolases, including **elastases** and **alkaline protease.** Allow facile spread of the organism through infected tissues.
- Through different mechanisms, *Pseudomonas* is **resistant to multiple antibiotics,** and therapy must be carefully chosen. The organism rapidly acquires resistance by mutation.

CLINICAL SYMPTOMS

Pseudomonas has a predilection for causing certain diseases in certain populations with decreased immune function (see Table 5-16).

TREATMENT

Pseudomonas can acquire resistance to many commonly used antibiotics, including aminoglycosides, penicillins, and fluoroquinolones. Appropriate therapy is **multiagent** for synergy and generally consists of a parenteral aminoglycoside coupled with an antipseudomonal penicillin such as piperacillin/tazobactam (Zosyn) or ticaricillin/sulbactam (Timentin). Ciprofloxacin and the third-/fourth-generation cephalosporins ceftazidime, cefoperazone, and cefipime as well as the carbapenem agents imipenem and meropenem are also usually active against *Pseudomonas.*

The cornerstones of prevention of pseudomonal infection are **sterilization of medical equipment** and prevention of overgrowth of resistant organisms via **appropriate use of broad-spectrum antibiotics,** since elimination of the pathogen from all contaminated surfaces is usually not feasible.

BACTEROIDIACEAE

Although there are several medically relevant members of the anaerobic Bacterioidiaceae family, the most important is *Bacteroides fragilis*, commonly implicated in visceral abscesses. Other members of the family include organisms causing periodontal disease and aspiration pneumonia such as *Bacteroides* spp., *Fusobacterium* spp., and *Porphyromonas* spp. In general, anaerobic

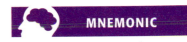

MNEMONIC

PSEUDO*monas causes:*

Pneumonia
Sepsis/**S**kin infections
Endocarditis
Urinary tract infection/corneal **U**lcers
Diabetic infections
Osteomyelitis

TABLE 5-16. Diseases Caused by *Pseudomonas aeruginosa*

DISEASE	SUSCEPTIBLE POPULATION(S)	CLINICAL SYNDROME
Pneumonia	Cystic fibrosis (CF).	Almost all CF patients are colonized with Pseudomonas, and exacerbations of the underlying disease are often associated with a necrotizing, destructive Pseudomonas pneumonia.
	Prior therapy with broad-spectrum antibiotics, or respiratory instrumentation.	Diffuse, bilateral necrotizing pneumonia with high mortality.
Urinary tract infections	Urinary instrumentation, broad-spectrum antibiotics.	Typical urinary tract infection symptoms of dysuria, pyuria, and urgency.
Osteomyelitis	Diabetics.	Pseudomonas is often the causative agent of infected diabetic foot ulcers.
	Children after puncture trauma.	Through-and-through puncture into the foot can lead to the introduction of Pseudomonas from the moist shoe environment into the wound.
Malignant otitis externa (OE)	Diabetics.	Typical OE is characterized by pain on ear traction and sometimes discharge; malignant OE is characterized by spread into the mastoid, with resultant destruction of bone and cranial nerves.
Wound infections	Burn patients.	The moist environment of the burn surface is an ideal breeding ground for Pseudomonas. One of the most feared complications of topical burns, it can lead to gram-negative sepsis.
Hot tub folliculitis	Anyone.	Inflammation of hair follicles with characteristic rash after immersion in warm, contaminated water.
Sepsis	Neutropenia, diabetics, extensive burns, leukemia.	Extremely high mortality rate for gram-negative sepsis.
Endocarditis	Intravenous drug abusers.	Infects right-sided heart valves.
Corneal ulcers	Contact lens wearers.	Usually occurs after incidental trauma to the eye; can rapidly progress if untreated.

infections tend to be polymicrobial, with a number of different organisms responsible for pathology.

Culture of obligate anaerobic bacteria presents a special problem; specific culture media as well as an O_2-free atmosphere are required. Treatment of these infections must include clindamycin, metronidazole, or other antibiotics with activity against anaerobes.

BACTEROIDES FRAGILIS

CHARACTERISTICS

This obligate anaerobe is a gram-negative commensal that lives within the alimentary and female reproductive tracts. When there is interruption of the wall of these areas (e.g., surgery, septic abortion, pelvic inflammatory disease, intestinal rupture), these organisms seed the intraperitoneal cavity, forming **abscesses** (see Figure 5-23).

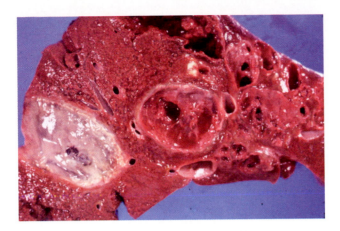

FIGURE 5-23. **Gross liver section with multiple *Bacteroides fragilis* abscesses.** This woman had a partial hepatectomy for metastatic colon cancer, and died of infectious complications from these abscesses. (Image courtesy of PEIR Digital Library [http://peir.net].)

CLINICAL SYMPTOMS

Fever and localized pain are the presenting symptoms of *B. fragilis* abscesses, and systemic hematogenous spread can result.

OTHER IMPORTANT BACTERIA

Several other groups of medically important bacteria do not have a definitive Gram's stain because of the makeup (or utter lack) of their cell walls or their obligate localization within the phagosomes of eukaryotic cells.

Mycobacterium

Mycobacteria are small, nonmotile, aerobic rods with a complex cell wall that differs from both gram-positive and gram-negative organisms. The cell walls of mycobacteria possess complex lipids called **mycosides**—**mycolic acid** residues on the most external surface—and various additional membrane proteins and cross linkages of the peptidoglycan layer. This cell wall structure causes mycobacteria to stain positive with **acid-fast stains,** as described previously. It also acts as a virulence factor, resulting in resistance to common antimicrobial agents, such as β-lactam and cephalosporin antibiotics.

There exist many pathogenic mycobacteria, most of which are either very slow-growing or unable to be grown in bacterial cultures. The two most important members of the genus are *M. tuberculosis*, the causative agent of **tuberculosis,** and *M. leprae,* the culprit behind **Hansen's disease** (formerly known as leprosy).

MYCOBACTERIUM TUBERCULOSIS

CHARACTERISTICS

M. tuberculosis infection is a major, life-threatening chronic condition affecting individuals in both impoverished and developed countries.

- *M. tuberculosis* is a small, acid-fast, obligate aerobe that resides inside macrophages and can establish lifelong infection.
- It is found worldwide—primarily in Southeast Asia, Africa, and Eastern Europe—and is spread by infectious aerosols from person-to-person (without animal reservoirs).

FLASH FORWARD

Zoonotic bacteria are covered in the zoonotic section on page 355.

KEY FACT

Acid-fast bacteria: *Mycobacterium* spp. and *Nocardia* spp.

- One third of the world's population carries some form of infection, but because of efficacious treatment regimens and strict reporting of cases, disease burden in the United States has been steadily decreasing.
- Risk factors for tuberculosis (in the United States) include:
  - Incarceration
  - Immunodeficiency, especially active, untreated HIV infection
  - Homelessness
  - Travel to endemic areas
  - Exposure to individuals with known active tuberculosis
  - Drug and alcohol abuse
  - Employment in a health care setting

FLASH FORWARD

Tuberculosis is the prototypical example of a T_H1-based infection. HIV patients with decreased CD4+ T-cell counts are especially susceptible to this infection.

PATHOGENESIS

Primary *M. tuberculosis* infection usually begins when infectious particles are inhaled and phagocytosed by alveolar macrophages. The microbe evades intravesicular killing by lysosomes by inhibition of lysosomal fusion; however, a chronic inflammatory response is produced. This inflammatory response damages tissue parenchyma, especially the lungs, resulting in the soft, deliquescent **caseous granulomas** composed of multiple infected macrophages and debris. Eventual control of the infection is achieved with **cell-mediated** (T_H1-based) immunity, but viable *M. tuberculosis* bacteria continue to exist within the granulomas and can **reactivate** when host immune function is depressed.

CLINICAL SYMPTOMS

The first exposure to the pathogen, termed **primary tuberculosis,** usually results in nothing more than an asymptomatic lung infection. The infection generally takes root in **central (perihilar) lung fields** (see Figure 5-24). The characteristic finding on chest radiograph is a **Ghon complex**, which consists of enlarged perihilar lymph nodes adjacent to a calcified granuloma. Symptomatic infection can occur in the elderly, pediatric, or immunosuppressed populations.

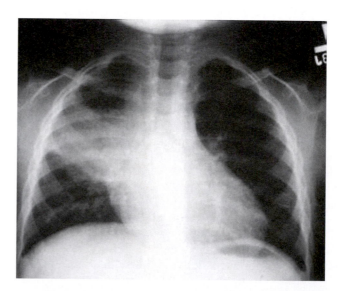

FIGURE 5-24. **Primary tuberculosis in a 3-year-old child.** There is no visible Ghon complex in this chest radiograph, but hilar lymphadenopathy and lobar consolidation are present. (Image courtesy of PEIR Digital Library [http://peir.net].)

- **Latent tuberculosis** is an asymptomatic state wherein the *M. tuberculosis* bacterium lies dormant inside caseous granulomas.
- **Reactivation (secondary) tuberculosis** occurs when the host undergoes a transient decrease in immune function, allowing escape of the organism from the granuloma and seeding of end organs. Most commonly, the apices of the lungs are affected because of the microbe's predilection for areas of high O_2 concentration.
    - Symptoms in this case are highly suggestive and include **fever, night sweats, weight loss,** and **hemoptysis.**
    - Without treatment, the bacteria and resultant inflammatory response slowly erode the lung parenchyma.

Tuberculosis can also reactivate in a number of **extrapulmonary organs:** The CNS (causing lymphocytic meningitis), vertebra (causing compression fractures and referred to as **Pott's disease**), kidneys, lymphoreticular system, and gastrointestinal tract.

- **Miliary tuberculosis** occurs when tubercular bacteremia causes distal seeding. This is seen mainly in immunosuppressed populations and has a high mortality rate. The radiographic and pathologic presentations of this disease are unforgettable (see Figure 5-25).

Diagnosis of active tuberculosis is usually clinical and radiographic, but the **purified protein derivative (PPD)** skin test provides a measure of whether individuals can mount a cell-mediated response to *M. tuberculosis*. Purified protein particles from killed *M. tuberculosis* bacteria are injected intradermally; a few days later, the area of induration (hard, raised bump; not the area of redness) is measured. Positive tests correlate with active, latent, or resolved infection; unfortunately, false-positive (due to cross-reactivity in recipients of the BCG vaccine) and false-negative (due to anergy in immunosuppressed patients) results are common.

TREATMENT

The mainstay of treatment for active tuberculosis is **prolonged multidrug therapy** to prevent the onset of resistance.

- Generally, a four-drug regimen consisting of isoniazid (INH), ethambutol, pyrazinamide, and rifampin for 2 months followed by INH/rifampin for 4–6 more months is used, although alternative combinations are required if resistance or drug intolerance develops.

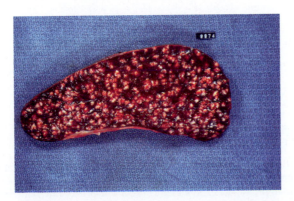

FIGURE 5-25.   Miliary tuberculosis of the spleen. Innumerable metastatic foci of *Mycobacterium tuberculosis* bacteria and inflammatory cells riddle the spleen and, presumably, other organs as well. (Image courtesy of PEIR Digital Library [http://peir.net].)

- Chemoprophylaxis for exposure to active tuberculosis or a positive PPD test without symptoms is generally nine months of INH; again, alternative regimens are possible depending on resistance patterns. The BCG (bacillus Calmette-Guerin) vaccine is given in some endemic countries to prevent primary infection. It prevents major sequelae of tuberculosis (disseminated or miliary) without actually preventing spread.

MYCOBACTERIUM LEPRAE

CHARACTERISTICS

M. *leprae* is an acid-fast, aerobic rod that causes the disfiguring disease known as **leprosy** or **Hansen's disease.** Humans and armadillos are the only known hosts. The disease is spread through contact with infected lesions. Better control of Hansen's disease has caused a 90% reduction in its incidence since 1985. M. *leprae* cannot be grown in artificial culture.

PATHOGENESIS

M. *leprae* has a predilection for cool surfaces, and therefore most of its pathogenic features occur in superficial tissues such as the skin and the peripheral nerves.

CLINICAL SYMPTOMS

Two clinical forms of leprosy are known: Tuberculoid leprosy and lepromatous leprosy (see Figure 5-26). They develop based on differential responses of the immune system to the bacteria (see Table 5-17).

TREATMENT

Therapy for the tuberculoid variant involves the antibiotics **dapsone** and **rifampin** for six months. Longer therapy of 12 months and the addition of clofazimine are required for the lepromatous variant.

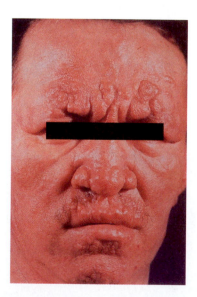

FIGURE 5-26. **Lepromatous leprosy.** Thickened and nodular facial skin produces the characteristic leonine facies and saddle-nose deformity. (Reproduced, with permission, from Kasper DL, Braunwald E, Fauci AS, et al. *Harrison's Principles of Internal Medicine*, 16th ed. New York: McGraw-Hill, 2005: 968.)

TABLE 5-17. **Pathogenesis and Clinical Features of Lepromatous and Tuberculoid Leprosy**

FEATURE	LEPROMATOUS LEPROSY	TUBERCULOID LEPROSY
Immunopathogenesis	Failed cell-mediated (T_H1) immunity; primarily ineffective humoral response.	Successful cell-mediated immunity; lesions contained.
Skin lesions	Many nodular growths with tissue compromise; stocking-and-glove peripheral neuropathy but no anesthesia around lesions; skin thickening.	Few, hypopigmented macules; complete sensory loss in/around lesions; presence of granulomas and vigorous chronic inflammatory response.
Organism presence in skin lesions.	Always, innumerable.	Few to none.
Infectivity of skin lesions	Highly.	Minimal.
Prognosis	Poor; can lead to death, if untreated.	Can be self-limiting.

ATYPICAL MYCOBACTERIA

CHARACTERISTICS

The atypical mycobacteria tend to cause disease in specific populations.

- *M. avium-intracellulare* (MAI) (also known as *M. avium* complex) is a ubiquitous organism present in soil and water.
- *M. kansasii* is a rare cause of a syndrome clinically identical to pulmonary tuberculosis.
- *M. scrofulaceum* is the etiologic agent of the pediatric disease **scrofula,** a chronic cervical lymphadenitis.
- *M. marinum* inhabits standing water and can cause ulceration and granulomas at sites of open wounds.

CLINICAL SYMPTOMS

Rarely, *M. avium-intracellulare* can cause pulmonary infections or lymphadenitis in immunocompetent individuals. More important, it has become a major cause of chronic disseminated disease in **patients with active AIDS.** This disease generally afflicts patients who have CD4+ T-cell counts below 10/mm^3. The disease manifests as an overwhelming, disseminated infection in virtually all tissues.

TREATMENT

Multidrug resistance is common. Susceptible AIDS patients are routinely prophylaxed for MAI with macrolide antibiotics (usually azithromycin).

Chlamydiae and Rickettsiae

Chlamydiae and rickettsiae are tiny organisms (between the size of viruses and bacteria) that are **obligate intracellular**—they are unable to live outside eukaryotic cells because they do not produce their own ATP. They stain gram-negative and possess a modified gram-negative cell wall, but the organisms are so small that they are invisible under conventional microscopy. *Chlamydia* spp. cause a variety of **respiratory and mucosal diseases** because of its tropism to ciliated columnar epithelial cells, whereas *Rickettsia* spp. (and the closely related pathogens Coxiella and Ehrlichia) tend to cause **fever and rash syndromes** owing to a predilection for endothelium. Diseases caused by these organisms are also commonly treated with macrolides, tetracyclines, or (rarely) chloramphenicol.

Chlamydia species

Chlamydia spp. are distinguished from all other bacteria because of their unique replicative cycle. The infectious particle associated with *Chlamydia* infection is the **elementary body (EB),** which is structurally similar to a spore in that much of its exterior peptidoglycan is cross-linked, protecting it from the elements. This peptidoglycan does not possess **muramic acid** and is not susceptible to disruption by penicillin antibiotics.

Once this form is taken up by the host cell, the cross-linkages are lost, and it transforms into a **reticulate body** (RB, also known as an **initial body**). In this form, the microbe is metabolically active and amplifies its DNA, RNA, and protein production, using host ATP. These RBs are visible under microscopy as **cytoplasmic inclusions.** Intracellular EBs are produced when the number of RBs is sufficient to sustain production; these are extruded from the host cell and the cycle begins again.

The three medically important members of the *Chlamydia* genus are *C. trachomatis*, which causes optic, genital tract, and neonatal pulmonary infections and *C. pneumoniae* and *C. psittaci*, both of which cause atypical pneumonia.

The EB of *C. trachomatis* is capable of infecting only certain types of cells—generally columnar or transitional epithelium, depending on the **serovar** or **serologic variant** of the organism. Different serovars have different epidemiologic and disease patterns (see Table 5-18).

Rickettsia species and Related Organisms

Like *Chlamydia* spp., *Rickettsia* spp. and the closely related organisms *Coxiella burnetii*, *Orientia tsutsugamushi*, and *Ehrlichia chaffeensis* are tiny obligate intracellular organisms with structures similar to gram-negative rods. As with *Chlamydia* infections, treatment is almost always with doxycycline, or with chloramphenicol in children. However, these organisms differ from *Chlamydia* spp. in several ways:

- Unlike *Chlamydia* infections, which affect only humans, these organisms generally have **arthropod vectors (tick, mite, louse)** (except for *Coxiella*).
- Reproduction is performed via conventional (**binary fission**) means.
- Intracellular localization is within the **cytoplasm** and **nucleus.**
- Diseases usually consist of headache, fever, and rash, resulting from the **vasculitis** (damage to blood vessels) secondary to the replication of the rickettsiae inside endothelial cells (see Table 5-19).

Mycoplasma

Mycoplasmas are the smallest free-living bacteria in nature—because of their small size, they were originally thought to be viruses. They are also unique in that they possess **no cell wall** and instead have a plasma membrane reinforced with **sterols.** Mycoplasmas can be grown (very slowly) on artificial media in the lab and assume a **fried-egg** appearance after a few weeks of culture.

? CLINICAL CORRELATION

Cases of mucopurulent urethritis and cervicitis are usually treated with ceftriaxone and doxycycline because of the high rate of gonococcal and chlamydial coinfection!

TABLE 5-18. Disease Patterns of *Chlamydia* Infections

SYMPTOMS	SUSCEPTIBLE POPULATIONS	TRANSMISSION PATTERN	CLINICAL SYMPTOMS	SEROVAR
Trachoma	Impoverished children in endemic areas (Middle East, India).	Hand-to-eye, eye-seeking flies, and contaminated clothing.	Follicular conjunctivitis, repeated infections leading to scarring and blindness.	A, B, C
Inclusion conjunctivitis	Neonates.	Passage through infected birth canal.	Purulent conjunctivitis occurring about 1 week after birth.	D–K
Infantile pneumonia	Neonates.	Passage through infected birth canal.	Rhinitis and cough without fever, about 2–3 weeks after birth.	D–K
Urethritis	Sexually active males and females.	Sexual transmission.	Asymptomatic, or dysuria with mucoid urethral discharge; can be a polymicrobial infection with *N. gonorrhoeae*.	D–K
Cervicitis	Sexually active females.	Sexual transmission.	Mostly asymptomatic, may progress to PID, may have purulent cervical discharge.	D–K
Pelvic inflammatory disease (PID)	Females with untreated cervicitis.	Ascending infection.	Vaginal bleeding or discharge, suprapubic pain, cervical motion tenderness, fever, nausea, vomiting; can lead to infertility or ectopic pregnancies.	D–K
Lymphogranuloma venereum	Sexually active individuals.	Sexual transmission.	Painless inguinal papule progressing to painful unilateral lymphadenopathy.	L1–L3
Psittacosis	Individuals with close contact with birds.	Aerosolized dust and feathers from birds.	Atypical pneumonia (fever, headache, dry nonproductive cough) 1–3 weeks after exposure.	*C. psittaci*
Chlamydial pneumonia	Common.	Person-to-person via aerosolized droplets.	Atypical pneumonia.	*C. pneumoniae*

The most important *Mycoplasma* is *M. pneumoniae*, which causes atypical pneumonia. *Ureaplasma urealyticum* can cause nongonococcal urethritis (like *C. trachomatis*).

MYCOPLASMA PNEUMONIAE

CHARACTERISTICS

This bacterium is actually smaller than some large viruses in nature. Its plasma membrane has two unique features. It possesses the **P1 protein,** which is capable of binding specifically to respiratory epithelial cells, and human anti-*Mycoplasma* cell membrane antibodies cross-react with erythrocyte antigens and agglutinate the cells **only at low temperatures.** Thus, the

TABLE 5-19. Rickettsial Diseases

ORGANISM/DISEASE	AFFECTED LOCATIONS	VECTOR/RESERVOIR	CLINICAL SYMPTOMS	RASH
R. rickettsii: Rocky Mountain spotted fever.	Southeastern and south central U.S.	"Hard" *Dermacentor* ticks.	High fever, chills, headache, myalgias.	Macular, centripetal spread (extremities to trunk) and palms/soles.
R. akari: Rickettsialpox.	Rare in U.S.	Mites that live on field mice.	Fever, chills, headache; mild.	Vesicular, generalized.
R. prowazekii: Epidemic typhus.	Latin America, Africa in areas of poor hygiene.	*Pediculus* body louse.	Fever, chills, myalgias, headache, arthralgias, mental status changes.	Petechial or macular, centrifugal spread (trunk to extremities).
R. typhi: Endemic typhus.	Warm areas.	Fleas that live on rodents.	Gradual onset of fever, chills, myalgias, nausea.	Maculopapular, restricted to chest/abdomen.
Orientia tsutsugamushi: Scrub typhus.	Asia, Pacific islands.	Larvae (chiggers) of mites.	High fever, headache, myalgias.	Maculopapular, centrifugal spread.
Coxiella burnetii: Q fever.	Worldwide.	Endospore inhalation.	Headache, high fever, chills, myalgias, atypical pneumonia.	None.
Ehrlichia chaffeensis: Ehrlichiosis.	Southern U.S., Asia.	*Amblyomma* ticks.	Headache, fever, chills, myalgias; GI symptoms; leukopenia.	Macular, centripetal spread.

cold agglutinin test is a simple (but nonspecific) test for an anti-*Mycoplasma* immune response.

CLINICAL SYMPTOMS

M. pneumoniae is a common cause of **atypical pneumonia** in young adults, and manifests as persistent low fever with a hacking, nonproductive cough and associated pharyngitis and malaise. Chest radiograph usually reveals patchy bilateral infiltrates that appear much worse than the clinical picture.

TREATMENT

Tetracyclines, macrolides, or fourth-generation fluoroquinolones.

KEY FACT

Atypical "walking" pneumonia can be caused by **Legionella, Mycoplasma,** or **Chlamydia.**

Spirochetes

Spirochetes are spiral-shaped bacteria with an internal flagellum:

MNEMONIC

BLT–
Borrelia
Leptospira
Treponema

- Technically gram-negative (i.e., contain endotoxin), but not well visualized with light microscopy. Seen with **darkfield** or fluorescent microscopy.
- Treated with tetracyclines or β-lactams.
- Three clinically important genera: *Borrelia, Treponema,* and *Leptospira* (see Table 5-20).

TABLE 5-20.   Summary of Spirochete Diseases

PATHOGEN	GENERAL	TRANSMISSION	DIAGNOSIS	INFECTION	TREATMENT
Treponema pallidum (syphilis)	Microaerophilic, extracellular.	Skin-skin contact Transplacental (TORCHES).	Serology: VDRL, then FTA-ABS.	*Primary:* Painless chancre. *Secondary:* Condylomata lata, palm and sole rash. *Tertiary:* Aortitis, gummas, Argyl-Robertson Pupil, tabes dorsalis.	Penicillin G.
Borrelia (Lyme)	Most common vector-borne disease. Microaerophilic, intracellular.	Deer tick (*Ixodes scapularis*).	Clinical, serology.	*Stage 1:* Erythema, chronicum migrans, flulike symptoms. *Stage 2:* Bell's palsy, AV block. *Stage 3:* Chronic arthritis, encephalopathy.	Doxycycline.
Borrelia recurrentis	Antigenic variation.	Human body louse.	Blood samples during fever.	Sudden onset of fever, etc. Spontaneous resolution and relapse.	Tetracycline, penicillin.
Leptospira interrogans	Aerobic.	Animal urine.	Microscopy.	*Initial:* Flulike symptoms, photophobia. *Later:* Liver damage with jaundice, renal failure.	Penicillin G; doxycycline for prophylaxis.

Treponema pallidum (Syphilis)

CHARACTERISTICS

- Gram-negative.
- Microaerophilic.
- Extracellular.
- Typically spiral-shaped, with an internal flagellum between outer membrane and cell wall.
- Diagnosed using darkfield microscope.
- Transmitted through sexual contact, contact with open chancre, or transplacentally.
- Humans are only host.

PATHOGENESIS

- Outer membrane carries endotoxin-like lipids.
- Spirochete penetrates mucous membranes, leading to bacteremia and seeding of organs throughout the body.

CLINICAL SYMPTOMS

There are three clinical stages of syphilis (see Table 5-21):

- **Primary syphilis** (following a 3- to 6-week incubation period).
    - A single nonpainful, indurated ulcer with smooth margins (**chancre**) that heals in 3–6 weeks (see Figure 5-27).
    - Early spread to regional lymph nodes and early bacteremia.
    - Self-limited primary stage, but highly contagious.

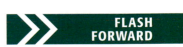

FLASH FORWARD

Symptoms of congenital syphilis:
- May result in stillbirth.
- Early rhinitis and mucocutaneous lesions.
- Late (more than two years) deafness and recurrent arthropathies.
- Affects organ systems: Skin, mucous membranes, lymph nodes, aorta, CNS.

TABLE 5-21. Summary of Syphilis

GENERAL	TRANSMISSION	DIAGNOSIS	INFECTION	TREATMENT
Microaerophilic, extracellular	Skin-skin contact, transplacental (TORCHES).	Serology: VDRL, then FTA-ABS.	■ *Primary:* Painless chancre. ■ *Secondary:* Condylomata lata, rash on palms and soles. ■ *Latent:* Usually asymptomatic. ■ *Tertiary:* Aortitis, ascending aortic aneurysm, gummas, Argyll-Robertson pupil, tabes dorsalis, neurosyphilis.	Penicillin G

- **Secondary syphilis** (1–3 months later; rarely coexists with primary syphilis):
  - Presents with flulike symptoms and a maculopapular rash on palms, soles, and mucous membranes.
  - May include condylomata lata (highly infectious wartlike lesions on perianal skin).
  - May involve any organ or part of body (e.g., hepatitis, arthritiis, meningitis, etc.).
  - Relapsing and remitting course, with cyclic symptoms and episodes of latency (i.e., latent syphilis).
- **Tertiary syphilis** (decades later):
  - **Aortitis**—aortic insufficiency, ascending aortic aneurysm.
  - Neurosyphilis—**tabes dorsalis** (posterior column disease); **Argyll-Robertson pupil** (accommodates but does not react to light), paralysis, and meningitis.
  - **Gummas**—granulomas of bone, skin, viscera.

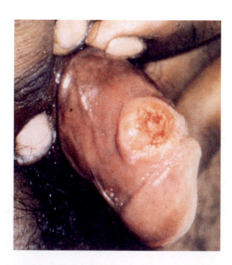

FIGURE 5-27. **Chancre of primary syphilis.** (Reproduced, with permission, from Kasper DL, Braunwald E, Fauci AS, et al. *Harrison's Principles on Internal Medicine*, 16th ed, New York: McGraw-Hill, 2005: 978)

DIAGNOSIS

Based on clinical presentation, microscopy, and especially **serology**:

- ***T. pallidum* ELISA (TP IgG).**
- **VDRL** (Venereal Disease Research Laboratories) or **RPR** (rapid plasma reagin):
  - High sensitivity, low specificity.
  - Turns positive 1 week after infection.
  - Is actually a nontreponemal antibody (reagin) that reacts with cow heart cardiolipin-lecithin in vitro.
  - False-positive in systemic lupus erythematosus, Epstein-Barr virus infection, and many others.
- **FTA-ABS** (fluorescent treponemal antibody-ABSorption test)
  - Confirmatory test—used to follow up positive VDRL/RPR:
  - Highly sensitive and specific.
  - Tests for antitreponemal antibody, which is the earliest to appear after infection.
  - Expensive.

TREATMENT

- Penicillin G for primary or secondary or prophylaxis to contacts.
- No vaccine.
- Complication of treatment due to lysis of treponeme = Jarisch-Herxheimer reaction (fevers, chills, myalgias).

PROGNOSIS

Depends on stage of infection and affected organs. Early syphilis and neurosyphilis tend to resolve well; however, aortitis may result in permanent structural defects.

Borrelia

Generally, microbes of the *Borrelia* genus are more loosely coiled than then treponemes, and are arthropod-borne (not sexually or transplacentally transmitted).

BORRELIA BURGDORFERI (LYME DISEASE)

CHARACTERISTICS

- Most common vector-borne disease in the United States.
- Can sometimes live intracellularly. As a result, body fluid samples may be PCR-negative.
- Some patients have coinfection with *Ehrlichia* or *Babesia*.
- Transmission via bite of *Ixodes scapularis* (deer or black-legged tick).
- Successful transmission requires more than 24 hours of feeding.
- **Reservoir** is the **white-tailed deer, white-footed mice.**

PATHOGENESIS

- Antigenic variation.
- Invades skin and spreads hematogenously; leads to immune complex deposition.
- Can access immunoprivileged sites such as CNS, tendons, and synoviae.

CLINICAL SYMPTOMS

There are three clinical stages of Lyme disease:

- **Primary (early):**
  - Erythema chronicum migrans (spreading, red target lesion, see Figure 5-28) and constitutional symptoms—fever, chills, fatigue, headache, myalgias, arthralgias.
- **Secondary,** disseminated phase (days to weeks after infection):
  - Bell's palsy (CN VII), aseptic meningitis, peripheral neuropathy.
  - AV block, carditis.
  - Multiple erythema migrans (secondary lesions).
  - Migratory myalgias, transient arthritis.
  - Other: Fever, stiff neck, headache, limb numbness or pain, malaise, fatigue.
- **Tertiary,** late (months to years after infection):
  - Chronic polyarthritis.
  - Neurologic impairment, fatigue.
  - Acrodermatitis chronicum atrophicans (skin atrophy).

DIAGNOSIS

Often clinical, based on history of tick bite with characteristic erythema chonicum migrans. Serology may also be tested, although many false-negatives result owing to antigenic variation and intracellular location. Skin biopsy can also be performed and is positive if motile spirochetes are visible under darkfield microscopy. Other diagnostic tests include PCR and culture (modified Kelly medium).

TREATMENT

Doxycycline (oral) for primary-stage Lyme disease and **ceftriaxone (IV)** for later-stage disease.

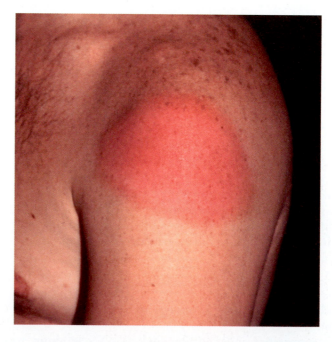

FIGURE 5-28. **Erythema chronicum migrans, stage 1 Lyme disease.** (Reproduced, with permission, from Wolff K, Johnson RA, Suurmond D, *Fitzpatrick Dermatology Atlas & Synopsis of Clinical Dermatology*, 5th ed, New York: McGraw-Hill, 2006: 679.)

BORRELIA RECURRENTIS (RELAPSING FEVER)

PATHOGENESIS

Antigenic variation allows new variants to evade the immune system and proliferate in the bloodstream, which then stimulates a subsequent immune response.

CLINICAL SYMPTOMS

- Inoculation: Transmitted by human body louse.
- Infection: Sudden onset of shaking chills, fever, myalgias, headache, delirium, cough, lethargy, hepatosplenomegaly.
- Spontaneous resolution and recurrence (less severe) due to antigenic variation and recurrent septicemia.
- Diagnosis blood sample when febrile; darkfield microscopy shows spirochete (Giemsa stain).
- Serology for serum antibodies against *Borrelia*.

TREATMENT

Penicillin, tetracycline. May cause Jarisch-Herxheimer reaction via lysis of bacteria and release of antigens.

Leptospira interrogans (Leptospirosis, Icterohemorrhagic Fever)

CHARACTERISTICS

- Aerobic.
- Two periplasmic flagella.
- Fine spirochete with hooked ends (see Figure 5-29).

PATHOGENESIS

Transmission is fecal-oral through animal urine (variety of wild and domesticated animals, especially rodents, dogs, fish, birds). Most common modes of transmission: Puddle stomping, recreation in contaminated water, working in sewers (rat urine).

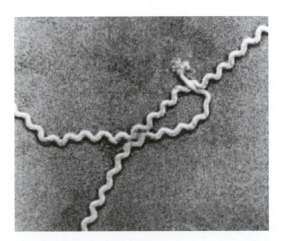

FIGURE 5-29.   **Scanning electron micrograph of *Leptospira interrogans.*** (Reproduced, with permission, from Kasper DL, Braunwald E, Fauci AS, et al, *Harrison's Principles on Internal Medicine,* 16th ed, New York: McGraw-Hill, 2005: 988.)

CLINICAL SYMPTOMS

- Disease syndrome is called leptospirosis.
- Leptospiremic phase: Flulike symptoms, photophobia.
- Immune phase: Increasing antileptospira IgM.
  - Mild → anicteric leptospirosis: Aseptic meningitis.
  - Severe → Weil's disease: Hemorrhagic vasculitis leading to kidney damage (renal failure) and hepatic damage (jaundice).
- Mortality is high in cases of severe infection (Weil's disease). Otherwise, prognosis is generally good and most patients recover.

DIAGNOSIS

Microscopy (spirochetes in blood, CSF, urine), serology.

TREATMENT

- Penicillin G
- Doxycycline prophylaxis

Mycology

FUNGI

General Characteristics

- Nonmotile organisms that form hyphae or spores.
- Cause an array of diseases including skin, lung, opportunistic, and systemic infection.
- Grows in Sabaroud's agar.
- Membrane contains ergosterol and chitin.

Life Forms

Fungi exist in two forms: yeast and molds. Many fungi can be found in either life form, depending on the temperature at which they are growing (see Figure 5-30 and Table 5-22).

Systemic

- Inhaled particles disseminate system-wide through the bloodstream producing systemic symptoms involving several organs.
- Includes **Histoplasma, Coccidioides, Blastomyces.**
- All are dimorphic fungi (existing in two forms), can cause disseminated disease, and can be treated with **fluconazole.**
- All can be diagnosed with sputum cytology, sputum cultures on blood agar, special media, and peripheral blood cultures (*Histoplasma*, particularly).

COCCIDIOIDES IMMITIS

CHARACTERISTICS (see Figure 5-31):

- Found in the southwestern United States, known as "desert rheumatic fever" or "valley fever."
- Dimorphic—arthroconidia and endospores.
- At 25°C (room temperature), grows as cylindrical arthroconidia.
- At 37°C (body temperature), grows as spherules in endospore (spores with spherules).

KEY FACT

Antifungals target ergosterol synthesis and function and are safe to use in humans because human cells do not contain ergosterol.
Antibiotics that target peptidoglycans do not affect fungi because fungi lack peptidoglycans.

KEY FACT

Important dimorphic fungi include *Coccidioides immitis, Histoplasma capsulatum, Blastomyces dermatitidis.*

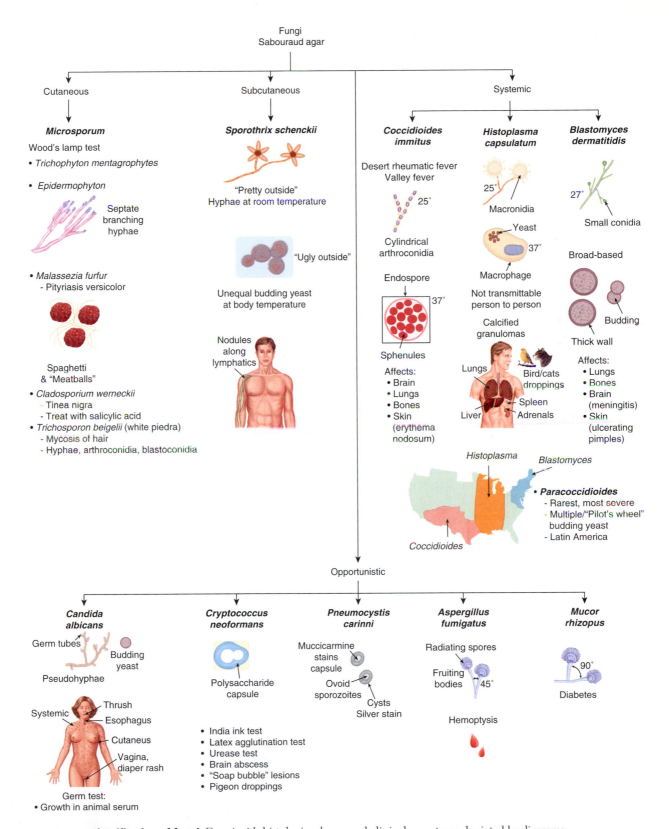

FIGURE 5-30. Classification of fungi. Fungi with histologies shown and clinical symptoms depicted by diagrams.

TABLE 5-22.   **Life Forms of Fungi**

	YEAST	**MOLDS**
Cellularity	Unicellular.	Multicellular.
Form	Budding cells.	Hyphae (elongated tubes of cells attached end to end).
Other forms	Pseudohyphae (long chains of cells formed by incomplete budding).	Septate hyphae—membranes separate cells. Nonseptate hyphae—no membranes between cells, multinucleate cells.

PATHOGENESIS

- Reservoir: Soil.
- Transmission: Airborne. Arthroconidia inhaled, become endospores in body.

CLINICAL SYMPTOMS

- Erythema nodosum
- Pneumonitis
- CNS involvement
- Arthritis
- AIDS patients: Meningitis, mucocutaneous lesion
- Pregnancy: Disseminated in third trimester

DIAGNOSIS

- Dimorphic yeast (no hyphae).
- Thick-walled spores.
- Granulomas.
- Biopsy showed **endospores inside spherules** all inside giant cells.

TREATMENT

- Cell-mediated immunity is required.
- Itraconazole for mild infections.
- Amphotericin B for severe without CNS involvement.
- Fluconazole for CNS involvement (good CNS penetration).

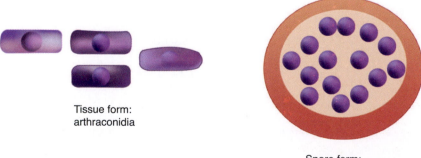

Tissue form:
arthraconidia

Spore form:
endospores, spherules

FIGURE 5-31.   ***Coccidioides* forms.**

PROGNOSIS

Fair, but may be fatal for elderly.

HISTOPLASMA CAPSULATUM

CHARACTERISTICS (see Figure 5-32):

- Found in Mississippi River Valley carried in bird and cat droppings.
- At 25°C, grows as hyphae with macronidia and micronidia.
- At 37°C, found as yeast inside macrophages in the body.
- Not transmittable from person to person.

PATHOGENESIS

- Reservoir: Soil and bird and bat droppings contain spores.
- Transmission: Spores are inhaled from dust and not transmittable person to person.
- Macrophages phagocytose spores and carry them systemically.
- Budding yeast form inside macrophages causing local infections throughout the body.
- Infections are contained within granulomas and calcify.

CLINICAL SYMPTOMS

- Asymptomatic in immunocompetent patient.
- Systemic infection in immunocompromised patient.
- Calcified granulomas in tissues involved.
- Pneumonitis that appears similar to milliary TB.
- May involve liver, spleen, adrenals in immunocompromised patients.

DIAGNOSIS

- Dimorphic yeast
- Thick-walled spores
- Granulomas
- Small budding cells within macrophages on biopsy.
- Calcified lung lesions; may become cavitary in chronic progressive form.

KEY FACT

Histoplasma capsulatum is named as such because it is found in histiocytes (macrophages). However, despite the name, it is *not* encapsulated.

TREATMENT

- Cell-mediated immunity required.
- Itraconazole for moderate infection.
- Amphotericin B for severe infection

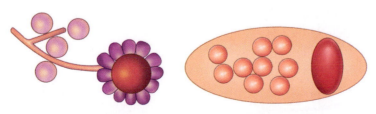

Tissue form   Intracellular form in a
                     reticuloendotheial cell

FIGURE 5-32.   *Histoplasma* forms.

MNEMONIC

BBB:

Blastomyces are found as **B**udding yeast with **B**road **B**ase.

BLASTOMYCES DERMATITIDIS

CHARACTERISTICS (see Figure 5-33):

- Found on the East Coast of the United States and Mexico.
- Rarest of all systemic mycoses.
- At 27°C, found as hyphae with small conidia.
- At 37°C, found as budding yeast with broad base in tissue.

PATHOGENESIS

- Reservoir: Soil, rotten wood contains spores.
- Transmission: Inhaled spores.
- Spores form yeast in the body, causing local infections.
- Yeast spread systemically over time and granulomas throughout the body (lungs, bones, skin).

KEY FACT

Remember **Blastomyces dermatitidis** as the only systemic fungus with ulcerating pimples.

CLINICAL SYMPTOMS

- Ulcerating pimples, verrucous.
- Pneumonitis, night sweats, weight loss.
- Meninigitis
- Arthritis
- Does **not** reactivate

DIAGNOSIS

- Dimorphic yeast
- Thick-walled spores
- Lung lesions do **not** calcify
- Granulomas

TREATMENT

KEY FACT

Systemic infection often occurs in the absence of lung disease.

- Cell-mediated immunity required.
- Itraconazole for moderate infection or meningeal involvement.
- Amphotericin B for severe infection without meningeal involvement.

PROGNOSIS

Poor, most severe of systemic mycoses.

PARACOCCIDIODES

CHARACTERISTICS (see Figure 5-34):

- Found in Latin America
- Appears as multiple budding yeast often described as "pilot's wheel"
- Affected population 90% male

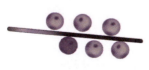
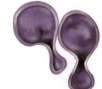
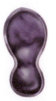

Endemic form   Budding yeast forms in tissue

FIGURE 5-33. *Blastomyces* forms.

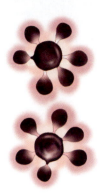

FIGURE 5-34. *Paracoccidioides—"pilot's wheel."*

PATHOGENESIS

- Reservoir: Spores found in soil.
- Transmission: Inhalation of spores.

CLINICAL SYMPTOMS

Symptoms are similar to those of *Coccidiodes*.

DIAGNOSIS

- Dimorphic yeast
- Multiple buds, like "spokes of a wheel" or "pilot's wheel".

TREATMENT

- Bactrim
- Amphotericin B
- Itraconazole

PROGNOSIS

Good.

Opportunistic

These fungi often cause symptoms only in immunocompromised hosts.

CANDIDA ALBICANS

CHARACTERISTICS (see Figure 5-35).

- Found in natural flora of skin.
- Appear as pseudohyphae and budding yeast in tissue biopsy.
- Common cause of yeast infection and skin infection in immuno-compromised.

PATHOGENESIS

- Reservoir: GI flora, endogenous to mucous membrane and normal skin flora in moist areas.
- Growth: Forms germ tubes at 37°C and pseudohyphae/true hyphae when invading tissue grows rapidly if not controlled.
- Antibiotic use, immunocompromise, and cancer increases risk of infection.

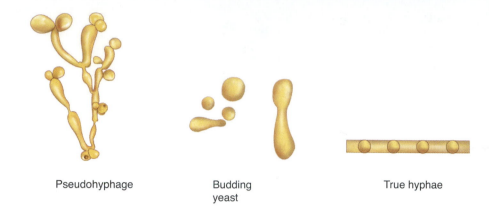

Pseudohyphage

Budding yeast

True hyphae

FIGURE 5-35. *Candida* **forms.**

CLINICAL SYMPTOMS

- In immunocompetent hosts
  - Oral thrush
  - Vaginiitis (yeast infection in diabetic women).
  - Diaper rash
- In immunocompromised hosts
  - Esophagiitis
  - Cutaneous infection—often found in moist areas like underneath breasts or in skin folds (i.e., diaper rash).
  - Disseminated systemic infection and septicemia.
  - Endocarditis in IV drug users.

DIAGNOSIS

- Silver stain
- KOH stain for pseudohyphae, budding yeast.
- Germ test—grow in animal serum.

TREATMENT

- Nystatin/fluconazole for cutaneous infection.
- Amphotericin B for systemic infection.

PROGNOSIS

Good.

CRYPTOCOCCUS NEOFORMANS

CHARACTERISTICS

- Appears as budding yeast in India ink stain.
- Urease-positive.
- Thick polysaccharide capsule.
- Affects AIDS patients and SLE patients.

PATHOGENESIS

- Reservoir: Pigeon and bird droppings.
- Transmission: Inhaled yeast from droppings, leading to lung infection.
- Spread hematogenously to CNS, causing meningitis, abscess formation, and increased intracranial pressure.

- Growth within Virchow-Robinson space (space between vessel wall and surrounding connective tissue).
- Affects people with poor T-cell–mediated Ab immunity.

CLINICAL SYMPTOMS

- Pneumonia.
- Fungemia.
- Meningitis—forms abscesses, also increases intracranial pressure.

DIAGNOSIS

- Latex agglutination test for capsular antigen in blood.
- "Soap bubble lesions".
- Budding yeast on India ink stain.
- Urease-positive.

TREATMENT

- Amphotericin B plus flucytosine for meningitis.
- Fluconazole for lifetime suppression in AIDS patients.

PROGNOSIS

Poor.

PNEUMOCYSTIS JIROVECI

CHARACTERISTICS (see Figure 5-36):

- Appears as dark ovoid sporozoites within cysts on silver stain.
- Frequently affects AIDS patients.
- Also may affect premature infants.

PATHOGENESIS

- Transmission: Cyst is inhaled by most people in childhood, leading to an asymptomatic or mild pneumonia, then a latent infection in the lungs.
- In immunocompromised hosts: Uncontrolled growth and an inflammatory response, leading to pneumonia.

CLINICAL SYMPTOMS

- Pneumonitis.
- Classically may cause pneumothorax.

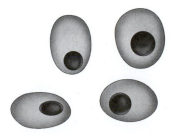

FIGURE 5-36. ***Pneumocystis jiroveci*** **in tissue with silver stain.**

DIAGNOSIS

Silver stain showing cysts containing dark oval bodies.

TREATMENT

- Bactrim or pentamidine.
- Bactrim, aerosolized pentamidine, or dapsone for prophylaxis.

PROGNOSIS

Fair.

ASPERGILLUS FUMIGATUS

CHARACTERISTICS (see Figure 5-37):

- Found in wheat stacks.
- Branching hyphae that branch at a 45° angle.
- Fruiting bodies at ends of hyphae.
- Affects neutropenic patients.

PATHOGENESIS

- Reservoir: Mold grows on decaying vegetation.
- Transmission: Spores are inhaled.
- May stimulate IgE response leading to bronchospasm and allergic bronchopulmonary aspergillosis.
- May deposit in existing lung cavity and form aspergillous ball (aspergilloma).
- May invade lung tissue and bloodstream in the immunocompromised host and occlude blood vessels leading to pulmonary infarction.

CLINICAL SYMPTOMS

- Various lung diseases, including fungus ball, acute and chronic pneumonitis, and disseminated systemic disease.
- Pneumonitis often with hemoptysis.

DIAGNOSIS

- Tissue biopsy reveals branching hyphae (branching at a 45° angle) with septae.
- Sputum culture shows radiating chains of spores.
- X-ray may detect aspergilloma.
- Overall, diagnosis is difficult.

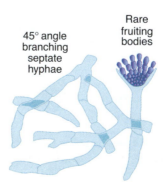

45° angle branching septate hyphae

Rare fruiting bodies

Aspergillus

FIGURE 5-37. *Aspergillus.*

TREATMENT

- Allergic bronchopulmonary aspergillosis: Corticosteroids, no antifungals needed.
- Aspergilloma: Surgery.
- Invasive aspergillosis: Amphotericin B.

PROGNOSIS

Depends on type of disease. For disseminated disease, prognosis is poor.

RHIZOPUS MUCOR

CHARACTERISTICS (see Figure 5-38)

- Branching hyphae that branch at 90° angle.
- Nonseptate hyphae.
- Afflicts diabetics and leukemia patients.

PATHOGENESIS

- Reservoir: Spores in the environment.
- Transmission: Spores inhaled.
- In immunocompromised hosts, colonizes tissue and invades blood vessels, leading to necrosis (similar to *Aspergillus*).

CLINICAL SYMPTOMS

- Invasive rhinocerebral infection.
- Pneumonitis similar to *Aspergillus*.

DIAGNOSIS

- Tissue biopsy shows branching hyphae (branching at 90° angle) without septae.
- Shows a broad ribbon-like growth pattern.

TREATMENT

- Control of diabetes
- Surgery for rhinocerebral infections
- Amphotericin

PROGNOSIS

Fair

> **KEY FACT**
>
> *Aspergillus fumigatus* and *Rhizopus mucor* appear very similar but Aspergillus branches at 45 degrees while Rhizopus branches at 90 degrees.

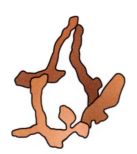

FIGURE 5-38. ***Rhizopus mucor.*** Irregular broad (empty-looking) nonseptate hyphae, wide-angle branching.

Cutaneous

MICROSPORUM

CHARACTERISTICS

- Includes multiple types of fungi that infect the skin.
- *Trichophyton* and *Epidermophyton* affect the nails specifically.
- *Trichophyton mentagrophytes* affects the feet.
- Branching hyphae that are septate with arthroconidia and cross-walls.

PATHOGENESIS

- Reservoir: Soil, animals, humans.
- Transmission: Spread by contact with infected individuals or animals.
- Colonizes keratinized epithelium (dead, horny layer) in warm, moist areas.
- Infection spreads centrifugally with curvy worm-like borders ("ringworm").
- Fungal antigens are released from the hyphae and may induce delayed-type hypersensitivity reaction (dermatophytoses: Inflammation, itching, scaly skin, pustules).
- Fungal antigens may diffuse systemically and cause dermaphytid reactions: Hypersensitivity responses (vesicles) at distant sites such as fingers.

CLINICAL SYMPTOMS

- Ringworm (tinea corporis): Ring lesion on the skin that appears to be spreading centrifugally.
- Athlete's foot (tinea pedis).
- Jock itch (tinea cruris).
- Oncomycoses (tinea unguium): Nail infection, discoloration of nails.
- Body infection (tinea corporis).

DIAGNOSIS

- Skin scrapings allow keratin to be removed. Hyphae can be observed on KOH prep.
- Wood's lamp (UV) detects *Microsporum*.

TREATMENT

- Topical antifungal creams for skin infections (imidazole).
- Oral antifungals for hair follicle and nail infections.

PROGNOSIS

Good

MALESSEZIA FURFUR

CHARACTERISTICS (see Figure 5-39):

- Appears as "spaghetti and meatballs" on KOH prep.
- Causes pityriasis versicolor.

PATHOGENESIS

- Reservoir: Animals, humans, soil.
- Transmission: Contact.

CLINICAL SYMPTOMS

- Pityriasis versicolor: Pale spots on the skin, often on the back.

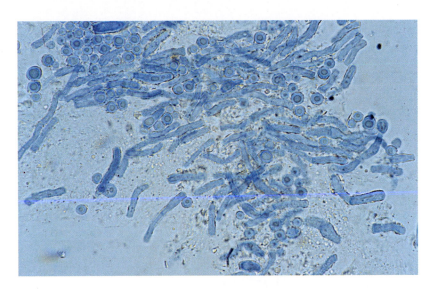

FIGURE 5-39. *Malassezia furfur,* **"spaghetti and meatballs," on KOH prep.** (Reproduced, with permission, from Wolff K, Johnson RA, Suurmond D. *Fitzpatrick's Color Atlas & Synopsis of Clinical Dermatology*, 5th ed. New York: McGraw-Hill, 2006: 732.)

DIAGNOSIS

- KOH prep.
- Short, unbranched hyphae.
- Spherical yeast.
- "Spaghetti and meatballs."

PROGNOSIS

Good.

TREATMENT

Topical antifungals: Imidazole.

Subcutaneous

SPOROTHRIX SHENCKII

CHARACTERISTICS (see Figure 5-40)

- Found in soil.
- "Gardener's nodule": Often transmitted via prick of finger on rose thorns.
- At 25°C, appears as branching hyphae with macronidia shaped–like flowers.
- At 37°C, appears as unequally budding yeast.

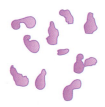

FIGURE 5-40. *Sporothrix schenckii.* **Yeast forms, unequal budding.**

PATHOGENESIS

- Reservoir: Spores in soil.
- Transmission: Spores enter skin through cuts and puncture wounds such as puncture of rose thorn.
- Slow local infection forms primary nodule that becomes necrotic and ulcerates.
- Secondary nodules form along lymphatic tracts draining primary infections.

CLINICAL SYMPTOMS

Subcutaneous nodules form along lymphatics usually in the upper extremity that was infected via break in the skin.

DIAGNOSIS

- Culture at different temperatures reveals branched hyphae at 25°C and single cells (cigar-shaped budding yeast) at 37°C.
- Produces black pigment.
- Rosette conidia.
- Neutrophilic microabscesses in skin.

TREATMENT

- Oral potassium iodide (mechanism unclear).
- Antifungals for extracutaneous involvement: Aphotericin B, itraconazole.

PROGNOSIS

Good

Helminths

Helminths are multicellular parasites (worms) often associated with **eosinophilia**. Three general types of helminths include nematodes (roundworms), cestodes (tapeworms), and trematodes (flukes) (see Figure 5-41).

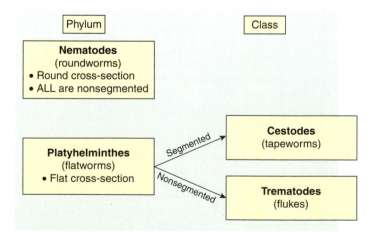

FIGURE 5-41. **Helminth classification scheme.**

CESTODES (TAPEWORMS)

Cestodes are segmented flatworms, and **all** are transmitted by ingestion. In general, infected persons are treated with albendazole, praziquantel, or niclosamide (see Table 5-23).

Taenia saginata (Beef Tapeworm)

CHARACTERISTICS

Composed of scolex and proglottids, with a body plan similar to that of *Taenia solium*. *T. saginata* can grow to several meters long.

PATHOGENESIS

Adheres to mucosa via scolex and absorbs nutrients from host.

CLINICAL SYMPTOMS

- Ingestion of larvae in undercooked beef leads to colonization of the intestinal tract.
- Infection may be asymptomatic or may present with abdominal discomfort and/or malnutrition.
- Diagnosis is by proglottids/eggs in stool.

TREATMENT

Niclosamide or praziquantel.

Taenia solium (Pork Tapeworm)

CHARACTERISTICS

Has scolex and proglottids, with a body plan similar to that of *T. saginata*. *T. solium* can grow to several meters long. Egg versus larval ingestion causes different diseases (see Figure 5-42).

TABLE 5-23. Summary of Cestodes

MODE OF TRANSMISSION	TYPE OF INFECTION	WORM	SYMPTOMS	BUZZWORDS/ ASSOCIATIONS	LAB FINDINGS
Ingestion of larvae	GI	*Taenia saginata* (beef tapeworm)	None, abdominal discomfort, malnutrition.	Undercooked beef, proglottids.	Eggs in stool.
	GI	*Taenia solium* (pork tapeworm)	None, abdominal discomfort, malnutrition.	Undercooked pork, proglottids.	Eggs in stool.
Ingestion of eggs	Tissue	*Taenia solium* (pork tapeworm)	Cysticercosis, seizures, blindness.	Worm can be seen in vitreous humor!	Tissue calcs on X-ray.
	GI	*Diphyllobothrium latum* (broadfish tapeworm)	None, B_{12} deficiency, macrocytic anemia.	Undercooked or pickled fish.	Eggs in stool.
	GI	*Echinococcus granulosus* (dog tapeworm)	Right upper quadrant pain, hepatomegaly, anaphylaxis.	Liver cysts, hydatid cyst disease, sheep, dogs.	Cysts on X-ray or CT.

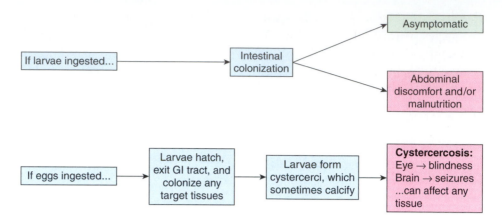

FIGURE 5-42. Mechanisms of *Taenia solium* infection.

PATHOGENESIS

Larval form ingested through contaminated pork leads to infestation of intestines. The egg form is ingested through fecal contamination, and hatches in the intestines. The larvae then penetrate the intestinal wall to enter the bloodstream. From there, they may infect any tissue.

CLINICAL SYMPTOMS

Diagnosis rests on calcified cystercerci on X-rays and serology.

TREATMENT

GI infection: Niclosamide or praziquantel. Cystercercosis: Albendazole with prednisone.

Diphyllobothrium latum (Fish Tapeworm)

CHARACTERISTICS

Can grow to several meters long.

PATHOGENESIS

Ingestion of infected undercooked or pickled freshwater fish results in intestinal colonization. May absorb nutrients and outcompete host for vitamin B_{12}.

CLINICAL SYMPTOMS

Diagnosis is based on finding eggs in stool. Infection is often asymptomatic, but can also cause B_{12} deficiency with a megaloblastic macrocytic pernicious anemia.

TREATMENT

Praziquantel.

Echinococcus granulosus (Dog Tapeworm)

CHARACTERISTICS

Smaller than other tapeworms.

PATHOGENESIS

Ingestion of eggs from canine fecal contamination allows larvae to hatch in the GI tract. They can then penetrate the intestinal wall and migrate to target tissues, where they form **hydatid cysts**.

CLINICAL SYMPTOMS

- **Diagnosis** is based on X-ray or CT visualization of cysts in tissue. Clinical manifestations of infection include **hydatid cyst disease,** which can affect the liver, lungs, and brain, resulting in organ **dysfunction.**
- Ruptured cysts can release high levels of antigen and may cause anaphylaxis.
- **Liver cysts** can present with **right upper quadrant pain** and **hepatomegaly.**

TREATMENT

Albendazole followed by cyst aspiration.

TREMATODES (FLUKES)

The trematode genera (flukes) consist of **non**segmented flatworms. Their life cycles are complex and involve **snails** as an intermediate host. They are most often treated with **praziquantel** (see Table 5-24).

Clonorchis sinensis (Chinese Liver Flukes)

CHARACTERISTICS

Endemic in Southeast Asia.

PATHOGENESIS

Encysted larvae are ingested in **raw or undercooked freshwater fish.** The larvae migrate through the GI tract and mature in the **biliary tree.**

CLINICAL SYMPTOMS

Diagnosis is by eggs in stool. Manifestations range from asymptomatic to vague right upper quadrant pain, cholangitis, and/or biliary obstruction. Associated with **cholangiocarcinoma.**

TREATMENT

All flukes are treated with praziquantel.

KEY FACT

Modes of transmission:
- Undercooked seafood: *Clonorchis sinensis, Paragonimus westermani, Diphyllobothrium latum*
- Undercooked beef: *Taenia saginata*
- Undercooked pork: *Taenia solium, Trichinella spiralis*
- Human feces: *Ascaris lumbricoides, Enterobius vermicularis, Trichuris trichuria*
- Dog feces: *Toxocara, Echinococcus*
- Drinking water: *Dracunculus*

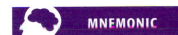

MNEMONIC

Clonorchis **cl**imbs the biliary tree.

TABLE 5-24. Summary of Trematodes

MODE OF TRANSMISSION	TYPE OF INFECTION	WORM	SYMPTOMS	BUZZWORDS/ ASSOCIATIONS	LAB FINDINGS
Ingestion of encysted larvae	GI	*Clonorchis sinensis* (Chinese liver fluke).	Biliary tree infection.	Undercooked fish, cholangiocarcinoma.	Eggs in stool.
Ingestion of eggs	Lung	*Paragonimus westermani.*	Hemoptysis, cough, fever.	Shellfish (crab meat).	Eggs in stool and sputum.
Larval penetration of skin	Tissue	*Schistosoma mansoni* and *Schistosoma japonicum.*	Pruritus at entry sites, constitutional symptoms (Katayama fever).	Portal HTN, intestinal polyps, snails.	Eggs in stool.
	Tissue	*Schistosoma haematobium.*	Pruritus at entry sites, constitutional symptoms (Katayama fever), hematuria.	Squamous cell carcinoma of bladder, snails.	Eggs in stool and urine.

Paragonimus westermani (Lung Fluke)

CHARACTERISTICS

Endemic in Asia, Africa, and South America.

PATHOGENESIS

Ingestion of eggs from infected shellfish.

CLINICAL SYMPTOMS

Diagnosis is via eggs in sputum and stool. Clinical manifestations of infection include **hemoptysis,** cough, and fever.

TREATMENT

All flukes are treated with praziquantel.

Schistosomes (Blood Flukes)

CHARACTERISTICS

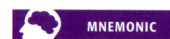

Paragonimus causes hemo**P**tysis, eggs in s**P**utum, and **P**ulmonary disease.

- Male folds its body ventrally to hold female in **permanent copulation.**
- Eggs are highly immunogenic, resulting in chronic inflammation and erosion of tissues.
- Transmission: Larvae released into freshwater penetrate through the skin. They then enter the bloodstream to reach target tissues.
- Clinical manifestations of infection: May be asymptomatic, or may present with constitutional symptoms (Katayama fever) and/or early dermatitis with pruritus at the entry site. Late manifestations are due to chronic inflammation of target tissue.
- **Three species:**
    - *Schistosoma **japonicum*** and ***mansoni***
        - Diagnosis. Eggs in stool.
        - Clinical manifestations: These schistosomes can mature in the portal circulation, resulting in periportal fibrosis and portal hypertension. They can also affect mesenteric circulation, resulting in intestinal polyps.
    - *Schistosoma **hematobium***
        - Diagnosis. Eggs in the urine and stool.
        - Clinical manifestations: Schistosomes can mature in the blood vessels supplying the bladder, resulting in **hematuria,** dysuria, frequency, and urgency. Long-term infection is associated with **squamous cell carcinoma of the bladder,** presumably as a result of chronic inflammation. (Note that most primary bladder cancers are transitional cell carcinoma.)

TREATMENT

All flukes are treated with praziquantel.

NEMATODES (ROUNDWORMS)

Nematodes are nonsegmented worms with a circular cross-section and complete digestive system. Table 5-25 contains a summary of cestodes.

Ascaris lumbricoides

CHARACTERISTICS

Ascaris is a large nematode that can grow up to 13 inches long. It is the **most common helminthic infection in the world** and is especially prevalent in tropical areas with poor sanitation.

TABLE 5-25.   Summary of Nematodes

Mode of Transmission	Type of Infection	Worm	Symptoms	Buzzwords	Lab Dx
Ingestion of eggs	GI	*Ascaris lumbricoides*	None, pneumonia, malnutrition	Bowel obstruction, bile obstruction	Eggs in stool
	GI	*Enterobius vermicularis* (pinworm)	Anal pruritus		Scotch tape test
	GI	*Trichuris trichuria* (whipworm)	None, diarrhea w/o pruritus		
Ingestion of larvae	Tissue	*Trichinella spiralis* (pork roundworm)	Diarrhea, myalgias, periorbital edema	Pork, wild game	
	Tissue	*Dracunculus medinensis* (Guinea worm)	Painful subcutaneous nodules	Copepods	Roll on a stick, surgery
Ingestion of eggs	GI	*Toxocara canis* (dog ascaris)	Hepatosplenomegaly, blindness	Visceral larva migrans	
Larvae penetrate skin (usually feet)	GI	*Strongyloides stercoralis* (threadworm)	None, pneumonitis, gastroenteritis		Larvae in stool, string test
	GI	*Necator americanus* (New World hookworm)	Pneumonitis, gastroenteritis, microcytic anemia		Eggs in stool
	GI	*Ancylostoma duodenale* (Old World hookworm)	Pneumonitis, gastroenteritis, microcytic anemia		Eggs in stool
	GI	Cat or dog hookworm	Itching along worm's path	Cutaneous larva migrans	
Arthropod bite					
Blackfly	Systemic	*Onchocerca volvulus*	River blindness, skin nodules, rash, hyperpigmentation		
Mosquito	Systemic	*Wuchereria bancrofti*	Elephantiasis, edema, fever, scaly skin	Enter bloodstream at night	
Deer fly	Systemic	*Loa loa* (eye worm)	Blindness, swelling in skin.		

PATHOGENESIS

Transmission is fecal-oral via ingestion of eggs from contaminated soil. Eggs hatch in the digestive tract, and larvae then penetrate the intestinal wall and enter the vasculature.

CLINICAL SYMPTOMS

Ascariasis may be **asymptomatic.** However, larvae often migrate through the vasculature into the lungs, which can result in **pneumonia.** From the lungs, the larvae can migrate up the trachea and into the pharynx where they are subsequently swallowed. These larvae mature into adults in the intestines and consume food eaten by the host. As a result, they may cause **malnutrition,** bowel obstruction, or biliary obstruction. Diagnosis is made by eggs in the stool and **esoinophilia.**

TREATMENT

Pyrantel pamoate, mebendazole, albendazole.

Enterobius vermicularis (Pinworms)

CHARACTERISTICS

Pinworms are small nematodes, about 1 cm long. Pinworm infection is the **most common helminthic infection in the United States.**

PATHOGENESIS

Transmission is fecal-oral via ingestion of eggs from contaminated surfaces or household dust. Eggs hatch in the digestive tract, where the larvae then mature and mate. Adult females migrate out through the anus and lay eggs in perianal skin.

CLINICAL SYMPTOMS

Pinworms most often affect **children,** and the eggs cause **intense perianal itching.** Diagnosis is made using the **Scotch tape test,** in which a piece of tape is pressed against the perianal skin and then examined for eggs.

TREATMENT

Pyrantel pamoate, mebendazole, albendazole.

Trichuris trichuria (Whipworm)

CHARACTERISTICS

Adult worms are typically 3–5 cm long, with a whip-like shape (narrow anterior, wide posterior).

PATHOGENESIS

Similar to pinworms, whipworm transmission is fecal-oral via ingestion of eggs. Eggs hatch in the digestive tract, where the larvae then mature and mate. Adult whipworms attach to the superficial mucosa.

CLINICAL SYMPTOMS

Usually **asymptomatic,** but heavier worm burdens may result in malnutrition, abdominal pain, **bloody diarrhea,** tenesmus, and/or rectal prolapse. Unlike with pinworms, there is **no** anal pruritus. Diagnosis of whipworm is made by eggs in the stool.

TREATMENT

Mebendazole, albendazole.

Trichinella spiralis (Pork Roundworm)

CHARACTERISTICS

Most common cause of parasitic myocarditis.

PATHOGENESIS

Transmission occurs by ingestion of encysted larvae in **undercooked pork** or wild game. Larvae mature in the human digestive tract and then mate. Eggs also hatch in the digestive tract, and larvae may subsequently penetrate the intestinal wall to enter the bloodstream. From the blood, larvae often migrate to skeletal muscle.

CLINICAL SYMPTOMS

Trichinosis is characterized by different stages of symptoms that correlate to the worm's life cycle. Early symptoms occur while the larvae are still within the digestive tract and include **nausea, vomiting, diarrhea,** and other constitutional symptoms. Migrating larvae that have entered the bloodstream and reached peripheral tissues may then cause both a local and a systemic response. Symptoms may include high **fever, eosinophilia, periorbital edema,** conjunctival and splinter hemorrhages, and urticarial rash. Once the larvae have migrated to skeletal muscle, **myalgias** may occur. Over time, these larvae may become surrounded by calcified fibrous tissue, thus forming **calcified cysts.** Higher innocula may lead to larval infiltrations of the heart and brain, leading to myocarditis and encephalitis, respectively. Diagnosis is confirmed by **muscle biopsy** and/or positive anti-*Trichinella* **serology.** Note that there are **no eggs in the stool** because they hatch in the intestinal submucosa.

TREATMENT

Mebendazole, albendazole, and thiabendazole are effective for the intestinal stages of infection. Although there is no effective treatment for muscle cysts, **glucocorticoids** may be beneficial in cases of severe myositis or myocarditis.

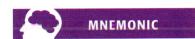

MNEMONIC

Don't get tricked by **trich**uris and **trich**inella. Just remember that trichine**LL**a is he**LL**a worse and affects your musc**L**es.

Dracunculus medinensis (Guinea Worm)

CHARACTERISTICS

Larvae live in tiny aquatic crustaceans (called **copepods**).

PATHOGENESIS

Copepods are ingested in drinking water. *Dracunculus* larvae are then free to mature and mate in the human host.

CLINICAL SYMPTOMS

Adult worms migrate to the skin to release their eggs back into the environment. They form painful subcutaneous nodules and can reach lengths up to 3 feet.

TREATMENT

Nodules can be removed surgically or by slowly pulling out the worm by rolling it on a stick. If the worm were to break during this process, **anaphylaxis** may result.

MNEMONIC

The Rod of Asclepius is a symbol of **MED**Icine, and depicts **D. MED**Inensis wrapped around a stick.

Toxocara canis (Dog Ascaris)

CHARACTERISTICS

Similar to *A. lumbricoides*, but can complete its life cycle only in dogs. Humans are a dead-end host.

PATHOGENESIS

Transmission is fecal-oral via ingestion of eggs soil contaminated with dog feces. Eggs hatch in the digestive tract, and larvae penetrate the intestinal wall and enter the vasculature.

CLINICAL SYMPTOMS

Larvae can migrate to many different organs. Therefore this disease is known as **visceral** larva migrans. Common manifestations include **hepatospleno-megaly** and **blindness**. Diagnosis is made by eosinophilia and anti-*Toxocara* serology.

TREATMENT

Infection is usually self-limited, but glucocorticoids may be helpful in severe cases.

Strongyloides stercoralis (Threadworm)

PATHOGENICITY

Larvae in contaminated soil are able to directly penetrate the skin, usually through the feet.

CLINICAL SYMPTOMS

Strongyloidiasis can be **asymptomatic.** However, **local itching** may occur at the site of entry, and larvae are transported through the vasculature to the lungs, where they may result in **pneumonia.** From the lungs, they can migrate up the trachea and into the pharynx where they are subsequently swallowed. Larvae can then mature and mate in the digestive tract. Females lay their eggs in the intestinal wall, which may cause abdominal pain and **diarrhea.** Once the eggs hatch, larvae may exit with feces or may penetrate the abdominal wall and reenter the bloodstream. In the latter case, larvae can then travel to the lungs and repeat the life cycle (**autoinfection**). Diagnosis is made by eosinophilia and **larvae in the stool.** Serology is highly sensitive and specific and has replaced the **"string test,"** in which a patient swallows a long string that reaches the duodenum, after which larvae can then be pulled out via the string.

TREATMENT

Ivermectin, thiabendazole.

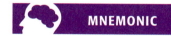

MNEMONIC

Use **iver**mectin to **over**come the strong strongyloides.

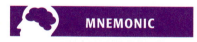

MNEMONIC

STrongyloides is the only helminth whose larvae are **ST**rong enough to get into the **ST**ool.

Necator americanus and *Ancylostoma duodenale* (New World Hookworm and Old World Hookworm)

CHARACTERISTICS

Both species of hookworms have characteristic "hooks" in their mouth that allow them to attach to the intestinal mucosa.

PATHOGENICITY

Similar to *Strongyloides*, larvae in contaminated soil are able to directly penetrate the skin, usually through the feet.

CLINICAL SYMPTOMS

Similar to *Strongyloides*, **local itching** may occur at the site of entry. Larvae are then transported through the vasculature to the lungs, where they may result in **pneumonia.** From the lungs, they can migrate up the trachea and into the pharynx, where they are subsequently swallowed. Larvae can then mature into adults in the GI tract. The adult form attaches to the intestinal mucosa using characteristic hooks. It can then feed off of the host's blood. Adults can also mate in the intestines and release eggs into the stool.

- Initial symptoms may include abdominal pain and **diarrhea.**
- Over time, the host may develop a **hypochromic microcytic anemia.**
- Diagnosis is made by eggs in the stool, along with **eosinophilia.**

TREATMENT

Mebendazole, pyrantel pamoate. Treat anemia with iron and folic acid.

Cat or Dog Hookworm

CHARACTERISTICS

Lacks the necessary collagenase to be able to penetrate through the epidermal basement membrane in humans. The infection is especially prevalent in warm, humid climates and usually affects children.

PATHOGENESIS

Larvae reside in soil contaminated with dog or cat feces. Similar to human hookworms, they are able to directly penetrate the skin, usually through the feet.

CLINICAL SYMPTOMS

Because the larvae cannot penetrate human skin, they are only able to migrate along the dermal-epidermal junction. Their path is marked by a serpiginous erythematous rash that is intensely pruritic. This is known as **cutaneous larva migrans** (see Figure 5-43).

TREATMENT

Infection is usually self-limited, and larvae usually die within several weeks.

Onchocerca volvulus (River Blindness)

CHARACTERISTICS

Arthropod-borne, endemic near rivers.

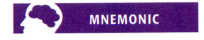

MNEMONIC

Remember that both hookworms can cause anemia:
Dracula sucks blood from your **Nec**(ator).
Ancylostoma forms an **an**astomosis with your gut.

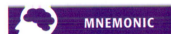

MNEMONIC

vi**SC**eral larvae migrans is caused by dog a**SC**aris (*T. canis*).
Kutaneous larvae migrans is caused by cat or dog hoo**K**worm.

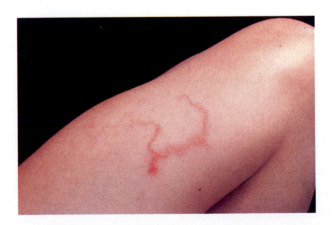

FIGURE 5-43. Cutaneous larva migrans. (Reproduced, with permission, from Wolff K, Johnson RA, Suurmond D. *Fitzpatrick Dermatology Atlas & Synopsis of Clinical Dermatology,* 5th ed. New York: McGraw-Hill, 2005: 863.)

PATHOGENESIS

Larvae migrate through skin and mature into adults. Adults can mate and release microfilariae into subcutaneous tissues. To complete their life cycle, microfilariae are ingested via a second fly bite and then mature into larvae.

CLINICAL SYMPTOMS

- A bite from the **black fly** releases larvae into the **skin.**
- Fibrosis can occur around adults, resulting in **subcutaneous nodules.**
- Migrating microfilariae result in an inflammatory response consisting of a thick, hyperpigmented, pruritic **rash.**
- If microfilariae reach the eye, local inflammation can also cause blindness (**river blindness**).
- Diagnosis can be made with a skin biopsy of a subcutaneous nodule.

TREATMENT

Ivermectin is effective against microfilariae only. Subcutaneous nodules (i.e., adults) must be surgically removed.

Loa loa (Eye Worm)

CHARACTERISTICS

Arthropod-borne, similar to *Onchocerca*. Found in Africa.

PATHOGENESIS

A bite from the **Chrysops fly** releases larvae into the skin.

CLINICAL SYMPTOMS

Infection is most often asymptomatic, but can lead to episodic swelling (Calabar swellings). Adult worms can sometimes be seen **migrating through the subconjunctiva.**

TREATMENT

Diethylcarbamazine.

Wuchereria bancrofti (Elephantiasis)

CHARACTERISTICS

Arthropod-borne, endemic in tropical areas.

PATHOGENESIS

A **mosquito** bite releases microfilariae into the **blood.**

CLINICAL SYMPTOMS

Microfilariae reach the lymphatic system and mature into adults. Fibrosis around adults results in obstruction, leading to edema and scaly skin (**elephantiasis**) which usually involves the **genitalia** and **lower extremities** (see Figure 5-44). Other signs and symptoms of infection may include fever, chills, lymphadenopathy, and eosinophilia. Diagnosis can be made by detecting microfilariae in the blood at **night.**

TREATMENT

Diethylcarbamazine treats the parasite; however, doxycycline treats an obligate intracellular parasite and has a high cure rate alone.

KEY FACT

In **Malay**sia and the Far East, *Brugia* ***malay****i* causes a disease similar to wuchereriasis and is also transmitted by mosquitoes.

MNEMONIC

Arthropod-borne nematodes—

OWL
Onchocerca
Wuchereria
Loa loa

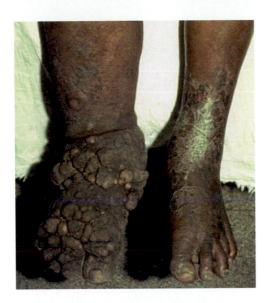

FIGURE 5-44. **Elephantiasis of the lower extremity.** (Reproduced, with permission, from Kasper DL, Braunwald E, Fauci AS, et al. *Harrison's Principles on Internal Medicine*, 16th ed. New York: McGraw-Hill, 2005: 1261.)

Zoonotic Bacteria

GRAM-NEGATIVE ZOONOTIC BACTERIA

Zoonotic infections are, by definition, acquired from reservoirs principally existing in animals; humans are usually accidental hosts. Wild or domesticated animals are the principal sources of infection of the following organisms. Transmission usually occurs by direct contact with the animal in question.

Yersinia pestis

CHARACTERISTICS

Y. pestis is the causative organism of the **plague**, the "Black Death" that decimated the population of Europe during the 1300s. As a gram-negative, lactose-fermenting rod, it is related to the enteric pathogen *Y. enterocolitica* but produces a markedly different clinical syndrome. It is a facultatively intracellular organism and is disseminated throughout the body by macrophages following phagocytosis.

The natural reservoirs of *Y. pestis* are rats in the urban setting and other wild rodents in more rural areas. Transmission is accomplished either by the bite of an infected rodent or by a secondary vector such as fleas. Currently, very few cases are reported in the United States, with most cases restricted to the American Southwest.

PATHOGENESIS

Y. pestis possesses an antiphagocytic **protein** capsule (called **F1**) as well as the **V** and **W** antigens, whose function is unknown. Together, these allow for the organism to remain resident in the phagosomes of macrophages without destruction. Very few organisms are required for infection to occur.

CLINICAL SYMPTOMS

Two syndromes are associated with Y. *pestis* infection: **bubonic plague** and **pneumonic plague.**

- **Bubonic plague** occurs after direct contact with an infected rodent or flea and is characterized by the presence of **buboes**, erythematous, painful, and swollen inguinal or axillary lymph nodes that become indurated about 1 week after exposure (see Figure 5-45). High fever and cutaneous hemorrhage follows, and bacteremia and multiorgan involvement are inevitable without treatment. Mortality is approximately 75% if untreated.
- **Pneumonic plague** has an incubation period of only three days and represents an instance in which the microorganism is aerosolized, causing the exhalations of affected humans to be infectious. Constitutional and respiratory symptoms predominate, and the mortality rate is even higher (90% if untreated) than that of bubonic plague.

TREATMENT

Appropriate treatment for plague involves the administration of a parenteral aminoglycoside: Streptomycin or gentamicin. Rodent control and vaccination of at-risk populations can help control the spread of this disease.

Francisella tularensis

CHARACTERISTICS

Another rare zoonotic bacterium, which is the causative agent of **tularemia.** It is an extremely small gram-negative coccobacillus that, like Y. *pestis*, is a facultative intracellular bacterium that spreads from the point of entry into the body via macrophage phagosomes. It is fastidious to culture and requires either "chocolate" or buffered charcoal yeast extract agar and an extended incubation period for growth in the lab.

The animal reservoirs for *F. tularensis* are wild rodents, especially rabbits, voles, and the like. Humans are usually infected either by contact with a domestic animal that has killed an infected rodent or by a tick bite. In the United States, tularemia is seen mostly in Central Plains states, although most

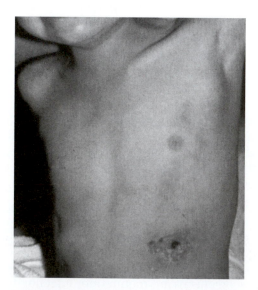

FIGURE 5-45. **Bubonic plague.** Note the bubo in the left axilla. The ulcer is an unusual manifestation at the initial site of infection. (Reproduced, with permission, from Kasper DL, Braunwald E, Fauci AS, et al. *Harrison's Principles of Internal Medicine*, 16th ed. New York: McGraw-Hill, 2005: 923.)

states have reported cases. The species is highly virulent; only a few organisms are required to produce infection.

PATHOGENESIS

F. tularensis has an antiphagocytic polysaccharide capsule, which protects against opsonization. It is resistant to intracellular killing in the phagosomes of macrophages.

CLINICAL SYMPTOMS

Tularemia can manifest as a variety of different syndromes.

- The **ulceroglandular** variant is the most common form. Lesions resemble bubo formation at the site of initial infection except that the skin surface ulcerates as well; the bacteria can spread from there to the bloodstream.
- **Pneumonic** tularemia results from contact with aerosolized bacteria and can lead to a bilateral pneumonia.
- **Oculoglandular** tularemia affects the eye and cervical lymph nodes.
- **Typhoidal** tularemia has gastrointestinal and systemic symptoms.

TREATMENT

Streptomycin and gentamicin are standard therapies for tularemia. Tick prophylaxis (light-colored clothing, insect repellents, long sleeves) and avoidance of known reservoirs of infection serve to decrease the incidence of disease in endemic areas.

Brucella

CHARACTERISTICS

Brucella spp. (*B. melitensis*, *B. abortus*, *B. suis*, and *B. canis*) are facultatively intracellular, small, nonmotile, encapsulated gram-negative organisms that infect mammals such as cows, goats, and pigs. Spread to humans is usually through contact with infected meat, aborted placentas, or unpasteurized milk products. *Brucella* infection is rare in the United States owing to cattle immunization and milk pasteurization.

CLINICAL SYMPTOMS

Brucellosis generally presents with nonspecific symptoms; one common finding is an intermittent fever (**undulant fever**), which rises during the day and resolves at night. Progressive involvement of the gastrointestinal or respiratory tracts or skeleton is possible.

TREATMENT

A combination of doxycycline and rifampin are used to eradicate the organism.

Pasteurella multocida

CHARACTERISTICS

Pasteurella is a nonmotile, encapsulated gram-negative organism distantly related to *Haemophilus*, which asymptomatically colonizes the mouths of dogs and especially cats.

CLINICAL SYMPTOMS

Common cause of localized wound infection, cellulitis, and lymphadenopathy following a bite or scratch from an infected cat or dog.

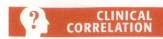
TREATMENT

Doxycycline or penicillin as well as appropriate wound care.

Bartonella Spp.

CHARACTERISTICS

Bartonella spp. are short, aerobic gram-negative rods recently discovered and poorly characterized to date. They are found in a number of animal reservoirs, often with insects as intermediate vectors. The most clinically important member of the genus is *Bartonella henselae*, the causative agent of **cat-scratch fever**. However, worth mentioning is *Bartonella quintana*, which causes **trench fever**, a 5-day illness frequently seen during World War I, characterized by fever and bone pain. *B. quintana* has no known animal reservoir; transmission occurs via the bite of the human body louse.

Bartonella henselae is often transmitted to humans via the scratch or bite of a cat; hence the name **cat-scratch fever**.

CLINICAL SYMPTOMS

Cat-scratch fever is a chronic lymphadenitis occurring mainly in children after being scratched by an infected cat. Lymph nodes near the site of infection become enlarged and painful, and chronic, low-grade fevers may develop.

TREATMENT

The infection is worrisome to parents but self-limited and does not respond to antibiotic therapy.

Virology

BASIC STRUCTURE

Virus Particles: Virions

Viruses are obligate intracellular parasites and can only replicate inside an appropriate host cell. They are composed of a genome encased in a protein coat (**capsid**). Depending on the life cycle of the virus, the capsid may or may not be surrounded by a lipoprotein envelope (see Figure 5-46).

Viral genome + Capsid ± Virus-Encoded Enzymes = Nucleocapsid = Naked Virus

Nucleocapsid + Host Membrane with Virus-Encoded Glycoproteins = Enveloped Virus

Viral Genome

The genome is composed of a nucleic acid sequence made up of either DNA or RNA. There is great variation in genomic structure:

- Double-stranded (**ds**)
- Single-stranded (**ss**)
- Segmented
- Nonsegmented
- Linear, circular, or helical.

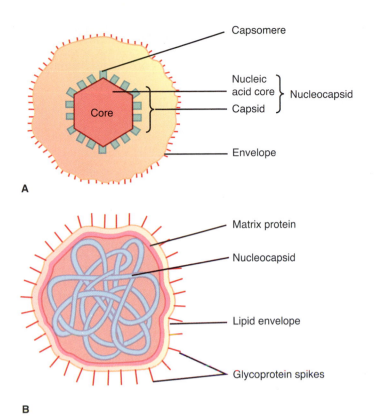

A

B

FIGURE 5-46. **Schematic diagram of the components of the complete virus particle (the virion).** (A) Enveloped virus with icosahedral symmetry. (B) Virus with helical symmetry. (Modified, with permission, from Brooks GF, Carroll KC, Butel JS, et al. *Jawetz, Melnick, & Adelberg's Medical Microbiology*, 24th ed. New York: McGraw-Hill, 2007.)

A virus with a **single-stranded genome** can either be:

- **Positive-stranded–positive sense RNA:** Genome exhibits mRNA-like characteristics; thus it can be directly translated by the host cell.
- **Negative-stranded–negative sense RNA:** The virus must first make a complementary copy of its genome before it can undergo translation. Negative-stranded viruses must carry their own enzymes, such as **RNA-dependent RNA polymerases** to transcribe the complement strand after infecting a host cell.
- **Ambisense:** Genome contains both positive strand and negative strand. This arrangement requires two rounds of transcription to be carried out.

Capsid (Capsomere)

Capsomere forms an outer shell which holds and protects the viral genome and virus-encoded enzymes. It is composed of structural proteins and serves as antigenic stimulus for antibody production. The capsid contains receptor-specific sites necessary for initiating infection. Capsomere exhibits several shapes:

- **Icosahedral** (symmetric sided symmetric polygon—polyhedron with 20 triangular faces)
- **Helical**
- **Complex**

ENVELOPED VERSUS NAKED VIRUSES

General characteristics of viral species important to human pathology are depicted in Figure 5-47.

Enveloped Viruses

Enveloped viruses are surrounded by a lipoprotein membrane acquired upon **nonlytic release** of the virus from the host cell. **Virus-encoded glycoproteins speckled throughout the envelope** are essential for attachment to the host

Positive-strand RNA viruses

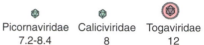
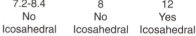

	Picornaviridae	Caliciviridae	Togaviridae	Flaviviridae	Coronaviridae
Genome size (kb)	7.2–8.4	8	12	10	16–21
Envelope	No	No	Yes	Yes	Yes
Capsid symmetry	Icosahedral	Icosahedral	Icosahedral	Icosahedral	Helical

Negative-strand RNA viruses

	Rhabdoviridae	Filoviridae	Paramyxoviridae
Genome size (kb)	13–16	13	16–20
Envelope	Yes	Yes	Yes
Capsid symmetry	Helical	Helical	Helical

Segmented negative-strand RNA viruses   **Segmented double-strand RNA viruses**

	Orthomyxoviridae	Bunyaviridae	Arenaviridae	Reoviridae
Genome size (kb)	14	13–21	10–14	16–27
Envelope	Yes	Yes	Yes	No
Capsid symmetry	Helical	Helical	Helical	Icosahedral

Retroviruses

	Retroviridae
Genome size (kb)	3–9
Envelope	Yes
Capsid symmetry	Icosahedral

DNA viruses

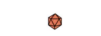

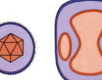

	Parvoviridae	Papovaviridae	Adenoviridae	Herpesviridae	Poxviridae
Genome size (kb)	5	5–9	36–38	100–250	240
Envelope	No	No	No	Yes	Yes
Capsid symmetry	Icosahedral	Icosahedral	Icosahedral	Icosahedral	Complex

├──┤
100 nm

FIGURE 5-47. Schematic diagrams of the major virus families including species that infect humans. The viruses are grouped by genome type and are drawn approximately to scale. (Modified, with permission, from Kasper DL, Braunwald E, Fauci, et al. *Harrison's Principles of Internal Medicine*, 16th ed. New York: McGraw-Hill, 2005: 1021.)

cell and initiation of infection. The glycoproteins also serve as viral antigens and stimulate antibody production.

- **Most DNA** viruses acquire their envelopes from the host's nuclear membrane as the virus exits the nucleus.
- **Exceptions** are **poxviruses**, because they replicate and acquire their envelope (through "Golgi wrapping") in the cytoplasm.

In addition to their primary function, viral glycoproteins also serve as **viral attachment proteins (VAPs)** that bind to host cell structures. Some examples are:

- **Hemagglutinin (HA):** Binds erythrocytes.
- **Neuraminidase (NA):** Facilitates release of virion from host cells.
- **Fusion proteins (F):** Facilitates fusion of virion and the host cell.

Enveloped viruses are susceptible to damage by dehydration, organic solvents, detergents, and extreme pH or temperature. These characteristics determine their **mode of transmission:**

- **Direct contact** with bodily fluids: Respiratory droplets, blood, mucus, saliva, and semen.
- Injections or organ transplants.

Naked Viruses

Naked viruses have no envelopes and are usually more stable than enveloped viruses because they are better equipped to withstand injury from the damaging agents mentioned above. Enteric viruses such as reoviruses and picornaviruses are transmitted via the **fecal-oral** route. Other viruses are transmitted via respiratory droplets and contact with fomites.

There are three families of **naked DNA** viruses:

- Parvoviridae
- Adenoviridae
- Papovaviridae

There are four families of **naked RNA** viruses:

- Astroviridae
- Reoviridae
- Picornaviridae
- Caliciviridae

DNA VERSUS RNA VIRUSES

DNA Viruses

There are **six families** of viruses **with DNA genomes** (see Figure 5-48):

These viruses share the following common characteristics (see Figure 5-48):

- **Double-stranded genome** with the exception of:
    - Parvoviridae (B-19)—**single-stranded** DNA genome.
    - Hepadnavirus—**incomplete double-stranded** genome.

KEY FACT

Many naked viruses are able to survive the harsh, acidic environment of the stomach and the detergent-like bile found in the intestines.

MNEMONIC

Naked DNA viruses: A woman needs to be naked for a **PAP** smear.

Parvovirus
Adenovirus
Papovavirus

MNEMONIC

Naked RNA viruses: **DR. P**olitical **C**orrectness does not approve of nudity.

Deltavirus
Reovirus
Picornavirus
Calcivirus

MNEMONIC

For **DNA** viruses—Think **HHAP-PP**y:

Herpesviridae
Hepadnaviridae
Adenoviridae
Papovaviridae
Parvoviridae
Poxviridae

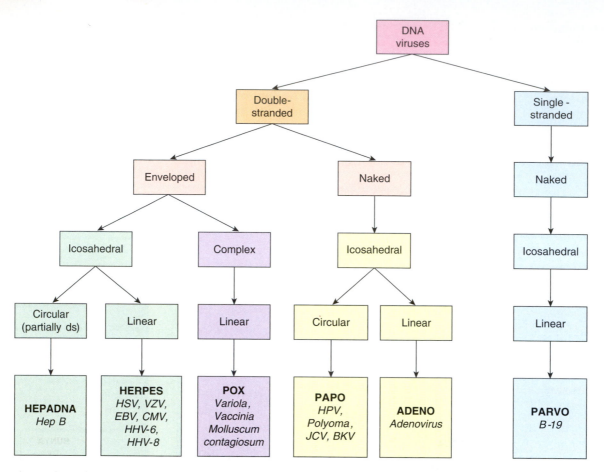

FIGURE 5-48. **Flowchart of DNA viruses.** Each family is categorized by the type of viral genome and capsid shape. Important examples of each viral family are highlighted.

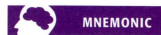

MNEMONIC

Single-stranded DNA genome:

Like a one **par** hole in golf.
Parvoviridae.

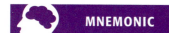

MNEMONIC

PhD's are egg-heads (circular).
PH: Papova, **H**epadna

KEY FACT

RNA viruses have the ability to produce great genetic diversity, which is generated by both **mutation** and **reassortment**.

2. **Linear** viral genomes with the exception of:
   ▪ Papovaviruses and hepadnavirus—**circular**.
3. **Icosahedral capsid** with the exception of:
   ▪ Poxviruses, which have a complex, **bullet-shaped capsid**.
4. **Replication** in the nucleus with the exception of:
   ▪ Poxviruses, which carry their own DNA-dependent RNA polymerase and can replicate in the cytoplasm.

RNA Viruses

There are **16** families of medically important **RNA viruses** (see Figure 5-49), which are generally categorized into **three** major groupings: Positive-sense (positive strand), negative-sense (negative strand), and ambi-sense RNA viruses. Terms "sense" and "strand" are used interchangeably.

▪ Genomes of **positive-sense RNA** viruses act as mRNA and can be directly translated once the virus invades the host cell.
▪ **Negative-sense RNA** viruses carry their own **RNA-dependent RNA polymerase** and makes positive-sense copy once the virus infects the host cell. The copy is then used as both a genomic template and as mRNA for protein synthesis.
▪ The genomes of **ambi-sense RNA** viruses have portions that are both positive- and negative-sense.
▪ **Segmented viral genomes** are seen mostly in human RNA viruses. After replication, these viral genomes are cleaved into two or more smaller,

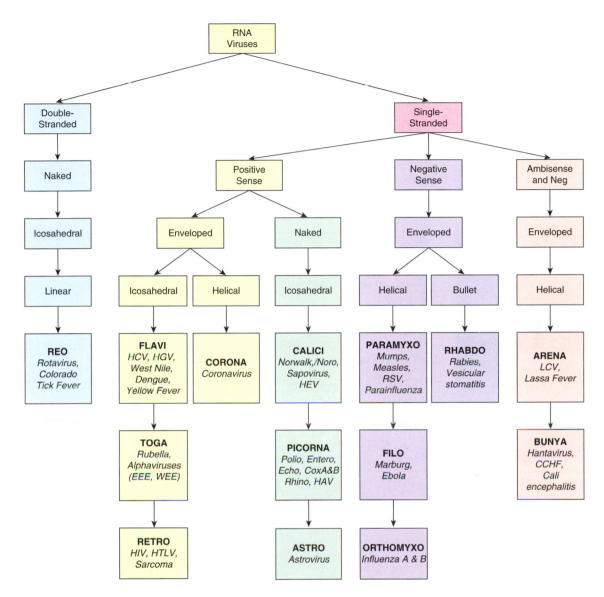

FIGURE 5-49. **Flowchart of RNA viruses.** Each family is categorized by the type of viral genome and capsid shape. Important examples of each viral family are highlighted.

physically separate segments of nucleic acid. When the virion attaches to and infects another cell, these segments come together, reassemble, and join to form a complete genome.

Because of the great number and diversity of the RNA viruses, they have fewer shared characteristics than the DNA viruses. However, they do share a few **common traits** (see Table 5-26):

- Single-stranded genome—except for reoviruses, which have a double-stranded RNA genome.
- Replicate in the cytoplasm—except for orthomyxoviruses and retroviruses, both of which replicate in the nucleus.

PATHOGENESIS

General Considerations

By definition, viral **pathogenesis** describes the interaction of viral and host factors that leads to disease production. A virus is considered **pathogenic** for a

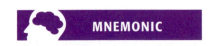

MNEMONIC

Viruses with segmented genomes: BOAR

Bunyaviruses: 3 segments
Orthomyxoviruses: 8 segments
Arenaviruses: 2 segments
Reoviruses: 10 or 11 segments

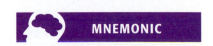

MNEMONIC

All RNA viruses divide in the cytoplasm… OR not.

Orthomyxo
Retro

TABLE 5-26. **Common Traits of RNA Viruses**

TRAIT	HELICAL AND SINGLE-STRANDED; REPLICATE IN CYTOPLASM, EXCEPT AS NOTED
Positive sense	Picornaviridae, Flaviviridae, Togaviridae, Calicivirus, Coronaviridae, Retroviridae
Negative sense	Paramyxoviridae, Filoviridae, Orthomyxoviridae, Rhabdoviridae
Ambisense	Arenaviridae, Bunyaviridae
Replicate in nucleus	Orthomyxoviridae, *Retro*viridae
Double-stranded genome	*Reoviridae*

KEY FACT

The virulence level of a virus is variable and genetically determined.

KEY FACT

Cell tropism and the virulence determine the target organ of each virus

KEY FACT

A virus that binds only to a specific receptor may only be able to infect a specific number of species.

CLINICAL CORRELATION

Arboviruses generally cause hemorrhagic fevers and encephalitis.
Roboviruses are another common cause of hemorrhagic fevers.

specific host if it can infect and cause disease-specific symptoms in that host. Several key properties determine viral infectivity, the cells /tissues affected, and the outcome of an infection.

- **Virulence:** Ability of the virus to cause disease by avoiding or otherwise overcoming the host's defense mechanisms.
- **Cellular tropism:** The specificity of a virus for a given host cell or host tissue, determined by surface receptors and intracellular content within the host cell. Infection by a certain virus tends to affect a specific organ or group of organs (**target organs**), causing classic symptoms for that particular virus.
- **Host range:** Range of cells (or species) that can become a host to a virus or bacteriophage; dictated by the presence or absence of specific receptors that enable active viral infection.

Infection

To produce a disease, viruses must enter the host, interact with susceptible cells/tissues, replicate, and produce cell injury. Humans are infected with viruses by the same basic mechanisms that allow the spread of other microorganisms. Common **modes of transmission** include:

- Direct contact with bodily fluids and/or an infected source.
- Vertical transmission (transplacental—mother to child).
- Direct inoculation through injections or trauma; organ transplant.
- Genetic modifications or mutations, such as those generated by retroviruses and oncogenic viruses.
- **Vectors,** such as insects and small rodents. Humans can become infected through bites of vector species or inhalation of viral particles from the vector's hair, fur, or feces.
    - **Arthropod-borne viruses—arboviruses:** Mainly belong to four families of viruses—Flaviviridae, Togaviridae, Bunyaviridae, and Reoviridae. The most common arthropod vectors are mosquitoes and ticks.
    - **Rodent-borne viruses—roboviruses:** Belong to the Arenavirdiae and Bunyaviridae families. These viruses are generally transmitted by rats and mice.
- **Reinfection:** Secondary infection that occurs upon recovery from a previous infection and is caused by the same agent.
- **Coinfection:** Concurrent infection of a host (single cell/tissue) by two or more viruses.

- **Superinfection:** Process by which a host previously infected by one virus acquires coinfection with another virus at a later point in time. Superinfection can also be caused by other microorganisms owing to the host's compromised immune system or the microorganisms' resistance to previous antibiotics.

Replication

Viruses are obligate intracellular parasites, and in order to survive, they must infect host cells, and replicate, thus causing disease. Replication is a complex process following infection and involves multiple steps:

- **Attachment to host cell:** Binding of viruses to host cells is mediated through the interaction of viral surface proteins with specific host cell surface-receptor sites.
- **Penetration and entry:** Differences between the naked and enveloped viruses.
    - Most naked viruses enter host cells through **receptor-mediated endocytosis.**
        - **Viropexis:** Upon attachment to the host cell surface, hydrophobic (lipophilic) structures of certain naked viruses' capsid proteins are exposed, thus enabling them to directly penetrate the host cell.
    - **Enveloped viruses** enter host cells by **fusing** with the cell membrane, thus allowing the nucleocapsid or the viral genome to be delivered directly into the cytoplasm.
    - The fusion activity can be mediated by **VAPs, fusion proteins,** or **other glycoproteins** found in the viral envelope.
    - Optimal **fusion pH** is specific to each type of virus.
        - If the optimal **pH** is **neutral,** the enveloped virus can fuse with the outer cell membrane.
        - If the optimal **pH** is **acidic,** the virus must first be internalized by endocytosis and fuse with an endosome to reduce the pH.
- **Uncoating of the virion:** Once a virus is internalized, the nucleocapsid must be brought to the site of replication and removed. Uncoating of a virion results in the loss of infectivity. Shedding of the capsid can be initiated by:
    - Attachment to a specific receptor.
    - Conformational changes resulting from an acidic environment.
    - Enzymatic activity of endosomal or lysosomal proteases.

REPLICATION OF DNA VIRUSES

DNA viruses (except for poxviruses; Figure 5-48) enter the nucleus and utilize the host cell's DNA-dependent RNA polymerase to transcribe its mRNA from the negative-strand template. There is a specific **temporal pattern of transcription:** immediate early, delayed early, and late mRNA transcripts.

Key steps in DNA virus replication:

- mRNA transcripts undergo modification: Addition of poly A tail and methylated cap takes place in the host cell's **nucleus.**
- Transcripts then are transported to the **cytoplasm** and translated on cytoplasmic polysomes.
- Newly synthesized proteins are then transported **back** to the nucleus, where the capsid is assembled and the viral genome and enzymes are packaged before the virus is released.

Genomic replication is performed by a **DNA-dependent DNA polymerase.**

KEY FACT

Enveloped viruses mediate host cell attachment through their glycoproteins (**VAPs**—viral attachment proteins)

Naked viruses use **capsid surface proteins** to attach to host cells.

KEY FACT

Papovaviruses and **picornaviruses** gain entry through **viropexis.**

KEY FACT

Early transcripts encode proteins important for viral replication, gene transcription, and takeover of the host cell.

Later transcripts commonly encode structural proteins, which serve to build new virions later released to infect other cells.

KEY FACT

Adenoviruses use the host cell's enzymes.
Herpes viruses carry their own.

Hepatitis B virus is a **unique DNA virus** because the genome is partially double-stranded with single-stranded regions scattered throughout. Before it can be delivered to the nucleus and replicate, this virus must first generate a fully double-stranded genome. Hepatitis B virus carries a **RNA-dependent DNA polymerase** with reverse transcriptase properties that uses a RNA template to synthesize the DNA.

REPLICATION OF RNA VIRUSES

Both replication and transcription of RNA viruses (except for orthomyxoviruses and retroviruses) occur **in the cytoplasm** (see Figure 5-50). This is possible because RNA viruses encode for their own **RNA-dependent DNA polymerases (replicases** and **transcriptases).**

- Positive-sense RNA viruses synthesize these proteins once inside the host cell.

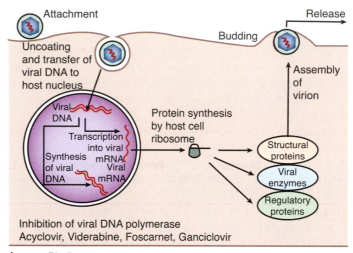

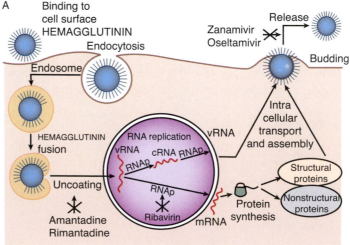

FIGURE 5-50. Replicative cycles of DNA (A) and RNA (B) viruses. The replicative cycles of herpes virus (A) and influenza A virus (B) are examples of DNA-encoded and RNA-encoded viruses, respectively. Sites of action of antiviral agents also are shown. An X on top of an arrow indicates a block to virus growth. The neuraminidase inhibitors zanamivir and oseltamivir specifically inhibit release of progeny virus. Small capitals indicate virus proteins. mRNA, messenger RNA; cDNA, complementary DNA; vRNA, viral RNA; RNAp, RNA polymerase; cRNA, complementary RNA. (Modified, with permission, from Brunton LL, Parker KL, Buxton ILO, Blumenthal DK. *Goodman & Gilman's The Pharmacological Basis of Therapeutics,* 11th ed. New York: McGraw-Hill, 2006.)

- Negative-sense RNA viruses carry these enzymes in their capsids. The **genomes of positive-sense RNA** viruses can **serve as mRNA.** Once inside the host cell, the genome can be directly translated to synthesize proteins (see Table 5-27).

RELEASE OF NEWLY SYNTHESIZED VIRUS

The process of releasing newly synthesized viruses differs in naked and enveloped viruses.

- **Naked viruses** kill the host cell through cytolysis in order to be released; thus, they are unable to establish persistent productive infections because infected cells are lysed in the process.
- **Enveloped viruses** are released from infected host cells through a process referred to as **"budding"**; thus, the infected host cell survives and budding can lead to **cell senescence.**
  - Virally encoded glycoproteins are synthesized and anchored in the host cell's membrane.
  - The nucleocapsid is surrounded by the glycoprotein-studded membrane, creating the "envelope."
  - The virus is released through **exocytosis.**

Once viruses are surrounded by the lipoprotein membrane and are released from the host cell, they are considered infective.

KEY FACT

The viral genomes of naked positive-sense RNA viruses can be infectious in and of themselves

CLINICAL CORRELATION

Naked viruses can only cause cytolytic productive or latent infections.

CLINICAL CORRELATION

Hepatitis B virus can establish **persistent productive infections;** that is, infected cells can produce low levels of virus over a period of years.

TABLE 5-27. Specifics of Genomic Replication of the RNA Viruses

VIRUS	GENOME	REPLICATION PROCESS	ENZYMES
Negative-sense RNA viruses	Complementary to mRNA.	Must generate positive-sense copy before translation.	Carry RNA-dependent RNA polymerase used to make mRNA transcript.
Positive-sense RNA viruses	Acts as mRNA transcript.	Genome is directly translated.	None
Ambi-sense RNA viruses	Some portions are positive-sense and others are negative-sense.	Similar to negative-sense RNA virus replication.	
Retroviruses	Positive-sense genome, but cannot be used as mRNA transcript.	Must synthesize circular complementary DNA (cDNA) copy in cytoplasm, which is brought into nucleus and integrated into host DNA.	Carry reverse transcriptases that synthesize cDNA.
Delta virus	Single-stranded RNA genome.	Most unique replication process; replicates in nucleus using host cell's DNA-dependent RNA polymerase II.	None

Patterns of Infections

Patterns of infection can be divided as follows (see Figure 5-51):

SUBCLINICAL INFECTIONS

Are either asymptomatic or cause a less severe, nonspecific illness that may not be recognized or identified as the result of a specific virus.

- The virus inoculum is small, or only a few host cells are infected.
- The virus is unable to reach its target tissue.

ACUTE INFECTIONS

Develop apparent clinical symptomatology within a short period of time after the incubation period of the virus. Infections can be **localized** or **disseminated**. In addition, these types of infections can be **rapidly cleared** or they can develop into either **persistent** or **latent** infection.

- **Localized infections** develop near the site of viral entry, where the primary replication and cell damage take place. These types of infections have short incubation periods.
  - Localized infections mostly affect the respiratory, gastrointestinal, and genitourinary tracts, as well as the eye.
  - Symptoms may include systemic response (e.g., fever).
  - The immune response is weaker than one that is mounted against a disseminated infection.
- **Disseminated infections** tend to have longer incubation periods (weeks rather than days) and generally cause **viremia.**
  - Disseminated infections affect multiple organ systems.
  - Symptoms are systemic, reflecting affected organ(s).
  - The immune response is usually greater than in localized infections; however, they also usually take longer to eradicate the virus and clear the infection.

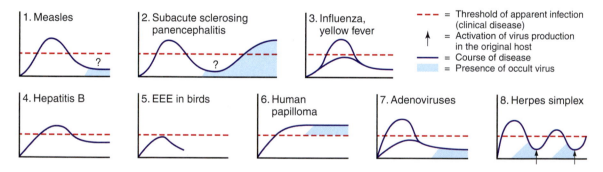

FIGURE 5-51. **Types of virus-host interactions: Apparent (clinical disease), inapparent (subclinical), chronic, latent, occult, and slow infections.** (1) Measles runs an acute, almost always clinically apparent course resulting in long-lasting immunity. (2) Measles may also be associated with persistence of latent infection in subacute sclerosing panencephalitis. (3) Yellow fever and influenza follow a pattern similar to that of measles except that infection may be more often subclinical than clinical. (4) In hepatitis B, recovery from clinical disease may be associated with chronic infection in which fully active virus persists in the blood. (5) Some infections are, in a particular species, always subclinical, such as eastern equine encephalomyelitis (EEE) in some species of birds that then act as reservoirs of the virus. (6) In human papilloma, the course of infection is chronic; when cervical cancer develops, the virus present is occult (not replicating). (7) Infection of humans with certain adenoviruses may be clinical or subclinical. There may be a long latent infection during which virus is present in small quantity; virus may also persist after the illness. (8) The periodic reactivation of latent herpes simplex virus, which may recur throughout life in humans, often follows an initial acute episode of stomatitis in childhood. (Modified, with permission, from Brooks GF, Carroll KC, Butel JS, et al. *Jawetz, Melnick, & Adelberg's Medical Microbiology*, 24th ed. New York: McGraw-Hill, 2007: 400.)

- **Congenital malformations** result from acute maternal infections that result in viremia. The virus can cross the placental barrier (**vertical transmission**) and easily infect the fetus because of its immature immune system.
- **Persistent infections** refer to continued presence of the infectious virus over an extended period of time (months, years, or possibly a lifetime).
  - **Carriers** live with a persistent viral infection (*hepatitis B virus*), and may or may not have clinical manifestations.
  - Other viruses (e.g., **herpes virus**) are able to establish persistent infections in patients in a noninfectious form (no symptoms, viral antigen or viral cytopathology are detected), and periodically reactivate into an infectious form (full-blown symptomatology/disease).

SLOW INFECTIONS

Have extremely long incubation periods (months or years). Although the virus is replicating and can cause cell damage during this time, no clinical symptoms are observed during the incubation. These types of infections are usually associated with **progressive, fatal viral diseases** affecting the central nervous system such as Creutzfeldt-Jakob disease and kuru.

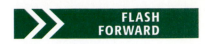

Congenital infections—

TORCHeS
Toxoplasmosis
Other infections
Rubella
Cytomegalovirus
Herpes, **H**IV
Syphilis

KEY FACT

Persistent infection = recurring disease with cycles of symptomatic outbreaks and silent periods.

VIRAL GENETICS

Viral variations and alterations that lead to new strains can result from a number of different processes:

- Changes directly affecting the genome: **Genetic drift,** and genetic reassortment resulting in **genetic shift.**
- Strictly phenotypic changes that do not modify viral genomes: **Complementation, phenotypic mixing,** and **phenotypic masking.**

Many of these processes occur when a single cell is infected by multiple strains of a virus or by multiple viruses.

Genetic Reassortment

When two strains of a segmented virus infect the same cell, respective segments can intermingle in the cytoplasm during replication.

- As viral particles undergo assembly, genomic segments of the respective strains can be packaged together in the capsid, thus creating a new (progeny) strain with a genome containing sequences from both (parental) strains.
  - Changes in the **genome** resulting from genetic reassortment are referred to as **genetic shift.**
  - Genetic shift alters the antigenic properties (gene expression profiles) of the affected viruses; hence the term **antigenic shift** (see Figure 5-52).
- Generated changes in the genome are drastic, yet stable, thus providing a source for major viral outbreaks and epidemics/pandemics.
- Prototypic example of a virus with ability to produce great genetic diversity via genetic reassortment is **influenza A** virus. This ability is secondary to its wide host range (see Figure 5-53). Influenza B and C viruses do not exhibit antigenic shift because few related viruses exist in animals.

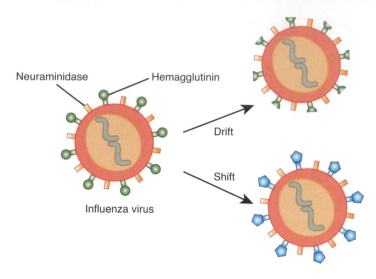

FIGURE 5-52. **Antigenic shift** generates viruses with entirely novel antigens (develops within a short period of time; source for epidemics/pandemics), whereas antigenic drift creates influenza viruses with moderately modified antigens (developed over years). (This image is a work of the U.S. Food and Drug Administration, part of the United States Department of Health and Human Services. As a work of the U.S. federal government, the image is in the public domain.)

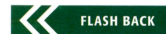

FLASH BACK

Antigenic drift should not be confused with **random genetic drift;** an important process in **population genetics.**

Genetic (Antigenic) Drift

Genetic drift comprises spontaneous mutations in viral genomes that create slight antigenic changes, which may or may not alter the virulence of the virus (see Figure 5-52).

■ **Most notable in RNA viruses,** especially in **HIV** and **orthomyxoviruses,** because their replication processes have no proof-reading step to weed out these mutations.

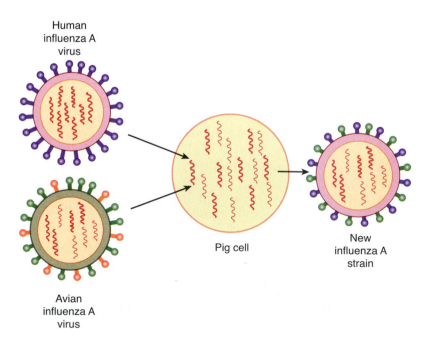

FIGURE 5-53. **New influenza A strain generated via genetic reassortment of human and avian strains of the virus.**

Complementation

A defective mutant strain of a virus may be missing a gene encoding an enzyme or factor necessary for replication. Complementation refers to the **rescue** of such a mutant via **co-replication** with **another mutant** or cell line that can replace the missing protein.

- The newly established (**rescued**) genome, though still defective, is able to replicate and form progeny.
- The progeny derived from the original (**mutant**) genome still lack the same gene and are not able to replicate unless they, too, are rescued.

Phenotypic Mixing

When two related, yet **antigenically distinct** viruses infect a **single host cell**, their proteins can mingle. Capsid proteins can merge during the assembly process, resulting in a capsid composed of a mixture of structural and surface proteins from both strains. The **genomes** remain **unchanged**, but the **capsids** are **hybrids** of the two strains, which may then alter the host range or develop resistance to antibody neutralization (see Figure 5-54).

Phenotypic Masking (Transcapsidation)

Similar to phenotypic mixing, phenotypic masking occurs when a **single** host cell is infected with **two related viral strains.**

- The genome of one strain is packaged in the capsid of the other.
- **Unlike** phenotypic mixing, the capsid is completely composed of proteins encoded by one strain.
- Phenotypic masking can occur with two completely different types of viruses and can result in what is called "**pseudotypes.**"

Viral Vectors

With the use of recombinant DNA technology, viruses can be manipulated to serve as vectors which deliver foreign genes into human cells. Viral vectors

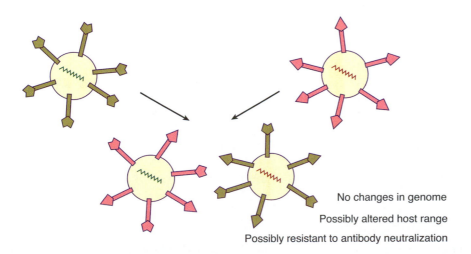

No changes in genome

Possibly altered host range

Possibly resistant to antibody neutralization

FIGURE 5-54.   Phenotypic mixing.

can be used to transfer DNA for gene therapy, as vaccines, and as killers that target specific tumor cells.

- **Defective viruses** are usually used as vectors because they cannot replicate, but they can infect and deliver genetic material into a targeted cell.

VACCINES

Active immunization with virus vaccines exposes patients to a virus or its antigenic proteins. This induces an immune response that results in the generation of memory cells.

Live Virus Vaccines

Live vaccines incorporate **attenuated** viral strains that are relatively nonvirulent. These viral vaccines are very effective against enveloped viruses, which require cell-mediated immune response to clear the infection.

- The **immune response** to a live virus vaccine mimics natural infection by generating TH1 and TH2 response, thus stimulating humoral, cellular, and memory immune responses.
- **Routes of application** can be parenteral, oral, or by inhalation to mimic the natural route of infection.
- **Immunity** derived from a live virus vaccine is generally long-lasting.

Immunization with a live virus vaccine carries a greater risk than when using an inactivated virus vaccine. Live virus vaccines carry the **potential to revert** to a virulent form of the virus and may actually cause disease.

Inactivated Vaccines

Contain either killed (inactivated) virus or viral subunits. Once killed vaccine is injected into the patient, the body mounts a response to the immunogenic surface antigens found on the viral capsid or envelope.

- The **immune response:**
  - Predominantly a TH2 (antibody) response, generating immunoglobulin G (IgG) that neutralizes and opsonizes the inactive virus.
  - Local secretory immunoglobulin A (IgA) response is not sufficient.
  - There is not a strong cell-mediated response.
- **Routes of application:** Generally parenteral.
- **Immunity:** Not as long lasting as live vaccines; **boosters** are usually required to maintain immunity.

Killed virus vaccines are generally very safe. However, they can stimulate a hypersensitivity reaction in some people.

Advantages and disadvantages of the respective types of vaccines are depicted in Table 5-28.

Future Developments in Viral Vaccines

There are several viruses that cannot be properly attenuated so that a live vaccine may be developed.

TABLE 5-28. Comparison of Advantages and Disadvantages of Live and Killed/Inactived Vaccines

	LIVE	KILLED/INACTIVED
Immunity duration	Longlasting	Short-term
Doses	Single	Multiple (boosters)
Antibody response	IgG, IgA	IgG
Cell-mediated response	Good	Poor
Side effects	Mild symptoms	Soreness around injection site
Temperature-sensitive	Yes	No
Reversion to virulence	Possible	Never

Portions of viral genomes can be inserted into the genomes of "safe" viruses, such as vaccinia or attenuated adenovirus, thereby generating **hybrid** virus vaccines. They have a potential for developing **polyvalent** vaccines.

Plasmids are also being studied as possible vectors to create viral DNA vaccines. Specific viral genes encoding for proteins that elicit a protective response (usually envelope proteins) are cloned into a plasmid. They have a potential to mount solid TH1 and TH2 response.

DIAGNOSTIC TESTS

Although the history and clinical signs and symptoms are often used to diagnose many viral illnesses, collected specimens can be used in the laboratory to confirm or to diagnose atypical or unusual cases. Most commonly used tests are described below.

- **Cytology** is a rapid detection method. Direct microscopic examination of collected specimens or monolayer cell culture samples are used to detect viruses.
- **Cytopathic effects (CPE).** Viruses can be also characterized and identified by the type of cells they infect, the rate of viral growth, and specific patterns of cellular changes caused by infection.
  - **Syncytia** (multinucleated giant cells) form when individual infected cells fuse together. They are often observed with **HSV, HIV, paramyxoviruses**, and **VZV.**
  - **Inclusion bodies** can also be seen in the cytoplasm or nucleus of infected cells.
- Other viral properties of diagnostic significance: **Heterologous interference.**
- **Detection of viral genetic material:** Northern and Southern blot analyses, restriction endonuclease fragment lengths, **genetic probes** and **PCR** can all be used to detect viral genetic material.
- **Detection of viral proteins:** Immunohistochemistry is used to detect and quantify viruses or their antigens in clinical specimens or culture samples. **Immunofluorescence**, enzyme-linked immunosorbent assays (**ELISA**), radioimmunoassay (**RIA**), and latex agglutination (**LA**) tests are commonly used methods.

KEY FACT

Inactivated vaccines:

HBV
Influenza
Adenovirus

KEY FACT

Owl's eye inclusion body = **CMV.**
Negri bodies = rabies infected brain tissue.
Cowdry type A inclusion = individual cells or syncytia of tissues infected with **HSV** or **VZV.**

- **Serologic tests:** Virus-specific antibodies may be detected, identified, and quantified in blood or serum samples.
  - **Seroconversion** indicates current infection and is determined by observing at least a fourfold increase in the antibody titer between serum collected during the acute phase and the convalescent phase of an infection.
  - Virus-specific **IgM**—usually present during the first 2–3 weeks of a **primary infection.**
  - High titers of **IgG** are usually detected a few weeks after infection; they may be detected earlier in a **reinfection.**
  - In patients who experience frequent recurrence of disease, antibody titers tend to remain high.
  - Additional serologic tests include **viral neutralization tests and hemagglutination.**

DNA VIRUSES

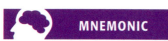

MNEMONIC

All DNA viruses are icosahedral except Pox. **PoX** is com**PleX.**

All viruses have a protein capsid. The capsid of all known DNA viruses is either icosahedral or complex. In addition to their capsid, some DNA viruses also have an outer phospholipid envelope; those that do not are known as naked viruses. DNA viral genomes are either single-stranded or double-stranded and can be linear or circular (see Table 5-29).

Parvovirus B19

Erythema infectiosum, fifth disease, slapped-cheek fever.

KEY FACT

Enveloped DNA viruses:
Herpes viruses
Hepadnavirus

CHARACTERISTICS

This is the **smallest** clinically important virus, with a size of 20–25 nm. It is also one of the **five** most common pediatric viral exanthems (diseases that cause a **rash**).

PATHOGENESIS

Transmitted via aerosolized droplets that inoculate the nasal cavity; infects erythroid precursor cells.

KEY FACT

Parvovirus B19:
ssDNA, linear, naked, icosahedral

CLINICAL SYMPTOMS

Immune complex deposition results in a lacy red rash (also called erythema infectiosum, fifth disease, or slapped-cheek fever) and arthralgias. Patients with thalassemia or sickle cell anemia may develop a **transient aplastic crisis.** Immunocompromised individuals may develop a **severe chronic anemia.** Infants may develop **hydrops fetalis** and severe anemia. Diagnosis can be confirmed with serology and CBC.

TREATMENT

Supportive care with blood transfusions as needed. Immunocompromised patients may require intravenous immunoglobulins.

Papovavirus Family

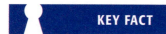

KEY FACT

Papovaviruses: dsDNA, **circular,** naked, icosahedral.

PAPILLOMAVIRUSES—HUMAN PAPILLOMAVIRUS (HPV)
CHARACTERISTICS

Infects squamous epithelial cells.

TABLE 5-29. **Summary of DNA Viruses**

Family	Structure	Disease	Route of Transmission	Important Facts
Hepadnaviridae				
Hepatits B	Partially dsDNA, ssDNA gap, enveloped, icosahedral, circular.	Infectious hepatitis.	Blood, blood products, sexual activity, shared needles.	Cause of primary hepatocellular carcinoma.
Herpesviridae				
Herpes simplex virus	dsDNA, enveloped, icosahedral, linear.	Cold sores, genital herpes, encephalitis.	Mucous membranes, breaks in skin.	Most common diagnosed cause of acute sporadic encephalitis in the United States.
Varicella-zoster virus	dsDNA, enveloped, icosahedral, linear.	Chickenpox, shingles, pneumonia.	Airborne.	Remains latent in sensory nerve ganglia throughout the body after infection.
Epstein-Barr virus	dsDNA, enveloped, icosahedral, linear.	Fever, phayngitis, lymphadenopathy.	Airborne.	Associated with malignancies, e.g., Burkitt's lymphoma, nasopharyngeal carcinoma, oral hairy leukoplakia.
Cytomegalovirus	dsDNA, enveloped, icosahedral, linear.	Causes infectious mononucleosis syndrome.	Close contact (perinatal, venereal), transfusion, transplacental organ transplantation.	One of the TORCHES viruses; causes teratogenic symptoms in fetus.
Human herpes virus 6 (HHV-6)	dsDNA, enveloped, icosahedral, linear.	Fever, rash, adenopathy, chemical hepatitis.	Saliva.	90% of all humans infected by age 3.
HHV-8	dsDNA, enveloped, icosahedral, linear.	Primary infection asymptomatic; causes Kaposi's sarcoma in AIDS patients.	Sexual and body fluids.	Causes purple lesions on the body.
Poxviridae				
Variola	dsDNA, enveloped complex, linear.	Smallpox.	Respiratory droplets or direct contact.	Lesions develop at the same pace and so are all at the same stage of development.
Vaccinia	dsDNA, enveloped complex, linear.	Pox-like Syndrome.	Contact.	Used to make smallpox vaccination.

(continues)

TABLE 5-29. Summary of DNA Viruses *(continued)*

FAMILY	STRUCTURE	DISEASE	ROUTE OF TRANSMISSION	IMPORTANT FACTS
Molluscum contagiosum	dsDNA, enveloped complex, linear.	Small flesh-colored poxes.	Contact	Common among wrestlers.
Papovaviridae				
Human papillomavirus	Naked, dsDNA icosahedral, circular.	Human cervical carcinoma and ano-genital cancers.	Sex, contact	Highly restricted in tissue tropism and replicates only in epithelial cells.
Polyomavirus	Naked, dsDNA icosahedral, circular.	Causes no disease in humans.	Sex, contact	Causes no human malignancy.
JC virus	Naked, dsDNA icosahedral, circular.	Progressive multifocal leukoencephalopathy (PML).	Sex, contact	Fatal disorder of CNS that can occur in immunodeficient patients.
BK virus	Naked, dsDNA icosahedral, circular.	Hemorrhagic cystitis, ureteral stenosis, and urinary tract infections.	Sex, contact	Oncogenic in animal models.
Adenviridae				
Adenovirus	dsDNA, naked, icosahedral, linear.	Respiratory diseases (pharyngitis, pharyngoconjuctival fever, acute respiratory disease), conjunctivitis, keratoconjuctivitis, gastroenteritis and diarrhea, bladder infection, urethritis/cervicitis.	Fecal-oral, aerosal	51 known serotypes of human adenoviruses.
Parvoviridae				
Parvovirus B19	ssDNA, linear, naked, icosahedral.	Erythema infectiosum (fifth disease), aplastic anemia, hydrops fetalis.	Respiratory droplets, oral secretions, parenterally	The only parvovirus known to cause human disease.

PATHOGENESIS

Transmitted by close contact.

CLINICAL SYMPTOMS

Varies depending on the strain.

- HPV 6 and 11 cause benign warts, including anogenital and laryngeal warts.

- HPV serotypes 16, 18, 31, 33, and 45 are associated with cervical cancer (see Figure 5-55).
- These strains produce two proteins that inactivate known tumor suppressor genes: E6 inhibits p53, E7 inhibits Rb.
- Diagnosis can be made by PCR, Pap smear, and/or biopsy.

TREATMENT

Most warts regress spontaneously after 1 or 2 years. Warts can also be ablated or surgically removed. With respect to cervical abnormalities, low-grade squamous intraepithelial lesions often regress and are monitored by regular Pap smears; higher-grade lesions are evaluated with a biopsy. Cervical cancer is managed according to stage (surgery and/or radiation).

PREVENTION

Vaccination.

POLYOMAVIRUSES: BK AND JC VIRUSES

CHARACTERISTICS

Both BK and JC viruses are common in the general population; most people are asymptomatic carriers by the age of 18.

PATHOGENICITY

Only cause clinical disease in immunocompromised individuals (e.g., those with AIDS, chemotherapy, immunosuppressants).

CLINICAL SYMPTOMS

Reactivation of latent **JC virus** in immunocompromised individuals results in progressive multifocal leukoencephalopathy (**PML**). PML is a demyelinating disease that affects oligodendrocytes (i.e., CNS) and is characterized by deficits in speech, coordination, and memory. Diagnosis is largely clinical, but can be confirmed by imaging and PCR of the CSF. **BK virus** causes kidney disease and can be found in patients with solid organ (kidney) and bone marrow transplants.

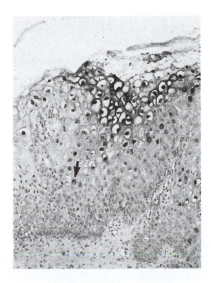

FIGURE 5-55. **Cervical biopsy stained for HPV 18 DNA.** Darker regions indicate cells infected with human papillomavirus (HPV). Most cells are located on the surface, with a single cell located deeper (*arrow*). (Image courtesy of PEIR Digital Library [http://peir.net].)

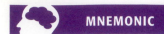

KEY FACT

Adenoviruses: dsDNA, linear, naked, icosahedral.

KEY FACT

Herpes viruses: dsDNA, linear, enveloped, icosahedral, includes: HSV-1 and 2, VZV, CMV, EBV, and HHV-6, 7, and 8.

TREATMENT

Only treatment available is improving immune function or treating the underlying HIV/AIDS.

ADENOVIRUSES

CHARACTERISTICS

One of the **most common causes of the common cold;** also causes nonpurulent **conjunctivitis.**

PATHOGENESIS

Transmitted via aerosolized droplets, contact, or fecal-oral route.

CLINICAL SYMPTOMS

There are over 40 serotypes, each of which has different manifestations, including rhinitis, pharyngitis, atypical pneumonia, conjunctivitis, hematuria, dysuria, and gastroenteritis with nonbloody diarrhea. Diagnosis can be confirmed by serology or viral cultures.

TREATMENT

None.

Herpesvirus Family

GENERAL CHARACTERISTICS

Herpesviruses are unique in that they are assembled in the nucleus and are the only viruses whose envelope is derived from the **nuclear** membrane. Because they are assembled in the nucleus, infected cells can often be identified histologically by the presence of **intranuclear inclusion bodies.** Infections may also become **latent.**

HERPES SIMPLEX VIRUS 1 (HSV-1)

CHARACTERISTICS

Most adults have been infected. HSV-1 is also the **most common cause of sporadic encephalitis** in the United States.

PATHOGENESIS

Transmitted by saliva. The virus invades mucous membranes and can cause a local infection. HSV may also invade nearby sensory nerve endings; it is then transported back to the cell body and becomes latent.

CLINICAL SYMPTOMS

Most infections are **asymptomatic.** Initial symptoms may include vesicular ulcerating lesions of the mouth (**gingivostomatitis**) or eye (**keratoconjunctivitis**). HSV can also infect the hand, causing a vesicular lesion called **herpetic whitlow.** HSV-1 may become latent in the **trigeminal** ganglia and can be reactivated under conditions of stress. Reactivation can result in recurring gingivostomatitis, keratoconjunctivitis, or **herpes labialis** (cold sores or fever blisters, see Figure 5-56). Recurrent keratoconjunctivitis may lead to blindness. In some cases, the virus can be transported into the brain (via cranial nerves), where it characteristically infects the temporal lobe. Symptoms of **temporal lobe encephalitis** include fever, headache, neck stiffness, and **olfactory hallucinations.** Permanent neurologic damage or death may ensue. Diagnosis of HSV encephalitis can be made by **PCR** of the CSF. Diagnosis of cutaneous

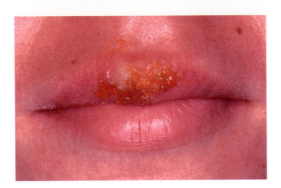

FIGURE 5-56.   **Herpes labialis due to HSV-1 infection.** (Image courtesy of PEIR Digital Library [http://peir.net].)

lesions can be made by direct fluorescent antibody test (DFA), demonstration of multinucleate giant cells on a **Tzank** smear, or by the presence of intranuclear inclusion bodies on skin **biopsy.**

TREATMENT

Acyclovir for active infection. No treatment for latent infections.

HERPES SIMPLEX VIRUS 2 (HSV-2)

CHARACTERISTICS

Like HSV-1, most adults have been infected. HSV is one of the **ToRCHeS**!

PATHOGENESIS

Transmitted by sexual contact. Like HSV-1, HSV-2 invades mucous membranes and can cause a local infection (see Figure 5-57). It may also invade nearby sensory nerve endings, where it is then transported back to the cell body and can become latent.

CLINICAL SYMPTOMS

Most infections are **asymptomatic.** Initial symptoms may include vesicular ulcerating lesions of the genitals and perianal area. HSV can also infect the hand, causing a vesicular lesion called **herpetic whitlow.** HSV-2 may become latent in the **lumbosacral** ganglia and can be reactivated under conditions

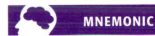
KEY FACT

HSV-1 above the waist; HSV-2 below.

MNEMONIC

Tzank goodness if you don't have herpes!

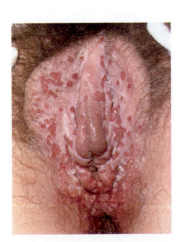

FIGURE 5-57.   **Multiple genital lesions due to HSV-2 infection.** (Reproduced, with permission, from Wolff K, Johnson RA, Suurmond D. *Fitzpatrick Dermatology Atlas & Synopsis of Clinical Dermatology,* 5th ed. New York: McGraw-Hill, 2005: 900.)

of stress, resulting in recurring genital lesions. **Neonatal HSV** can occur via transplacental transmission (ToRCHeS) or during delivery. Infection may be local (mouth, eyes, skin), may affect multiple organs and cause congenital defects, or result in spontaneous abortion. HSV-2 can also cause **neonatal encephalitis.** Diagnosis of cutaneous lesions can be made by direct DFA by demonstration of multinucleate giant cells on a **Tzank** smear or by visualization of intranuclear inclusion bodies on skin **biopsy.**

TREATMENT

Acyclovir for active infection. No treatment for latent infections. **Cesarean section** is indicated for mothers with active lesions.

VARICELLA-ZOSTER VIRUS (VZV, CHICKENPOX, ZOSTER, SHINGLES)

CHARACTERISTICS

Highly contagious.

PATHOGENESIS

Transmitted by respiratory secretions or contact with active lesions. Like HSV, VZV also causes local infection and can invade sensory nerve endings, where it is then transported back to the cell body and can become latent.

CLINICAL SYMPTOMS

- In **children,** VZV typically causes a mild, flulike illness with characteristic skin lesions (**varicella** or **chickenpox**).
- Often described as **"dew drops on a rose petal,"** these lesions appear initially as discrete papules on a macular erythematous base (see Figure 5-58). The papules then vesiculate, become pustules, and eventually rupture and release additional virus particles.
- The lesions tend to spread distally from the trunk and are characteristically **asynchronous** (i.e., multiple lesions at different stages of infection).
- Infection is usually self-limited and resolves after a few weeks. In **adults,** primary infection can be much more severe and lead to **pneumonia** and **encephalitis.**

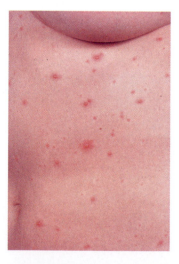

FIGURE 5-58. **Varicella-zoster virus (VZV) lesions characterized by multiple papules and vesicles on an erythematous base.** (Reproduced, with permission, from Wolff K, Johnson RA, Suurmond D. *Fitzpatrick Dermatology Atlas & Synopsis of Clinical Dermatology,* 5th ed. New York: McGraw-Hill, 2005: 819.)

- **Reactivation** of latent VZV (**herpes zoster** or **shingles**) can also occur under conditions of stress.
- Zoster is often characterized by extremely **painful** vesicular lesions in a **unilateral dermatomal** distribution (due to reactivation of latent VZV in a single sensory nerve). In **immunocompromised** patients, both primary and reactivated VZV infections are much more severe.
- Diagnosis of cutaneous lesions can be made by direct fluorescent antibody test (DFA), demonstration of multinucleate giant cells on a **Tzank** smear, or by the presence of intranuclear inclusion bodies on skin **biopsy.**

TREATMENT

Usually supportive. In severe cases, acyclovir can be given. In immunocompromised patients, anti-VZV Ig (VZIG) can be given intravenously. **Reye's syndrome** has often been associated with the use of aspirin to treat chickenpox in children. There are two **VZV vaccines**–one for children to prevent chickenpox and one for adults to prevent shingles. However, long-term efficacy has not been proven.

EPSTEIN-BARR VIRUS (EBV, INFECTIOUS MONONUCLEOSIS)

CHARACTERISTICS

Symptomatic infections typically affect teenagers and young adults.

PATHOGENESIS

Transmitted by saliva and respiratory secretions. EBV binds to CD21 on B cells. This selective transformation causes B cells to proliferate abnormally. The host's response to these infected B cells results in the clinical presentation.

CLINICAL SYMPTOMS

EBV can cause **infectious mononucleosis (kissing disease)**, which presents with **flulike** symptoms, profound **fatigue**, painful **pharyngitis, lymphadenopathy,** and **hepatosplenomegaly.** Patients are at risk for splenic rupture and should avoid contact sports. Infection is usually self-limited. In immunocompromised patients, sustained B-cell proliferation may result in mutations that predispose to future neoplasms (**Burkitt's lymphoma** and **nasopharyngeal cancers**).

DIAGNOSIS

- The presence of **atypical T lymphocytes** in the blood (these are the cytotoxic T cells responding to the infection, not the proliferating B cells).
- **Monospot test** detects **heterophile antibodies** in the blood.
- Heterophile antibodies are produced during an active EBV infection and are able to agglutinate animal RBCs.

TREATMENT

Supportive.

CYTOMEGALOVIRUS (CMV)

CHARACTERISTICS

Very common. Also can cause neonatal infection (one of the **ToRCHeS**).

PATHOGENESIS

Transmitted by close contact, body fluids, organ **transplantation,** and through the placenta. Infects many cell types.

CLINICAL SYMPTOMS

Most infections are **asymptomatic** and become **latent**.

- Primary infections in **adults** can be similar to infectious mononucleosis, but do not result in the production of heterophile antibodies (**heterophile negative mononucleosis**).
- In **newborns**, primary infection results in **cytomegalic inclusion disease**. Symptoms include microcephaly, hepatosplenomegaly, and CNS deficits.
- In **immunocompromised** patients, latent CMV can reactivate and cause severe infections such as retinitis, pneumonia, and esophagitis.
- **Diagnosis** can be made with a tissue biopsy, based on the visualization of large cells with characteristic purple intranuclear inclusion bodies surrounded by a halo (**owl's eye inclusion bodies**). See Figure 5-59.
- CMV infections are **monospot negative**.

TREATMENT

Ganciclovir (not acyclovir) and foscarnet (in the rare case of a ganciclovir resistant virus).

HUMAN HERPESVIRUSES 6 AND 7 (HHV-6, HHV-7, ROSEOLA)

CHARACTERISTICS

Affects infants or bone marrow transplant recipients (encephalitis).

PATHOGENESIS

Infects B and T cells.

CLINICAL SYMPTOMS

Roseola is characterized by a fever and a rash on the trunk.

TREATMENT

Foscarnet.

HUMAN HERPESVIRUS 8 (HHV-8, KSHV OR KAPOSI'S SARCOMA-ASSOCIATED HERPES VIRUS)

CHARACTERISTICS

Affects patients with **HIV**, especially men.

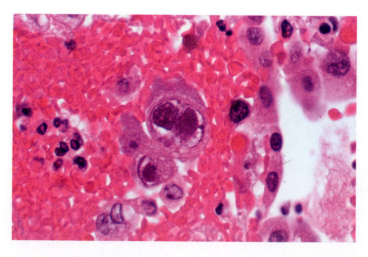

FIGURE 5-59.   Cytomegalovirus infection. Owl's eye inclusion bodies can be seen here in lung tissue. (Courtesy of PEIR Digital Library [http://peir.net].)

PATHOGENESIS

HHV-8 interacts with HIV to produce angioproliferative lesions.

CLINICAL SYMPTOMS

Kaposi's sarcomi (KS) lesions can affect any organ, but are often seen as raised violaceous skin nodules containing extravasated RBCs.

TREATMENT

Antiretroviral drugs can be effective by treating underlying HIV disease.

HEPADNAVIRUS (HEPATITIS B VIRUS, HBV)

CHARACTERISTICS

HBV has a complicated life cycle. After infecting host cells, the partial dsDNA genome is completed by viral DNA polymerase, thus becoming a fully double-stranded genome. Viral genes are then transcribed into mRNA. Viral mRNA is used both to make viral proteins **and** to regenerate the partially dsDNA viral genome through the action of a **viral reverse transcriptase.** Replicated genomic DNA and viral proteins are then repackaged into virion particles.

PATHOGENESIS

Transmitted through blood (**transfusions**), sexual contact, and the placenta (one of the **ToRCHeS**). Initial viremia leads to hepatocyte infection.

CLINICAL SYMPTOMS

Infection may be acute or chronic, depending on the host response. Infected hepatocytes can be killed by cytotoxic T cells; therefore, a robust immune response may result in a severe but acute course that ultimately clears the infection. A weaker immune response results a milder course, but the infection may not be cleared. Liver function tests are elevated in both cases. Acute infection is characterized by **jaundice** and **fever** (see Figure 5-60). Chronic infection may result in an asymptomatic **carrier** state. However, if a chronic inflammatory response is present, the host may develop **cirrhosis** and/or **hepa-**

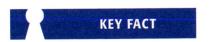

KEY FACT

HBV: **Partially** ds DNA, **circular,** enveloped, icosahedral

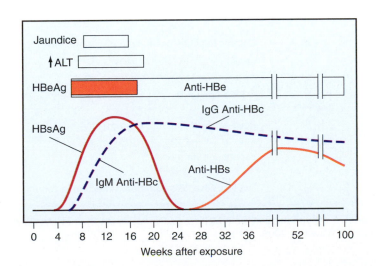

FIGURE 5-60. **Typical clinical and laboratory features of acute hepatitis B virus (HBV) infection.** (Modified, with permission, from Kasper DL, Braunwald E, Fauci AS, et al. *Harrison's Principles on Internal Medicine,* 16th ed. New York: McGraw-Hill, 2005: 1825.)

tocellular carcinoma. Different stages of infection can be diagnosed based on **serology** (see Table 5-30).

TREATMENT

INF-α, adefovir, tenofovir, lamivudine. There is also an HBV **vaccine** that contains HBsAg. Passive immunization with anti-HBsAg Ig can be used in some cases (needlesticks, and immediately after delivery of infants from infected mothers).

Poxvirus Family

Poxviruses are the **largest human viruses.** They are also the only viruses that **make their own envelope** and the only DNA viruses that replicate in the **cytoplasm.** Infected cells often have characteristic **cytoplasmic inclusion bodies** (in contrast to nuclear inclusion bodies in herpes virus infections).

SMALLPOX (VARIOLA)

PATHOGENESIS

Transmitted as aerosolized droplets.

CLINICAL SYMPTOMS

Smallpox (variola) is characterized by constitutional symptoms and a disseminated rash that is initially maculopapular, then forms vesicles, and later pustules (see Figure 5-61). The rash begins on the face and extremities and spreads to the trunk (centripetal). Systemic illness results in a 10%–30% mortality rate during the second week of symptoms.

TABLE 5-30. Serologic Patterns and Interpretation of HBV Infection

HBsAg	Anti-HBs	Anti-HBc	HBeAg	Anti-HBe	INTERPRETATION
+	–	IgM	+	–	Acute hepatitis B.
+	–	IgG[a]	+	–	Chronic hepatitis B with active viral replication.
+	–	IgG	–	+	Chronic hepatitis B with low viral replication.
+	+	IgG	+ or –	+ or –	Chronic hepatitis B with heterotypic anti-HBs (about 10% of cases).
–	–	IgM	+ or –	–	Acute hepatitis B.
–	+	IgG	–	+ or –	Recovery from hepatitis B (immunity).
–	+	–	–	–	Vaccination (immunity).
–	–	IgG	–	–	False-positive; less commonly infection in remote past.

[a]Low levels of IgM anti-HBc may also be detected. (Reprinted, with permission, from McPhee SJ, Papadakis MA, Tierney LM. *Current Medical Diagnosis & Treatment 2008,* 47th ed. New York: McGraw-Hill, 2008: 571.)

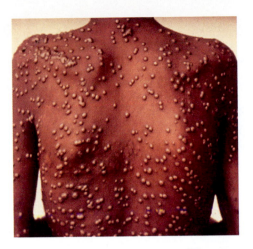

FIGURE 5-61. **Multiple pustules of smallpox can be seen on the back of this patient.** Note that all lesions are at the same stage of development. (Reproduced, with permission, from Wolff K, Johnson RA, Suurmond D. *Fitzpatrick Dermatology Atlas & Synopsis of Clinical Dermatology*, 5th ed. New York: McGraw-Hill, 2005: 771.)

TREATMENT

Supportive. The smallpox vaccine successfully eradicated smallpox infections in 1977. The vaccine contained an attenuated virus similar to smallpox (**vaccinia**) that served as the antigen.

MOLLUSCUM CONTAGIOSUM

PATHOGENESIS

Transmitted by close contact.

CLINICAL SYMPTOMS

Most often seen in children and immunocompromised patients and is characterized by benign **umbilicated** papules on the skin that are small and flesh-colored (see Figure 5-62). Infection is usually self-limited.

TREATMENT

None.

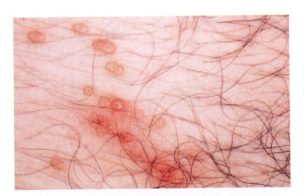

FIGURE 5-62. **Multiple umbilicated lesions, characteristic of molluscum contagiosum infection.** (Reproduced, with permission, from Kasper DL, Braunwald E, Fauci AS, et al. *Harrison's Principles on Internal Medicine*, 16th ed. New York: McGraw-Hill, 2005: 1053.)

POSITIVE (SINGLE)-STRANDED RNA VIRUSES—SS (+) RNA

GENERAL CHARACTERISTICS

All positive, single-stranded RNA viruses have an icosahedral capsid with the exception of the coronavirus, which has a helical capsid. RNA can either be enveloped or naked (exits host cells through budding or lysis, respectively; see Table 5-31). All replicate in the cytoplasm with an exception of HIV, which replicates in the nucleus (carries its own RNA-dependent DNA polymerase— reverse transcriptase—RT).

- RNA of ss-RNA viruses is polyadenylated at the 3' end, which makes it infectious itself.
- Removal of the poly A tail decreases the infectivity of the RNA.

Hepatitis E (Enteric Hepatitis)

CHARACTERISTICS

Unique 30-nm hepatitis virus. It does not appear to cause chronic infection and is serologically distinct from hepatitis A virus (HAV).

PATHOGENESIS

Transmitted enterically and can cause water-borne outbreaks (water contamination with fecal material).

CLINICAL SYMPTOMS

It resembles HAV in its incubation, course, and severity; typically causes mild hepatitis in healthy individuals. It is self-limited but can cause **fulminant hepatitis in pregnant women.**

TREATMENT

Supportive; no merit in administering INF-α. **Vaccine is in development.**

Polioviruses

Abortive poliomyelitis, paralytic poliomyelitis, postpolio syndrome

CHARACTERISTICS

Very small virus (20–30 nm), which usually causes a subclinical syndrome. It is important, however, because it can also cause paralysis, which is completely preventable.

PATHOGENESIS

The portal of entry is the mouth, and viral replication occurs in the gut. Active virus is excreted in the feces for several weeks.

CLINICAL SYMPTOMS

- Most common outcome is **abortive poliomyelitis,** which is a mild febrile syndrome.
- **Paralytic poliomyelitis** occurs in 1% of all cases. Paralysis results from viral damage to **anterior horn motor neurons.**
- Many years after resolution, some patients can develop **postpolio syndrome**, which causes further muscle atrophy.
- Diagnosis can be confirmed by serology, virus isolation or RT-PCR (reverse transcriptase-polymerase chain reaction), and DNA hybridization.

TABLE 5-31.   **Positive-Stranded RNA Viruses**

FAMILY	STRUCTURE	DISEASE	ROUTE OF TRANSMISSION	IMPORTANT FACTS
Caliciviridae				
Hepatitis E (HEV)	Naked, icosahedral, linear	Enteric hepatitis.	Fecal-oral.	Self-limiting disease.
Norwalk and Norovirus (Norwalk agent)	Naked, icosahedral, linear	Epidemic adult gastroenteritis.	Fecal-oral.	Vomiting more frequent than diarrhea.
Sapovirus	Naked, icosahedral, linear	Epidemic outbreaks of gastroenteritis.	Fecal-oral.	Associated with pediatric gastroenteritis.
Picornaviridae				
Polioviruses	Naked, icosahedral, nonsegmented	Paralysis.	Fecal-oral.	Immunization: Natural infection confers lifelong immunity.
Echoviruses	Naked, icosahedral, nonsegmented	Can cause mild or febrile illnesses, rashes, and aseptic meningitis.	Infection by viral invasion of nasopharyngeal mucosa.	*High incidence during summer-fall.
Enteroviruses	Naked, icosahedral, nonsegmented	Common cause of mild or febrile illness, aseptic meningitis. Enterovirus 70 can cause conjunctivitis.	Fecal-oral.	High incidence during summer-fall.
Rhinoviruses	Naked, icosahedral, nonsegmented	Number 1 cause of common cold.	Often spread by self-inoculation nose/throat.	Clinical diagnosis from symptoms.
Hepatitis A (HAV)	Naked, icosahedral, nonsegmented	Infectious hepatitis.	Fecal-oral.	Anti-HAV IgG: Indicates person had a previous infection.
Coxsackieviruses	Naked, icosahedral, nonsegmented	Group A viruses can cause herpangina, hand-foot-mouth disease, and pharyngitis. Group B viruses can cause myocarditis and pleurodynia.	Infection by viral invasion of nasopharyngeal mucosa.	High incidence during summer-fall.
Flaviviridae				
Hepatitis C (HCV)	Enveloped, icosahedral	Acute, usually subclinical hepatitis; ~80% chronic.	Parenteral; sexual.	Associated with hepatocellular carcinoma; cirrhosis.

(continues)

TABLE 5-31. **Positive-Stranded RNA Viruses** *(continued)*

FAMILY	STRUCTURE	DISEASE	ROUTE OF TRANSMISSION	IMPORTANT FACTS
Sr. Louis encephalitis	Enveloped, icosahedral	Most common encephalitis in elderly in the United States.	Mosquito vector	
West Nile virus	Enveloped, icosahedral	Fever, nausea, vomiting, and rash.	Mosquito vector	Peaks in summer.
Japanese encephalitis virus	Enveloped, icosahedral	Mild febrile illness, acute menigoencephalitis.	*Culex* mosquito	Reservoirs in pigs and birds.
Yellow fever virus	Enveloped, icosahedral	Chills, fever, black vomit, headaches.	*Aedes* mosquito	If liver affected, patients have jaundice.
Dengue fever	Enveloped, icosahedral	Mild fever, headache, bone aches, hemorrhagic fever.	*Aedes* mosquito	Biggest arbovirus problem.
Togaviridae				
Rubella	Enveloped, icosahedral, linear	Maculopapular rash, fever, conjunctivitis, sore throat.	Respiratory droplets	Congenital rubella syndrome prevented if mother is vaccinated.
Western equine **encephalitis** virus	Enveloped, icosahedral, linear	Flulike illness, encephalitis.	Mosquito vector	Can travel through placenta to fetus.
Venezuelan equine **encephalitis** virus	Enveloped, icosahedral, linear	Flulike illness, encephalitis.	Mosquito vector	Neurologic symptoms in 0.05% of adults and 4% of children.
Eastern equine **encephalitis** virus	Enveloped, icosahedral, linear	Flulike illness, encephalitis.	Mosquito vector	Neurologic symptoms in 1:23 cases.
Coronaviridae				
Coronaviruses	Enveloped, helical, nonsegmented	Second leading cause of common cold. Implicated in infant gastroenteritis.	Aerosols and respiratory droplets	Human disease caused by 229E and OC43 strains.
Astroviridae				
Astroviruses	Naked, icosahedral, linear	Endemic gastroenteritis in neonates and young kids.	Fecal-oral	Outbreaks similar to rotavirus; peaks in winter in temperate climates and during rainy season in tropics.

(continues)

TABLE 5-31.   Positive-Stranded RNA Viruses *(continued)*

FAMILY	STRUCTURE	DISEASE	ROUTE OF TRANSMISSION	IMPORTANT FACTS
Retroviridae				
Human immunodeficiency virus (HIV)	Enveloped, icosahedral, linear; *diploid* ss(+) RNA RNA-dependent DNA polymerase	Primary infection: Mono-like syndrome. As disease progresses, virus infects and kills more CD4+ T cells; without these cells both humoral and cell-mediated arms of the immune system are weakened. (CDC criteria).	Vertical, perinatal via breast milk, sex, blood transfusions, and needles.	Common opportunistic infections. At risk for thrush when CD4+ T cells < 400. At risk for *Pseudomonas carinii* pneumonia when CD4+ T cells < 200. At <100, risk of cytomegalovirus, *Mycobacterium avium* complex, and toxoplasmosis.
Human T-cell lymphotrophic virus type I (HTLV-I)	Enveloped, icosahedral, linear	Causes adult T-cell leukemia and tropical spastic paraparesis (TSP).	Vertical, perinatal via breast milk, sex, blood transfusions, and needles.	TSP/HTLV-1–associated myelopathy: Demyelination of the spinal cord pyramidal tract. Rapid onset.

TREATMENT

Supportive care.

- Prevention: Two types of vaccines are available: Killed (**Salk; IPV**) and live attenuated (**Sabin; OPV**) vaccinations.
    - The IPV is given to immunocompromised patients.
    - There are three serotypes of poliovirus in OPV. This vaccine has also been known to cause **vaccine-associated paralytic poliomyelitis (VAPP)** as a result of reversion to wild-type virus.

Hepatitis A (HAV)

Enteric hepatitis; short incubation hepatitis.

CHARACTERISTICS

Positive sense, single-stranded RNA virus of 27 nm associated with poor sanitation. Common childhood infection in developing countries.

PATHOGENESIS

Acquired by **fecal-oral route**.

- Incubation is between 2 and 6 weeks, with shedding of virus occurring during late incubation period and the prodrome.
- The virus is shed in stool and thus can be contracted through exposure to contaminated water, food, and shellfish.
- The **highest prevalence** is in densely populated areas and developing countries.

KEY FACT

Young children receive **four doses of Salk (IPV) vaccine. Sabin (OPV) is no longer available in the United States.**

KEY FACT

Hepatitis A: ssRNA, linear, naked, icosahedral

CLINICAL SYMPTOMS

Often asymptomatic and anicteric; experienced as flulike illness. Presentation is often with jaundice and GI disturbances (watery diarrhea is most common). Fulminant hepatitis or carrier states are rare. The infection is usually self-limited and is **not** associated with chronic hepatitis or hepatocellular carcinoma. Diagnosis can be confirmed with ELISA tests for HAV antigen and antibody.

TREATMENT

Supportive care. Prevention involves hand washing.

- **Vaccine.** HAV vaccine is given to all patients with chronic liver disease (especially hepatitis C), travelers to high-risk countries, those with high-risk behavior, and those from high-risk communities. Anti-HAV antibody is 90% effective if given within 2 weeks of exposure.

Coxsackieviruses

Herpangina, hand-foot-and-mouth disease.

CHARACTERISTICS

This small 20- to 30-nm virus is the most common cause of meningitis (far more than all bacterial forms). It is highly contagious and presents with rash.

PATOGENESIS

Fecal-oral transmission.

CLINICAL SYMPTOMS

- **Group A** coxsackievirus is responsible for **herpangina** (see Figure 5-63), hand-foot-and-mouth disease, and acute hemorrhagic conjunctivitis (enterovirus 70 in particular).
- **Group B** coxsackievirus is responsible for mild or fatal encephalitis in infants, cardiomyopathy (acute myocarditis and pericarditis), aseptic meningitis, and pleurodynia.

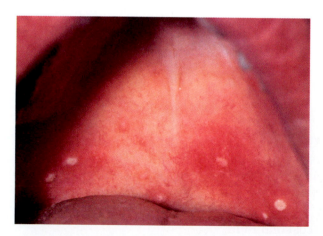

FIGURE 5-63. **Infectious enanthem: Herpangina.** Multiple, small vesicles and erosions with erythematous halos on the soft palate. (Reproduced, with permission, from Wolff K, Johnson RA, Suurmond D. *Fitzpatrick's Color Atlas & Synopsis of Clinical Dermatology,* 5th ed. New York: McGraw-Hill, 2005: 784.)

TREATMENT

Supportive care.

Hepatitis C (HCV, Infectious Hepatitis)

CHARACTERISTICS

The HCV genome is a 10-kB positive-sense RNA genome, with a 42-nm capsid. It is a major cause of non-A, non-B (NANB) hepatitis worldwide.

PATHOGENICITY

Mainly acquired through IV drug use or blood products. It can also be transmitted perinatally or sexually.

CLINICAL SYMPTOMS

Presentation is similar to that of hepatitis B, but less severe. Persistent infections may progress to chronic active hepatitis, cirrhosis, and hepatocellular carcinoma. Enzyme immunoassay (EIA) detects the antibodies to HAV, which indicate acute or chronic infection. RT-PCR and bDNA assays are also used to determine the viral load.

TREATMENT

Supportive care and INF-α (or pegylated-α) + ribavirin.

Rubella (German Measles)

CHARACTERISTICS

This togavirus can persist in humans for years with no detectable signs or symptoms. Rubella virus readily crosses the placenta and is highly teratogenic, causing deafness, blindness, and/or heart or brain defects in fetuses of mothers infected in the first trimester.

PATHOGENESIS

Spreads primarily through aerosolized particles. The mucosa of the upper respiratory tract is the portal of viral entry and initial site of virus replication.

CLINICAL SYMPTOMS

Clinically apparent rubella is characterized by a maculopapular rash, lymphadenopathy, low-grade fever, conjunctivitis, sore throat, and arthralgias.

TREATMENT

Supportive care.

PREVENTION

Live vaccine is available and confers long-term immunity to rubella. However, **the vaccine is not given to pregnant women.**

Human Immunodeficiency Virus (HIV)

CHARACTERISTICS

The genome consists of two identical subunits of (ss) RNA (**diploid linear**), surrounded by a conical truncated capsid (see Figure 5-64). These compo-

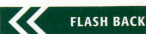

FLASH BACK

Cowdry type A inclusions in HSV lesions help to differentiate between HSV lesions and herpangina

KEY FACT

Hepatitis C: ssRNA, linear, enveloped, icosahedral.

KEY FACT

Most hepatitis C viral infections develop into chronic hepatitis.

KEY FACT

Rubella: ssDNA, linear, enveloped, icosahedral.

KEY FACT

Human immunodeficiency virus (HIV): Positive (ss) RNA, **diploid linear,** enveloped, icosahedral.

KEY FACT

The core nucleocapsid proteins (p6, p7, and p9) are associated with the genomic RNA, thus preventing its digestion by nucleases**.**

Structural genes:
- *Gag*—group-specific antigen; encodes p24; p6, p7, and p9; p17.
- *Pol*—encodes RT; integrase; protease.
- *Env*— encodes gp120; gp41.

Regulatory genes:
- *Tat*—encodes transactivator proteins.
- *Rev*—encodes regulatory virion proteins.
- *Nef*—encodes negative factor.

Major **risk factors** for contracting HIV:
- Unprotected sexual intercourse.
- Sharing contaminated needles.
- Birth from an infected mother.
- In underdeveloped countries, blood products and transfusions still pose major risk factors.

gp 24 and gp 120 are primary target antigens for early detection.

CD4+ T-lymphocyte categories
- Category 1: ≥ 500 cells/mcL
- Category 2: 200–499 cells/mcL
- Category 3: < 200 cells/mcL

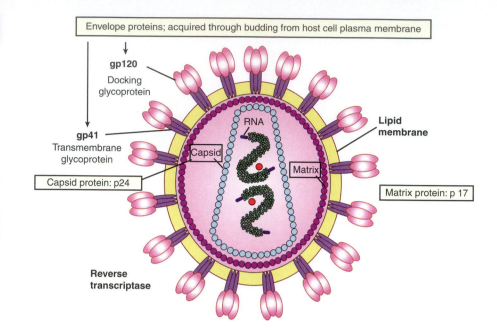

Envelope proteins; acquired through budding from host cell plasma membrane

gp120
Docking glycoprotein

gp41
Transmembrane glycoprotein

Capsid protein: p24

RNA

Capsid

Matrix

Lipid membrane

Matrix protein: p 17

Reverse transcriptase

FIGURE 5-64. **Diagram of the HIV virus.**

nents are surrounded by a plasma membrane of host-cell origin, formed when the capsid buds from the host cell.

- (ss) RNA: Tightly bound to the nucleocapsid proteins and enzymes, such as reverse transcriptase (**RT**), **integrase**, and **protease**.
- The main **matrix protein (p17)** surrounds the capsid (**p24–capsid protein**) and maintains the integrity of the virion particle.
- The **envelope** includes glycoproteins **gp120** and **gp41**.

The HIV genome is very complex and includes several major genes coding for **structural proteins** (expressed in all retroviruses), and several **regulatory genes,** unique to HIV.

PATHOGENESIS

Transmission of HIV may occur secondary to sexual contact (semen, vaginal secretions), blood transfusions, IV drug use, and contact with other infected bodily fluids (plasma, CSF). HIV can also be transmitted through the placenta (intrauterine transmission), perinatally, and through breast milk.

HIV primarily infects macrophages and CD4+ T cells. Macrophages are thought to play a key role in primary HIV-1 infection. Infection of and replication in monocytes/macrophages results in the spread of HIV to other tissues.

- Viral entry to **CD4+ T cells** and macrophages is **initiated** through **interaction** of the envelope glycoproteins (**gp120**) with **CD4** molecules of target cells.
- Fusion with target cells is further facilitated through their own chemokine receptors (**CCR5** or **CXCR4**)

HIV invades CD4+ T cells, impairing both the humoral and cell-mediated arms of the immune system (see Figure 5-65).

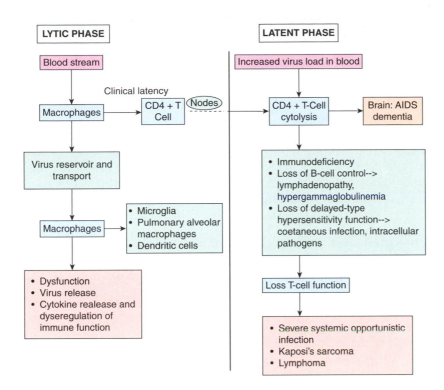

FIGURE 5-65. **HIV/AIDS cycle and evasion.**

PRESENTATION

The hallmarks of initial infection with HIV are an abrupt drop in the CD4+ T-cell count and rapid viral replication (increased **viral load**). Typical course of an HIV-infected individual is as follows (see Figure 5-66):

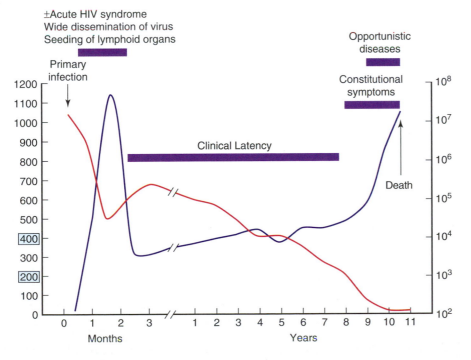

FIGURE 5-66. **Typical course of an HIV-infected individual.** Red line = CD4+ T lymphocyte count (cells/mm³); blue line = HIV RNA copies per mL plasma.

KEY FACT

Although 40%–70% of infected patients experience symptoms in the acute stage, the symptoms are rather nonspecific; most HIV cases are not detected at this time.

KEY FACT

Clinical latency is an extremely variable stage, which can last from a few weeks to over 20 years, depending on the patient.

KEY FACT

Mutations in **CCR5** can lead either to immunity (homozygous) or to slower progression to AIDS (heterozygous).
Mutations in **CXCR4** lead to rapid progression to AIDS.

CLINICAL CORRELATION

HIV-positive patients are said to be at risk for developing **candidiasis** (thrush) and **tuberculosis** once their **CD4+** T-cell count drops **below 400.**

KEY FACT

CD4+ T-cell count below 200: Patients are at increased risk for developing *Pneumocystic jiroveci* pneumonia (formerly referred to as *Pneumocystic carinii* pneumonia [PCP]).

CD4+ T-cell count below 100: Severe CMV infections, which can result in blindness from retinitis, and *Mycobacterium avium* complex infections.

- **Primary infection; acute HIV syndrome (CDC category A):** Patients may experience mononucleosis-like syndrome, which usually occurs 4–8 weeks after initial infection. Major symptoms include, but are not limited to, **fever, generalized lymphadenopathy, headache, myalgia,** and **pharyngitis.**
- **Clinical latency stage:** CD4+ T-cell count rebounds, and most symptoms of the acute infection subside. However, lymphadenopathy can be present throughout the entire course of an HIV infection.
- **Disease progression:** Dictated by the number of viable CD4+ T cells. As they decline over time, patients have an increased risk of acquiring common and not so common infections **(CDC category B).**
  - **Constitutional symptoms:** Moderate, unexplained weight loss, fever (38.5°C lasting more than 1month), chronic diarrhea.
  - **Infectious conditions:** Oropharyngeal and persistent vulvovaginal candidiasis, herpes zoster (shingles), frequent respiratory infections, pelvic inflammatory disease.
  - **Precancer/cancer lesions:** Most common are oral hairy leukoplakia and cervical dysplasia/cervical carcinoma in situ.
  - **Other:** Peripheral neuropathy may develop.
- **Later stages (AIDS):** Broad spectrum of clinical entities (AIDS-defining conditions; depicted in Table 5-32), as defined under CDC category C. Patients may also suffer **neurologic complications** (HIV/AIDS encephalopathy and AIDS dementia).
- Complications of these severe systemic opportunistic infections may result in death.

DIAGNOSIS

Involves initial screening and follow-up detection methods:

- **ELISA** tests for initial screening: Target HIV antigens **p24, p17, gp120,** and **gp41.**

TABLE 5-32.   AIDS-Defining Conditions—CDC Category C

FUNGAL INFECTIONS	CARCINOMAS	VIRAL INFECTIONS	PARASITIC INFECTIONS	BACTERIAL INFECTIONS
Candidiasis of oral cavity, esophagus, trachea, bronchi, or lungs.	Invasive cervical carcinoma	Cytomegalovirus retinitis or disease.	Cryptosporidiosis	*Mycobacterium tuberculosis*
Coccidioidomycosis, disseminated or extrapulmonary.	Kaposi's sarcoma	Herpes simplex: Chronic ulcers, bronchitis, pneumonitis, or esophagitis.	Isosporiasis	*Mycobacterium avium* complex
Cryptococcosis (extrapulmonary).	Burkitt's lymphoma	Progressive multifocal leukoencephalopathy.	Toxoplasmosis of the brain	Recurrent *Salmonella* septicemia
Histoplasmosis, disseminated or extrapulmonary[a].	Immunoblastic lymphoma	Wasting syndrome (due to HIV).		
Pneumocystis carinii pneumonia.	Primary CNS lymphoma			

[a]1993 Revised classification system for HIV infection and expanded surveillance case definition for AIDS among adolescents and adults. MMWR 992;41(Dec. 18):RR-17.

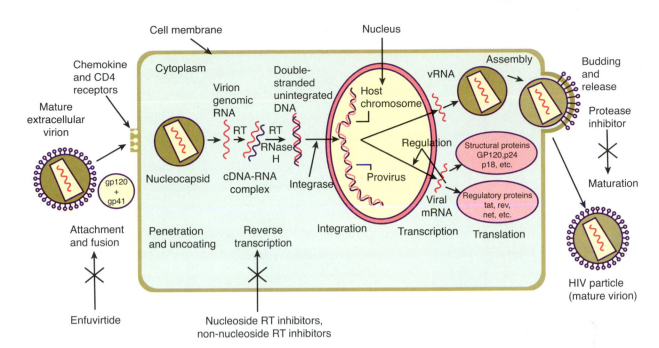

FIGURE 5-67. **Replicative cycle of HIV-1 showing the sites of action of available antiretroviral agents.** Available antiretroviral agents are shown in blue; cDNA, complementary DNA; gp120 + gp41, extracellular and intracellular domains, respectively, of envelope glycoprotein; mRNA, messenger RNA; RNase H, ribonuclease H; RT, reverse transcriptase. (Modified, with permission, from Brunton LL, Parker KL, Buxton ILO, Blumenthal DK. *Goodman & Gilman's The Pharmacological Basis of Therapeutics*, 11th ed. New York: McGraw-Hill, 2006: 1274.)

- **Western blot:** Warranted if ELISA test yields positive results. HIV infection is confirmed if antibodies to **at least two HIV antigens are positive.**
- **HIV DNA–PCR:** To determine viral load and monitor the effects of the treatment. Also used to screen for HIV infection in newborns of HIV-positive mothers
- **CD4+ T-cell count:** Assess treatment progress.

TREATMENT

Patients are usually placed on highly active antiretroviral therapy (**HAART**).

- HAART includes at least two reverse transcriptase inhibitors combined with a protease inhibitor (see Figure 5-67).
- Pregnant women are prescribed zidovudine (AZT), which has been shown to prevent perinatal transmission of the virus.

PROGNOSIS

There is no cure for AIDS. All patients with HIV/AIDS eventually die from complications of the disease or from opportunistic infections.

NEGATIVE (SINGLE)-STRANDED RNA VIRUSES–SS (-) RNA

GENERAL CHARACTERISTICS

Negative, single-stranded RNA viruses have the largest variety in structure (see Table 5-33). All are enveloped and replicate in the host cell cytoplasm with the exception of ortomyxoviruses, which replicates in both nucleus and cytoplasm, and influenza, which replicates in the nucleus. They all carry their own virion-associated polymerase. The capsid shape varies from icosahedral to helical. There are also linear, circular, segmented, and nonsegmented genomes among the negative single-stranded RNA viruses.

> **KEY FACT**
>
> Antigen **p24** is detectable shortly after initial infection, so it is often used as an **early sign of HIV infection.**

> **KEY FACT**
>
> Definitive diagnosis of HIV infection can be made only when there are antibodies to at least two viral antigens, as confirmed by Western blot analysis.

> **MNEMONIC**
>
> *For the negative-sense RNA viruses, think **P**airing **R**ats **Fi**ght **O**ver **Bun**ny's **Are**a:*
>
> **Pa**ramyxoviridae
> **R**habdoviridae
> **Fi**loviridae
> **O**rthomyxoviridae
> **Bun**yaviridae
> **Are**naviridae
> And remember, fighting is a **negative** thing to do!

TABLE 5-33. **Negative-Stranded RNA Viruses**

FAMILY	STRUCTURE	DISEASE	ROUTE OF TRANSMISSION	IMPORTANT FACTS
Paramyxoviridae				
Parainfluenza	Enveloped, helical, linear.	Croup, bronchiolitis, pneumonia.	Aerosol/airborne.	Self-limiting disease.
Measles	Enveloped, helical, linear.	Cough, coryza, conjunctivitis, rash.	Aerosol/airborne.	Symptoms due to immune response.
Mumps	Enveloped, helical, linear.	Aseptic meningitis, meningoencephalitis, parotitis, unilateral nerve deafness, orchitis.	Aerosol/airborne.	Infection confers lifelong immunity.
Respiratory syncytial virus	Enveloped, helical, linear.	Bronchiolitis, pneumonia.	Aerosol/airborne.	Can be deadly to infants.
Rhabdoviridae				
Rabies	Enveloped, bullet/helical, linear.	Fever, nausea, hydrophobia, delirium, paralysis, and coma.	Animal bite.	Evidence of infection, including symptoms and the detection of antibody; does not occur until too late for intervention.
Filoviridae				
Ebola virus	Enveloped, helical, linear.	Viral hemorrhagic fevers, flulike symptoms, death in ~90%.	Contact with body fluids.	Most deadly hemorrhagic fevers.
Marburg virus	Enveloped, helical, linear.	Viral hemorrhagic fevers, flulike symptoms, death in ~90%.	Contact with body fluids.	Most deadly hemorrhagic fevers.
Orthomyxoviridae				
Influenza	Enveloped, helical, segmented (8 segments).	Fever, arthalgias, malaise.	Aerosol/airborne.	Undergoes antigenic shift and antigenic drift.
Bunyaviridae				
Hantavirus	Enveloped, helical, linear→circular, segments.	Hantavirus disease (HVD), HV pulmonary syndrome (HPS).	Inhale rodent feces.	Treat with ribavirin.

(continues)

TABLE 5-33. Negative-Stranded RNA Viruses *(continued)*

FAMILY	STRUCTURE	DISEASE	ROUTE OF TRANSMISSION	IMPORTANT FACTS
Rift Valley fever virus	Enveloped, helical, linear→circular, segments.	Acute febrile illness (saddle-back fever), myalgias, low back pain, headache, anorexia, retroorbital pain.	Tick borne	Military—important.
La Crosse virus	Enveloped, helical, linear→circular, segments.	Viral encephalitis.	Mosquito vector	Most important cause of insect encephalitis in the Midwest.
Arenaviridae	Ambi-sense			
Lymphocytic choriomeningitis virus (LCMV)	Enveloped, helical, circular, segmented.	Aseptic meningitis orencephalitis; often asymptomatic to mild febrile illness most common.	Rat	No human–human transmission except mother to fetus.
Lassa fever	Enveloped, helical, circular, segmented.	Fever, retrosternal pain, sore throat, back/abdominal pain, cough, vomit, diarrhea, conjunctivitis, *facial swelling*, proteinuria, mucosal bleeding.	Rat	High death rates in pregnant women in 3rd trimester and fetuses (~95% mortality rate). *Complications:* Most common is deafness in ~1/3 of cases.

PARAMYXOVIRIDAE

GENERAL CHARACTERISTICS

Large, enveloped, ss (-) RNA, nonsegmented.

Major cause of diseases of upper respiratory tract (URT), lower respiratory tract (LRT; parainfluenza and RSV), and systemic diseases (measles, mumps). Paramyxoviruses are the most important causes of respiratory infections in infants and young children (under five years). Typical virus organization is depicted in Figure 5-68.

- Major structural proteins are **M** matrix protein, **NP** nucleocapsid protein, and **L** and **P** phosphorylated protein; the latter dictates viral RNA polymerase activity.
- Major virulence factors are larger glycoproteins:
  - **Attachment** to host cell via **hemagglutinin** and **neuraminidase** activity: **HN, H** only in measles (no N). **G** only in RSV (no HN). They enable attachment to sialic acid receptors of host cells.
  - **Membrane fusion** and hemolysin activities are carried out by **F**, fusion glycoprotein. It exists as inactive **F0,** which is cleaved to the active **F1** form by cellular proteases. Also responsible for large syncytia formation in cells infected with paramyxoviruses.

KEY FACT

Viral envelopes can fuse with cell membranes only at **neutral** or **alkaline pH.**

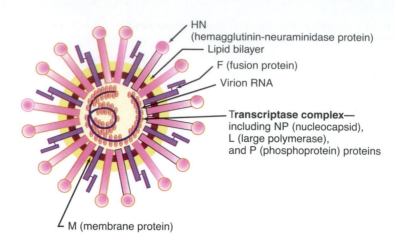

FIGURE 5-68. **Schematic diagram of a paramyxovirus showing major components (not drawn to scale).** The lipid bilayer is shown as the gray concentric circle; underlying the lipid bilayer is the viral matrix protein (*black concentric circle*). Inserted through the viral membrane are the hemagglutinin-neuraminidase (HN) attachment glycoprotein and the fusion (F) glycoprotein. (Not all paramyxoviruses possess hemagglutinin and neuraminidase activities; those glycoproteins are designated H or G.) Inside the virus is the negative-strand virion RNA, which is encased in the nucleocapsid protein (N/NP). Associated with the nucleocapsid are the L and P proteins, and together this complex has RNA-dependent RNA transcriptase activity. (Modified, with permission, from Brooks GF, Carroll KC, Butel JS, Morse SA. *Jawetz, Melnick, & Adelberg's Medical Microbiology*; 24th ed. New York: McGraw-Hill, 2007: 549.)

Parainfluenza

CHARACTERISTICS

Primarily affects young children (3–8 years of age), manifesting through upper (**common cold**) and lower respiratory tract infections. Parainfluenza viruses (PIVs) are also a common cause of community-acquired respiratory tract infections in adults. Reinfection with PIV can occur throughout life, with elderly and immunocompromised persons being at a greater risk of serious complications of infections.

PATHOGENESIS

Disease is airborne, and virus invades the mucosa of the upper respiratory tract. It may progress to the lower segments and does not disseminate.

CLINICAL SYMPTOMS

Clinical manifestations include:

- **Common cold:** Upper respiratory infection, may last 2–3 days to 1 week. Disease has an acute onset and subsides after 7–10 days if uncomplicated.
  - **Symptoms** include runny nose, nasal congestion, and sneezing. In addition, sore throat, cough, and headache are not uncommon. Adults and older children with colds generally have minimal to no fever. Young children, however, may have fever of 38° to 39°C.
- **Croup:** Affects the larynx, trachea, and bronchi (laryngotracheobronchitis). Mild cold usually persists for several days before the barking cough becomes evident.
  - **Symptoms** include fever, hoarse barking cough, laryngeal obstruction, and inspiratory stridor.

KEY FACT

Parainfluenza: ssRNA, linear, enveloped, helical.

KEY FACT

- **PIV-1 =** croup in children ages 6 months to 5 years; prevalent in autumn.
- **PIV-3 =** second only to respiratory syncytial virus (RSV) as a cause of **pneumonia** and **bronchiolitis** in infants (under 6 months)

CLINICAL CORRELATION

Most common conditions associated with PIVs:
- Common cold with fever.
- Croup.
- Bronchiolitis and pneumonia.

- **Bronchiolitis:** Begins as a mild upper respiratory infection that, over a period of 2–3 days, can develop into increasing respiratory distress with wheezing and a **tight, wheezy cough.** The peak incidence of bronchiolitis is during the first year of life, it dramatically declines until it virtually disappears by school age.
  - **Signs and symptoms** include fever, expiratory wheezing, tachypnea, retractions, rales, and air trapping.
- **Pneumonia** is usually a complication of parainfluenza virus, is prevalent in infants, very young children, elderly, and immunocompromised patients. It is associated with all viral subtypes:
  - **Signs and symptoms** include fever, rales, and evidence of pulmonary consolidation.

In addition, **PIVs routinely cause** otitis media, pharyngitis, and conjunctivitis coryza, occurring separately or in combination with a lower respiratory infection.

TREATMENT

Mainly supportive. Antivirals and antibiotics as needed. No vaccine available.

- **Ribavirin** aerosol or systemic therapy has been used to treat PIV infections in children and adults who are severely immunocompromised. Broader use at this time is of uncertain clinical benefit.
- **Antibiotics** are used only when bacterial complications (e.g., otitis, sinusitis) develop.
- **Corticosteroids** and **nebulizers** are used to treat respiratory symptoms and to help reduce the inflammation and airway edema of croup.

Respiratory Syncytial Virus (RSV)

CHARACTERISTICS

Acute viral infection with short incubation period and recovery occurring within 7–12 days. RSV is the most important cause of lower respiratory tract disease in young children. It infects almost all infants by the age of 2.

PATHOGENESIS

Disease is airborne, transmitted via aerosols. The virus invades the mucosa of the upper respiratory tract and replicates only within respiratory epithelium. RSV does not have HN or NA attachment proteins; only F (fusion) glycoprotein.

CLINICAL SYMPTOMS

In most infants, the virus causes **symptoms resembling** those of the **common cold.** In infants born prematurely and/or with chronic disease, RSV can cause a severe or even life-threatening disease.

- **Signs and symptoms** include low-grade fever, cough, tachypnea, cyanosis, retractions, wheezing, and rales.
- Most common **complications** are ear infections. Less common, but serious complications include pneumonia (0.5%–1%) and respiratory failure (2%).

KEY FACT

PIV-1 infection has been associated with secondary bacterial pneumonias in elderly persons.

KEY FACT

Because of its high potency and prolonged intramuscular half-life, dexamethasone is the preferred anti-inflammatory drug for croup.

KEY FACT

RSV: ssRNA, linear, enveloped, helical.

TREATMENT

Mostly supportive with airway management (most important). **Ribaviran** is a nucleoside analog and is the only antiviral approved for use. However, it is not used routinely. Its main use is in infants at serious risk for lower respiratory tract infections.

- **Prevention. Synagis (palivizumab)**, monoclonal anti-F-reactive antibody, is indicated for the **prevention** of serious lower respiratory tract disease caused by RSV in pediatric patients and prematurely born infants (at less than 32 weeks' gestation).
- **No vaccine available.** Strict hygiene and no contact with diseased individuals are imperative.

Measles (Rubeola)

CHARACTERISTICS

Highly infectious **childhood febrile exanthema.** Has long incubation period of about 2 weeks followed by a classic viral prodrome and virus-specific immune response. Complete recovery ensues 7–10 days after onset of measles rash. The clearance of virus coincides approximately with fading of the rash.

PATHOGENESIS

Disease is airborne, transmitted by aerosolized particles. It infects the respiratory tract and replicates locally in the respiratory epithelium before spreading to regional lymphatic tissue (further replication). Ultimately, viremia develops and the virus disseminates throughout the body.

CLINICAL SYMPTOMS

Clinical picture develops in relation to above-described pathogenic characteristics (see Figure 5-69):

- **Classic viral prodrome** occurs following the incubation period. It is commonly referred to as the **3 C's: Cough, Coryza, and Conjunctivitis** with photophobia.
  - Pathognomonic **Koplik's spots** typically arise on the buccal, gingival, and labial mucosae within 2–3 days of initial symptoms. The Koplik's spots are 1- to 2-mm blue-gray macules on an erythematous base (see Figure 5-70).
  - **Giant cell pneumonia**, characterized by **Warthin-Finkeldey cells** (multinucleated giant cells with eosinophilic nuclear and cytoplasmic inclusion bodies) found in the lungs and sputum.
  - Additional **prodromal symptoms** may include fever, malaise, myalgias, photophobia, and periorbital edema.
- **Virus-specific immune response** is characterized by the appearance of the **rash.** Measles rash is a **maculopapular erythematous.**
  - Typically begins at the hairline and spreads caudally over the next 3 days as the prodromal symptoms resolve.
  - Lasts 4–6 days and then fades from the head downward. Lesion density is greatest above the shoulders, where macular lesions may coalesce.
  - Desquamation may be present but is generally not severe.
- **Complete recovery** from measles generally occurs within 7–10 days from onset of the rash.

TREATMENT

Mainly supportive care; intravenous hydration, antipyretics. Secondary infections such as pneumonia and otitis media should be treated with antibiotics.

KEY FACT

Measles: ssRNA, linear, enveloped, helical.

CLINICAL CORRELATION

Patients with compromised cell-mediated immunity do not develop rash, but will develop measles giant cell pneumonia.

CLINICAL CORRELATION

Measles may also cause:
- Croup
- Pneumonia
- Diarrhea with protein-losing enteropathy
- Keratitis with scarring and blindness
- Encephalitis
- Hemorrhagic rashes (black measles) in malnourished children with poor medical care

---

FLASH BACK

Immunosuppression develops as a result of measles' viral hemagglutinin protein binding to CD46 and signaling lymphocytic activation molecule (SLAM).

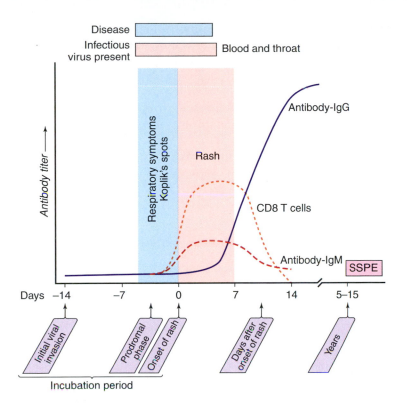

FIGURE 5-69. **Natural history of measles infection.** Viral replication begins in the respiratory epithelium and spreads to monocyte-macrophages, endothelial cells, and epithelial cells in the blood, spleen, lymph nodes, lung, thymus, liver, and skin and to the mucosal surfaces of the gastrointestinal, respiratory, and genitourinary tracts. The virus-specific immune response is detectable when the rash appears. Clearance of virus is approximately coincident with fading of the rash. SSPE, subacute sclerosing panencephalitis. (Modified, with permission, from Brooks GF, Carroll KC, Butel JS, Morse SA. *Jawetz, Melnick, & Adelberg's Medical Microbiology*; 24th ed. New York: McGraw-Hill, 2007: 559.)

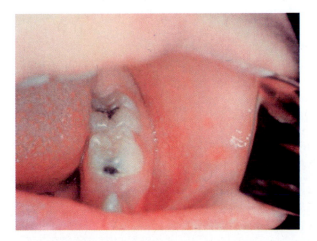

FIGURE 5-70. **Koplik's spots.** The spots manifest as white or bluish lesions with an erythematous halo on the buccal mucosa. They usually occur in the first 2 days of measles symptoms and may briefly overlap the measles exanthem. The presence of the erythematous halo differentiates Koplik's spots from Fordyce's spots (ectopic sebaceous glands), which occur in the mouths of healthy individuals. (Reproduced, with permission, from Kasper DL, Braunwald E, Fauci AS, et al. Harrison's Principles of Internal Medicine, 16th ed. New York: McGraw-Hill; 2005: 1148.)

- **Postexposure prophylaxis** with immune globulin may be given within 6 days of exposure to high-risk patients such as immunocompromised children and pregnant women.
- **Prevention.** There is one serotype worldwide; all cases are clinically apparent. The **MMR vaccine (3-in-1)** protects against measles, mumps, and rubella and consists of live attenuated virus. Infection produces lifelong immunity. Maternal antibody can protect newborns.
- **Complications:**
  - **Common:** Respiratory complications in up to 15% of cases.
  - **Uncommon and severe:** Postinfectious encephalomyelitis, subacute sclerosing panencephalopathy (SSPE), and bacterial super-infection due to immunosuppression.

Mumps

CHARACTERISTICS

A systemic infection usually affecting unvaccinated children between the ages 2 and 12, but can occur in other age groups. Mumps usually spreads from person to person by saliva droplets or by direct contact with contaminated articles.

PATHOGENESIS

The upper respiratory tract is the point of initial entry via the inhalation of respiratory droplets. The virus then spreads to draining lymph nodes and replicates in lymphocytes, after which it disseminates hematogenously to the salivary gland, as well as other glands.

- Long incubation period (an average of 16–18 days with a range of 12–29 days).
- No clinical indication of infection in ~one-third of infected individuals, however, they can still transmit the disease
- The **period of communicability** (transmissibility) is usually from nine days before onset of parotid edema to 1–2 days after onset of swelling and occasionally lasting as long as seven days after swelling.

CLINICAL SYMPTOMS

- **Parotid glands:** After initial presentation of fever, headache, and earache, the parotid gland enlarges and rapidly progresses to maximum size in 1–3 days, displacing the lobe of the ear, resulting in increased pain and tenderness. Symptoms rapidly subside after swelling reaches its peak. The parotid gland gradually decreases in size in 3–7 days.
- **Epididymo-orchitis** is the second most common manifestation of adult mumps. Symptoms include:
  - Acute onset of fever, chills, nausea, vomiting, and lower abdominal pain following parotitis.
  - After the acute syndrome, the testes begin to swell rapidly. As the fever decreases, the pain and edema subside. A loss of turgor demonstrates atrophy. The sequela of absolute sterility is rare; a few patients have impaired fertility.

TREATMENT

Supportive.

KEY FACT

Mumps: ssRNA, linear, enveloped, helical.

KEY FACT

Parotid glands are commonly, but not always, affected by mumps.

KEY FACT

Post-pubertal males who develop mumps have a 15%–20% risk of developing orchitis.

PREVENTION

There is only one serotype worldwide. Infection confers lifelong immunity (both humoral and cell-mediated immune response are induced). Infants are protected for approximately 6 months by maternal antibodies. The **MMR vaccine (3-in-1)** protects against measles, mumps, and rubella and consists of live attenuated virus.

COMPLICATIONS

Mumps infection can invade the epithelial cells of multiple organs, including the testes, ovaries, pancreas, meninges, kidneys, thyroid, bladder, and kidney.

- **Meningoencephalitis** is the most common complication in **children,** and results from a primary infection of the neurons and/or postinfection encephalitis with demyelination.
- **Aseptic meningitis** is usually indistinguishable from other causes. The mumps virus can be isolated in the CSF.
- **Unilateral deafness,** permanent or transient, is uncommon. However, mumps is the leading cause of deafness worldwide.
- **Pancreatitis** is a severe but fortunately rare manifestation.
  - **Elevated amylase** is seen, regardless of the presence of pancreatitis.
  - **Lipase** is a more specific indicator of pancreatic involvement and should be tested if this complication is suspected.

ORTHOMYXOVIRIDAE (INFLUENZA A, B, AND C VIRUSES)

GENERAL CHARACTERISTICS

Large, enveloped, ss (-) RNA, segmented. Unlike most RNA viruses, influenza **replicates** in the host cell's **nucleus.** However, it acquires its envelope from the host cell membrane through budding. It has nine structural and functional proteins (see Table 5-34). There are three known serotypes of influenza viruses: A, B, and C.

- Types A and B exhibit continual antigenic changes; type C appears to be antigenically stable.
- Influenza A has human and zoonotic hosts (aquatic birds, chickens, ducks, pigs, horses, and seals), whereas B and C types have human hosts only.

PATHOGENESIS

Influenza causes protracted illness with short incubation period (1–4 days) and exhibits both respiratory and systemic symptoms. It spreads by respiratory droplets or contact with contaminated surfaces and hands. It colonizes the respiratory epithelium and replicates locally. There is no viremia; systemic symptoms are ascribed to interferon and cytokines produced by the host. Antigenic variants of influenza virus are caused by **antigenic shift** and **antigenic drift** (see Figure 5-71). Influenza A is the only type prone to antigenic shift, which is the principal cause of flu epidemics.

CLINICAL SYMPTOMS

Major cause of local infections of respiratory tract with constitutional symptoms.

- Uncomplicated influenza typically presents with cough, sore throat, runny or stuffy nose, fever, muscle aches and pains, headache, and fatigue.
- Gastrointestinal symptoms such as nausea, vomiting, and diarrhea also can occur but are more common in children than in adults.

KEY FACT

Influenza: ss (-) RNA, **segmented** (eight segments), enveloped, helical.

KEY FACT

Influenza replicates in the nucleus; carries cell membrane-acquired envelope.

FLASH BACK

Antigenic drift: Gradual change in antigenicity due to point mutations that affect major antigenic sites on the glycoprotein.
Antigenic shift: Abrupt change due to genetic reassortment with an unrelated strain.

TABLE 5-34.   **Structural and Functional Proteins of Influenza Viruses**

ENCODED PROTEIN	FUNCTION
HA (hemagglutinin) **Envelope glycoprotein**	▪ Mediator of viral attachment to host cells ▪ Binds to sialic acid ▪ Fusion activity at acid pH ▪ Host range determinant ▪ Vaccine/drug target; 95% of outer spikes
NA (neuraminidase) **Envelope glycoprotein; enzyme**	▪ Cleaves sialic acid from HA–host cell complex; promotes virus release from cells ▪ Vaccine/drug target; 5% of outer spikes
M1 (matrix protein)	▪ Involved in viral assembly ▪ Binds RNP complex for export to cytoplasma
M2 (membrane protein) **Membrane protein; ion channel** **Present in the envelope**	▪ Essential for virus uncoating ▪ Lowers pH in viral particle; removes M1 from RNP complexa ▪ Drug target (amantadine/rimantadine)
NP (nucleocapsid protein)	▪ Forms nucleocapsid ▪ Protects viral RNA from degradation
NS (nonstructural protein, NS1/NS2) **NS2 present in the envelope**	Reduces interferon response?
PB2/PB1/PA	Polymerase components of RNP[a]

[a]Nucleoprotein (NP) associated with viral RNA forms RNP complex.

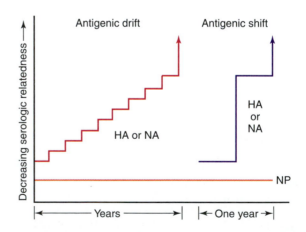

FIGURE 5-71.   **Antigenic drift and antigenic shift account for antigenic changes in the two surface glycoproteins (HA and NA) of influenza virus.** Changes in HA and NA occur independently. Internal proteins of the virus, such as the nucleoprotein (NP), do not undergo antigenic changes. (Modified, with permission, from Brooks GF, Carroll KC, Butel JS, Morse SA. *Jawetz, Melnick, & Adelberg's Medical Microbiology*, 24th ed. New York: McGraw-Hill, 2007: 537.)

TREATMENT

- **Amantadine** (24–48 hours after onset of symptoms) and **rimantidine** target the M2 ion channel responsible for the alteration of pH required for viral uncoating and assembly. Both are specific for **influenza A virus**.
- **Zanamivar (Relenza)** and **oseltamivir phosphate (Tamiflu)** are neuraminidase inhibitors for **both** influenza **A** and **B**.

VACCINE

Natural immunity toward **single** influenza **strain** is long lasting and is provided by IgA of the respiratory tract. The single best way to prevent the flu is the flu vaccine. There are two types of vaccines:

- Intramuscular **flu shot** is an inactivated vaccine. It contains three influenza strains (2A's and 1B), and is approved for use in individuals over 6 months, both healthy people and those with chronic medical conditions.
- The **nasal-spray** flu vaccine is a live, attenuated flu virus. It is approved for use in healthy people 5 years to 49 years of age who are not pregnant.

Antibodies develop within approximately 2 weeks following vaccination. Flu vaccines do not protect against flulike illnesses caused by noninfluenza viruses.

COMPLICATIONS

Rare, affects specific populations.

- **Pneumonia:** Young children, immunocompromised patients and elderly people in nursing homes are particularly susceptible. In some epidemics (depending on the viral strain), pregnant women are at high risk as well.
  - Can be primary influenza, bacterial, or a combination of the two. Infection with *staph aureus* is common.
- **Reye's syndrome.**
- **Interstitial myocarditis.**

Rhabdoviridae (Rabies)

CHARACTERISTICS

Simple bullet-shaped virus with enveloped virions; diameter of 50–95 nm.

PATHOGENESIS

The virus is secreted in the animal's saliva, and infection results from a bite of the rabid animal. Following local inoculation, the virus progresses to the peripheral nervous system and reaches the central nervous system by way of **retrograde axonal transport.** The incubation period may be 3 months or longer, hence, the rabies virus is considered a **slow virus.**

CLINICAL SYMPTOMS

The initial symptoms of rabies are fever, malaise, headache, pain or paresthesia at the bite site, GI symptoms, fatigue, and anorexia. After the initial "flulike" syndrome, the patient develops **hydrophobia,** seizures, disorientation, and hallucinations. The final symptoms are paralysis, which may lead to respiratory failure, and coma. Unfortunately, rabies cannot be diagnosed until it is too late to treat. **Negri bodies** in the affected neurons are the hallmark diagnostic finding.

KEY FACT

Immune response to first infection overrides the immune response to subsequent infections with different antigenic flu variants.

FLASH FORWARD

Reye's syndrome:
Hepatoencephalopathy resulting from the use of salicylates in children with upper respiratory infections, influenza A or B, or varicella.

KEY FACT

Rabies: ssRNA, negative sense, enveloped, bullet/helical, linear.

TREATMENT

Postexposure prophylaxis (PEP) is used to prevent overt clinical illness in an affected person. The wound is cleaned and the patient is administered human rabies immunoglobulin and the rabies vaccination, which is a killed-virus vaccine.

DOUBLE-STRANDED RNA VIRUSES

Double-stranded RNA viruses all lack an envelope and have an icosahedral capsid and segmented genome (see Table 5-35). The segmented genome allows for switching of various segments among viruses within the same family. This is called **antigenic shift.**

Rotavirus

CHARACTERISTICS

This double-stranded segmented RNA virus is a common agent of diarrhea in children. Human disease is caused by group A and, occasionally, group B and C rotaviruses.

PATHOGENESIS

The virus is spread via the fecal-oral route and possibly the respiratory route.

> **KEY FACT**
>
> Rotavirus: dsRNA, naked, icosahedral, segmented.

TABLE 5-35. Overview of Double-Stranded RNA Viruses

FAMILY	STRUCTURE	DISEASE	ROUTE OF TRANSMISSION	IMPORTANT FACTS
Reoviridae				
Reovirus	Naked, icosahedral, segmented	Causes mild, self-limiting infections of the upper respiratory or GI tracts.	Aerosol and fecal-oral.	Very stable and have been detected in sewage and river water.
Colorado tick fever virus	Naked, icosahedral, segmented	Causes serious hemorrhagic disease due to vascular endothelial infection. Symptoms of acute disease include fever and muscle/joint pain; can have subclinical cases.	Transmitted by wood tick *Dermacentor andersoni.*	Found in western and northwestern U.S., as well as West Canada.
Rotavirus	Naked, icosahedral, segmented	Diarrhea.	Fecal-oral.	Most common agent of infantile diarrhea worldwide.

CLINICAL SYMPTOMS

The major clinical findings are vomiting, diarrhea, fever, and dehydration. Because most patients have large quantities of virus in stool, the direct detection of viral antigen is the method of choice for diagnosis.

TREATMENT

Supportive care. The **Rota Teq (PRV) vaccine** is a pentavalent human–bovine reassortment and is currently recommended for infants in the United States. The previous version, Rotashield, was removed from the market after being linked to **intusseption in children.**

SLOW VIRUSES AND PRION DISEASES

Slow Viruses

Etiologically associated with diseases that exhibit slow and progressive course, spanning months to years. Many involve the central nervous system and ultimately lead to death. Medically important entities are described elsewhere in the text.

Prion Diseases

Prion diseases are a related group of rare, fatal brain diseases that affect animals and humans. These diseases were previously classified as slow virus diseases.

Prion diseases are also known as **transmissible spongiform encephalopathies (TSE)** and include bovine spongiform encephalopathy (BSE, or mad cow disease) in cattle, Creutzfeldt-Jakob disease (CJD) in humans, and scrapie in sheep (see Table 5-36).

TABLE 5-36.   Overview of Prion Diseases

FAMILY	STRUCTURE	DISEASE	ROUTE OF TRANSMISSION	IMPORTANT FACTS
Prion				
Animal Disease				
Scrapie	Proteinaceous infectious particle (PrP).	Sheep: Chronic, progressive fatal ataxia and pruritus.	Digesting prions	Name came from sheep scraping their hind legs.
Bovine spongiform encephalopathy	PrP	Mad cow disease.	Digesting prions	Attributed to feeding cows parts of sheep that have scrapie.
Human Disease				
Creutzfeldt-Jakob disease (CJD)	PrP	Spongiform encephalitis, usually sporadic.	Digesting prions	Dementia, with spongiform change in gray matter. Reactive astrocytosis, amyloid plaques.
Kuru	PrP	Spongiform encephalitis in cannibals.	Digesting prions	Ataxia and shivering with spongiform change in gray matter. Reactive astrocytosis, amyloid plaques.

PRION HYPOTHESIS

Prion is an abbreviation for proteinaceous infectious particle (PrP). According to early studies, the protein thought to be responsible for the TSEs did not differ in amino acid sequence from that of a normal protein expressed on cell membranes throughout the CNS. This led to the proposal that this protein exists in two alternative structural forms:

- The first (cellular type) form contains a large proportion of α-helix (approximately 40%) and only 3% β-pleated sheet and is termed PrPc.
- The second (pathogenic variation; PrPsc) form contains a much higher proportion of β-sheet and less α-helix. Based on this, it was proposed that:
  - PrP is an infectious agent (as a result of anucleation).
  - Abnormal-folded (β-sheets) PrP associate with normal-folded proteins, inducing normal-folding proteins to adopt β configuration (become pathogenic).
  - Sequence-folded protein into amyloid → produce more protein → further nucleation.

Microbiology: Systems

NORMAL FLORA

Although bacteria are commonly associated with infection, even healthy individuals are colonized by a variety of organisms, as described in Table 5-37.

TABLE 5-37. Location of Normal Flora and Potential Associated Pathogens

LOCATION	NORMAL FLORA	POTENTIAL PATHOGENS
Skin	*Staphylococcus epidermidis, Propionibacterium.*	*Staphylococcus aureus.*
Nasopharynx	Viridans streptococci (group D), *Neisseria.*	*Streptococcus pneumoniae.* *N. meningitides.* *H. influenzae.* Group A streptococci. *S. aureus* (found in anterior nares of 25%–30% of healthy people).
Mouth	Viridans streptococci.	*Candida albicans.*
Dentition		*S. mutans.*
Colon	*Bacteroides fragilis, Escherichia coli.*	*B. fragilis, E. coli, Pseudomonas, Clostridium.*
Vagina	*Lactobacillus acidophilus* May be colonized by *E. coli* and group B streptococci.	*Candida.*
Upper urinary tract and bladder	Normally sterile.	*E. coli.*

In fact, the average person's body contains 10 times more bacterial cells than human cells. This colonization begins when membrane rupture allows flora from the vagina and surrounding environment to migrate into the previously sterile fetus.

Beneficial Effects

By competing with pathogens, indigenous flora play an important role in providing **defense against infection.** Anaerobic bacteria in the intestines are a major source of **vitamin K,** help make **B vitamins,** and break down cellulose to aid digestion.

Role in Infection

Although usually harmless in their native environment, normal flora can cause infection if they migrate to otherwise sterile locations in the body or areas to which they are not indigenous. If the overall composition of the normal flora is altered, as by antibiotic use or immune deficiency, overgrowth of particular organisms can lead to disease.

Urinary tract infections in sexually active women are often caused by intestinal *E. coli* that spreads to the urinary bladder.

Endocarditis can occur when viridans streptococci enter the bloodstream following dental procedures and lodge on susceptible heart valves.

Peritonitis can occur when ruptured viscera from conditions such as appendicitis, diverticulitis, or a penetrating abdominal wound introduce fecal anaerobes like *B. fragilis* into the peritoneal cavity.

C. difficile **(pseudomembranous) colitis** develops when the composition of the normal flora of the gastrointestinal tract is altered by **antibiotic therapy.** This results in overgrowth of the opportunistic pathogen *C. difficile,* causing illness.

Candidiasis is a fungal infection, commonly caused by *Candida albicans.* Vaginal candidiasis is a common complication of antibiotic therapy in women. Oral candidiasis (thrush) may be an early sign of an immune deficiency, such as HIV/AIDS.

MICROBIAL DISEASES OF THE RESPIRATORY TRACT

Upper Respiratory Infections

Result from invasion of the oral and nasal cavities, sinuses, pharynx, and tonsils. Middle respiratory tract infections involve the larynx, epiglottis, and trachea. Viruses are the most common cause of upper respiratory tract infections. Bacteria may secondarily infect these tissues as a complication of a viral infection.

Dental caries are caused by *Streptococcus mutans.*

Periodontal disease is associated with anaerobic bacteria such as *Bacteroides, Actinomyces,* and *Prevotella.*

Rhinitis is most often caused by viruses such as **adenovirus,** rhinovirus, coxsackievirus A, echovirus, coronavirus, influenza, and respiratory syncytial virus (RSV).

KEY FACT

Vitamin K is essential for the production of clotting factors II, VII, IX, and X, as well as the anticoagulant proteins C and S.

CLINICAL CORRELATION

Patients who are immunocompromised for any reason (as from HIV/AIDS, diabetes, chemotherapy, or vitamin deficiencies) are more susceptible to infection by normal flora.

Sinusitis can be acute or chronic. Acute sinusitis is usually caused by *S. pneumoniae* or *H. influenzae*. Chronic sinusitis is more likely to involve anaerobic organisms.

Pharyngitis is most often caused by viruses such as adenovirus, rhinovirus, coronavirus, influenza, and Epstein-Barr virus. "Strep throat" is caused by *S. pyogenes* (group A). Key clinical manifestations of strep throat include a **sore erythematous throat, fever, tonsillar exudates, and tender cervical lymphadenopathy.** Patients typically have **no cough.** Treatment of strep throat with antibiotics is important because of the potential for dangerous sequelae, such as rheumatic fever and acute poststreptococcal glomerulonephritis.

Epiglottitis is becoming less common since the implementation of vaccine programs for *H. influenzae,* formerly the most common cause of epiglottitis in children. Today, this inflammatory disease of the epiglottis is more likely to be caused by *S. aureus.* The young patient usually prefers to sit upright with neck extended to ease breathing. Lateral cervical spine X-ray reveals a swollen epiglottis, dubbed the "thumbprint sign" (see Figure 5-72).

Lower Respiratory Infections

Involve the bronchi, bronchioles, alveoli, and extra-alveolar lung tissues. Bronchitis and bronchiolitis are, like upper respiratory infections, more commonly caused by viruses than bacteria.

KEY FACT

In a young adult with pharyngitis, suspect infectious mononucleosis caused by Epstein-Barr virus (EBV). Diagnosis is with the Monospot heterophile test.

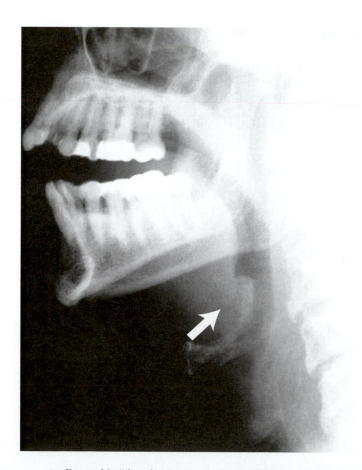

FIGURE 5-72. **Radiographic "thumbprint sign" of epiglottitis in a child.** (Reproduced, with permission, from Tintinalli JE, Kelen DG, Stapczynski JS. *Tintinalli's Emergency Medicine: A Comprehensive Study Guide,* 6th ed. New York: McGraw-Hill, 2004: 1497.)

Laryngotracheal bronchitis (croup) is most often caused by parainfluenza virus. It classically presents as a child with a seal-like **barking cough.**

Pneumonia is most often caused by bacteria. Viruses, fungi, mycobacteria, and parasites may also cause infection. Clues to the causative organism can be found in the patient's age (see Table 5-38), where the infection was acquired (i.e., community versus hospital), the patient's immune status, and other risk factors.

COMMUNITY-ACQUIRED PNEUMONIA

Typical causes include:

- *Streptococcus pneumoniae*
- *H. influenzae*
- *Moraxella catarrhalis*

Atypical causes of community-acquired pneumonia include:

- *Mycoplasma pneumoniae* ("walking pneumonia")
- *Chlamydophila pneumoniae*
- *Legionella* (associated with contaminated aerosolized water, classically in air-conditioning systems)

Hospital-acquired (nosocomial) pneumonia is most likely to be caused by *S. aureus*. Also suspect *P. aeruginosa* and other gram-negative rods.

Some population-specific agents of pneumonia are summarized in Table 5-39.

KEY FACT

Typical community-acquired pneumonia is heralded by an abrupt onset of fever, chills or rigors, respiratory distress, and purulent or bloody sputum. Radiographs often demonstrate **lobar consolidation** (see Figure 5-73).

KEY FACT

Atypical organisms cause diffuse interstitial disease, rather than lobar disease, and are characterized by a dry cough.

TABLE 5-38. Causes of Pneumonia by Age Group

AGE GROUP	MOST LIKELY PATHOGEN	OTHER CAUSES
Neonates (0–6 wk)	*Streptococcus agalactiae* (group B)	*Escherichia coli* *Chlamydia trachomatis*
Children (6 wk–18 yr)	Viruses like respiratory syncytial virus (RSV)	*Mycoplasma pneumoniae* *Chlamydophila pneumoniae* *Streptococcus pneumoniae*
Young adults (18–40 yr)	*M. pneumoniae*	*C. pneumoniae* *S. pneumoniae*
Older adults (40–65 yr)	*S. pneumoniae*	*H. influenzae* Anaerobes and viruses *M. pneumoniae*
Elderly (> 65 yr)	*S. pneumoniae*	*Moraxella catarrhalis* Anaerobes and viruses *H. influenzae* Gram-negative rods *M. tuberculosis* (reactivation)

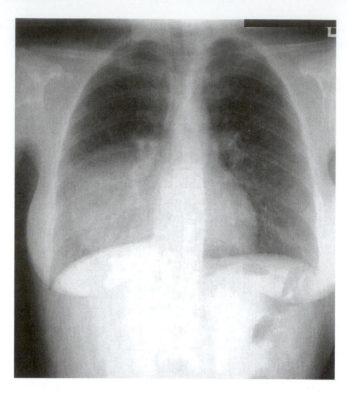

FIGURE 5-73. **Right lobar pneumococcal pneumonia.** (Courtesy of Dr. Diane Twickler.)

MICROBIAL DISEASES OF THE CARDIOVASCULAR SYSTEM

Infective Endocarditis

Occurs when endothelial damage to the heart valves or other cardiac surfaces allows circulating organisms to colonize the damaged tissue. Colonization leads to **vegetation** and subsequent inflammatory, embolic, and immunologic complications. Clinical manifestations can include fever, heart murmur, painful indurated nodules on the fingers and toes (**Osler nodes**), painless erythematous macules on the palms and soles (**Janeway lesions**), red linear

TABLE 5-39. **Common Pneumonial Pathogens Associated with Specific Populations**

POPULATION AFFECTED	COMMON PATHOGENS CAUSING PNEUMONIA
Aspiration	Mixed anaerobes
Immunocompromised hosts	*Staphylococcus*, gram-negative rods, fungi, viruses, *Aspergillus*, *Cryptococcus*, tuberculosis, cytomegalovirus (CMV)
HIV/AIDS	*Pneumocystis carinii* (*P. jiroveci*)
Cystic fibrosis	*Pseudomonas aeruginosa*
Alcoholics/IV drug users	*Streptococcus pneumoniae*, *Klebsiella pneumoniae*, *Staphylococcus aureus*
Postviral infections	*S. aureus*, *Haemophilus influenzae*, *S. pneumoniae*

lesions in the nailbeds (**splinter hemorrhages**), and retinal hemorrhages with clear centers (**Roth spots**) (see Figure 5-74).

CLASSIFICATION OF ENDOCARDITIS

Endocarditis can be divided into **acute, subacute,** or **chronic,** depending on the virulence of the causative organism and the progression of the disease if no treatment is initiated (see Table 5-40).

SPECIAL POPULATIONS

IV drug users tend to get **right-sided** endocarditis, with vegetations on the **tricuspid** valve. Typical organisms in this population include S. *aureus,* enterococci, gram-negative enteric bacilli, and C. *albicans.*

Hospital-acquired endocarditis is usually associated with gram-positive cocci such as S. *aureus,* coagulase-negative staphylococci, and enterococci.

Gastrointestinal malignancy is often associated with endocarditis caused by *Streptococcus bovis* and *Clostridium septicum.*

KEY FACT

Acute endocarditis affects previously **normal** valves.
Subacute endocarditis affects previously **abnormal** valves.

MNEMONIC

HACEK

Haemophilus aphrophilus, H. parainfluenzae, and H. paraphrophilus
Actinobacillus actinomycetemcomitans
Cardiobacterium hominis
Eikenella corrodens
Kingella kingae

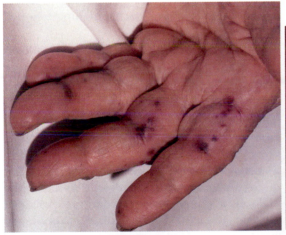

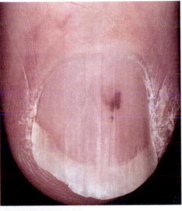

A   B

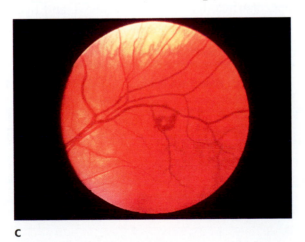

C

FIGURE 5-74.   **Infective endocarditis.** (A) Janeway lesions; (B) splinter hemorrhage; (C) Roth spot. (Parts A and B reproduced, with permission, from Wolff, K, Johnson RA, Suurmond D. *Fitzpatrick's Color Atlas & Synopsis of Clinical Dermatology,* 5th ed. New York: McGraw-Hill, 2005: 636 and 1010. Part C courtesy of William E. Cappaert, MD as printed in Knoop KJ, Stack LB, Storrow AB. *Atlas of Emergency Medicine,* 2nd ed. New York: McGraw-Hill, 2002: 80.)

TABLE 5-40.   Types of Endocarditis

Type of Endocarditis	Incubation Time	Most Common Cause
Acute	Days to weeks	*Staphylococcus aureus*
Subacute	Weeks to months	Viridans streptococci
Chronic	Months	*Staphylococcus epidermidis*

HACEK organisms are a group of gram-negative bacilli that are part of the normal oropharyngeal flora. They are difficult to culture and have a tendency to produce endocardial infections. These organisms cause infections in IV drug users who contaminate the needle or injection site with saliva, as well as in patients with poor dental hygiene or preexisting valvular damage.

Bacteremia

The presence of viable bacteria in circulating blood. Transient bacteremia can occur during tooth brushing and during menstruation, but usually resolves quickly secondary to macrophage clearance of the bacteria.

KEY SOURCES OF BACTEREMIA

One of the most common causes of bacteremia is an indwelling urinary catheter, which provides easy access for *E. coli* to invade via the urinary tract. Other possible organisms include *S. pneumoniae, H. influenzae,* and *S. pyogenes* from the respiratory tract; *S. aureus* from the skin (especially through an IV); and *Salmonella typhi* or *Enterobacter* from the GI tract.

MICROBIAL DISEASES OF THE GI TRACT

Food-Poisoning Syndromes

Caused by eating food contaminated with bacterial toxins (see Table 5-41) or live organisms (see Table 5-42). Symptoms may include nausea, vomiting, abdominal cramps, diarrhea, fever, chills, weakness, and headache. Onset of

KEY FACT

Sepsis is a life-threatening condition resulting from the immune response to bacteremia, characterized by fever, chills, and hypotension (shock).

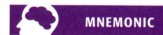

MNEMONIC

Reheated rice? Be serious! (B. *cereus*)

TABLE 5-41.   Food-Poisoning Syndromes Caused by Preformed Toxins

Organism	Associated Food	Points to Remember
Staphylococcus aureus	Potato salad, custard, mayonnaise left at room temperature.	Severe vomiting and diarrhea appear 2–6 hours after ingestion.
Bacillus cereus	Reheated rice and other starchy foods, undercooked meat or vegetables.	May cause emetic or diarrheal disease.
Clostridium botulinum (adults)	Inadequately preserved canned foods.	Neurotoxin binds synaptic vesicles in cholinergic nerves, blocks acetylcholine release, causes paralysis and death.

TABLE 5-42.   **Food-Poisoning Syndromes Caused by Bacterial Infection**

ORGANISM	ASSOCIATED FOOD	POINTS TO REMEMBER
Salmonella enteriditis	Meat, poultry, fish, eggs.	Most common cause of noninvasive food poisoning in the United States; may cause watery or mucous diarrhea.
Campylobacter jejuni	Poultry, milk, contaminated water.	Most common invasive bacterial enterocolitis, produces crypt abscesses and ulcers resembling ulcerative colitis, causes explosive diarrhea with blood and/or mucus, may cause Guillain-Barré syndrome.
Clostridium perfringens	Meat that is unrefrigerated or cooled too slowly.	Causes cramps and watery diarrhea lasting 24 hours.
Clostridium botulinum (infants)	Honey.	Spores contaminate honey and germinate in infant's GI tract; neurotoxin blocks acetylcholine release, causes constipation and "floppy baby."
Enterohemorrhagic *E. coli* strain 0157:H7	Hamburger meat, spinach.	Shiga-like toxin causes severe inflammatory diarrhea, can lead to hemolytic uremic syndrome.
Vibrio parahaemolyticus	Raw or undercooked seafood (usually oysters).	Causes vomiting and watery diarrhea that are self-limited.

symptoms varies with etiology—from as few as 2–6 hours to 1 or 2 days after ingestion.

Bacterial Causes of Diarrhea Not Associated with Food

Cholera is an acute disease of the small intestine caused by *V. cholerae*. This gram-negative curved bacillus is spread by the fecal-oral route, usually via contaminated water. The bacteria attach to intestinal epithelial cells and release the cholera toxin, which activates adenylate cyclase, increasing intracellular cAMP and stimulating hypersecretion of Na^+, K^+, Cl^-, HCO_3^- and water. This produces secretory "**rice water**" diarrhea, with volume depletion, normal gap metabolic acidosis, and hypokalemia. Treatment is supportive, including oral rehydration solutions.

Shigella is spread by the fecal-oral route, usually from hand-to-hand contact. Bacteria invade the epithelial cells lining the colon and release Shiga toxin, which destroys the cells by inhibiting the 60S ribosome. The disease is characterized by fever, abdominal pain and inflammatory diarrhea that may contain specks of bright red blood and pus. Treatment is with ciprofloxacin.

C. difficile (**pseudomembranous**) **colitis** occurs iatrogenically as a result of antibiotic administration, which alters the intestinal flora and allows overgrowth of *C. difficile*. The bacteria produce an enterotoxin and a cytotoxin,

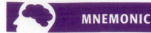

leading to the formation of creamy to greenish exudates (pseudomembranes) in the colon. Clinical manifestations include fever, cramping, and severe diarrhea. Diagnosis is with **toxin assay of stool.** Treatment is with metronidazole or oral vancomycin.

E. coli **gastroenteritis** occurs when this component of the normal intestinal flora acquires virulence factors (see Table 5-43).

Parasitic Causes of Diarrhea

Amebiasis is an infection caused by amebas; *Entamoeba histolytica* is the primary pathogenic ameba in humans. It is spread by cysts in fecally contaminated food and can lead to asymptomatic passage of cysts, non-dysenteric infection characterized by watery diarrhea, or dysenteric infection characterized by **bloody diarrhea** and tenesmus.

Giardiasis is caused by the protozoan parasite *Giardia lamblia*, which is a single-celled parasite with a prominent ventral sucking disk and flagella (see Figure 5-75). Patients may ingest cysts from mountain spring water. In the small intestine, each cyst develops into two trophozoites that use their sucking disks to attach themselves to the columnar cells of the duodenum, mechanically impairing duodenal function. Half of patients remain asymptomatic; however, symptomatic disease can range from a self-limited acute diarrhea to severe chronic diarrhea. Treatment is with metronidazole.

Cryptosporidiosis is caused by protozoa of the genus *Cryptosporidium*, predominantly *C. parvum* and *C. hominis*. Ingestion of oocysts from fecally contaminated water results in infection of the brush border of the intestine, leading to a self-limited diarrheal illness in immunocompetent patients. In immunocompromised patients, the diarrhea is often severe and unrelenting. Paromomycin can be used for suppressive therapy in patients with AIDS.

TABLE 5-43. Types of *E. coli* Causing Gastroenteritis

Organism	Virulence Factor	Clinical Features
Enteropathogenic *Escherichia coli*	Bacteria adhere to intestinal epithelial cells and prevent fluid absorption.	Secretory diarrhea associated with epidemics in infants.
Enteroaggressive *E. coli*	Aggregates of bacteria adhere to intestinal epithelial cells and prevent fluid absorption.	Secretory diarrhea—one cause of traveler's diarrhea.
Enterotoxigenic *E. coli*	Heat-stable enterotoxin activates guanylate cyclase, inhibiting intestinal fluid uptake; heat-labile enterotoxin activates adenylate cyclase, stimulating hypersecretion of fluids (just like cholera toxin).	Secretory diarrhea (up to 20 L/day), most common cause of traveler's diarrhea.
Enteroinvasive *E. coli*	Bacteria invade the epithelial cells lining the colon, then replicate and destroy the cells; also produces small amounts of Shiga-like toxin.	Inflammatory diarrhea.

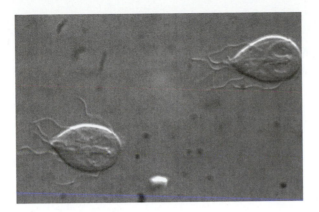

FIGURE 5-75.   ***Giardia lamblia* trophozoites.** (Reproduced, with permission, from Kasper DL, Braunwald E, Fauci AS, et al. *Harrison's Principles of Internal Medicine*,16th ed. New York: McGraw-Hill, 2005: 1249.)

Viral Causes of Diarrhea

Viral gastroenteritis is spread via the fecal-oral route. Viruses cause diarrhea by invading the intestinal epithelial cells and multiplying intracellularly. As they subjugate host cell metabolism, fluid transport is disrupted and cell destruction occurs, leading to decreased fluid resorption. The resulting nausea, vomiting, and watery diarrhea are usually self-limited but can lead to life-threatening dehydration in patients who are very young, malnourished, or immunocompromised.

Rotavirus is the most common cause of diarrhea in children. Its incidence increases during the winter. Diagnosis is made by stool antigen testing.

Norwalk virus is a common cause of diarrheal outbreaks among adults and children, particularly on cruise ships, in nursing homes, and at camps.

Astrovirus is an important cause of diarrhea in children younger than 1 year.

Cytomegalovirus is an important cause of colitis, which produces chronic watery diarrhea in patients with HIV/AIDS.

MICROBIAL DISEASES OF THE URINARY AND REPRODUCTIVE SYSTEMS

Infections commonly occur as a result of fecal contamination, sexual transmission, or as a complication of medical instrumentation (e.g., catheterization).

Urinary Tract Infections (UTIs)

Defined by the presence of bacteria in the urine (bacteriuria) in combination with symptoms such as dysuria, urgency, and frequency. The urinary tract is normally sterile, but infection is frequently caused by ascension of coliform bacteria such as *E. coli* into the bladder via the urethra. Any cause of urinary stasis, such as a tumor, stone, enlarged prostate or neurogenic bladder, or the presence of a foreign body can predispose to UTI. Common causative organisms are listed in Table 5-44.

Women, especially sexually active young women, are at risk for developing UTIs because of the short length of the female urethra and the small distance between the urethra and the anus. UTIs are 10 times more common in women than in men. Uncomplicated UTIs in the outpatient setting can be

 MNEMONIC

SSEEK PP

Serratia marcescens
Staphylococcus saprophyticus
Escherichia coli
Enterobacter cloacae
Klebsiella pneumoniae
Pseudomonas aeruginosa
Proteus mirabilis

TABLE 5-44. Bacteria Causing Urinary Tract Infections

ORGANISM	DISTINCTIVE FEATURES
Serratia marcescens	Some strains produce a red pigment.
Staphylococcus saprophyticus	Second leading cause of community-acquired urinary tract infection (UTI) in sexually active women.
Escherichia coli	Leading cause of UTI. Colonies have a metallic sheen on EMB (eosin–methylene blue) agar.
Enterobacter cloacae	Often hospital-acquired and drug-resistant.
Klebsiella pneumoniae	Large mucoid capsule and viscous colonies.
Pseudomonas aeruginosa	Blue-green pigment and fruity odor.
Proteus mirabilis	Motility causes "swarming" on agar. Produces urease; associated with struvite calculi.

KEY FACT

Urinalysis findings in UTI:
- White blood cells (pyuria).
- Red blood cells may be present.
- Positive leukocyte esterase indicates bacterial infection.
- Positive **n**itrite test indicates colonization by gram-**n**egative organisms.

KEY FACT

- Clinical manifestations of **UTI** include dysuria, frequency, urgency, suprapubic pain, and sometimes hematuria.
- Fever, nausea, vomiting, or costovertebral angle (CVA) tenderness suggests **pyelonephritis.**

KEY FACT

In many cases, a newly diagnosed STI should be reported to the health department. It is also important to notify the patient's partner(s) of possible infection. These public health responsibilities override the physician's usual responsibility to maintain patient confidentiality. Details of reporting and notification laws vary by state.

treated empirically with trimethoprim-sulfamethoxasole (TMP-SMX) or fluoroquinolones. Causative organisms include:

- Uropathogenic *E. coli* (70%–95%)
- *Staphylococcus saprophyticus* (10%–15%)
- *K. pneumoniae*

Hospitalized patients are at increased risk for developing UTIs, typically secondary to the presence of a Foley catheter. This is the most common hospital-acquired infection. *E. coli* remains the most common causative organism, but other causative organisms are seen increasingly, such as *Proteus*, *Klebsiella*, *Serratia*, and *Pseudomonas*. Urine culture should be performed in hospitalized patients to determine the specific bacteria causing the infection.

Pregnancy is commonly associated with asymptomatic bacteriuria. UTIs during pregnancy are more likely to develop into pyelonephritis and also increase the risk for preterm labor and low birth weight. Pregnant women should be screened for bacteriuria early in pregnancy and should always be treated, regardless of the presence of symptoms.

Children with recurrent UTIs should be evaluated for vesicoureteral reflux and other congenital abnormalities. Frequent UTIs or other pelvic infections in children raise the suspicion of child abuse.

Sexually Transmitted Infections

Sexually transmitted infections (STIs) are among the most common infectious diseases in the United States today. Because they share a common mechanism of transmission, it is not uncommon for a patient to present with more than one infection simultaneously. In many cases, individuals are asymptomatic while carrying (and transmitting) these infections. Women in particular are at risk for developing serious complications, such as pelvic inflammatory disease (PID), from even asymptomatic STIs. These infections are summarized in Table 5-45.

TABLE 5-45.   Sexually Transmitted Infections

DISEASE	ORGANISM	CLINICAL FEATURES	TREATMENT
Chlamydia	*Chlamydia trachomatis* (D–K)	Urethritis, cervicitis, conjunctivitis, pelvic inflammatory disease (PID).	Doxycycline for 7 days or single-dose azithromycin.
Lymphogranuloma venereum	*Chlamydia trachomatis* (L1–L3)	Ulcers, lymphadenopathy, rectal strictures.	Doxycycline for 21 days.
Gonorrhea	*Neisseria gonorrhoeae*	Urethritis, cervicitis, prostatitis, arthritis, PID, creamy purulent discharge.	Ceftriaxone (also treat for possible *Chlamydia*).
Primary syphilis	*Treponema pallidum*	Painless chancre.	Single dose of benzathine penicillin G IM.
Secondary syphilis	*Treponema pallidum*	Rash (affecting palms and soles), fever, lymphadenopathy, condylomata lata.	Single dose of benzathine penicillin G IM.
Tertiary syphilis	*Treponema pallidum*	Gummas, aortitis. Meningitis, tabes dorsalis, general paresis, Argyll-Robertson pupils.	Three doses of benzathine penicillin G IM. 10–14 days of aqueous crystalline penicillin G IV.
Genital herpes	Herpes simplex virus (usually HSV-2)	Painful penile, vulvar or cervical ulcers.	Acyclovir, famciclovir, or valacyclovir.
Trichomoniasis	*Trichomonas vaginalis*	Vaginitis, frothy vaginal discharge, "strawberry cervix."	Metronidazole (for patient and partners).
AIDS	Human immunodeficiency virus (HIV)	Opportunistic infections, Kaposi's sarcoma, lymphoma.	Highly active antiretroviral therapy (HAART).
Condylomata acuminata	Human papillomavirus, types 6 and 11	Genital warts.	Cryotherapy or surgical excision.
Hepatitis B	Hepatitis B virus	Jaundice, liver failure.	INF-α, lamivudine, adefovir, or entecavir.
Chancroid	*Haemophilus ducreyi*	Painful genital ulcer, inguinal lymphadenopathy.	Azithromycin, ceftriaxone, or ciprofloxacin.
Granuloma inguinale (donovanosis)	*Calymmatobacterium granulomatis*	Small papule or painless ulcer with rolled edges that bleeds easily.	Doxycycline twice daily for 21 days.

Chlamydia is the most commonly reported STI in the United States and is a leading cause of infertility in women. The causative organism, *C. trachomatis*, is an obligate intracellular bacterium with 15 immunotypes. Immunotypes D-K cause genital tract infections and immunotypes L1–L3 cause genital ulcers (lymphogranuloma venereum). Most cases of chlamydia are **asymptomatic**, but the disease may cause dysuria and mucopurulent discharge from the urethra.

Gonorrhea is a common STI characterized by acute **purulent urethral discharge** and painful or difficult urination. It is caused by *N. gonorrhoeae*, aerobic gram-negative cocci that are characteristically coffee bean-shaped and form pairs. Because coinfection with *C. trachomatis* is common, patients diagnosed with gonorrhea should also be treated for chlamydia.

Pelvic inflammatory disease (PID) can be a serious complication of sexually transmitted infections in women. Chlamydia and gonorrhea are the most common causes, either alone or in combination. Organisms infecting the vagina and cervix ascend the female genital tract and cause disease in the uterus, fallopian tubes, and ovaries. The infection progresses to form scar tissue and adhesions. Sequelae can include **ectopic pregnancy, infertility,** and **chronic pelvic pain.**

Vaginal Infections

Often present with symptoms including itching, burning, irritation and abnormal discharge. The three most common types of vaginitis are bacterial vaginosis, candidiasis, and trichomoniasis, which together account for more than 90% of cases. Several diagnostic criteria used to differentiate these infections are listed in Table 5-46.

Bacterial vaginosis is the most common cause of vaginitis. It is caused by an overgrowth of organisms such as *Gardnerella vaginalis, Mobiluncus, Mycoplasma hominis,* and *Peptostreptococcus.* It is often asymptomatic, but can present with a thin, white, adherent vaginal discharge, which releases a fishy odor when mixed with KOH (positive whiff test). Diagnosis is confirmed by saline wet mount showing epithelial cells covered in bacteria (**clue cells**), as seen in Figure 5-20.

Candidiasis is a fungal infection that can be associated with antibiotic use or immune deficiency.

Trichomoniasis is an STI that produces a frothy vaginal discharge and a characteristic "strawberry cervix." The bacterium can be isolated from up to 80% of male partners of infected women; therefore, both the patient and her partner(s) should be treated.

TABLE 5-46. Diagnostic Characteristics of Common Vaginal Infections

	NORMAL	**BACTERIAL VAGINOSIS**	**CANDIDIASIS**	**TRICHOMONIASIS**
Vaginal pH	3.8–4.2	> 4.5	< 4.5	> 4.5
Discharge	White, clear, flocculent	Thin, adherent, white-gray, homogeneous.	White, curd-like	White to yellow-green, frothy.
Amine odor	Absent	Present (fishy).	Absent	Variable (fishy).
Microscopic	Lactobacilli	Clue cells, cocci.	Budding pseudohyphae	Trichomonads.
Complaints	None	Discharge, odor.	Discharge, itching	Frothy discharge, itching, odor.

Infections during Pregnancy

A number of infections can cause severe congenital problems if a patient contracts them during pregnancy. The acronym ToRCHeS (toxoplasmosis, rubella, cytomegalovirus, Herpes/HIV, syphilis) identifies infectious diseases commonly screened for during pregnancy.

Toxoplasmosis is a parasitic disease contracted by eating undercooked meat or being exposed to cat feces. It causes a mild flulike illness in healthy adults, but when transmitted to the fetus, can result in hearing loss, vision loss, mental retardation, or seizures.

Rubella is a viral infection that causes a mild rash and flulike illness in healthy adults. During the first trimester of pregnancy, however, it can lead to miscarriage, stillbirth, or serious birth defects. Congenital rubella syndrome can include **heart malformations** (including atrial septal defect, ventricular septal defect, and patent ductus arteriosus), deafness, mental retardation, cataracts, microcephaly, and hepatomegaly.

Cytomegalovirus is a viral infection that can be transmitted during delivery or via breast milk. Infected infants may develop hearing loss, mental retardation, pneumonia, hepatitis, or blood disorders.

Herpes is a common viral infection causing painful mucosal ulcers. An infant may acquire the infection while still in the uterus or while passing through the birth canal, leading to skin lesions, eye diseases, encephalitis, or death.

HIV should be screened for in all pregnant patients. Antiretroviral therapy greatly reduces the likelihood that the virus will be transmitted to the fetus during pregnancy and delivery. HIV positive women should be counseled not to breast feed their babies.

Syphilis is an STI with a wide variety of clinical manifestations. During pregnancy, treponemes can pass through the placenta to the fetus. Approximately 50% of these fetuses are aborted or stillborn. The remainder may present with the **Hutchinson triad** of notched teeth, eighth-nerve deafness, and interstitial keratitis. Infected infants may also present with other syphilitic stigmata such as a rash, anemia, hepatosplenomegaly, and blindness.

MICROBIAL DISEASES OF THE BONES, JOINTS, AND SKIN

Osteomyelitis

INFECTION OF THE BONE

Osteomyelitis can occur as a result of trauma, postsurgical infection, hematogenous spread of bacteria into the bone, invasion of the bone from a contiguous source of infection, or skin breakdown in the setting of vascular insufficiency. The most common cause of osteomyelitis overall is *S. aureus*, although certain groups may be predisposed to infection with other organisms.

- **Sexually active patients** may present with osteomyelitis caused by *N. gonorrhoeae*, although septic arthritis is a much more common manifestation of this infection.
- **Diabetics and drug addicts** may present with osteomyelitis caused by *P. aeruginosa*.
- **Sickle cell disease** is associated with *Salmonella* osteomyelitis.

- **Prosthetic joint replacements** are associated with osteomyelitis due predominantly to staphylococcal organisms, such as *S. aureus* or *S. epidermidis*.
- **Tuberculosis** can lead to **vertebral** osteomyelitis (Pott's disease).

Infectious Arthritis

Bacterial invasion of a joint. *S. aureus* and *N. gonorrhoeae* are the first and second most common causes in adults, respectively. The disease typically affects a single large joint, producing pain, tenderness, warmth, and erythema. The synovial fluid is thick and cloudy with many white blood cells, although bacteria may not be evident on Gram stains or cultures.

Lyme disease, caused by the spirochete *Borrelia burgdorferi*, is transmitted by *Ixodes* ticks in the United States. It produces a characteristic target-shaped rash (**erythema chronicum migrans**) at the site of the tick bite and arthritis.

Cellulitis

An acute, spreading infection of the skin extending into the subcutaneous tissues. Group A streptococci and *S. aureus* are the most common causes.

Erysipelas is a superficial cellulitis with prominent lymphatic involvement. It most commonly presents on the legs with lesions that are bright red, edematous and indurated with a sharp, raised border. It is almost always caused by group A streptococci.

MICROBIAL DISEASES OF THE EYE AND EAR

Conjunctivitis

Children and neonates are particularly susceptible to conjunctivitis. Neonatal conjunctivitis can be classified according to its temporal presentation after birth:

- **Day 1:** Silver nitrate susceptibility.
- **Days 1–4:** *N. gonorrhoeae.* Presents with **hyperpurulent exudates.**
- **Days 3–10:** *C. trachomatis.* Presents with purulent exudates. Microscopic evaluation reveals **inclusion bodies** in cells. This infection may progress to pneumonia if left untreated.

POSTNEONATAL AND CHILDHOOD

Purulent exudates suggest infection with *H. influenzae* or *S. pneumoniae.* Watery exudates and sore throat with recent swimming pool exposure suggest adenovirus ("pink eye"), a naked virus resistant to chlorination.

Contact lens wearers can develop conjunctivitis after leaving contacts in their eyes for long periods of time (Pseudomonas) or from using homemade saline (*Acanthamoeba*).

Parasitic causes of conjunctivitis include *Trypanosoma cruzi* (Chagas' disease) and *Trichinella.*

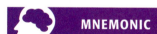
MNEMONIC

In chronologic order of presentation: Some Neonates Can Hardly See Anything:

Silver nitrate susceptibility
N. *gonorrhoeae*
C. *trachomatis*
H. *influenzae*
S. *pneumoniae*
Adenovirus

Conjunctivitis with vision loss may be caused by *C. trachomatis*, types A, B, and C. These immunotypes are uncommon in the United States, but chronic infection commonly causes corneal scarring and blindness in Africa.

Otitis

Otitis externa is most commonly caused by *P. aeruginosa*. It causes severe tenderness and pain. Swimmers and diabetics are at increased risk for this infection. Treatment is with antibiotic drops (typically an aminoglycoside or fluoroquinolone, with or without steroids).

Otitis media is an exceedingly common infection in children under the age of six. It usually arises as a complication of a viral upper respiratory infection. Secretions and inflammation cause a relative obstruction of the eustachian tubes. As the mucosa of the middle ear absorbs air that cannot be replaced because of this obstruction, negative pressure is generated, and a serous effusion develops. This provides a fertile medium for bacterial growth. Common causative organisms include *S. pneumoniae*, *H. influenzae*, and *Moraxella*.

MICROBIAL DISEASES OF THE NERVOUS SYSTEM

Meningitis

Inflammation of the leptomeninges and underlying CSF. Symptoms include headache, fever, and nuchal rigidity. As with pneumonia, the common causes of meningitis can be grouped according to the age of the patient (see Table 5-47). The incidence of *H. influenzae* type B meningitis, formerly the most common cause of meningitis in children, has declined significantly with the introduction of vaccine programs in the last 10–15 years. Bacterial, viral, and fungal causes of meningitis can be differentiated by characteristic patterns of the patient's CSF, as summarized in Table 5-48.

HIV/AIDS is associated with meningitis caused by opportunistic pathogens such as *Cryptococcus*, *Toxoplasma*, cytomegalovirus (CMV), and JC virus (progressive multifocal leukoencephalopathy).

TABLE 5-47   Causes of Meningitis by Age Group

Age Group	Most Common Pathogens	Other Causes
Newborn (0–6 months)	Group B Streptococci *Escherichia coli*	*Listeria*
Children (6 mo–6 yr)	*Streptococcus pneumoniae*	*N. meningitides* *Haemophilus influenzae* type B Enteroviruses
6–60 yr	*Neisseris meningitidis* *S. pneumoniae*	Enteroviruses Herpes simplex virus
Elderly (> 60 yr)	*S. pneumoniae*	Gram-negative rods *Listeria*

TABLE 5-48.   Cerebrospinal Spinal Fluid Findings in Meningitis

CAUSE	PRESSURE	CELL TYPE	PROTEIN	GLUCOSE
Bacterial	↑	↑ PMNs	↑	↓
Fungal/TB	↑	↑ Lymphocytes	↑	↓
Viral	Normal/↑	↑ Lymphocytes	Normal	Normal

PMNs = polymorphonuclear leukocytes.

NOSOCOMIAL INFECTIONS

Table 5-49 summarizes the pathogens commonly associated with various hospital-related risk factors.

KEY FACT

Using two drugs that are both either bactericidal or bacteriostatic is often **synergistic** (e.g., penicillin/aminoglycoside or trimethoprim-sulfonamide). Using a bacteriostatic drug with a bactericidal drug is often **antagonistic** (e.g., penicillin/tetracycline).

Antimicrobials

ANTIBACTERIAL DRUGS

Table 5-50 lists the site and mechanism of action of the major antibacterial drugs. It categorizes the drugs as either bactericidal or bacteriostatic, which is important for understanding the action of individual drugs as well as the synergistic or antagonistic effects of certain drug combinations. Figure 5-76 illustrates the sites of action of the drugs in the cell.

β-Lactams

Bacterial cell walls contain peptidoglycans, repeating disaccharides with amino acid side chains. The amino acid side chains are cross-linked with one another via covalent bonds, thus strengthening the cell wall.

MECHANISM

These compounds are so named because they have a β-lactam ring (see Figure 5-77), which binds to and irreversibly inactivates the bacterial **transpeptidase** enzyme responsible for peptidoglycan cross-linking. The inhibition

TABLE 5-49.   Risk Factors and Associated Pathogens Implicated in Nosocomial Infections

RISK FACTOR	PATHOGEN
Newborn nursery	Cytomegalovirus, respiratory syncytial virus
Urinary catheterization	*Escherichia coli, Proteus mirabilis*
Respiratory therapy equipment	*Pseudomonas aeruginosa*
Work in renal dialysis unit	HBV
Hyperalimentation	*Candida albicans*
Water aerosols	*Legionella*

TABLE 5-50. Antibiotics: Site of Action and Mechanism

SITE OF ACTION	MECHANISM OF ACTION	BACTERICIDAL	BACTERIOSTATIC
Cell wall	Inhibit peptidoglycan cross-linking	β-Lactams (penicillins, cephalosporins, aztreonam, imipenem).	
	Inhibit peptidoglycan polymerization	Vancomycin	
Outer membrane	Disrupt outer membrane in gram-negative bacteria.	Polymixins	
Nucleotide synthesis	Inhibit dihydropteroate synthetase		Sulfonamides
	Inhibit dihydrofolate reductase		Trimethoprim, pyrimethamine
DNA	Inhibit type II topoisomerase	Fluoroquinolones (ciprofloxacin)	
	Inhibit mRNA synthesis	Rifampin	
50S ribosomal subunit	Block initiation complex formation		Linezolid
	Block release of nascent peptides from the ribosome.	Quinupristin/dalfopristin	
	Block peptide bond formation and peptide release from the ribosome.		Clindamycin
	Inhibit peptide bond formation		Chloramphenicol
	Block release of nascent peptides from the ribosome.		Macrolides (erythromycin)
30S ribosomal subunit	Cause miscoding of mRNA and incorrect amino acid linking for peptide formation, blocking normal protein synthesis.	Aminoglycosides (gentamicin)	
	Block binding of tRNA and addition of amino acids to the peptide chain.		Tetracyclines
Various	Toxic metabolites	Metronidazole	
Other	Unknown		Nitrofurantoin

of transpeptidase (**penicillin-binding protein**) in turn inhibits cross-linking, leading to the arrest of cell wall synthesis, thus killing the dividing bacteria. Transpeptidase inhibition results in the activation of **autolytic enzymes** that dissolve the cell wall. β-Lactams are **bactericidal.**

RESISTANCE

Bacteria have evolved different ways of protecting themselves from β-lactam drugs.

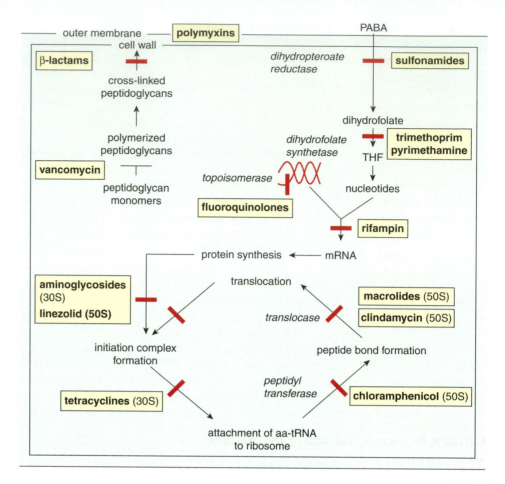

FIGURE 5-76. **Mechanism of action of major antibacterials.**

- **Inactivation via β-lactamase penicillinase:** Both gram-positive and gram-negative bacteria have enzymes that cleave the C-N bond in the β-lactam ring.
- **Changes in drug target through mutation of binding site:** Through mutations, bacteria can develop forms of transpeptidase to which β-lactams cannot bind.
- **Decreased permeability, restricting drug entry:** Because of their size and/or charge, some β–lactam drugs are unable to pass through the outer membrane of gram-negative bacteria. Note that this is not a mechanism of resistance for gram-positive bacteria because they do not have outer membranes.

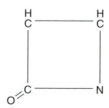

FIGURE 5-77. **The β-lactam ring, the chemical structure that inhibits peptidoglycan cross-linking.**

CLASSES

Listed below are the four classes of β-lactams, which differ in their susceptibility to bacterial β-lactamase, spectrum of coverage, and side-effect profiles.

- Penicillins
- Cephalosporins
- Monobactams
- Carbapenems

PENICILLIN

MECHANISM

See above (beta lactams).

USES

- Narrow spectrum; primarily effective against gram-positive bacteria.
- *N. meningitidis*
- *Clostridia*
- Most anaerobes except *B. fragilis*.
- Spirochetes: Drug of choice for syphilis.

SIDE EFFECTS

Hypersensitivity (urticaria, pruritus, fever, anaphylaxis, nephritis, joint swelling); rash; hemolytic anemia (Coombs'-positive).

NAFCILLIN, METHICILLIN, CLOXACILLIN, DICLOXACILLIN

MECHANISM

Same as penicillin, but are **β-lactamase-resistant** because of their bulky R groups and therefore can be used without clavulanic acid.

USES

- Narrow-spectrum gram-positive coverage, antistaphylococcal infections (e.g., cellulitis, impetigo).
- *N. meningitidis*
- Particularly effective for organisms that produce β-lactamase.

SIDE EFFECTS

Hypersensitivity; interstitial nephritis (especially methicillin when used in combination with aminoglycosides).

AMPICILLIN, AMOXICILLIN

MECHANISM

Same as penicillin. β-Lactamase-sensitive.

USES

- Broad-spectrum gram-positive and gram-negative coverage.
- Drug of choice for gram-positive organisms enterococcus and Listeria.
- When used in combination with clavulanic acid, provides extended coverage to gram-negative rods *H. influenzae*, *E. coli*, *P mirabilis*, *Salmonella*, *Shigella*.
- Amoxicillin is second-line treatment for Lyme disease.

SIDE EFFECTS

Hypersensitivity; rash; pseudomembranous colitis.

KEY FACT

Clavulanic acid, a β-lactam-like molecule, binds to and inactivates β-lactamase → confers broader activity to β-lactamase-susceptible penicillins.

KEY FACT

Pencillin G is given IM or IV; penicillin V is given PO.

MNEMONIC

Unlike other penicillins, **N**aficillin is **N**ot susceptible to β-lactamase.

MNEMONIC

Am**O**xicillin is an **O**ral form of ampicillin.

MNEMONIC

Ampicillin/amoxicillin coverage: Ampicillin/amoxicillin **HELPS** **S**laughter enterococcus.

Haemophilus influenzae
E. coli
Listeria
Proteus mirabilis
Salmonella
Shigella
Enterococcus.

TICARCILLIN, CARBENICILLIN, PIPERACILLIN, MEZLOCILLIN

MECHANISM

Same as penicillin. β-Lactamase-sensitive.

USES

- Extended spectrum for gram-negative rods, including *Pseudomonas*.
- Synergistic with aminoglycosides against *Pseudomonas*.

SIDE EFFECTS

Hypersensitivity; interference with platelet function can cause bleeding.

CLAVULANIC ACID, SULBACTAM

MECHANISM

Binds to β-lactamase and prevents its binding and destruction of the β-lactam ring on susceptible penicillins.

USES

- Expands the spectrum of activity for antibiotics that are susceptible to β-lactamases.
- Used in combination with pencillin, ampicillin, and ticarcillin.
- Confers activity against gram-positive cocci *S. aureus*, anerobe *B. fragilis*, and gram-negative rods *H. influenzae* and Klebsiella.

SIDE EFFECTS

None

CEPHALOSPORINS

MECHANISM

Same as penicillin.

USE

- First-generation (**cefazolin, cephalexin**): Gram-positive cocci; *P. mirabilis*, *E. coli*, *K. pneumoniae*. β-lactamase-sensitive.
- Second-generation (**cefotetan, cefuroxime**): Gram-positive cocci; extended gram-negative coverage includes *H. influenzae*, *Enterobacter*, Neisseria, *P. mirabilis*, *E. coli*, Klebsiella, *S. marcescens*. Moderate β-lactamase resistance.
- Third-generation (**cefoperazone, ceftazidime, ceftriaxone**): Broad-spectrum gram-negative coverage; most cross blood-brain barrier and are commonly used for treatment of meningitis and sepsis.
  - Ceftazidime for Pseudomonas.
  - Ceftriaxone for gonorrheal infections.
  - *N. meningitides*.
- Fourth-generation (**cefepime**): Increased activity against Pseudomonas and gram-positive cocci due to increased resistance to β-lactamase.

SIDE EFFECTS

Hypersensitivity; 10%–15% of patients with penicillin allergy have cross-reactivity with cephalosporins; increases aminoglycoside nephrotoxicity; cephalosporins containing a methylthiotetrazole group (cefotetan, cefoperazone) can cause disulfiram-like reaction with ethanol and increased risk of bleeding; cefaclor and cefalexin can cause a serum sickness–like reaction.

KEY FACT

Other antipseudomonal antibiotics include third- and fourth-generation cephalosporins, aztreonam, and imipenem.

MNEMONIC

*Organisms covered by first-generation cephalosporins—***PEcK**

P. *mirabilis*
E. *coli*
K*lebsiella*

MNEMONIC

*Organisms covered by second-generation cephalosporins—***HEN PEcKS**

H*aemophilus influenzae*
E*nterobacter*
N*eisseria*
P*roteus mirabilis*
E. *coli*
K*lebsiella*
S*erratia marcescens*

KEY FACT

Enterococci are resistant to all cephalosporins.

AZTREONAM

MECHANISM

Monobactam, same as penicillin.

USES

- Gram-negative rods, including Pseudomonas.
- No activity against gram-positive organisms or anaerobes.
- β-lactamase-resistant.
- Reserved for infections that are resistant to other antibiotics and for patients who cannot tolerate pencillins or aminoglycosides.
- Safe in pregnancy.

SIDE EFFECTS

Rash, GI distress, fevers, phlebitis, no penicillin cross-reactivity.

IMIPENEM/CILASTATIN, MEROPENEM

MECHANISM

Carbapenem, same as penicillin.

USES

- Broad-spectrum against gram-positives, gram-negatives, and anaerobes.
- Drugs of choice for *Enterobacter*.
- Effective against all bacteria except methicillin-resistant *S. aureus* (MRSA) and vancomycin-resistant enterococci (VRE).
- β-lactamase–resistant.
- Used with **cilastatin,** a renal dihydropeptidase inhibitor that decreases the metabolism of imipenem in the kidneys.
- **Meropenem** is degraded by renal dihydropeptidase and does not cause seizures.

SIDE EFFECTS

Hypersensitivity and rash; GI distress; drug fever; seizures at high serum levels, especially in patients with renal dysfunction; cross-reactivity with penicillin.

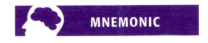

MNEMONIC

Make imipenem **EVER LASTIN'** with ci**LASTATIN.**

Peptidoglycan Synthesis Inhibitors

VANCOMYCIN

MECHANISM

Bactericidal. Prevents polymerization of peptidoglycans by binding D-alanine-D-alanine moiety of cell wall precursors and preventing the addition of murein units to the growing polymer chain.

RESISTANCE

Acquisition of an enzyme that changes D-alanine-D-alanine precursors to D-alanine-D-lactate precursors. This is the mode of resistance in vancomycin-resistant enterococcus.

USES

- Effective against all gram-positives but reserved for multidrug-resistant bacteria such as methicillin-resistant *S. aureus* (MRSA)
- Used orally for pseudomembranous colitis caused by *C. difficile,* along with metronidazole.

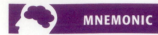
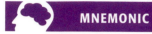
SIDE EFFECTS

Flushing caused by rapid infusion due to histamine release (red man syndrome); nephrotoxicity; ototoxicity; thrombophlebitis. Decreased dosage is needed for patients with renal dysfunction.

BACITRACIN

MECHANISM

Inhibits peptidoglycan precursors from being transported across the bacterial cell membrane.

USES

- Topical antibiotic for wound irrigation.
- Covers gram-positive bacteria.

SIDE EFFECTS

Nephrotoxicity prevents systemic use.

Drugs that Disrupt the Bacterial Cell Membrane

POLYMYXIN

MECHANISM

Polymyxins are basic proteins that act like detergents. They bind to and disrupt the cell membrane of gram-negative bacteria.

USES

- Resistant gram-negative infections.
- Resistant Pseudomonas in cystic fibrosis.

SIDE EFFECTS

When given systemically: Nephrotoxicity and neurotoxicity.

Nucleotide Synthesis Inhibitors

SULFONAMIDES (SULFAMETHOXAZOLE, SULFADIAZINE, SULFADOXINE, TRISULFAPYRIMIDINES)

MECHANISM

Bacteriostatic, synergistic with trimethoprim and pyrimethamine. PABA analogs inhibit **dihydropteroate synthetase,** the enzyme essential for synthesis of folate in bacteria. As a result, synthesis of purines, thymidine, and certain amino acids is impaired (see Figure 5-78).

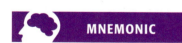
USES

- Treatment in combination for *Nocardia*.
- *Toxoplasma*.
- Used with trimethoprim (TMP-SMX) for uncomplicated UTIs, *Salmonella*, *Shigella*, Serratia, *Pneumocystis jirovecii* (PCP).
- Sulfadiazine—silver ointment for burn infection.

SIDE EFFECTS

Hemolytic anemia in glucose-6-phosphate dehydrogenase (G6PD) deficiency; kernicterus in neonates; hypersensitivity (including Stevens-Johnson syndrome); photosensitivity; interstitial nephritis.

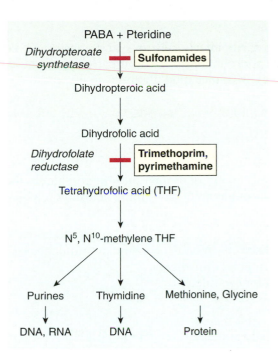

FIGURE 5-78. **Inhibitors of the folate pathway.**

TRIMETHOPRIM, PYRIMETHAMINE

MECHANISM

Bacteriostatic, synergistic with sulfonamides. Folic acid analog that inhibits dihydrofolate reductase (**DHFR**) and decreases synthesis of purines, thymine, and certain amino acids (see Figure 5-79).

USES

- Trimethoprim: See Sulfonamides.
- Pyrimethamine: Used with sulfadiazine to treat parasitic infections such as toxoplasmosis.

SIDE EFFECTS

Bone marrow suppression; GI distress; pruritus; rash.

DNA Topoisomerase Inhibitors

FLUOROQUINOLONES (CIPROFLOXACIN, NORFLOXACIN, OFLOXACIN, GATIFLOXACIN)

MECHANISM

Bactericidal. Inhibit DNA gyrase (topoisomerase II) and topoisomerase IV, two bacterial enzymes that unwind, sever, and re-anneal DNA during replication and transcription.

USES

- Gram-negative rods that cause UTIs and gastroenteritis (including Pseudomonas).
- N. gonorrhoeae
- Mycobacteria
- Atypicals such as Mycoplasma and Legionella.
- Some gram-positive bacteria.

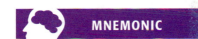

Trimethoprim (**TMP**): **T**reats **M**arrow **P**oorly.

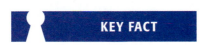

Marrow suppression caused by folate deficiency can be treated with folinic acid.

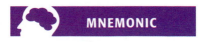

All **FL**uoroquinolones end in –**FL**oxacin.

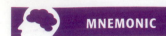
SIDE EFFECTS

GI distress; rash; CNS effects (seizures and insomnia); contraindicated in pregnant women and children because it causes cartilage damage; tendinitis and tendon rupture in adults; mild photosensitivity; prolonged QT interval.

Protein Synthesis Inhibitors at the 50S Ribosomal Subunit

CHLORAMPHENICOL

MECHANISM

Bacteriostatic. Binds to 50S ribosomal subunit and blocks the proper positioning of tRNA and the addition of new amino acids to the polypeptide chain.

USES

- Meningitis caused by meningococcus, pneumococcus, *H. influenzae* in individuals with penicillin allergy.
- Used topically for eye infections.

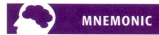
SIDE EFFECTS

Idiosyncratic aplastic anemia; reversible bone marrow suppression; gray baby syndrome (seen in premature infants with immature liver metabolic function). Limited use because of multiple severe toxicities. Crosses blood-brain barrier and placenta.

MACROLIDES (ERYTHROMYCIN, AZITHROMYCIN, CLARITHROMYCIN)

MECHANISM

Bacteriostatic. Binds reversibly to the 50S ribosomal subunit and blocks the translocation step.

USES

Broad spectrum of action. Sexually transmitted diseases (chlamydia, *N. gonorrhea*); pneumonia (*Mycoplasma, Legionella*); streptococcal infection in patients allergic to penicillin; *C. diphtheriae*.

SIDE EFFECTS

GI distress; cholestatic hepatitis; allergy—fever, eosinophilia, rashes.

CLINDAMYCIN, LINCOMYCIN

MECHANISM

Bacteriostatic. Binds the 50S ribosomal subunit and inhibits the aminoacyl translocation step by blocking the growth and release of the growing peptide chain.

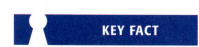
USES

- Narrow spectrum, covers anaerobes in mixed infections.
- Implicated as a causative agent in pseudomembranous colitis due to *C. difficile* infection.
- Drug of choice for anaerobic infections above the diaphragm (*B. fragilis* and *C. perfringens*).
- Safe in pregnancy.

SIDE EFFECTS

Pseudomembranous colitis (*C. difficile* superinfection); GI distress.

LINEZOLID

MECHANISM

Bacteriostatic. Binds to 50S ribosomal subunit and inhibits initiation complex formation.

USES

Effective against methicillin-resistant *S. aureus* (MRSA) and vancomycin-resistant enterococcus (VRE).

SIDE EFFECTS

Same as clindamycin; bone marrow suppression.

QUINUPRISTIN/DALFOPRISTIN

MECHANISM

Bactericidal. This combination of streptogramin antibiotics binds to the 50S ribosomal subunit and inhibits protein synthesis at two successive steps.

USES

Methicillin-resistant *S. aureus* (MRSA) and vancomycin-resistant enterococcus (VRE).

SIDE EFFECTS

Phlebitis; hyperbilirubinemia.

Protein Synthesis Inhibitors at the 30S Ribosomal Subunit

AMINOGLYCOSIDES (GENTAMICIN, NEOMYCIN, AMIKACIN, TOBRAMYCIN, STREPTOMYCIN)

MECHANISM

- Bactericidal.
- Enter bacteria via an O_2-dependent transporter.
- Exert effect by:
  - Inhibits formation of initiation complex.
  - Causes misreading of mRNA resulting in the creation of aberrant proteins.
  - Prevents all protein synthesis at high concentrations.
  - Causes breakup of polysomes.

USES

- Serious gram-negative rod infections.
- Used with β-lactams or vancomycin to treat serious gram-positive infections.
- Neomycin—given in the setting of bowel surgery and hepatic encephalopathy.
- Streptomycin—mycobacteria.
- Spectinomycin—second-line treatment for gonorrhea.

SIDE EFFECTS

Contraindicated in renal insufficiency due to reversible nephrotoxicity (especially when used with cephalosporins); irreversible ototoxicity (especially when used with loop diuretics); nondepolarizing neuromuscular blockade at high concentrations; contraindicated in pregnancy owing to teratogenicity; Fanconi's syndrome; neomycin—GI malabsorption and superinfection.

 KEY FACT

Linezolid is the drug of choice for VRE.

 MNEMONIC

Site of action of protein synthesis inhibitors: Buy **AT 30, CELL** at **50.**
Aminoglycosides and **T**etracyclines inhibit the **30**S ribosomal subunit.
Chloramphenicol, **E**rythromycin, **L**inezolid, and **Cl**indamycin inhibit the **50**S ribosomal subunit.

 MNEMONIC

Acronym for the aminoglycosides:
GNATS.

Gentamicin
Neomycin
Amikacin
Tobramycin
Streptomycin

 KEY FACT

Aminoglycosides are ineffective against anaerobes since O_2 is needed for drug uptake.

 KEY FACT

Aminoglycosides are the only protein synthesis inhibitors that are bactericidal.

MNEMONIC

Organisms covered by tetracyclines. **VACUUM** *your* **BedRooM Tonight.**

V. *cholerae*
Acne
Chlamydia
Ureaplasma **U**realyticum
Mycoplasma *pneumoniae*
Borrelia *burgdorferi*
Rickettsia
Multidrug-resistant **M**alaria
    (*P. falciparum*)
Tularemia

MNEMONIC

Antiprotozoal coverage: **GET** *on the* **Metro** *(nidazole).*

Giardia
Entamoeba
Trichomonas

MNEMONIC

H. pylori treatment. **BAM!** Use these three drugs and *H. pylori* is gone!

Bismuth
Amoxicillin
Metronidazole

MNEMONIC

Antibiotics contraindicated in pregnancy:

SAFE Moms **T**ake **R**eally **G**ood **C**are.

Sulfonamides–kernicterus
Aminoglycosides–ototoxicity
Fluoroquinolones–cartilage damage
Erythromycin–cholestatic hepatitis
    in mother (clarithromycin is
    embryotoxic, *but* azithromycin is
    safe in pregnancy)
Metronidazole–teratogenic
Tetracyclines–fatty liver in mother;
    impaired bone growth, and tooth
    discoloration in baby
Ribavirin (antiviral)–teratogenic
Griseofulvin (antifungal)–teratogenic
Chloramphenicol–gray baby
    syndrome

TETRACYCLINES (TETRACYCLINE, DOXYCYCLINE, MINOCYCLINE, DEMECLOCYCLINE)

MECHANISM

Bacteriostatic. Inhibit the 30S ribosomal subunit by preventing attachment of the aminoacyl-tRNA to the ribosome. Must be imported through the inner cytoplasmic membrane via an energy-dependent active transport system present in bacteria but not humans.

USES

Broad-spectrum: *V. cholerae*, acne, *Chlamydia*, *Ureaplasma urealyticum*, *Mycoplasma pneumoniae*, *Borrelia burgdorferi*, *Rickettsia*, multidrug-resistant malaria (*P. falciparum*), tularemia.

- Second line after penicillin for syphilis.

SIDE EFFECTS

- GI distress; tooth discoloration and bone growth abnormalities in young children; photosensitivity; fatty liver disease in women. Drugs past expiration date can cause Fanconi's syndrome (dysfunction of renal electrolyte reabsorption).
- Minocycline—reversible vestibular toxicity.
- Demeclocycline—used to treat syndrome of inappropriate antidiuretic hormone (SIADH) because it causes nephrogenic diabetes insipidus.

Drugs that Act Via Toxic Metabolites

METRONIDAZOLE

MECHANISM

Bactericidal. Bioactivation of the drug in aerobic environments produces toxic metabolites that react with bacterial DNA, protein, and bacterial and protozoal cell membranes.

USES

- Drug of choice for pseudomembranous colitis (due to *C. difficile*).
- Anaerobic infections below the diaphragm.
- Antiprotozoal: *Giardia, Entamoeba, Trichomonas*.
- Used with bismuth and amoxicillin (or tetracycline) for *H. pylori* "triple therapy."

SIDE EFFECTS

Headache; nausea; metallic taste in mouth; disulfiram-like reactions with ethanol; teratogen. Patients should be cautioned not to drink alcohol while taking metronidazole.

Antibacterial Coverage

Table 5-51 illustrates the spectrum of coverage for the antibacterial drugs. It is provided as a reference and is not meant to be memorized! Unless otherwise noted, all drugs within the same class have the same coverage. For example, nafcillin has the same coverage as oxacillin and methicillin.

Antimycobacterial Drugs

Other than dapsone, which is used to treat leprosy and *Pneumocystis jirovecii* (PCP), all antimycobacterial agents in this section are used to treat tuberculosis. Isoniazid is used for prophylaxis in addition to treatment of active infection. Figure 5-79 illustrates the mechanism of action of the antimycobacterial drugs, with the exception of pyrazinamide.

TABLE 5-51. Antibiotic Coverage

Drugs	\	Gram-Positive Bacteria						\	Gram-Negative Bacteria						\	Anaerobes	
	S. epidermidis	S. aureus	Listeria	Group B strep	Enterococcus	S. pneumoniae	Group A strep	N. meningitidis	H. influenzae	E. coli	Klebsiella	Enterobacter	Serratia	Pseudomonas	Mouth	Gut	B. fragilis
Penicillin			■	■	■	■	■	■							■		
Nafcillin	■	■	■	■	■	■	■	■									
Ampicillin			◆	■	◆	■	■	■	■								
Ticarcillin			■	■	■	■	■	■	■	■	■	■	■	■	■	■	■
Cephalosporins (1st gen.)	■	■	■	■	■	■	■	■	■	■	■						
Cephalosporins (2nd gen.)	■	■	■	■	■	■	■	■	■	■	■	■			*	*	*
Cephalosporins (3rd gen.)	■	■	■	■	■	■	■	■	■	■	■	■	■	■			
Cephalosporins (4th gen.)	■	■	■	■	■	■	■	■	■	■	■	■	■	■			
Aztreonam											■	■		■			
Imipenem		■	■	■	■	■	■	■	■	■	■	◆	■	■	■		■
Vancomycin	■	■	■	■	■	■	■									■	
Gentamicin					■					■	■	■	■	■			
Tobramycin					■					■	■	■	■	■			
Amikacin										■	■	■	■	■			
Erythromycin	■	■	■	■		■	■										
Clindamycin	■	■	■			■	■								◆	■	◆
Azithromycin	■	■	■			■	■	■	■						■	■	■
Tetracycline				■		■	■			■	■	■	■	■			
Chloramphenicol						■		■	■								■

■, coverage; ◆, drug of choice; *Cefotetan.

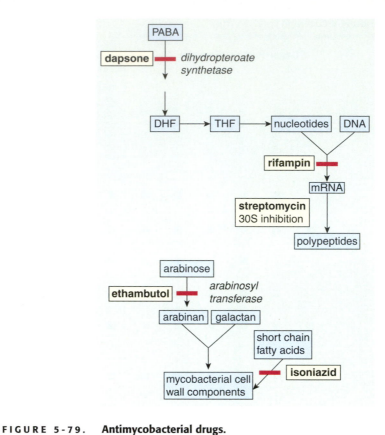

FIGURE 5-79. Antimycobacterial drugs.

DAPSONE

MECHANISM

PABA analog that inhibits dihydropteroate synthase. Humans don't synthesize folate de novo, so this drug is highly specific for microorganisms.

USES

- *M. leprae* (leprosy).
- *Pneumocystis* pnemonia prophylaxis and treatment.

SIDE EFFECTS

Hemolysis in patients with G6PD deficiency; methemoglobinemia.

RIFAMPIN

MECHANISM

Bactericidal against both intracellular and extracellular bacteria. Blocks mRNA synthesis by inhibiting DNA-dependent RNA polymerase.

USES

- *M. tuberculosis*, as component of combination therapy.
- *M. leprae*, as component of combination therapy.
- Prophylaxis for *H. influenzae* and *N. meningitidis*.

SIDE EFFECTS

Hepatotoxicity; turns urine and tears orange-red.

Isoniazid (INH)

Mechanism

Mycobactericidal. Following activation by mycobacterial enzyme Kat-G, INH inhibits an enzyme needed for the synthesis of mycolic acid, a component of the mycobacterial cell wall.

Uses

- *M. tuberculosis.*
- Only drug to be used alone as prophylaxis against TB.

Side Effects

Hepatitis; hemolysis in G6PD-deficient individuals; SLE-like syndrome; peripheral neuropathy.

Pyrazinamide

Mechanism

Mycobactericidal. A prodrug that is activated by a mycobacterial enzyme. It inhibits the synthesis of fatty acid precursors of mycolic acid.

Use

M. tuberculosis.

Side Effects

Hepatitis; asymptomatic hyperuricemia; arthralgias.

Ethambutol

Mechanism

Mycobacteriostatic. Inhibits arabinosyl transferase, an enyzme required for synthesis of arabinogalactan, a component of the mycobacterial cell wall.

Uses

Used in combination to treat *M. tuberculosis* and *M. avium-intracellulare.*

Side Effects

Hepatotoxicity; optic neuritis.

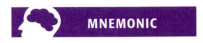

MNEMONIC

INH

Injures **N**eurons and **H**epatocytes

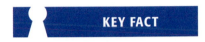

KEY FACT

Give pyridoxine (vitamin B_6) with INH to prevent neurotoxicity.

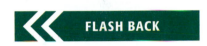

FLASH BACK

Fast acetylators degrade INH faster than slow acetylators.

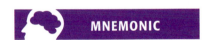

MNEMONIC

Ethambuto**L**: Affects **E**yes and **L**iver.

ANTIFUNGALS

Antifungal drugs target several sites critical to fungal viability and replication (see Figure 5-80 and Table 5-52).

Azoles (Ergosterol Synthesis Inhibitors)

Mechanism

Disrupt permeability of the fungal membrane by inhibiting ergosterol synthesis and incorporation into fungal membranes. Ergosterol is unique to fungi, and is a cholesterol molecule necessary for membrane stability.

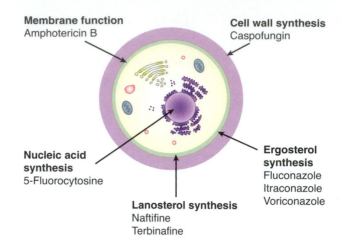

FIGURE 5-80. Fungal components targeted by antifungals.

USES

Systemic mycoses.
- Clotrimazole and miconazole are topical, and thus used for fungal skin infections.
- Fluconazole is used to treat cryptococcal meningitis in AIDS patients and all *Candida* infections.
- Ketoconazole is used for *Blastomyces, Coccidioides, Histoplasma, candida albicans* and hypercortisolism.

SIDE EFFECTS

Ketoconazole inhibits androgen and cortisol synthesis in the adrenal cortex, leading to gynecomastia in men, liver dysfunction secondary to inhibition of the cytochrome P-450 system (drug interactions).

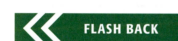

Ketoconazole may be used to treat Cushing's syndrome because it inhibits synthesis of cortisol in the adrenal gland.

TABLE 5-52. Antifungal Drugs

DRUG	MECHANISM	INDICATIONS FOR USE	SIDE EFFECTS
Azoles	Ergosterol synthesis inhibitors	Systemic mycoses.	Inhibition of cytochrome P-450
Terbinafine	Blocks fungal cell wall synthesis	Dermatophytoses.	
Flucytosine	Antimetabolite	Used with amphotericin to treat systemic mycoses.	Bone marrow suppression
Amphotericin, nystatin	Pore-forming	Systemic mycoses, oral candidiasis.	Nephrotoxicity
Caspofungin	Cell wall synthesis inhibitors	Invasive aspergellosis.	GI upset, flushing
Griseofulvin	Mitosis inhibitor	Dermatophytes.	Teratogenic, bone marrow suppression

Terbinafine (Fungal Squalene Peroxidase Inhibitor)

MECHANISM

Blocks fungal cell wall synthesis by blocking synthesis of precursor to ergosterol.

USES

Preferred treatment of dermatophytoses, especially onychomycosis because it accumulates in nails.

SIDE EFFECTS

Not metabolized by P-450 and therefore little potential for drug interactions.

Flucytosine (Antimetabolite)

MECHANISM

Inhibits DNA synthesis by conversion to fluorouracil, which competes with uracil.

USES

Treatment of systemic mycoses

SIDE EFFECTS

Bone marrow suppression, leading to leukopenia and thrombocytopenia, is a common side effect of the antimetabolites.

KEY FACT

In AIDS patients, do not treat fungal infections with flucytosine because bone marrow suppression may exacerbate the immunocompromised state.

AMPHOTERICIN B, NYSTATIN (Pore-Forming)

MECHANISM

Bind to ergosterol, thereby disrupting the fungal membrane and generating pores that allow leakage of electrolytes and disruption of homeostasis, causing lysis.

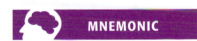

MNEMONIC

Ampho*terrible* "tears" holes in the fungal membrane by forming pores.

USES

- Amphotericin B—systemic mycoses. May be administered intrathecally for fungal meningitis (it does not cross blood-brain barrier).
- Nystatin—swish and swallow for oral candidiasis (there is no oral absorption).
- May be used topically for diaper rash or vaginal candidiasis.

SIDE EFFECTS

"Shake and Bake" fever and chills; nephrotoxicity measured as a reversible increase in BUN:creatinine ratio, along with increased excretion of metabolites (less when using lipid variant); arrhythmias.

Caspofungin (Cell Wall Synthesis Inhibitors)

USES

Invasive aspergillosis.

SIDE EFFECTS

GI upset, flushing.

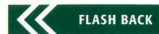
MNEMONIC

Griseofulvin: A greasy ol' fulcrum that prys the nail dermatophytes off.

◀◀ FLASH BACK

Recall that drugs that inhibit growth but do not primarily kill organisms are referred to as bacteriostatic drugs. Griseofulvin is an example.

KEY FACT

Corticosteroids must be given with albendazole in the treatment of cysticercosis to reduce symptoms resulting from the degenerating cysts, which typically elicit a strong host immune response.

Griseofulvin (Mitosis Inhibitors)

MECHANISM

Inhibits growth of dermatophytes by interfering with microtubule function and thereby disrupting mitoses. The drug concentrates in the stratum corneum in keratin-containing tissues (e.g., nails).

USES

Oral treatment of superficial infections. Represents a slow cure because it relies on keratin cells to divide—the fungus is shed along with the keratinized stratified squamous epithelium.

SIDE EFFECTS

Teratogenic, carcinogenic, increased warfarin metabolism (resulting in decreased INR), and bone marrow suppression.

ANTIPARASITICS

The antiparasitic class of drugs is best learned by determining the stage of the life cycle the parasite, in addition to the type of parasitic infection (see Table 5-53).

Antihelminthics

ALBENDAZOLE

MECHANISM

Prevents polymerization of parasite microtubules by inhibiting fumarate reductase.

USES

Cestode (tapeworm) infections in which the patient is an intermediate host (parasite in larval state migrates through patient)—*Taenia solium* neurocysticercosis, *Echinococcus* hydatid disease.

SIDE EFFECTS

Mild GI side effects.

PRAZIQUANTEL

MECHANISM

Blocks voltage-gated calcium channels, causing increased calcium influx into the helminth, which causes severe spasms and paralysis of the worms' muscles.

USES

Cestode, trematode (flukes) infections in which the patient is a definitive host (sexually mature helminth-laying eggs). Examples include *Taenia solium* contracted by ingesting undercooked pork tapeworm, schistosomiasis, clonorchiasis, *Paragonimus westermani*.

SIDE EFFECTS

Bloody diarrhea, GI discomfort.

TABLE 5-53. Antiparasitic Agents

Drug Name	Mechanism	Indications	Side Effects
Albendazole	Inhibits polymerization of parasitic microtubules.	Neurocysticercosis, echinococcus hydatid disease, cestode.	
Praziquantel	Blocks voltage-gated calium channels.	Cestode, trematode.	Bloody diarrhea.
Mebendazole/ pyrantel pomoate	Blocks glucose absorption, paralysis worms.	Intestinal nematode.	
Thiabendazole		Strongyloides, trichinosis.	Hallucinations, severe diarrhea, nausea/vomiting, numbness/ tingling hands or feet.
Ivermectin	Paralysis and kills offspring of adult nematode.	In combination with thiabendazole.	Arthralgias.
Diethylcarbamazine	Effective against microfilarial diseases.		Swelling/itching face, loss of vision and arthralgias with long-term use.
Metronidazole	Forms toxic metabolites in bacterial cell making it bactericidal.	*Gardnerella vaginalis* (bacterial vaginitis), Giardiasis, *Entamoeba histolytica* (amebic dysentery), *Trichomonas vaginalis*, anaerobes (*Bacteroides, Clostridium*).	Disulfiram-like reaction with alcohol, headache, metallic taste.
Chloroquine	Generates toxic heme byproducts that kill the parasite within infected RBCs.	Prophylaxis and treatment of malaria.	Severe hemolysis in G6PD-deficient patients, blurred vision.
Quinine		Prophylaxis and treatment for malaria.	Cinchonism (tinnitus, deafness), proarrhythmic, hemoloysis in G6PD-deficient patients; hypoglycemia.
Mefloquine		Prophylaxis and treatment of malaria, chloroquine-resistant malaria.	Mood changes, suicidality, unusual dreams.
Atovaquine and proguanil	Proguanil has synergy with atovaquine.	Prophylaxis and treatment of malaria, chloroquine-resistant malaria, treatment *Pneumocystis carinii* pneumonia.	Fever, skin rash.
Nifurtimox		Chagas' disease caused by *Trypanosoma cruzi*.	

(continues)

TABLE 5-53. Antiparasitic Agents *(continued)*

DRUG NAME	MECHANISM	INDICATIONS	SIDE EFFECTS
Suramin, melarsoprol	Act to deplete *T. gambiense and rhodiense* of energy by inactivating pyruvate kinase causing inhibition of ATP synthesis leading to their death.	African sleeping sickness (suramin when blood, melarsoprol when CNS); suramin also for river blindness.	Stinging sensation on skin.
Sodium stibogluconate/ pentavalent antimony		Leishmaniasis.	
Sulfadiazine + pyrimethamine	Pyrimethamine interrupts folate synthesis by inhibiting dihydrofolate reductase synergizing with sulfadiazine inhibition of dihydropteroate synthetase, thereby preventing DNA, RNA synthesis.	Toxoplasmosis, malaria.	Folate deficiency; therefore, add leucovorin (folate supplement that does not rely on dihydrofolate reductase) to drug regimen.

RBC = red blood cell; CNS = central nervous system.

MEBENDAZOLE/PYRANTEL PAMOATE

MECHANISM

Mebendazole prevents glucose absorption by the nematode eventually causing loss of energy and death of the worm. Pyrantel pamoate paralyzes the nematodes.

USES

Intestinal nematode infections.
- **Fecal-oral transmission**—*Enterobius vermicularis* (pinworm), trichuriasis (whipworm).
- **Fecal-oral + lung migration**—*Ascaris lumbricoides* (giant roundworm).
- **Skin penetration + lung migration**—*Ancylostoma duodenale* (hookworm).

SIDE EFFECTS

GI complaints.

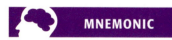

MNEMONIC

The "**thi**gh" (**thi**abendazole) is (used to treat) the **strong**est muscle **(Strongyloides).** No need for corticosteroids prior to treatment of **Strongyloides** with thiabendazole.

THIABENDAZOLE

USES

Skin penetration + lung migration
- *Strongyloides stercoralis* infections.
- Trichinosis (pork worms), *Toxocara canis* (cutanea larval migrans) and toxocariasis (visceral larval migrans).

SIDE EFFECTS

Hallucinations, severe diarrhea, nausea/vomiting, numbness/tingling in hands or feet.

IVERMECTIN

MECHANISM

Acts to paralyze and kill offspring of adult nematodes.

USES

In combination with thiabendazole for strongyloidiasis, onchocerciasis (river blindness).

SIDE EFFECTS

Arthralgias, painful glands neck, groin, tachycardia, ocular irritation.

DIETHYLCARBAMAZINE

MECHANISM

Effective against microfilaria.

USES

- Bancroft's filariasis (tropical pulmonary eosinophilia).
- Loiasis
- Onchocerciasis (river blindness).
- Toxocariasis

SIDE EFFECTS

Swelling/itching face, loss of vision, and arthralgias with long-term use.

ANTIPROTOZOA

Metronidazole

MECHANISM

Forms toxic metabolites in bacterial cell. Bactericidal.

USES

Gardnerella vaginalis (bacterial vaginitis), giardiasis, *Entamoeba histolytica* (amebic dysentery), *Trichomonas vaginalis*, anaerobes (*Bacteroides, Clostridium*).

SIDE EFFECTS

Disulfiram-like reaction with alcohol, headache, metallic taste.

ANTIMALARIALS

Chloroquine

MECHANISM

Generates toxic heme byproducts that kill the parasite within infected RBCs.

USES

Prophylaxis and treatment of malaria.

SIDE EFFECTS

Severe hemolysis in G6PD-deficient patients, blurred vision.

MNEMONIC

r**IVER** blindness is treated with **IVER**mectin.

FLASH BACK

Metronidazole is used with bismuth and amoxicillin/tetracycline as part of "triple therapy" for *H. pylori*.

MNEMONIC

GGET on the "Metro" to kill anaerobes below diaphragm.

Gardnerella vaginalis.
Giardiasis
Entamoeba histolytica.
Trichomonas vaginalis.

KEY FACT

Disulfiram-like reactions may also occur with chloramphenicol, third-generation cephalosporins, procarbazine, and first-generation sulfonylureas.

FLASH FORWARD

Recall that sulfonamides, isoniazid, aspirin, ibuprofen, nitrofurantoin, and fava beans are other drugs that cause hemolysis in **G6PD**-deficient patients by increasing oxidative stress in RBCs.

KEY FACT

PRIME-time ti**VO**
Primaquine is used to prevent relapse caused by *Plasmodium* **v**ivax and *P.* **o**vale hypnozoites latent in hepatocytes.

Quinine

USES

Prophylaxis and treatment of malaria.

SIDE EFFECTS

Cinchonism (tinnitus, deafness), proarhythmic, hemoloysis in G6PD-deficient patients, hypoglycemia.

Mefloquine

USES

Prophylaxis and treatment of malaria, chloroquine-resistant malaria.

SIDE EFFECTS

Mood changes, suicidality, unusual dreams.

Atovaquine and Proguanil

MECHANISM

Proguanil has synergy with atovaquine.

USES

Prophylaxis and treatment of malaria, chloroquine-resistant malaria, treatment of *Pneumocystis carinii* pneumonia.

SIDE EFFECTS

Fever, skin rash.

Nifurtimox

USES

Chagas' disease caused by *Trypanosoma cruzi*.

Suramin, Melarsoprol

MECHANISM

Inactivate pyruvate kinase, which inhibits ATP synthesis. This depletes *Trypanosoma gambiense and rhodiense* of energy, leading to their death.

USES

African sleeping sickness (suramin used for blood-based infections, melarsoprol for CNS infections), Suramin also for river blindness.

SIDE EFFECTS

Stinging sensation on skin.

Sodium Stibogluconate/Pentavalent Antimony

USES

Leishmaniasis.

Sulfadiazine + Pyrimethamine

MECHANISM

Pyrimethamine interrupts folate synthesis by inhibiting dihydrofolate reductase. Synergistic with sulfadiazine inhibition of dihydropteroate synthetase, thereby preventing DNA and RNA synthesis.

USES

Toxoplasmosis, malaria.

SIDE EFFECTS

Folate deficiency; therefore leucovorin (folate supplement that does not rely on dihydrofolate reductase) is added to drug regimen.

ANTIVIRALS

Understanding which sites are critical to viral activity will help to learn both viral function and how the antiviral agents disrupt viral infection and replication (see Table 5-54 and Figure 5-81).

Anti-influenza

AMANTADINE

MECHANISM

Blocks viral penetration/uncoating, may buffer pH of endosome. Causes the release of dopamine from intact nerve terminals.

USES

Prophylaxis and treatment for influenza A; Parkinson's disease.

SIDE EFFECTS

Ataxia, dizziness, slurred speech, hallucinations (exacerbated by anticholinergics).

ZANAMIVIR, OSELTAMIVIR

MECHANISM

Inhibits influenza neuraminidase.

USES

Shortens symptoms of influenza A and B infection by 1–2 days.

RIBAVIRIN

MECHANISM

Inhibits synthesis of guanine nucleotides by competitively inhibiting inosine monophosphate (IMP) dehydrogenase.

USES

Respiratory syncytial virus, chronic hepatitis C (in combination with IFN-α).

SIDE EFFECTS

Hemolytic anemia, severe teratogen.

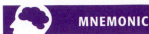

MNEMONIC

A-man-to-dine takes off his **coat**. **Amantadine** blocks viral uncoating.

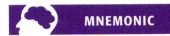

MNEMONIC

Amantadine blocks influenza **A** and rubell**A** and causes problems with the cerebell**a**.

KEY FACT

Rimantidine is a derivative with fewer CNS side effects.

FLASH BACK

Recall that neuraminidase cleaves neuramic acid to disrupt the mucin barrier in the upper respiratory tract. Removal of the mucin coat exposes sialic acid receptors for hemagglutinin binding, promoting viral adsorption.

FLASH BACK

Remember that Influenza A undergoes antigenic shift and infects humans, mammals (swine), and birds, whereas Influenza B infects only humans and therefore undergoes only antigenic *drift*.

FLASH FORWARD

Recall that IFN-α is a leukocyte product that inhibits viral replication.

TABLE 5-54. **Antiviral Drugs**

DRUG NAME	MECHANISM	INDICATIONS FOR USE	SIDE EFFECTS
Amantadine	Blocks viral penetration/uncoating, may buffer pH of endosome.	Prophylaxis and treatment for influenza A; Parkinson's disease.	Ataxia, dizziness, slurred speech, hallucinations (exacerbated by anticholinergics).
Zanamivir, oseltamivir	Inhibits influenza, neuraminidase.	Shortens symptoms from Influenza A and B infection by 1–2 days.	
Ribavirin	Inhibits synthesis of guanine nucleotides by competitively inhibiting inosine monophosphate dehydrogenase.	RSV, chronic hepatitis C (in combination with INF-α).	Hemolytic anemia, severe teratogen.
Acyclovir	Preferentially inhibits viral DNA polymerase when phosphorylated by viral thymidine kinase.	HSV, VZV, EBV. Relieves pain and discomfort of mucocutaneous and genital herpes lesions but does not eradicate the virus. Prophylaxis in immunocompromised patients and prevents recurrent genital herpes infections.	Deliruim, tremor, nephrotoxicity by crystallizing in renal tubules.
Ganciclovir	Phosphorylation by viral kinase, preferentially inhibiting CMV DNA polymerase.	CMV (especially in immunocompromised patients—AIDS, bone marrow transplant patients).	Leukopenia, neutropenia, thrombocytopenia —pancytopenia; renal toxicity; more toxic to host enzymes than acyclovir, impacting rapidly dividing cells.
Protease inhibitors Saquinavir, ritonavir, indinavir, nelfinavir, amprenavir	Inhibit assembly of new virus by blocking HIV protease.		GI intolerance (nausea, diarrhea), hyperglycemia, lipid abnormalities, thrombocytopenia (indinavir).
Nucleosides Zidovu**dine**, (azt), didanosine (**d**di), zalcitabine (**d**dc), stavudine (**d**4t), lamivudine (3tc), abacavir			Lactic acidosis, peripheral neuropathy (d's), megaloblastic anemia (AZT).
Non-nucleosides Nevirapine, delavirdine, efavirenz			Rash.

(continues)

TABLE 5-54.   **Antiviral Drugs** *(continued)*

DRUG NAME	MECHANISM	INDICATIONS FOR USE	SIDE EFFECTS
INF-α	Leukocyte product that inhibits viral replication.	Chronic hepatitis B and C, Kaposi's sarcoma (HHV-8).	All interferon Neutropenia
INF-β	Fibroblast product that inhibits viral replication.	Relapsing multiple sclerosis.	
INF-γ	Released by TH1 cells to stimulate macrophage to destroy phagocytosed contents.	NADPH oxidase deficiency.	

CMV = cytomegalovirus; EBV = Epstein-Barr virus; HSV = herpes simplex virus; VSV = varicella zoster virus.

Antiherpes

ACYCLOVIR

MECHANISM

Preferentially inhibits viral DNA polymerase when phosphorylated by viral thymidine kinase.

USES

HSV, VZV, EBV. Relieves pain and discomfort of mucocutaneous and genital herpes lesions but does not eradicate the virus. Used for prophylaxis in immunocompromised patients, prevents recurrent genital herpes infections.

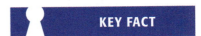

> **KEY FACT**
>
> Because ribavarin is a guanosine analog, it should be avoided in patients with hematologic disorders such as anemia and thalassemia major.

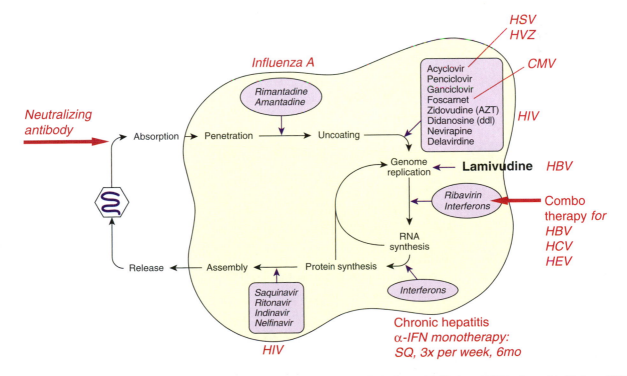

FIGURE 5-81.   **Antiviral agent sites of action.** CMV = cytomegalovirus; HBV = hepatitis B virus; HCV = hepatitis C virus; HEV = hepatitis E virus; HSV = herpes simplex virus; HVZ = herpes varicella zoster; IFN = interferon; SQ = subcutaneously.

FLASH FORWARD

Recall that cytomegalovirus (CMV) lacks thymidine kinase, rendering acyclovir ineffective against CMV infection because it requires activation by viral thymidine kinase.

MNEMONIC

A **"gang of cycles"** running over WBCs and platelets.

MNEMONIC

Never (-**navir**) tease a pro—**pro-tease** inhibitors all end in -navir.

KEY FACT

AZT is used during pregnancy to reduce risk of fetal transmission by first treating the mother, then the baby following delivery. AZT is also given within 72-hours of a needlestick from an HIV-positive patient. Transmission depends on the viral load of the patient and the amount of virus that may have been transmitted.

SIDE EFFECTS

Deliruim, tremor, nephrotoxicity by crystallizing in renal tubules.

GANCICLOVIR

MECHANISM

Phosphorylation by viral kinase, preferentially inhibiting CMV DNA polymerase.

USE

CMV, especially in immunocompromised patients such as those with AIDS, bone marrow transplantation.

SIDE EFFECTS

Pancytopenia (leukopenia, neutropenia, thrombocytopenia). Renal toxicity. More toxic to host enzymes than is acyclovir. Impacts rapidly dividing cells.

HIV Therapy

USE

Highly active antiretroviral therapy (HAART) entails a combination therapy using protease inhibitors and reverse transcriptase inhibitors. Initiated when patients have low CD4 counts (< 500 cells/mm^3).

PROTEASE INHIBITORS

(SAQUINAVIR, RITONAVIR, INDINAVIR, NELFINAVIR, AMPRENAVIR)

MECHANISM

Inhibit assembly of new virus by blocking HIV protease.

SIDE EFFECTS

GI intolerance (nausea, diarrhea), hyperglycemia, lipid abnormalities, thrombocytopenia (indinavir)

REVERSE TRANSCRIPTASE INHIBITORS

MECHANISM

Preferentially inhibit reverse transcriptase of HIV, thereby preventing incorporation of viral genome into host DNA.

SIDE EFFECTS

Bone marrow suppression (neutropenia, anemia) is common to both nucleosides and non-nucleosides.

NUCLEOSIDES

(ZIDOVUDINE [AZT], DIDANOSINE [DDI], ZALCITABINE [DDC], STAVUDINE [D4T], LAMIVUDINE [3TC], ABACAVIR)

SIDE EFFECTS

Lactic acidosis, peripheral neuropathy (ddl, ddC, D4T), megaloblastic anemia (AZT).

Non-Nucleosides (Nevirapine, Delavirdine, Efavirenz)

SIDE EFFECT

Rash.

Interferons

SIDE EFFECT

Neutropenia.

Interferon α

MECHANISM

Leukocyte product that inhibits viral replication.

USES

Chronic hepatitis B and C, Kaposi's sarcoma (HHV-8).

Interferon β

MECHANISM

Fibroblast product that inhibits viral replication.

USE

Relapsing multiple sclerosis.

Interferon-γ

MECHANISM

Released by TH1 cells to stimulate macrophages to destroy phagocytosed contents.

USE

NADPH oxidase deficiency.

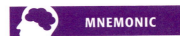

Interferons "interfere" with viral replication.

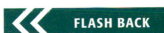

Remember that patients with NADPH oxidase deficiency are defective in generating the oxidative burst necessary to kill phagocytosed organisms—**chronic granulomatous disease.**

ANTIMICROBIAL TABLES

TABLE 5-55. Inhibition of Cell Wall Synthesis (Peptidoglycan/PG Biosynthesis)

Antibiotic	Binding Site	Mechanism of Action	Bactericidal or Bacteriostatic	Bacteria Affected	Advantages	Disadvantages
Inhibition of soluble enzymes located in cytoplasm (must get inside the bacteria to work)–blocking PG formation						
Fosfomycin	Active site of pyruvyl transferase.	PEP structural analog. Blocks PG synthesis (UDP-MurNAc formation).	Bactericidal	Broad spectrum.		High-frequency, single-dose resistance. Limited to UTIs.
D-Cycloserine	Active site of alanine racemase and D-alanine synthetase.	Competitive inhibitor of alanine racemase and D-alanine synthetase. Blocks PG synthesis (UDP-MurNAc pentapeptide formation).	Bacteriostatic	Broad spectrum.	Rigid ring structure causes high-affinity bonding to enzymes.	Neurotoxic side effects. Limited to TB and UTI.
Inhibition of membrane-bound enzymes (must get through peptidoglycan layer to work) blocking transpeptidation (cross-linking) of PG						
Vancomycin	D-Alanyl-D-alanine residues on pentapeptide.	Blocks GCL formation. Steric hindrance prevents precursor binding to synthetase. Binding occurs on *outer face,* after GCL translocation across membrane.	Bactericidal	Gram-positive (esp. staphylococci and enterococci).	NOT degraded by β-lactamase.	Resistance emerges when target (D-ala-D-ala) residue is modified.
Bacitracin	Lipid pyrophosphate of GCL-PP.	Blocks GCL formation on *outer face.* Final step of GCL synthesis (blocks dephosphorylation of GCL-PP → GCL-P).	Bactericidal	Gram-positive (esp. staphylococci).	*Not degraded by β-lactamase.*	Topical use only.

Antibiotic	Binding Site	Mechanism of Action	Bactericidal or Bacteriostatic	Bacteria Affected	Advantages	Disadvantages
β-Lactam antibiotics Penicillins Cephalosporins Cephamycins Carbapenems Monobactams	Terminal D-ala-D-ala-COOH region of pentapeptide.	Inhibit transpeptidases. Substrate analogs of terminal D-ala-D-ala-COOH region of pentapeptide.	Bactericidal	Older: Narrow spectrum, gram-positive. Newer: Broad-spectrum, gram-negative and *Pseudomonas aeruginosa.*	Very effective acylating agents for active sites of multiple transpeptidase enzymes (penicillin-binding proteins or PBPs). Activates autolytic enzymes that degrade old peptidoglycan.	Kills only *growing* cells (i.e., when crosslinking in progress). Can cause hypersensitivity reactions (anaphylaxis). Degraded by β-lactamase (penicillinase); cleavage of β-lactam ring inactivates drug. Most have to be administered with a β-lactamase inhibitor.

Bacteriostatic → microorganisms can overcome inhibition of cell wall synthesis by using an excess of D-alanine.

Murein is the principle PG layer, forming the rigid cell wall of most bacteria (except mycoplasma, and L-form mutants.).

GCL is a carrier molecule that anchors intermediates to the cytoplasmic membrane and facilitates their translocation from the cytoplasmic face of membrane to the outer face. Blocking its formation prevents the cell from completing synthesis of the cell wall.

GCL = glycosyl carrier lipid; PEP = phosphoenolpyruvate; PG = peptidoglycan TB = tuberculosis; UTI = urinary tract infection.

TABLE 5-56. Inhibition of Protein Synthesis

Inhibition of recognition step in polypeptide chain synthesis—all drugs act on 30S subunit

Antibiotic	Binding Site	Mechanism of Action	Bactericidal or Bacteriostatic	Bacteria Affected	Advantages and Basis for Selectivity	Disadvantages and Sources of Resistance
Streptomycin and aminoglycosides (gentamicin, tobramycin, kanamycin, etc.)	Specific proteins on 30S subunit. Strep. = S12 (no common site). Newer aminoglycosides target two proteins (30S & 50S).	**Misreading** of mRNA due to distortions of codons in recognition region of A-site. Cyclic polysomal blockade → kills by *destabilizing* 70S initiation complex (does *not* block formation).	Bactericidal	Broad spectrum (esp. gram-negative but also gram-positive).	Target binding sites absent in host. Streptomycin actively transported into bacterial cells and *not* human cells (selective toxicity). Newer aminoglycosides less susceptible to resistance (can't occur in single step).	*Older aminoglycosides:* High-frequency, single-dose resistance develops when target protein mutates. Nephrotoxicity and ototoxicity. Ineffective against intracellular bacteria (*Chlamydia, Rickettsia*). Ineffective against anaerobes (transport into microbe requires O_2).
Tetracyclines	30S subunit (specific target not known).	Inhibits aa-tRNA binding to A-site.	Bacteriostatic	Broad spectrum (*Chlamydia, Mycoplasma, Rickettsia,* other select gram +/−).	Active transport into bacterial cells and *not* human cells (some still gets in). Useful against intracellular microorganisms (hydrophobic).	Resistance develops by decreased entry into microbe, **active efflux** out, or **elongation factor** proteins that protect 30S subunit.
Spectinomycin	30S subunit.	Formation of unstable 70S complex only.	Bacteriostatic	Narrow spectrum.		Treat **gonorrhea** only.

Antibiotic	Binding Site	Mechanism of Action	Bactericidal or Bacteriostatic	Bacteria Affected	Advantages and Basis for Selectivity	Disadvantages and Sources of Resistance
Inhibition of peptidyl transfer step in polypeptide chain synthesis—both drugs act on 50S subunit						
Chloramphenicol	50S subunit. Preformed polysomes.	Alters P-site tRNA, blocking peptidyl transfer.	Bacteriostatic	Broad spectrum.	Unable to enter mitochondria (host).	Resistance by plasmid-encoded acetylation of tRNA or porin mutation.
Lincomycin and clindamycin	50S subunit. Only ribosomes w/*very short* polypeptide chains.	Similar to chloramphenicol (blocks peptidyl transfer).	Bacteriostatic	Narrow spectrum Gram-positive bacteria (both). Clindamycin w/ staphylococci and anaerobic gram-negative bacteria.	Esp. effective against *Bacteriodes* genus. Effective against anaerobic bacteria.	Resistance develops owing to methylation of 23S ribosomal RNA (also causes resistance to erythromycin).
Drugs that inhibit translocation step in polypeptide chain synthesis						
Erythromycin and other macrolides (azithromycin, clarithromycin).	50S subunit. L15 and L16 proteins.	Prevents ejection of tRNA from P-site after transfer. Prevents peptidyl-tRNA from returning to P-site from A site.	Bacteriostatic	Medium spectrum (*Legionella, Chlamydia, Camphylobacter*).		Resistance develops owing to methylation of 23S ribosomal RNA (also causes resistance to clindamycin). Hydrolysis of macrolide lactone ring and active efflux.

TABLE 5-57. Inhibition of Nucleic Acid Synthesis

ANTIBIOTIC	BINDING SITE	MECHANISM OF ACTION	BACTERICIDAL OR BACTERIOSTATIC	ORGANISM AFFECTED	ADVANTAGES	DISADVANTAGES
Drugs that inhibit precursor synthesis						
Sulfonamides	Active site of dihydropteroic acid synthetase.	Competitive inhibitor of dihydropteroic acid synthetase (inhibits folate synthesis). Structural analog of PABA.	Bacteriostatic	Broad spectrum. Bacterial and some parasitic infections.	Synergistic when used with trimethoprim.	Inhibits only *new* synthesis of tetrahydrofolic acid. Inhibition can be overcome by excess of PABA.
Trimethoprim	Active site of dihydrofolate reductase.	Competitive inhibitor of dihydrofolate reductase (inhibits folate synthesis). Structural analog of pteridine ring of dihydrofolic acid.	Bacteriostatic	Broad spectrum.	Synergistic when used with sulfonamides. Bacterial enzyme has much higher affinity for drug than for host.	Inhibits only *existing* pools of dihydrofolate.
Para-aminosalicylic acid (PAS)		Akin to sulfonamide. Competitive inhibitor of dihydrofolate reductase (inhibits folate synthesis).	Bacteriostatic	Broad, but different from sulfonamides. Effective against *Mycobacterium tuberculosis.*		

Antibiotic	Binding Site	Mechanism of Action	Bactericidal or Bacteriostatic	Organism Affected	Advantages	Disadvantages
Drugs that inhibit RNA synthesis						
Rifampin and rifabutin	β-Subunit of DNA-dependent RNA polymerase.	Inhibits mRNA synthesis. Inhibits *initiation* of transcription (but not ongoing transcription).	Bactericidal	Narrow spectrum (gram-positive bacteria, *Neisseria*, mycobacteria). Rifabutin for *Mycobacterium avium* infection.	Host RNA polymerase not sensitive to drug. Mitochondria RNA-sensitive but impermeable.	Does not inhibit transcription already in progress.
Drugs that inhibit DNA synthesis						
Quinolones (nalidixic acid, ciprofloxacin, norfloxacin, etc.)	DNA gyrase (topoisomerase).	Inhibit DNA gyrase (topoisomerase) of prokaryotic organisms only.	Bactericidal	Nalidixic acid narrow-spectrum; gram-negative. Newer quinolones broad-spectrum and *Pseudomonas*.	Newer quinolones effective against *Pseudomonas* spp.	*Pseudomonas* develops resistance rapidly. Resistance by altering gyrase subunit structure. Resistance by altering porins of gram-negative bacteria.

TABLE 5-58.   **Alteration of Cell Membranes**

ANTIBIOTIC	BINDING SITE	MECHANISM OF ACTION	BACTERICIDAL OR BACTERIOSTATIC	BACTERIA AFFECTED	ADVANTAGES	DISADVANTAGES
Polymyxins and colistin (polymyxin E)	Hydrophobic tail inserts into cell membranes. Hydrophilic head (a cyclic polypeptide) binds PE and LPS.	Binding disrupts cytoplasmic membrane, causes loss of inner components and cell death. Pore also creates leak in cells.	Bactericidal	Narrow spectrum (gram-negative).	UTIs caused by pseudomonads that do not respond to other antibiotics. Active against growing *and* nongrowing cells. Host cells do not have PE and LPS in their membranes.	Resistance by altering cell membrane (lipid A moiety of LPS).
Amphotericin B and nystatin (polyene antibiotics).	Hydrophobic portion binds ergosterols in fungal membrane.	Inserts into fungal membranes forming a channel/pore into cell.	Fungicidal (*not* effective against bacteria!)	Opportunistic mycoses (i.e., *Candida*, *Aspergillus*, etc.)	IV treatment of systemic mycoses and ointments. Ergosterol targets not in host membranes.	Absorbed poorly in gut. Toxicity (still binds cholesterol, but to lesser extent). Include nausea, anemia, vomiting, diarrhea, nephrotoxicity.

LPS = lipopolysaccarides; PE = phosphatidylethanolamine; UTIs = urinary tract infections.

Immunology

Principles of Immunology

The immune system distinguishes foreign molecules and potential **pathogens** from the body's own cells and removes these pathogens from the body. Cells of the immune system respond to **antigens**, molecular structures (such as peptides) capable of producing an immune response. Infection or autoimmune disease can result from the failure of these processes.

CONCEPTS OF IMMUNITY

Depending on how immune protection is acquired, immune processes can be classified as **passive immunity** or **active immunity**.

Passive Immunity

Protection provided by preformed antibodies from a source outside the body. Exposure to virulent pathogens or toxins can result in serious illness or death if the body's own immune system is unable to mount an adequate response. Preformed antibodies can be administered therapeutically to quickly neutralize the pathogens. However, the antibodies are short-lived, and the body is unable to respond to a subsequent exposure. Some examples of passive immunity include:

- Antibodies in mothers' milk for breast-fed infants
- Administered **antitoxins** for tetanus or botulinum toxins
- Administered **antibodies** to the hepatitis B or rabies virus

Active Immunity

The body's own active mechanisms to fight infection constitute active immunity. In general, active immunity has a slower onset than does passive immunity, but it has the capacity for immune **memory**, which results in a rapid response to a second exposure to a pathogen. Some important components of active immunity include:

- **Lymphocytes** and other immune cells
- Lymphoid organs

Immune processes can also be divided into those that are present at birth (**innate immunity**) and those that require antigen exposure before forming a precise response (**adaptive immunity**).

Innate Immunity

Rapid but nonspecific immunologic processes that recognize and destroy certain common antigens. The protein receptors involved in recognizing these antigens are germ line–encoded, so they do not require prior exposure for shaping the response. However, innate processes have no capacity for memory. Some components of innate immunity include:

- Physical barriers, such as skin and mucous membranes
- Cells, such as **neutrophils, macrophages,** and **dendritic cells**
- The complement system

Adaptive Immunity

The adaptive immune response is highly specific to individual pathogens, but is much slower than innate immunity on first exposure. This response has the capacity for memory. Cells of adaptive immunity have the ability to undergo

KEY FACT

Lymphocytes and their products are the key cells involved in the adaptive response and are responsible for the two key features of adaptive immunity: specificity and memory.

TABLE 6-1.   Subsets of Immunity

	PASSIVE	ACTIVE	INNATE	ADAPTIVE
Source	Outside the body	Within the body.	Within the body	Within the body.
Speed of protection	Rapid	Slow on first exposure, faster on next.	Rapid	Slow on first exposure, faster on next.
Specificity	Specific	Specific.	Nonspecific	Specific.
Memory	No	Yes.	No	Yes.

genetic rearrangements, resulting in a highly specific and powerful response to pathogens. Key components of adaptive immunity include:

- Cellular components, such as T lymphocytes (**cell-mediated immunity**)
- Antibody-producing B lymphocytes (**humoral immunity**)

Table 6-1 summarizes the characteristics of each subset of immunity.

ANATOMY OF THE IMMUNE SYSTEM

The immune system is composed of both primary and secondary lymphoid organs, as summarized in Table 6-2. The primary, or central, lymphoid organs include the bone marrow and thymus and are involved in lymphocyte production and development. The spleen and lymph nodes are considered secondary, or peripheral, lymphoid organs and are important sites of antigen interaction with cells of the immune system.

Bone Marrow

Location of **hematopoiesis**, or production of white and red blood cells. In addition, the development of immune cells occurs in the bone marrow. Some immunodeficiency syndromes, such as severe combined immunodeficiency (SCID), can be treated by bone marrow transplantation, thus providing a source of functional cells to protect the body.

Thymus

Encapsulated primary lymphoid organ located in the anterior mediastinum. It is derived from the third branchial pouch during development and is the site

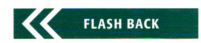
FLASH BACK

Chemotherapy or radiation treatment may result in anemia, leukopenia, and immunosuppression due to bone marrow damage.

TABLE 6-2.   Organs of the Immune System

	ORGAN	FUNCTION
Primary	Bone marrow	Production and maturation of immune cells.
	Thymus	Maturation of T cells.
Secondary	Spleen	Interaction of immune cells with antigen.
	Lymph nodes	Interaction of immune cells with antigen.

of **T-cell differentiation,** maturation, and selection. The thymus increases in size until adolescence, when it begins to involute and accumulate fat.

Following production in the bone marrow, immature T cells migrate to the thymic **cortex** early in their development to undergo the process of positive and negative selection (see Anergy and Tolerance later in chapter). Selection begins as the cells reach the **corticomedullary junction,** and continues as the T cells move into the inner **medulla.** Mature T cells are finally released into the bloodstream and travel to peripheral sites (see Figure 6-1).

Microscopically, the cortex stains darkly owing to the density of lymphocytes. The medulla is lighter, with fewer lymphocytes and a higher concentration of dendritic and epithelial reticular cells. Pale-staining **Hassall's corpuscles** are characteristic of the medulla. These structures contain flat, concentric epithelial cells that have become keratinized; their function is unknown.

Spleen

Secondary lymphoid organ located in the upper left quadrant of the peritoneal cavity. It is attached to the stomach by the **gastrosplenic ligament** and to the posterior abdominal wall by the **splenorenal ligament.** The splenic artery and vein are located within the splenorenal ligament.

The spleen contains many blood-filled sinuses that filter antigens and cells from the blood. Microscopically, the splenic parenchyma is divided into the red and white pulp. The **red pulp** is the location of red blood cell storage and turnover; it contains rich vasculature with fenestrated capillaries to allow blood cells to freely pass through.

The **white pulp** is the location of immune cell interaction. Blood flows into the white pulp through the central arteriole, which is surrounded by a **periarterial lymphatic sheath (PALS)** of T lymphocytes. Follicles of B cells are found more distant from the central arteriole; they have pale germinal centers when B cells are activated. The marginal zone surrounds the PALS and follicle and separates the white and red pulp. Antigen-presenting cells (APCs) in the marginal zone ingest pathogens by phagocytosis and present them to nearby lymphocytes. Blood is drained through the **marginal sinus** located

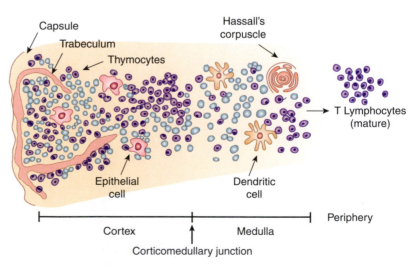

FIGURE 6-1. **Microscopic structure of the thymus.**

within the marginal zone. The microscopic structure of the spleen is shown in Figure 6-2.

Lymph Nodes

Encapsulated secondary lymphoid organs that receive lymph from multiple afferent vessels, thus providing for interaction between the stored immune cells and the lymphatic fluid. The fluid is returned to the lymphatic ducts through the efferent vessel after the antigens and pathogenic cells contained in the fluid encounter APCs, B cells, and T cells.

The microscopic structure of lymph nodes is maximized for antigen recognition and response, as shown in Figure 6-3. **Trabeculae** span the outer capsule into the medulla, separating the cortical **follicles** of B lymphocytes.

- Primary, or inactive, follicles are dense with stored lymphocytes awaiting antigen presentation.
- Secondary, or active, follicles have pale **germinal centers** within the cluster of lymphocytes. Here, B cells proliferate and produce antibodies in response to antigens.

T cells are found in the **paracortex** between the follicles and the medulla. The paracortex may become enlarged in severe infections, such as viral infections, that result in a cellular immune response.

Lymph nodes are supplied by their own capillary system. B and T lymphocytes enter and exit lymph nodes via **high endothelial venules** located in the paracortex. The medullary sinus drains cells and fluid in the medulla into the efferent lymphatic duct. APCs within the sinus filter the lymph by engulfing

> **KEY FACT**
>
> The presence of enlarged lymph nodes is helpful in determining whether an ill patient is mounting an immune response.

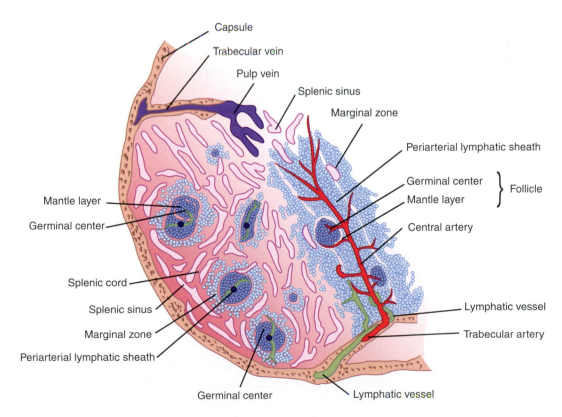

FIGURE 6-2. Anatomy of the Spleen. The presence of enlarged lymph nodes is helpful in determining whether an ill patient is mounting an immune response.

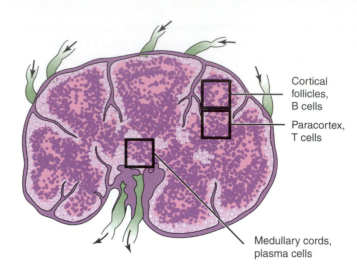

FIGURE 6-3. Lymph node architecture. (Modified, with permission, from Chandrasoma P, Taylor CR. *Concise Pathology*, 3rd ed. Originally published by Appleton & Lange. Copyright © 1998 by the McGraw-Hill Companies, Inc.)

pathogens and presenting them to lymphocytes, enhancing the response to pathogens.

Lymphatic System

Drains fluid from the body, filters it through lymph nodes, and returns it to the circulatory system. The **right lymphatic duct** drains the right arm and right half of the head and neck, whereas the **thoracic duct** drains all other body parts. The fluid from the thoracic duct and right lymphatic duct is returned to the left and right subclavian veins, respectively.

Peripheral Lymphoid Tissue

Collections of lymphocytes outside the spleen and lymph nodes that are at prime locations for antigen interaction. Some examples of peripheral lymphoid tissue include:

- Gut-associated lymphoid tissue (GALT), which includes the tonsils, appendix, and Peyer's patches of the intestines
- Mucosal-associated lymphoid tissue (MALT)
- Bronchial-associated lymphoid tissue (BALT)

CELLS AND MOLECULES OF THE IMMUNE SYSTEM

Innate Immunity

PHAGOCYTIC CELLS

Cells that engulf pathogens and debris. Key phagocytic cells include:

- **Neutrophils** are myeloid cells present in acute inflammatory responses. These cells contain multilobed nuclei and abundant cytoplasmic granules for killing pathogens. Neutrophils are short-lived.
- **Macrophages** are differentiated myeloid cells present in both pathologic and normal physiologic responses. These cells are very large, amorphous, and have high phagocytic capacity and a longer life span than neutrophils. Macrophages are derived from monocytes that leave the bloodstream and differentiate in response to cytokines.
- **Dendritic cells** are differentiated myeloid cells that engulf antigen in the epithelia of the skin, gastrointestinal, and respiratory tracts. Before antigen

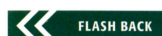

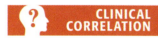

exposure, they can be identified by long, finger-like processes of cytoplasm. After taking up antigen and becoming activated, dendritic cells lose the finger-like processes and travel to lymph nodes, where they present antigen to T cells.

ANTIGEN-PRESENTING CELLS

Cells that process engulfed pathogens and express the resulting antigens to other immune cells. Some examples of APCs include:

- Macrophages
- B cells
- Dendritic cells

Following phagocytosis of extracellular pathogens, APCs break the pathogen into peptides within phagolysosomes. The peptides are loaded on to a major histocompatibility complex (MHC) II molecule within an endosome, which fuses with the cell membrane so the MHC II–antigen complex may be presented to T cells. In this way, APCs provide a link between innate and adaptive immunity.

NATURAL KILLER (NK) CELLS

Cells with lytic granules that attack and kill virus-infected or cancerous cells that lack MHC I. Unlike lymphocytes, NK cells lack specific antigen receptors. However, binding of antibodies to NK cell surface receptors triggers the release of lytic granules in a process known as **antibody-dependent cellular cytotoxicity (ADCC)**.

THE COMPLEMENT SYSTEM

A cascade of proteins, C1 through C9, which results in lysis of pathogenic cells, as shown in Figure 6-4. The complement system links innate immunity and the humoral branch of adaptive immunity.

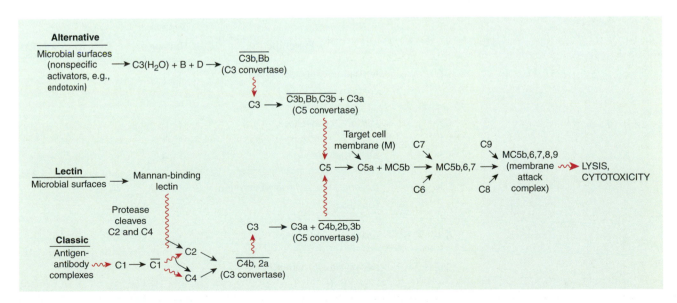

FIGURE 6-4. The complement system. (Modified, with permission, from Levinson W. *Medical Microbiology and Immunology: Examination and Board Review*, 8th ed. New York: McGraw-Hill, 2004: 432.)

There are three ways the complement cascade can be activated:

- The **classic pathway** is activated when C1 recognizes and binds an antigen-antibody complex, thus linking the innate and adaptive immune systems.
    - The constant fragments of IgG and IgM are important activators of the complement system.
    - Because this pathway recognizes antigen-antibody complexes, it is important in neutralizing viruses that have been targeted by B lymphocytes and their antibodies.
- The **alternative pathway** is triggered when activated C3 recognizes certain nonspecific antigens (such as endotoxin on gram-negative bacteria) on microbial surfaces.
- The **lectin pathway** is activated when mannose-binding lectin, a serum protein, recognizes carbohydrate antigens on the surface of microorganisms such as encapsulated bacteria or viruses.

The three activation pathways converge at the generation of **C3 convertase**, an enzyme that remains associated with the pathogen surface to trigger cleavage of other complement proteins. C3 convertase breaks down other C3 molecules to the enzymatically active **C3b** and the **anaphylatoxin** C3a, which mediates a local inflammatory response (recruitment of cells). C3b is also important in triggering phagocytosis of pathogens.

Binding of C3b to C3 convertase creates **C5 convertase**, which cleaves C5 into C5a (another anaphylatoxin) and C5b, which is inserted into the cell membrane of the pathogen. The binding of C6, C7, C8, and C9 to C5b soon follows, forming the **membrane attack complex (MAC)**, which perforates the pathogen's cell membrane and causes major damage to the cell.

A summary of the functions of complement proteins is shown in Table 6-3.

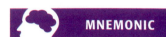

MNEMONIC

GM makes **classic** cars:
Ig**G** and Ig**M** are part of the **classic** complement pathway.

TABLE 6-3.   Complement System Proteins

	FUNCTION	PATHWAYS INVOLVED	DEFICIENCY RESULTS
C1	Recognize antigen-antibody complexes.	C	
C2	Part of C3 convertase.	C, L	
C3a	Anaphylatoxin.	C, A, L	Recurrent pyogenic infections (respiratory tract).
C3b	Opsonization, removal of immune complexes.	C, A, L	
C4a	Anaphylatoxin.	C, L	
C5a	Anaphylatoxin, neutrophil chemotaxis.	C, A, L	
C5b, C6, C7, C8, C9	Cytolysis (MAC).	C, A, L	Recurrent *Neisseria* infections (C6–C8).

MAC = membrane attack complex.

As with the coagulation system, the formation of a few active enzymes can lead to rapid activation and amplification of the complement cascade. Therefore, regulatory proteins are important in maintaining control of the cascade:

- **C1 esterase inhibitor** (C1INH) breaks apart the C1 enzyme, thus limiting its activation. Deficiency of C1INH results in **hereditary angioedema**, in which swelling occurs because of uncontrolled activation of the classic pathway and a resulting increase in C2 kinin. In addition, absence of C1INH leads to overproduction of bradykinin by kallikrein.
- **Decay-accelerating factor** (DAF) disrupts formation of C3 convertase, thus halting the complement cascade. In **paroxysmal nocturnal hemoglobinuria,** the protein that associates DAF with the red blood cell membrane is abnormal, thus making the RBCs more susceptible to complement-induced lysis.

Adaptive Immunity

Adaptive immunity can be divided into cell-mediated immunity and humoral immunity.

T Lymphocytes

Bone marrow–derived cells responsible for **cell-mediated immunity**, in which T cells directly kill target cells. T cells also stimulate the activation of macrophages and help B cells to produce antibody.

Within the thymus, T cells undergo differentiation to become mature CD4+ or CD8+ T cells. The mature T cells can also be divided into **helper T cells** (Th) and **cytotoxic T cells** (Tc).

- **Th** cells are CD4+ cells that "help" other immune cells perform their functions. Th cells differentiate into Th1 or Th2 cells, depending on the type of cytokine stimulation they receive from the local environment.
  - **Th1** cells are formed in the presence of **interleukin-12 (IL-12).** They are responsible for the activation of macrophages and cytotoxic T cells via IL-2 and interferon-γ (IFN-γ).
  - **Th2** cells are formed in the presence of **IL-4.** They stimulate the production of antibody by B cells by secreting IL-4 and IL-5.
- **Tc** cells are CD8+ cells that kill target cells infected with viruses or intracellular bacteria.

A summary of T-cell maturation is shown in Figure 6-5.

B Lymphocytes

Bone marrow–derived cells involved in **humoral immunity**. The function of B lymphocytes is to recognize extracellular pathogens and differentiate into **plasma cells** that produce antibodies to target pathogens for elimination from the body.

Antibodies

Proteins composed of two **heavy (H) chains** and two **light (L) chains**. Both heavy and light chains have a **constant (C_H or C_L) region** that is identical for all antibodies of the same **isotype**, or class, as well as a **variable region** (V_H or V_L) that has been designed by the B cell to specifically recognize an antigen. This general structure is shown in Figure 6-6.

Antibodies can be broken into fragments by enzymatic digestion. In the presence of the protease papain, the antibody molecule is broken into two anti-

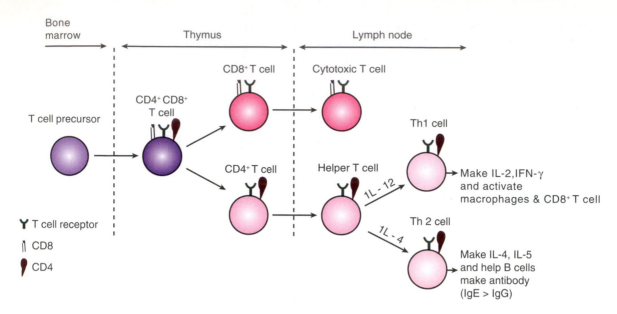

FIGURE 6-5. **T-cell maturation.**

gen-binding fragments (**Fab**) and one constant fragment (**Fc**). The Fab fragments are each composed of one light chain and one N-terminal end of the heavy chain, which are normally attached to each other by disulfide bonds. The Fc fragment is composed of the two C-terminal ends of the heavy chains.

Antibodies have three major functions:

- **Opsonization.** Binding of immunoglobulin, particularly **IgG,** to microbial surfaces enhances phagocytosis by making the antigen "tastier" to the phagocyte. Phagocytes have cell surface receptors that bind the Fc portion of antibodies.
- **Neutralization.** Binding to microbial surfaces can prevent adherence to and infection of host tissues. Furthermore, binding to antigens or inflammatory molecules can prevent an excessive immune response (as in passively administered anti-TNF-α antibodies).

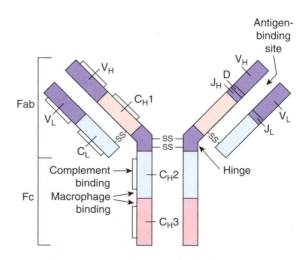

FIGURE 6-6. **Antibody structure.** (Modified, with permission, from Ganong WF. *Review of Medical Physiology,* 22nd ed. New York: McGraw-Hill, 2005: 528.)

■ **Complement activation.** Binding of IgG or IgM to antigens activates the complement system, leading to phagocytosis, anaphylaxis, and cytolysis, as described above.

Immunoglobulins with similar structures belong to the same class, or **isotype** ("same" type). There are five immunoglobulin isotypes, as determined by their heavy-chain constant regions. Please see Table 6-4 for a summary.

ANTIBODY DIVERSITY

Although B cells contain a limited number of antibody-encoding genes, they can produce a diverse number of antibody molecules by four mechanisms:

■ **Somatic recombination of VJ or VDJ genes.** Each B cell in an individual contains a given set of genes to transcribe and translate into antibody molecules. However, these genes have multiple exon segments in various regions (V and J regions for light chains and V, D, and J regions for heavy chains) that can be differentially spliced together. In this way, B cells can produce antibodies with different amino acid sequences, and thus different antigen specificities.

■ **Genetic recombination.** During VJ or VDJ recombination, various DNA segments are cut out of the genome. To repair the strand breaks, the enzyme **terminal deoxynucleotidyl transferase (TdT)** adds nucleotides to the sticky ends of the DNA strands.

TABLE 6-4. **Immunoglobulin Isotypes**

	EXPRESSED BY	STRUCTURE	COMPLEMENT FIXATION	CROSSES PLACENTA	FUNCTION
IgM	Mature B cell (surface or secreted).	Monomer or pentamer	Yes	No	Primary response.
IgD	Mature B cell (surface).	Monomer	No	No	Functions as B-cell receptor for early immune response.
IgG	Plasma cells (secreted; high concentration in serum).	Monomer	Yes	Yes	Important in secondary responses; opsonization and neutralization.
IgA	Plasma cells (secreted).	Monomer or dimer	No	No	Prevents pathogen attachment to mucous membranes; found in secretions.
IgE	Plasma cells (secreted; low concentration in serum).	Monomer	No	No	Type I hypersensitivity (induces mast cell degranulation); worm immunity.

- **Random combinations of heavy and light chains.** The differentially spliced heavy- and light-chain genes must then combine to form a functional antibody molecule.
- **Somatic hypermutation.** Once B cells have been activated (following the binding of their BCR [B-cell receptor] to antigen), the variable regions of the immunoglobulin genes are subject to a high rate of random point mutations. At some point, these mutations result in an antibody that is more specific to the initial antigen than was the original antibody molecule; these B cells are selected to differentiate into plasma cells in a process known as **affinity maturation.**

Cell Surface Proteins

In addition to their normal functions, cell surface proteins function as useful identifying markers of immune system components. Through flow cytometry, lymphocytes and other cells can be separated based on their membrane components. This is useful when attempting to count the number of B or T lymphocytes in a patient or to determine the level of differentiation of a population of cells (e.g., when evaluating for immunodeficiency or lymphoid cancers).

B-Cell Receptors (BCRs)

Membrane-bound antibody (IgM or IgD) that has been designed by the B cell for antigen recognition. Once the BCR binds antigen, and the appropriate costimulation is received, the B cell differentiates into an antibody-producing plasma cell that is capable of generating antibodies of all isotypes.

T-Cell Receptors (TCRs)

Two-component cell surface receptors responsible for T cell signaling upon binding antigen. Like BCRs, TCR components have both a constant region and a variable region that binds a particular antigen. Most TCRs have one α chain and one β chain (α:β TCR), but some are δ:γ.

TCRs interact with MHC molecules, as shown in Figure 6-7.

Major Histocompatibility Complexes (MHCs)

Surface proteins responsible for communication with T lymphocytes and NK cells. The **human leukocyte antigen (HLA) genes** encode the MHC proteins. The characteristics of MHC I and II molecules are listed in Table 6-5.

MHCs are the most important molecules pertaining to organ and tissue transplantation. By **HLA matching**, it can be determined whether a donor tissue is suitable for transplantation or whether it will be rejected by the recipient. There are multiple types of tissue grafting:

- **Autografts.** Transfer of an individual's own tissue to another location. Skin autografts are used when transferring healthy skin to a burned or damaged location on the same individual.
- **Allografts (homografts).** Transfer of tissue between genetically different members of the same species. These grafts are commonly used for organ and tissue transplantation.
- **Syngeneic grafts.** A transfer of tissue between genetically identical members of the same species, such as between identical twins.
- **Heterografts (xenografts).** Transfer of tissue between different species. For example, some heart valve replacements are performed with modified pig valves.

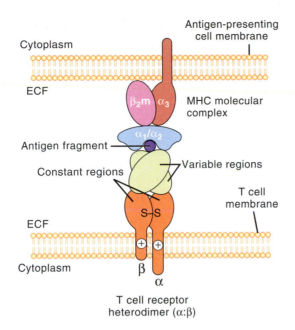

FIGURE 6-7. **T-cell and antigen-presenting cell interaction.** (Modified, with permission, from Ganong WF. *Review of Medical Physiology*, 22nd ed. New York: McGraw-Hill, 2005: 527.)

CLUSTERS OF DIFFERENTIATION (CDs)

Surface protein complexes widely found on cells of the immune system. There are hundreds of known CDs, with a wide variety of functions. Some of the most common and well-characterized CDs are described below.

T CELLS. Mature T cells express CD3 and either CD4 or CD8, as shown in Figure 6-8.

- CD3 is associated with the TCR and is required for signal transduction through the TCR.

TABLE 6-5. **Characteristics of Major Histocompatibility Complexes (MHCs)**

	MHC I	MHC II
Expressed by	All nucleated cells.	APCs.
Present	Intracellular peptides (self and viral peptides).	Extracellular peptides (engulfed pathogens).
Acquires peptide in	Rough ER.	Vesicles, after fusion with acidic endosomes.
Associated with	β_2 Microglobulin.	
Encoded by	α Chain: HLA-A, -B, and -C genes β Chain: Chromosome 15 (β_2-microglobulin).	HLA-DR, -DP, and -DQ genes.
Binds to	TCR, and CD8 coreceptor.	TCR, and CD4 coreceptor.

APC = antigen-presenting cell; ER = endoplasmic reticulum; HLA = human leukocyte antigen; TCR = T-cell receptor.

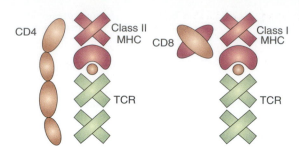

FIGURE 6-8. **Expression of costimulatory CDs on T cells (bottom) to interact with antigen-presenting cells (top).** MHC, major histocompatibility complex; TCR, T-cell receptor.

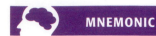

MNEMONIC

CD**4** × MHC **2** = **8** = CD**8** × MHC **1**

FLASH FORWARD

Rituximab is a monoclonal antibody used therapeutically as an immunosuppressant. The antibody binds CD20 on B cells.

KEY FACT

Abnormal expression of cell surface proteins may influence the prognosis of leukemias and lymphomas.

MNEMONIC

Hot T-Bone StEAk—

IL-1 (**hot** fever)
IL-2 (**T** cells)
IL-3 (**bone** marrow)
IL-4 (Ig**E**)
IL-5 (Ig**A**)

MNEMONIC

A cute, neu taxi 2 kill 1—

IL-6 (**acute**-phase reaction)
IL-8 (**neu**trophil chemo**taxi**s)
IL-10 (acts on Th**2**)
IL-12 (acts on natural **kill**er cells and Th**1**)

- CD4 on Th cells is a coreceptor for MHC II molecules on APCs. CD4 is also the receptor for human immunodeficiency virus (**HIV**).
- CD8 on Tc cells is a coreceptor for MHC I molecules on cells expressing abnormal intracellular peptides (typically virus-infected cells).

T cells also express **CD40** ligand, or CD40L, which is important in antibody isotype switching, and CD28, which is important in T-cell activation.

B CELLS. In addition to the BCR, **CD19** and **CD20** are markers for B lymphocytes. Another surface protein, **CD21,** is involved in the complement pathway and is the receptor for Epstein-Barr virus.

B cells also express **CD40,** which binds CD40L of helper T cells. This interaction is a crucial costimulatory signal for B cells, stimulating differentiation and isotype switching.

A summary of the most common cell surface proteins is found in Table 6-6.

Cytokines

Cytokines are intercellular communication signals that are crucial in immune system function. Some important cytokines include interleukins, interferons, and tumor necrosis factor-α (TNF-α).

INTERLEUKINS

Family of secreted proteins with a diversity of actions. The most common interleukins are summarized in Table 6-7.

INTERFERONS

Secreted proteins from virus-infected cells that promote the transition of local cells to an antiviral state. Interferons bind to interferon receptors on the target cell surface, signaling the uninfected cell to degrade viral mRNA and increase antigen presentation. Interferons also activate NK cells and stimulate them to kill infected cells. There are three types of interferons:

- **IFN-α** and **IFN-β** signal a cell to produce a protein that degrades viral (but not host) mRNA.

TABLE 6-6. Summary of Cell Surface Proteins

	CELL-SPECIFIC SURFACE PROTEINS	ADDITIONAL SURFACE PROTEINS
T lymphocytes	CD3, TCR.	CD28.
Helper T cells	CD4.	CD40L.
Cytotoxic T cells	CD8.	
B lymphocytes	IgM, CD19, CD20.	MHC II, B7, CD21, CD40.
Macrophages	—	MHC II, CD14, Fc receptors, C3b receptors.
Natural killer cells	CD56.	MHC I receptors, CD16.
Nucleated cells	—	MHC I.

MHC = major histocompatibility complex; TCR = T-cell receptor.

TABLE 6-7. Functions of Interleukins

	SECRETED BY	ACTS UPON	RESULTS IN
IL-1	Macrophages	T cells, B cells, neutrophils, fibroblasts, epithelial cells, hepatocytes.	Growth, differentiation of cells; endogenous pyrogen; production of acute phase proteins.
IL-2	Th cells	Th and Tc cells.	Growth of cells.
IL-3	Activated T cells	Bone marrow stem cells.	Growth and differentiation of cells.
IL-4	Th2 cells	B cells.	Growth of cells; class switching of IgE and IgG.
IL-5	Th2 cells	B cells, eosinophils.	Differentiation/activation of eosinophils; class switching of IgA.
IL-6	Th cells, macrophages	Hepatocytes, B cells.	Production of acute phase proteins and immunoglobulins; endogenous pyrogen.
IL-8	Macrophages	Neutrophils.	Chemotaxis.
IL-10	Th2 cells	Th2 and Th1 cells.	Turns off immune response; helps attenuate response to prevent autoimmunity.
IL-12	B cells, macrophages	NK and Th1 cells.	Activation of cells.

IL = interleukin; NK cell = natural killer cell.

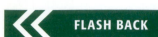
- **IFN-γ** signals for increased expression of MHC I and MHC II, thus increasing antigen presentation in all cells that receive the signal. IFN-γ is also secreted by helper T cells to stimulate phagocytosis by macrophages.

TNF-α

Protein secreted by macrophages and T cells. A key mediator of the inflammatory response during infection and autoimmune disease. Some functions of TNF-α are shown in Figure 6-9.

Immune System Interactions

ISOTYPE SWITCHING

Naïve (mature but inactive) B cells express IgM on their surface but do not secrete antibody until activation and **isotype switching** occurs. Once IgM binds antigen, antigenic peptides are presented via MHC II. The binding of MHC II to the TCR and CD4 of Th cells, along with the binding of the appropriate costimulatory molecules (CD40 on the B cell and CD40L on the T cell), triggers the T cell to produce cytokines. These cytokines induce isotype switching, which results in the production of all isotypes of immunoglobulin via changes in expression of the constant region of heavy-chain genes.

T-CELL ACTIVATION

Naïve T cells are not activated until they receive stimulation from an APC. In this process, the TCR binds antigen presented on the MHC molecule of the APC (the primary signal). A secondary signal is also required for T-cell activation; one example of a proper costimulatory signal is the binding of the B7 surface glycoprotein of the APC to CD28 on the T cell. These two interactions result in clonal expansion of the T cell. A summary of the interactions leading to T-cell activation is shown in Figure 6-10.

SUMMARY

Immune cells and the molecules they express or secrete are significantly interconnected to form a coordinated, efficient immune response to pathogens. These interactions are summarized in Figure 6-11.

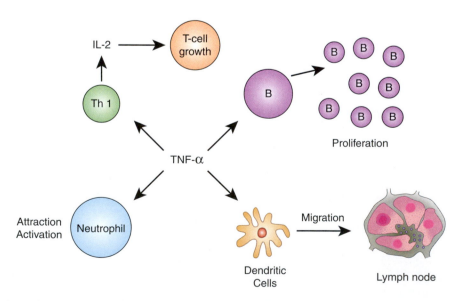

FIGURE 6-9. Functions of tumor necrosis factor (TNF)-α.

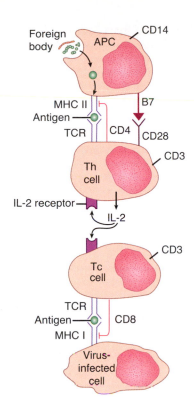

FIGURE 6-10. T-cell activation. Two signals are required for T-cell activation: Signal 1 and Signal 2. Th activation: (1) Foreign body is phagocytosed by APC; (2) Foreign antigen is presented on MCH II and recognized by TCR on Th cell (Signal 1); (3) "Costimulatory signal" is given by interaction of B7 and CD28 (Signal 2); (4) Th cell activated to produce cytokines. Tc activation: (1) Endogenously synthesized (viral or self) proteins are presented on MHC I and recognized by TCR on Tc cell (Signal 1), (2) IL-2 from Th cell activates Tc cell to kill virus-infected cell (Signal 2).

Immunizations

An effective vaccine induces sustained, protective immunity in the recipient without causing illness. In general, an effective vaccine must provide several years of protection, although multiple doses (boosters) may be neces-

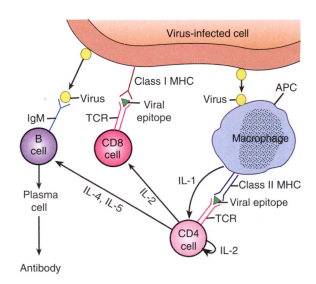

FIGURE 6-11. Immune cell interactions. MHC, major histocompatibility complex; TCR, T-cell receptor.

sary. Effective vaccines stimulate the production of neutralizing antibodies or induce cell-mediated immunity. There are multiple types of vaccines:

- **Killed vaccines** contain inactivated whole organisms or viruses.
- **Live attenuated vaccines** contain live organisms or virus particles that have been altered to reduce pathogenicity.
- **Toxoid vaccines** contain inactivated toxins isolated from the microorganisms that produce them.
- **Recombinant vaccines** contain engineered protein components (or subunits) that can stimulate production of protective antibodies to a pathogen.
- **Conjugate vaccines** contain synthetic compounds designed to induce a stronger immune response than the original pathogen or compound. For example, carbohydrates are weakly antigenic, but when combined with a protein fragment, the resulting compound is better able to stimulate the production of protective antibodies.

Important vaccines are listed in Table 6-8.

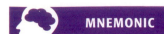

MNEMONIC

The Sal**K** polio vaccine is a **K**illed vaccine.

ANERGY AND TOLERANCE

Since B- and T-cell specificity is determined by random recombination events to create a large repertoire of antigen receptors, some developing immune cells react with self-antigen. These cells must be removed by one of the mechanisms discussed below to prevent autoimmune disease.

B Cells

CLONAL DELETION

B cells that react with self-antigen can either be deleted or undergo receptor editing of the light chain during their development in the bone marrow. Receptor editing changes the antigen specificity of the cell with the goal of preventing recognition and binding to self (innate) proteins. This receptor editing event serves as the last chance for the autoreactive B cell to escape deletion. Failing this, the cell is deleted. This process is termed **negative selection**.

ANERGY

Sometimes self-reacting B cells escape deletion and are accidentally released to the periphery. When these self-reactive cells encounter the antigen they recognize in the absence of costimulatory molecules, they are stimulated to become permanently **anergic**. Costimulatory molecules are "danger" signals expressed on APCs stimulated by the inflammatory response of the innate immune system. Anergic cells are detected by decreased IgM and increased IgD (see Figure 6-12).

CLONAL IGNORANCE

Other B cells bind only weakly to self antigen and so escape detection and deletion. These B cells are usually nonfunctional (since their binding is weak), but can become activated if the concentration of their antigen is unusually high.

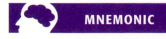

MNEMONIC

B-cell education and development occurs in the **B**one marrow.
T-cell maturation takes place in the **T**hymus

T Cells

CLONAL SELECTION

T cells undergo both positive and negative selection during development (see Figure 6-13). Like B cells, T cells that react to self-antigen are deleted in

TABLE 6-8.   Common Vaccines

Type of Vaccine	Prevents	Protects From
Killed	Polio[a]	Poliovirus
	Rabies	Rhabdovirus
	Influenza	An orthomyxovirus
	Hepatitis A	Hepatitis A virus
	Cholera	*Vibrio cholerae*
Live attenuated	Measles[b]	A paramyxovirus
	Mumps[b]	A paramyxovirus
	Rubella[b]	A togavirus
	Polio[c]	Poliovirus
	Chickenpox	Varicella-zoster virus
	Yellow fever	A flavivirus
	Smallpox	A poxvirus
	Pharyngitis, pneumonia	Adenovirus
	Tuberculosis (BCG)[d]	*Mycobacterium tuberculosis*
Toxoid	Diphtheria[e]	*Corynebacterium diphtheriae*
	Tetanus[e]	*Clostridium tetani*
	Whooping cough[e]	*Bordetella pertussis*
Recombinant	Hepatitis B	Hepatitis B virus
	Cervical cancer (HPV)	Human papillomavirus
Conjugate	Meningitis (Hib)	*Haemophilus influenzae* type b
	Meningitis	*Neisseria meningitidis*
	Pneumonia	*Streptococcus pneumoniae*

[a]The Salk intramuscular polio vaccine (IPV) contains inactive poliovirus.

[b]The measles, mumps, and rubella vaccines are often combined (MMR).

[c]The Sabin oral polio vaccine (OPV) contains mutated poliovirus.

[d]The BCG vaccine contains a different strain of the bacteria that causes tuberculosis. This vaccine is not used in the United States but is widely used in other countries.

[e]The diphtheria, tetanus, and pertussis vaccines are often combined (DTP or DTaP).

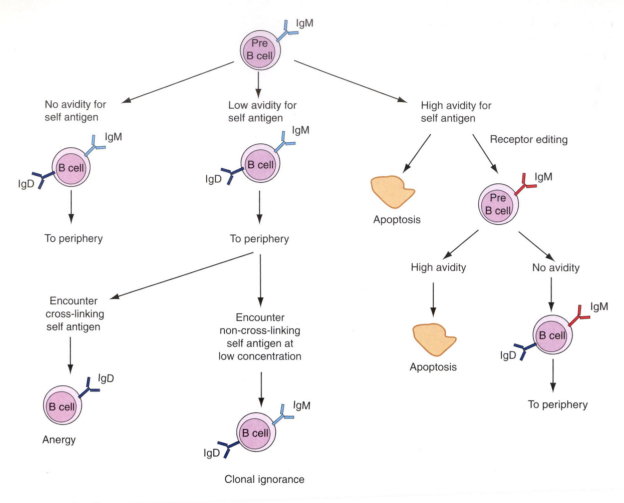

FIGURE 6-12. **B-cell anergy and tolerance.**

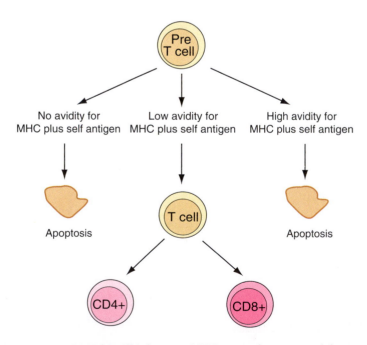

FIGURE 6-13. **Central T-cell tolerance.** MHC, major histocompatibility complex.

negative selection. Positive selection of T cells in the thymus occurs when the T cell binds self-MHC and receives a signal to proceed to the periphery. T cells must bind self-MHC to recognize antigen. Positive selection ensures that T cells that do not recognize self-MHC do not survive in the periphery. Clonal selection ensures that the mature T-cell population can react with foreign antigen (presented by MHC I and MHC II), but does not react with self-antigen.

PERIPHERAL TOLERANCE

Inevitably, there are self-antigens expressed at very low levels (or not at all) in the thymus, so that T cells reacting to these antigens do not undergo negative selection. These cells are released to the periphery (see Figure 6-14), where they must be controlled through the following processes:

- **Clonal deletion.** A T cell that binds repeatedly (e.g., because of a high concentration of self-antigen) will undergo programmed cell death.
- **Anergy.** Anergic T cells recognize self-antigen but remain inactive owing to a lack of the costimulatory molecules (CD80/CD86) required for activation of the T cell.
- **Active suppression.** Self-reactive T cells are kept nonfunctional when self-antigen is presented at low levels. The cells reacting at low levels differentiate into regulatory cells, which secrete regulatory cytokines to prevent other cells from reacting to that antigen. This is the most common mechanism for controlling peripheral T cells. Regulatory T cells (T suppressor cells) are recognized by their co-expression of both CD4 and CD25.
- **Ignorance.** Like any other T cell, if a self-reactive T cell never encounters its antigen, it will die from lack of stimulation.

Anergy and tolerance are very similar in B cells and T cells. Table 6-9 summarizes the key points related to each and allows for comparison between the two.

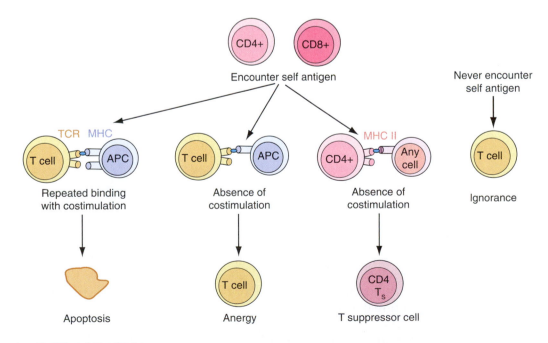

FIGURE 6-14. **Peripheral T-cell tolerance.**

TABLE 6-9.   Summary of Anergy and Tolerance in B Cells and T Cells

	ANTIGEN REACTIVITY	LOCATION	OUTCOME	REACTIVATION?
B cells				
Clonal deletion	Strong reaction to self-antigen.	Bone Marrow	Light-chain rearrangement or deletion.	No
Anergy	Strong reaction to self-antigen.	Periphery	Cell nonfunctional, lack of costimulation.	No
Clonal ignorance	Weak reaction to self-antigen.	Periphery	Cell nonfunctional, weak binding.	Yes
T cells				
Clonal selection	Normal signaling.	Thymus	Positive and negative selection.	-
Clonal deletion	Strong and repeated reaction to self-antigen.	Periphery	Cell death.	No
Anergy	Normal recognition of self-antigen.	Periphery	Cell nonfunctional, lack of costimulation.	Yes
Active suppression	Low frequency recognition of self-antigen.	Periphery	Cell differentiates to a regulatory T cell.	No
Ignorance	Never encounters self-antigen.	Periphery	Cell death from lack of stimulation.	No

Pathology

HYPERSENSITIVITY

There are four types of hypersensitivity, as seen in Table 6-10. Types I through III are antibody mediated, whereas type IV is mediated by T cells. The general effector mechanism of all four types is immune-mediated damage to otherwise normal, healthy tissue.

Type I: IgE-Mediated

Also called **immediate hypersensitivity**, the type I response can be **anaphylactic** (systemic) or **atopic** (local). After being sensitized to an antigen, the

TABLE 6-10. **Hypersensitivity**

Type I	Anaphylactic and atopic IgE mediated	First and **f**ast.
Type II	Cytotoxic IgM, IgG mediated	Cy-**2**-toxic.
Type III	Immune complex	**3** things in an immune complex: antigen-antibody-complement.
	Serum sickness	Mostly due to drugs.
	Arthus reaction	Antigen-antibody complexes.
Type IV	Cell-mediated (delayed type)	Delayed = **4th** and last **4 Ts** = **T** lymphocytes, **T**ransplant rejections, **TB** skin tests, **T**ouching (contact dermatitis).

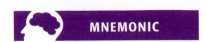

MNEMONIC

To remember the order of the types of hypersensitivity, remember ACID:

Anaphylactic and **A**topic
Cytotoxic
Immune Complex
Delayed

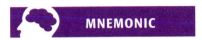

MNEMONIC

Type I (**F**irst) sensitized individuals have reactions that are **F**ast.

patient will experience an immune response to low concentrations of that same antigen. Genetic susceptibility plays a role in this reaction.

PATHOGENESIS

Figure 6-15 outlines the pathogenesis of type I hypersensitivity.

Example: Atopic reactions include urticaria, allergic rhinitis, and asthma. All three are characterized by local effects, and patients generally have consistently high circulating levels of IgE.

- **Urticaria**, or hives, is the mildest form of atopy. Histamine release causes vasodilation and a visible wheal and flare.
- **Allergic rhinitis and asthma** result from inhalation of allergens. This can cause inflammation of either the nasal mucosa leading to rhinitis or of the lower bronchi resulting in bronchial constriction and air trapping (asthma).

Anaphylaxis is the most severe form of type I hypersensitivity and occurs when histamine and other mediators are released systemically. Widespread vasodilation and increased vessel permeability can result in hypotension and shock.

Type II: Antibody-Mediated (Cytotoxic)

Antibody-mediated hypersensitivity occurs when antibodies are directed to cell surface antigens.

PATHOGENESIS

- Circulating antibody binds to its antigen on the intruding cell.
- Complement is activated.
- Cell falls victim to
  - Opsonization, followed by phagocytosis
  - Antibody-dependent cell-mediated cytotoxicity
  - Cell death mediated by NK or T cells
  - Immune response–mediated damage to healthy tissue

FLASH FORWARD

Epinephrine is used to treat anaphylaxis because it rapidly constricts blood vessels.

KEY FACT

In autoimmune hemolytic anemia, the patient makes IgM to his/her own RBC antigens.

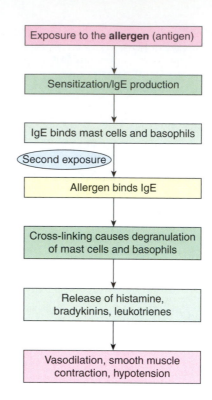

FIGURE 6-15. **Pathogenesis of type I hypersensitivity.**

Example: Blood transfusions. The most common example are incompatible blood transfusions. The recipient has preformed IgM antibodies to the donor's major RBC antigens, resulting in rapid destruction of the infused red blood cells.

Erythroblastosis fetalis results from an Rh mismatch between mother and fetus. Rh antibodies (from a sensitized Rh– mother) pass transplacentally and attack fetal (Rh+) erythrocytes. The by-products of red blood cell destruction can cause brain damage. The mother is treated with anti-Rh antibody (RhoGam) which binds the fetal Rh+ erythrocytes, thus removing them from circulation before the mother's immune system can respond to and mount an anti-Rh response, and preventing the formation of Rh antibodies.

Goodpasture's syndrome is caused by an antibody to the glomerular basement membrane (GBM) of the kidney. The antibody forms complexes in the kidney and lungs, resulting in glomerulonephritis and pulmonary hemorrhage.

KEY FACT

In type II reactions, the antigen is bound to the surface of a cell within tissue. Type III reactions result from soluble antigens.

Type III: Immune Complex–Mediated

Soluble antigen-antibody complexes form when antigen is abundant. Complex deposition in tissues causes type III hypersensitivity.

PATHOGENESIS

- Clearance of infections creates antigen-antibody complexes.
- Normally, the complexes aggregate into clusters that activate the complement system, which triggers an inflammatory response to clear the infection.
- Certain smaller complexes escape detection and are deposited in the walls of blood vessels. They accumulate on the endothelium and synovium of joints, leading to:

- Complement activation resulting in tissue inflammation which manifests as vasculitis (endothelium) or arthritis (synovium).
- Chemotaxis of neutrophils that cause significant tissue damage or arthritis.

Example: Immune complexes can form with antibodies to self-proteins. This is the mechanism underlying autoimmune disorders, such as systemic lupus erythematosus (SLE) (antinuclear antibody [ANA]). Kidney disease is a major consequence of SLE because the immune complexes are deposited in the glomerulus and cause inflammation and tissue damage.

Serum sickness occurs when serum or antibodies, such as horse antivenom for a snakebite victim, are administered to a patient. Approximately 1 week following the treatment, antibodies are formed to the foreign proteins; this leads to lymphadenopathy and systemic inflammatory symptoms such as fever and rash.

Arthus reaction is a local swelling at the site of injection of an antigen to which the patient has been immunized. The reaction occurs quickly and can be cleared within 24 hours. It is now most often seen at the site of desensitization allergy shots.

Type IV: Cell-Mediated (Delayed Type)

T cells are primed as effector cells specific to intracellular antigens or aberrant cells (foreign or mutated).

PATHOGENESIS

Initial exposure to an antigen or infection causes production of memory immune cells, among them effector T cells. On repeated exposure, effector T cells are drawn to the site, where they proliferate and activate a macrophage response to clear the infection (see Figure 6-16). This process generally takes 1–2 days.

Example: The **tuberculin skin test** uses hypersensitivity to determine whether a person has been previously exposed to *Mycobacterium tuberculosis*. Tuberculin purified protein derivative (ppd) is injected in the skin. If a T cell has been previously sensitized to the ppd antigen, its proliferation results in an erythematous induration at the site of injection, indicating previous exposure. It is important to note that with certain T-cell immunodeficiencies (i.e., HIV), induration may not be seen despite previous exposure.

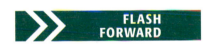

FLASH FORWARD

Remember, *M. tuberculosis* can hide in pulmonary granulomas.

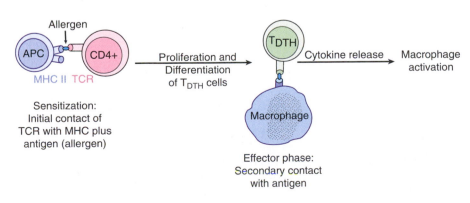

FIGURE 6-16. **Delayed-type hypersensitivity.** TCR, T-cell receptor.

Contact dermatitis results from a similar reaction, except that the T cells are sensitized to environmental antigens such as poison ivy. These reactions generally involve both CD4+ and CD8+ T cells and can be as widespread as the area of contact. Exposure to a large volume of antigen increases the magnitude of the immune response, which consequently can cause severe local tissue damage.

IMMUNODEFICIENCY

B-Cell Deficiencies

TRANSIENT HYPOGAMMAGLOBULINEMIA (OF INFANCY)

A naturally occurring deficiency of B cell–secreted immunoglobulins occurring in infants 3–6 months of age. At this age, maternal IgG is disappearing, but the infant's B cells are not yet producing sufficient quantities of antibodies to suppress infection. Although this occurs in all infants, some display a more profound depression and require treatment.

PRESENTATION

Recurrent and/or potentially severe bacterial infections.

DIAGNOSIS

Measure circulating antibody levels and confirm that the level is lower than age-matched standards.

TREATMENT

If the infections are threatening, intravenous immunoglobulin (IVIG) can be given to boost the immune response.

PROGNOSIS

Most infants go on to develop normal circulating immunoglobulin levels and have no lasting sequelae.

BRUTON'S AGAMMAGLOBULINEMIA

An X-linked defect in Bruton's tyrosine kinase (Btk), which functions in B-cell differentiation, maturation, and mature signaling. B cells fail to develop normally past the pre–B-cell stage, resulting in low levels of all classes of immunoglobulins.

PRESENTATION

Recurrent extracellular pyogenic and enterovirus infections.

DIAGNOSIS

B cells are absent on peripheral smear, immunoglobulin levels are low to undetectable, and the patient lacks tonsils. Lymph node biopsy showing lack of germinal centers is confirmatory.

TREATMENT

Intravenous gamma globulin from adult donors.

DYSGAMMAGLOBULINEMIA (SELECTIVE IMMUNOGLOBULIN DEFICIENCY)

Lack of any immunoglobulin class due to defective B-cell class switching or activation. The most common type is circulating IgA deficiency, affecting as many as 1 in 600 people. Affected individuals have decreased mucosal immunity and potentially increased susceptibility to autoimmune disease.

PRESENTATION

Often asymptomatic and diagnosed incidentally in patients with chronic lung disease.

DIAGNOSIS

Decreased serum titers of IgA.

TREATMENT

Antibiotics are given to symptomatic patients to help clear infections.

PROGNOSIS

IgA deficiency is not known to cause any significant morbidity or mortality.

See Table 6-11 for a summary of B-cell–related immunodeficiencies.

T-Cell Deficiencies

THYMIC APLASIA (DiGEORGE SYNDROME)

Characterized by the triad of hypocalcemia, tetany, and the absence of T cells. The defect is caused by defective formation of the third and fourth pharyngeal pouches early in gestation. Although not hereditary, thymic aplasia is associated with 22q11 chromosomal microdeletions. The syndrome results in a nondeveloping thymus and a lack of parathyroid glands, which cause T-cell and calcium deficiencies, respectively.

PRESENTATION

Neonatal tetany and recurrent opportunistic viral and fungal infections. A velocardiofacial syndrome, infants often also show facial abnormalities and/or cardiac malformations.

TABLE 6-11.   Summary of B-Cell Immunodeficiency Syndromes

	IMMUNE DEFECT	COMMON INFECTIONS
Transient hypogammaglobulinemia	Uniformly decreased immunoglobulins.	Recurrent bacterial sinopulmonary infections (i.e., otitis media, pneumonia and sinusitis).
Bruton's agammaglobulinemia	Loss of Btk tyrosine kinase leads to complete absence of B cells.	
Dysgammaglobulinemia	Defective class switching leads to decrease of immunoglobulin, most commonly IgA.	

DIAGNOSIS

Patients generally present with **cyanosis** or **tetany** due to the cardiac disease or hypocalcemia, respectively. Fluorescent *in situ* hybridization can be used to detect the 22q11 chromosomal deletion. Chest X-ray shows absent or greatly reduced thymic shadow. Low to undetectable circulating T cells are seen, as well as low circulating levels of immunoglobulin (due to lack of B-cell activation by T cells).

TREATMENT

If the patient possesses any fragments of thymus, immunomodulatory agents can be given to stimulate thymic growth. If not, fetal thymic transplantation can be performed if the patient remains symptomatic.

PROGNOSIS

Given proper treatment of cardiac disease and hypocalcemia, patients with thymic aplasia have a good prognosis. Many even survive without thymic transplantation, although the reason for this is unknown.

CHRONIC MUCOCUTANEOUS CANDIDIASIS

A selective lack of T-cell reactivity to *Candida* species. It commonly presents with associated endocrine disorders.

PRESENTATION

Recurrent *Candida* infections on skin and mucosal areas.

DIAGNOSIS

Laboratory studies show normal levels and functioning of both B and T cells. Diagnosis is made on highly specific T-cell challenge.

TREATMENT

Antimycotic agents can aid the patient in clearing the infection, but avoidance of potential sources of infection is more effective.

ACQUIRED IMMUNODEFICIENCY SYNDROME (AIDS)

The sequelae of infection with HIV, which directly infects and then kills CD4+ helper T cells. This immunosuppression manifests as a loss of cell-mediated immunity and can lead to opportunistic infections (see Table 6-12) and malignancies.

PRESENTATION

General wasting and constitutional symptoms (fever, weight loss, etc.). Affected individuals also have increased occurrence of opportunistic infections and rare malignancies, such as Kaposi's sarcoma.

DIAGNOSIS

Peripheral blood CD4+ T-cell count is an indicator that an HIV-positive patient has progressed to AIDS. HIV seropositivity is most frequently determined by enzyme-linked immunosorbent assay (ELISA) and Western blot.

TREATMENT

Control viral replication with highly active antiretroviral therapy (HAART) including reverse transcriptase inhibitors and/or protease inhibitors. Treat

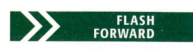

FLASH FORWARD

HIV and AIDS are discussed in more detail in the Microbiology chapter.

TABLE 6-12.   Most Common Opportunistic Infections in Untreated AIDS Patients

Protozoa	■ *Toxoplasma gondii* ■ *Isospora belli* ■ *Cryptosporidium* spp.
Fungi	■ *Candida albicans* ■ *Cryptococcus neoformans* ■ *Coccidiodes immitis* ■ *Histoplasma capsulatum* ■ *Pneumocystis jiroveci*
Bacteria	■ *Mycobacterium avium-intracellulare* ■ *Mycobacterium tuberculosis* ■ *Listeria monocytogenes* ■ *Nocardia asteroides* ■ *Salmonella* spp. ■ *Streptococcus* spp.
Viruses	■ Cytomegalovirus ■ Herpes simplex virus ■ Varicella-zoster virus ■ Adenovirus ■ Polyomavirus ■ JC virus ■ Hepatitis B virus ■ Hepatitis C virus

infections with appropriate antibiotics. Broad-spectrum antibiotics are often given prophylactically to decrease the occurrence of opportunistic infections.

See Table 6-13 for a summary of T-cell–related immunodeficiencies.

TABLE 6-13.   Summary of T-Cell Immunodeficiency Syndromes

	IMMUNE DEFECT	PRESENTATION
DiGeorge syndrome	Thymic aplasia due to defective formation of 3rd/4th pharyngeal pouches.	Cyanosis and/or tetany.
Chronic mucocutaneous candidiasis	Decreased T-cell reactivity to Candida species.	Recurrent Candida infections.
Acquired immunodeficiency syndrome	HIV-induced depletion of CD4+ T cells.	Opportunistic infections, see Table 6-12.

Combined Deficiencies

SEVERE COMBINED IMMUNODEFICIENCY (SCID)

Class of inherited disorders leading to malfunctioning of both B and T cells. Enzyme deficiencies in adenosine deaminase (ADA) or purine nucleotide phosphorylase can cause accumulation of toxic metabolites in the purine degradation pathways of lymphocytes. **Bare lymphocyte syndrome** is an autosomal recessive defect in MHC II gene regulatory proteins that leads to a complete deficiency of MHC II on APCs and in the thymic epithelium. This inhibits development of CD4+ T cells and severely impairs B-cell functioning. **X-linked SCID** is the most common and results from a defect in the common gamma chain. This chain is common to several cytokine receptors, including IL-2, which is important in T-cell development.

PRESENTATION

Failure to thrive and chronic viral infections in an infant with low lymphocyte counts.

DIAGNOSIS

Flow cytometry indicating lack of lymphocytes. More specific diagnosis is made by gene mutation analysis.

TREATMENT

Bone marrow transplantation, prophylactic antibiotics.

PROGNOSIS

In the absence of treatment, death occurs within 1 year of birth.

WISKOTT-ALDRICH SYNDROME

X-linked defect in Wiskott-Aldrich syndrome (WAS) protein (WASP) causing cellular defects in the actin cytoskeleton. This affects all hematopoietic cells, especially platelets and T cells. T cells lose the ability to stimulate B cells in response to capsular polysaccharides present on some bacteria.

PRESENTATION

Pyogenic infections, bleeding diathesis, and eczema. Affected individuals also have an increased incidence of autoimmune disorders and lymphoma.

DIAGNOSIS

Low serum IgM with normal levels of IgG and IgA, abnormally small platelets on peripheral smear.

TREATMENT

Bone marrow transplantation.

PROGNOSIS

In the absence of treatment, most patients do not live beyond the teenage years.

HYPER-IgM SYNDROME

An X-linked defect in T-cell CD40-ligand. The CD40-CD40 ligand interaction is required for full activation of B cells as well as antibody class switching.

PRESENTATION

Recurrent bacterial infections. May also have increased susceptibility to auto-immune disorders or lymphoma.

DIAGNOSIS

Serum antibody titers reveal increased IgM and decreased IgA and IgG.

TREATMENT

Bone marrow transplantation. If no donor, immune function is augmented with IVIG antibodies and the administration of appropriate antibiotics to treat infections.

PROGNOSIS

Varies, but is significantly better with early diagnosis and/or bone marrow transplantation.

ATAXIA-TELANGIECTASIA

Autosomal recessive defect in the ATM protein that leads to insufficient cellular responses to DNA damage. Lymphocytes are targeted because of high rates of proliferation and the need to rapidly divide. It is associated with IgA deficiency and malignancies.

PRESENTATION

Cerebellar ataxia and oculocutaneous telangiectasias in early childhood; increased susceptibility to mucosal infections.

DIAGNOSIS

Clinical presentation in addition to identified genetic defects on both alleles of ATM.

TREATMENT

Antibiotics for infection.

PROGNOSIS

Most patients die of infections, cancer, or advanced neurodegenerative disease in their mid-20s.

See Table 6-14 for a summary of the combined immunodeficiencies.

Phagocyte Deficiencies

LEUKOCYTE ADHESION DEFICIENCY SYNDROME

Autosomal recessive group of defects in the integrin receptor responsible for phagocyte binding to endothelium (LFA-1). This prevents phagocytic infiltration at the site of infection or injury.

PRESENTATION

Increased frequency of **bacterial infections** in the first year of life, often preceded by delayed separation of the umbilical cord.

DIAGNOSIS

Leukocytosis, flow cytometric analysis of integrins, or phagocyte functional studies.

TABLE 6-14. **Summary of Combined Immunodeficiency Syndromes**

	CAUSE	PRESENTATION	TREATMENT
Severe combined immunodeficiency	Multiple genetic associations; see text.	Failure to thrive in infancy.	Bone marrow transplantation
Wiskott-Aldrich syndrome	X-linked defective WASP gene.	Pyogenic infections, bleeding diathesis, eczema.	
Hyper-IgM syndrome	X-linked defect in T-cell CD40 ligand.	Recurrent bacterial infections.	
Ataxia-telangiectasia	Autosomal recessive defect in ATM.	Cerebellar ataxia, oculocutaneous telangiectasia, mucosal infections.	Antibiotics for infections

TREATMENT

Bone marrow transplantation is the only treatment with documented benefit. Other options include prophylactic administration of antibiotics and regular leukocyte transfusions.

PROGNOSIS

Without treatment, patients die within 1 year. Success varies with treatments.

CHRONIC GRANULOMATOUS DISEASE (CGD)

Defective NADPH oxidase system (mutation in any of the four enzymes) impairs the production of reactive oxygen intermediates required for phagocyte killing. As a result, phagocytes can internalize bacteria but are unable to kill certain classes. This malfunction causes accumulations of immune cells in granulomas, which form at the site of infection. Myeloperoxidase deficiency is often considered a milder form of CGD (see next section).

PRESENTATION

Severe catalase-positive bacterial infections (e.g., *Staphylococcus aureus*) and/or fungal infections, especially of the skin; hepatosplenomegaly; and lymphadenopathy.

DIAGNOSIS

Phagocyte function is determined using a test of the ability to reduce nitroblue tetrazolium dye. The specific defect is determined by genetic testing.

TREATMENT

Bone marrow transplantation can be curative. IFN-γ and prophylactic antibiotics are the current standard of care.

PROGNOSIS

Depends on severity of disease; highest mortality is seen in children.

MYELOPEROXIDASE DEFICIENCY

The myeloperoxidase pathway is not critical for phagocyte function, and affected individuals are often asymptomatic and undiagnosed; it can present as a somewhat milder form of CGD. This deficiency may be inherited or acquired. Acquired forms are generally transient.

CHÉDIAK-HIGASHI SYNDROME

Autosomal recessive mutation in lysosomal trafficking regulator (LYST) causes a failure of vesicle fusion in neutrophils (impaired phagosome-lysosome fusion), platelets, and melanocytes, among others.

PRESENTATION

Recurrent infections, partial albinism, prolonged bleeding times, and widespread lymphoproliferation. Peripheral neuropathy may also be seen.

DIAGNOSIS

Microscopic analysis of peripheral blood shows large granules in leukocytic cells.

TREATMENT

Bone marrow transplantation ameliorates all symptoms except peripheral neuropathy.

PROGNOSIS

Death resulting from infection or excess lymphoma-like states usually occurs within the first decade of life.

IL-12 RECEPTOR/IFN-γ RECEPTOR DEFICIENCIES

IL-12 and IFN-γ are involved in phagocyte signaling through Toll-like receptors. Deficiencies in these receptors cause increased susceptibility to *Mycobacterium*, including the strain used in tuberculosis vaccination.

See Table 6-15 for a summary of phagocyte immunodeficiencies.

TABLE 6-15. Summary of Major Phagocyte Deficiency Syndromes

	DEFECT	PRESENTATION	TREATMENT
Leukocyte adhesion deficiency	Autosomal recessive defect in LFA-1.	Recurrent pyogenic infections, delayed wound healing.	Bone marrrow transplantation
Chronic granulomatous disease	Mutation in any of 4 NADPH oxidase enzymes.	Catalase+ bacterial infections.	
Chédiak-Higashi disease	Autosomal recessive mutation in LYST.	Recurrent infections, partial albinism.	

MNEMONIC

TAP D3

Antibodies that cross the placenta:
Anti-**T**SH, Anti-**A**Ch, Anti-**P**latelet,
and Anti-**D**esmoglein-**3**.

KEY FACT

Goodpasture's syndrome is an
example of type II hypersensitivity.

MNEMONIC

DR**2**= MS (**2** letters)
DR**3**= SLE (**3** letters)
DR**4**= RA (affects **all 4** extremities)

MNEMONIC

HLA-B27 is associated with the PAIR diseases:

Psoriasis
Ankylosing spondylitis and **A**cute
anterior uveitis
Inflammatory bowel disease
Reiter's syndrome and **R**eactive
arthritis

AUTOANTIBODIES AND ASSOCIATIONS

Although autoimmune disease is discussed in detail in the immunopathology section, it is important to note key autoantibody associations, as found in Table 6-16.

HLA ASSOCIATIONS

HLA associations are important when considering familial inheritance of disease or disease susceptibility. Table 6-17 lists important HLA-linked disorders.

GENERAL AUTOIMMUNE PATHOLOGY

Under ordinary circumstances, the body is able to distinguish between its own normal cells and abnormal cells or infectious organisms. Immature B lymphocytes that strongly react to self-antigens in the bone marrow are either destroyed or undergo alteration of receptor specificity. Mature B lymphocytes encounter high concentrations of self-antigens in the peripheral lymphoid tissues, learn to recognize these antigens, and do not mount an immune response against them. If these natural mechanisms of immunologic tolerance to self fail, then autoimmune pathology may develop. This development can be influenced by a number of factors, including genetics and infections.

Genes may predispose individuals to particular autoimmune diseases. **HLA genes** are an important type of gene frequently associated with autoimmunity. Individuals who inherit certain HLA alleles are at an increased risk of developing certain autoimmune diseases. However, autoimmune diseases are not *caused* by HLA alleles, and the majority of patients with a particular allele associated with disease never develop that disease. The exact mechanism of autoimmunity is frequently unknown, but particular HLA alleles may be inefficient at displaying self-antigens or may fail to stimulate T-cell regulation. Non-HLA genes may also be associated with particular autoimmune diseases.

Infections may activate self-reactive lymphocytes, leading to an autoimmune response. Many mechanisms can be involved in this activation; an infection may induce a local immune response and promote the survival of self-reactive T lymphocytes, infections may injure tissues and release self-antigens that are normally isolated from the immune system, or infectious organisms may produce peptides that are similar to self-antigens and trigger an autoimmune response via cross-reactivity (**molecular mimicry**).

SYSTEMIC AUTOIMMUNE DISEASES

Systemic Lupus Erythematosus

A chronic inflammatory autoimmune disorder characterized by immunologic abnormalities, such as the presence of **ANAs.** ANAs are polyclonal IgG, IgM, and IgA autoantibodies that are reactive with antigens in the cell nucleus. They are not organ-specific and are not cytotoxic to intact, viable cells. However, they are deposited as immune complexes, thus triggering inflammatory changes and tissue damage. ANAs are found in the serum of patients with SLE, but they may also be seen with other autoimmune disorders, such as rheumatoid arthritis (RA) and systemic sclerosis. Ninety percent of patients with SLE are females between the ages of 14 and 45. It is most common and severe in **black females.**

TABLE 6-16. **Autoantibodies and Their Associations**

DISEASE	ANTIBODY	COMMENTS
Autoimmune hemolytic anemia	Anti-RBC	Rh and I antigens are the targets.
Celiac disease	Anti-gliadin Anti-tissue transglutaminase	For diagnosis, anti-tissue transglutaminase IgG and IgA (both) are key.
Crohn's disease	Anti-desmin	
Goodpasture's syndrome	Anti-basement membrane	Antigen is type IV collagen; also found in the lungs.
Graves' disease	Anti–thyroid-stimulating hormone receptor	Crosses placenta; antibody is stimulatory at the receptor.
Hashimoto's thyroiditis	Anti-thyroid peroxidase, antithyroglobulin	
Multiple sclerosis	Anti-myelin	
Myasthenia gravis	Anti-acetylcholine	Crosses placenta, antibody is inhibitory at the nicotinic ACh-receptor.
Pemphigus vulgaris	Anti-desmoglein-3	Crosses placenta.
Pernicious anemia	Anti-intrinsic factor, Anti-parietal cell	Results in vitamin B_{12} deficiency.
Polymyositis, dermatomyositis	Anti-Jo 1	
Primary biliary cirrhosis	Anti-mitochondrial Anti-actin	
Rheumatoid arthritis	Anti-IgG (rheumatoid factor)	Also found in 30% of SLE.
Scleroderma	Anti-centromere	Associated with CREST syndrome (calcinosis, Raynaud's phenomenon, esophageal dysmotility, sclerodactyly, telangiectasias).
	Anti-Scl-70	Diffuse, specific.
Systemic lupus erythematosus (SLE)	Anti-nuclear	Thought to be microbially induced.
	Anti-dsDNA, Anti-Smith	Specific and diagnostic.
	Anti-histone	Only seen in drug-induced cases.
Thrombocytopenic purpura	Anti-platelet	Crosses placenta.
Type I diabetes mellitus	Anti-islet cell Anti-insulin	
Vasculitis	Anti-neutrophil	
Miscellaneous	Anti-microsomal	Found in SLE, rheumatoid arthritis, Sjögren's syndrome, and Hashimoto's thyroiditis, among others.

TABLE 6-17. **HLA-Linked Disorders**

HLA TYPE	ASSOCIATED DISEASE
A1	Graves' disease, dermatitis herpetiformis.
B8	Graves' disease, celiac disease, autoimmune hepatitis, primary sclerosing cholangitis, dermatitis herpetiformis.
B13	Psoriasis.
B17	Psoriasis.
B27	Psoriasis, ankylosing spondylitis, acute anterior uveitis, inflammatory bowel disease, reactive arthritis.
DR2	Goodpasture's syndrome, multiple sclerosis, narcolepsy, systemic lupus erythematosus (SLE), hay fever, cicatricial pemphigoid (*decreases* risk of diabetes mellitus type I).
DR3	Celiac disease, myasthenia gravis, SLE, Graves' disease, type I DM, autoimmune hepatitis, primary sclerosing cholangitis, dermatitis herpetiformis.
DR4	Rheumatoid arthritis, type I DM, pemphigus vulgaris, giant cell (temporal) arteritis, autoimmune hepatitis, cicatricial pemphigoid.
DR5	Hashimoto's thyroiditis, pernicious anemia.
DR7	Steroid-responsive nephrotic syndrome.
DR8	Primary biliary cirrhosis.
Dw3	Sjögren's syndrome.
Dw4	Rheumatoid arthritis.

PRESENTATION

Many manifestations of SLE are possible. Symptoms often wax and wane over time. **Arthritis** and muscle pain are the most common complaints. The arthritis associated with SLE is symmetric and affects the small joints of the hands, feet, wrists, knees, and elbows. Other common findings in this disease can include:

- **Malar rash,** a butterfly-shaped rash that may erupt on the face, as shown in Figure 6-17.
- **Nephritis** occurs in about half of patients, and can lead to nephrotic syndrome, renal failure, and death. As the renal disease progresses, a characteristic "wire loop" pattern can be seen on biopsy caused by the thickening of the capillaries.
- **Hematologic abnormalities** can include anemia (due to both chronic disease and circulating anti-RBC antibodies), thrombocytopenia (due to anti-platelet antibodies), and recurrent thromboses (particularly in association with antiphospholipid syndrome).
- **Cardiac manifestations** can include pericarditis, myocarditis, valvulitis, or characteristic vegetations affecting both sides of cardiac valves (Libman-Sacks endocarditis).

KEY FACT

Lupus nephritis produces a **wire loop** pattern on biopsy.

KEY FACT

The presence of antiphospholipid antibodies in patients with SLE may result in false-positive results on syphilis tests (RPR and VDRL).

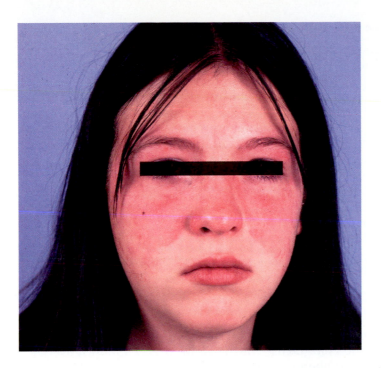

FIGURE 6-17.   Malar rash in young woman with systemic lupus erythematosus. (Reproduced, with permission, from Wolff K, Johnson RA, Suurmond D. *Fitzpatrick's Color Atlas & Synopsis of Clinical Dermatology*, 5th ed. New York: McGraw-Hill, 2005: 385.)

- **Neurologic disturbances,** such as strokes and seizures.
- **Pulmonary abnormalities,** such as fibrosis and pulmonary hypertension.
- **Mucositis,** with ulcers in the nose and mouth.
- **Photosensitivity.**

DIAGNOSIS

Diagnostic criteria for SLE include a history of at least four of the findings summarized by the mnemonic **I'M DAMN SHARP.**

Laboratory tests may be useful for confirming the diagnosis. ANA is over 95% *sensitive* for SLE, but not very specific. Antibodies to double-stranded DNA (**anti-dsDNA**) are very *specific* and are associated with a poor prognosis. Anti-Smith (**anti-Sm**) antibodies are also very *specific* to SLE, but not prognostic. **Anti-histone** antibodies are seen in cases of drug-induced lupus.

TREATMENT

The treatment for lupus depends on its manifestations. NSAIDs are the typical treatment for arthritis, and sunscreen can be used for photosensitivity. **Steroids** are often given if there is major organ involvement, but chronic use carries a risk of avascular necrosis, osteoporosis, diabetes, and ocular disease. Hydroxychloroquine is used for skin disease and arthritis. The cytotoxic agent cyclophosphamide and the antimetabolites mycophenolate mofetil and azathioprine are particularly useful for treating lupus nephritis.

PROGNOSIS

SLE is an unpredictable disease, and outcomes vary drastically. It is typical for patients to experience a series of relapses and remissions, although symptom-free periods may last for years. Prognosis is improved with early detection and treatment for kidney disease. Death can occur secondary to renal failure, infection, stroke, or other complications.

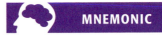
MNEMONIC

I'M DAMN SHARP

Immunologic disorder
Malar rash
Discoid rash
Antinuclear antibodies
Mucositis
Neurologic disturbances
Serositis (pleuritis, pericarditis)
Hematologic abnormalities
Arthritis
Renal disorders
Photosensitivity

KEY FACT

Drug-induced lupus is associated with anti-histone but not anti-dsDNA or anti-Sm.

KEY FACT

Drug-induced lupus is associated with the use of procainamide, hydralazine, chlorpromazine, isoniazid, methyldopa, quinidine, and other drugs. Symptoms resolve when the causative drug is discontinued.

Systemic Sclerosis (Scleroderma)

A generalized rheumatologic disorder of connective tissue characterized by degenerative and inflammatory changes leading to fibrosis and collagen deposition. The disease is more common in females and typically manifests between the ages of 30 and 50. The overall cause is unknown, but several pathogenic mechanisms have been proposed, including endothelial cell injury, fibroblast activation, and immunologic derangement. T cells sensitized to collagen and other skin antigens infiltrate the skin of patients with systemic sclerosis. **Anti-topoisomerase** (formerly anti-Scl-70) antibodies are associated with diffuse systemic sclerosis and **anti-centromere** antibodies are associated with limited systemic sclerosis (CREST syndrome).

PRESENTATION

Skin involvement is almost universal in patients with systemic sclerosis. Skin may be edematous or indurated early in the disease, but progresses to sclerosis with hair loss, decreased sweating, and loss of the ability to make a skin fold. This gives the skin a characteristic tight and shiny appearance. Other common manifestations of the disease include:

- **Raynaud's phenomenon,** episodic attacks of vasospasm which cause tingling and color change in the digits, is also almost universal (see Figure 6-18). This phenomenon can be precipitated by cold weather, emotional upset, and cigarette smoking.
- **Telengiectasias,** punctate macular lesions representing dilated small vessels just beneath the dermis can be seen on the face, palms, and digits (see Figure 6-19).

In the GI tract, systemic sclerosis can present with dilation and impaired motility of the lower esophagus, atony of the small bowel with bacterial overgrowth and malabsorption, or dilation of the large intestine with formation of pseudodiverticula. In the lungs, pulmonary interstitial fibrosis and pulmonary

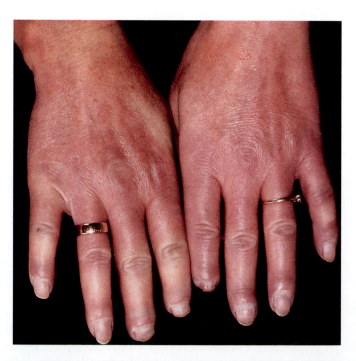

FIGURE 6-18. **Hands of a patient with systemic sclerosis showing sclerodactyly and Raynaud's phenomenon.** (Reproduced, with permission, from Wolff K, Johnson RA, Suurmond D. *Fitzpatrick's Color Atlas & Synopsis of Clinical Dermatology*, 5th ed. New York: McGraw-Hill, 2005: 399.)

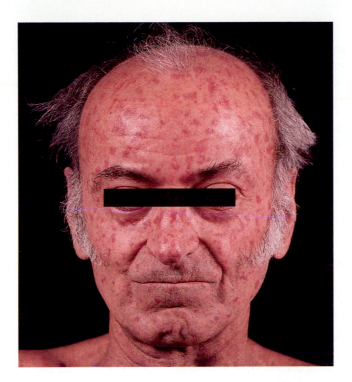

FIGURE 6-19. **Telangiectasias covering the face of a man with CREST syndrome.** (Reproduced, with permission, from Wolff K, Johnson RA, Suurmond D. *Fitzpatrick's Color Atlas & Synopsis of Clinical Dermatology*, 5th ed. New York: McGraw-Hill, 2005: 401.)

hypertension can occur. Patients with rapidly progressive disease may experience the sudden onset of malignant hypertension leading to acute renal failure.

There are multiple subtypes of systemic sclerosis, with differing presentations and prognoses.

- **Diffuse systemic sclerosis** is characterized by widespread skin involvement, rapid progression, and early visceral involvement. Skin changes appear rapidly following the development of Raynaud's phenomenon. This subtype of systemic sclerosis is associated with anti-topoisomerase antibodies (formerly anti-Scl-70).
- Limited systemic sclerosis, or **CREST syndrome**, is associated with a more benign clinical course characterized by **calcinosis, Raynaud's phenomenon, esophageal dysmotility, sclerodactyly,** and **telangiectasias.** Skin changes typically appear years after Raynaud's phenomenon and are often limited to the face and distal extremities. This subtype of systemic sclerosis is associated with anti-centromere antibodies.
- **Localized scleroderma,** or morphea, is confined to the skin, with no visceral involvement.

DIAGNOSIS

History and physical evaluation are typically the basis for a diagnosis of scleroderma. Serologic testing for anti-topoisomerase or anti-centromere antibodies can be used to support the diagnosis but not exclude it. ANAs are present in about 95% of patients. Skin biopsy demonstrating atrophy and thinning of the epidermis, fibrosis and focal collections of lymphocytes in the deep dermis, and loss of dermal appendages such as hair follicles and sweat glands can be helpful in some cases.

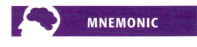

MNEMONIC

CREST syndrome:

Calcinosis
Raynaud's phenomenon
Esophageal dysmotility
Sclerodactyly
Telangiectasias

TREATMENT

There are no FDA-approved treatments for systemic sclerosis. D-penicillamine may be used to treat the skin manifestations. Severe Raynaud's phenomenon may be treated with calcium channel blockers. Angiotensin-converting enzyme (ACE) inhibitors are used to treat hypertension and prevent progression to renal crisis. Cyclophosphamide may be used for fulminant presentations or in cases of active alveolitis.

PROGNOSIS

Diffuse systemic sclerosis is a serious disease with a 10-year survival rate of about 20%. Prognosis is improving with increased use of ACE inhibitors to prevent renal crisis, which was formerly the leading cause of death. Pulmonary involvement is now the primary cause of mortality.

CREST syndrome is a more benign disease with a 10-year survival rate of > 70%.

Sjögren's Syndrome

A chronic autoimmune disorder characterized by lymphocytic infiltration of the exocrine glands. It is the second most common rheumatologic disorder (after RA) and is much more common in women than in men. It can occur either as a primary disease or secondary to other autoimmune disorders, such as RA and SLE. The pathogenesis of the disease involves circulating autoantibodies that cause activated T and B lymphocytes to accumulate around blood vessels and ducts, particularly in the salivary and lacrimal glands. These autoantibodies target the **muscarinic acetylcholine receptor,** chronic stimulation of which ultimately causes parenchymal tissue to lose the ability to produce fluid (e.g., saliva and tears). As the disease progresses, it may affect other major organ systems and can rarely evolve into malignant lymphoma.

PRESENTATION

The hallmark symptoms of Sjögren's syndrome are dry mouth (**xerostomia**) and dry eyes (**xerophthalmia**). This combination of symptoms can lead to difficulty chewing, dysphagia, dental caries, periodontal disease, keratoconjunctivitis, impairment in vision, and corneal ulcerations. Parotid gland enlargement is common. Other symptoms can include arthralgias, myalgias, Raynaud's phenomenon, and nonthrombocytopenic purpura.

KEY FACT

The combination of xerostomia and xerophthalmia is known as the **sicca complex.**

DIAGNOSIS

The damaged corneal epithelium can be visualized using the **Rose Bengal stain.** Decreased tear production can be confirmed with the **Schirmer test.** Both ANA and rheumatoid factor (RF) are usually present. **Anti-Ro (SS-A)** and **anti-La (SS-B)** are associated with earlier onset, longer duration, and more extraglandular manifestations. Salivary gland biopsy reveals a **lymphocytic infiltrate.**

TREATMENT

Treatment of patients with Sjögren's syndrome focuses on relieving symptoms and includes artificial tears, lozenges, and oral hygiene.

PROGNOSIS

Primary Sjögren's syndrome generally has a very good prognosis unless significant extraglandular manifestations develop. The prognosis for secondary disease depends on the primary autoimmune disorder. Patients have a small risk of developing lymphoma.

Reactive Arthritis

An autoimmune disease characterized by urethritis, conjunctivitis, arthritis, and mucocutaneous lesions. The disease occurs in two forms. The **postvenereal** (endemic) form is triggered following urethritis or cervicitis, usually caused by *Chlamydia trachomatis* or *Mycoplasma pneumoniae*. The **post-dysenteric** (epidemic) form is triggered following infectious diarrhea, usually due to *Shigella flexneri*, *Salmonella*, or *Yersinia*. The postvenereal form occurs almost exclusively in males, whereas the postdysenteric form affects both sexes equally. HLA-B27 is present in 80% of patients.

PRESENTATION

Symptoms generally appear 1–3 weeks after the inciting episode of urethritis/cervicitis or diarrhea. **Urethritis** ultimately occurs regardless of the inciting infection. **Arthritis** mainly affects the lower extremities and is asymmetric. **Conjunctivitis** is usually accompanied by mucopurulent discharge, lid edema, and anterior uveitis. **Mucocutaneous lesions** can include painless superficial ulcers of the palate and buccal mucosa, painless ulcers on the penis (balanitis circinata), and a hyperkeratotic rash affecting the soles, palms, scrotum, trunk, and scalp (keratoderma blennorrhagica).

DIAGNOSIS

History and physical evaluation are sufficient to make the diagnosis of reactive arthritis. Aspirates of joint fluid are usually sterile, and biopsy of the rash is indistinguishable from psoriasis.

TREATMENT

NSAIDs are the mainstay of treatment for joint symptoms. Sulfasalazine is an alternative for patients who have a contraindication to or do not experience relief from NSAIDs.

PROGNOSIS

The disease is usually self-limited, lasting between 2 and 6 months. Symptoms recur in about 50% of patients, but permanent joint damage is uncommon.

Sarcoidosis

A multisystemic disorder characterized by an exaggerated cellular immune response to an unknown antigen, leading to the formation of **noncaseating granulomas** in affected tissues. It is most common in black females between the ages of 20 and 40.

PRESENTATION

Sarcoidosis can occur in any organ system, but most commonly affects the lungs and lymph nodes. It is asymptomatic in about 50% of patients, and is often diagnosed incidentally after radiographic imaging for other reasons. **Dyspnea** is the most common complaint. Patients may also present with vague constitutional symptoms such as fever, malaise, weight loss, and fatigue.

DIAGNOSIS

Chest radiography is an important tool in differentiating sarcoidosis from other granulomatous diseases involving the lung, as described in Table 6-19. Definitive diagnosis is made by biopsy, often requiring 5–10 samples from the lung parenchyma. Histologic characteristics of sarcoidosis in comparison with other granulomatous diseases are described in Table 6-20.

KEY FACT

The **seronegative spondyloarthropathies** are a group of related inflammatory joint diseases associated with HLA-B27. These include the **PAIR** diseases:

- **P**soriatic arthritis
- **A**nkylosing spondylitis
- **I**nflammatory bowel disease with enteropathic arthritis
- **R**eactive arthritis

Serologic testing for RF is typically negative in these diseases.

MNEMONIC

Hurts to see (conjunctivitis)
Hurts to pee (urethritis)
Hurts to bend your knee (arthritis)

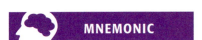

CLINICAL CORRELATION

The **Kveim-Siltzbach test** involves intradermal injection of a tissue suspension from the spleen or lymph node of a patient with known sarcoidosis into a patient suspected of having the disease. A biopsy is taken from the area 2–7 weeks after injection and is examined for the presence of noncaseating granulomas. This test is not commonly performed in the United States.

TABLE 6-20. **Differentiating Granulomatous Diseases by Histology**

	SARCOIDOSIS	TUBERCULOSIS	HYPERSENSITIVITY PNEUMONITIS
Caseation	Absent	Present	Rare
Necrosis	Rare	Present	Rare
Inclusions	Present (70%)	Rare	Rare
Eosinophils	Present	Minimal	Prominent
Bronchiolitis	Rare	Rare	Present

TREATMENT

Steroids are the mainstay of therapy for patients with symptomatic sarcoidosis, although exact regimens vary drastically according to the location and severity of the disease.

PROGNOSIS

Most cases of sarcoidosis resolve spontaneously, usually over a period of about 2–5 years. One third of cases persist for longer than 5 years and 5% result in death. Pulmonary fibrosis and extrapulmonary manifestations such as chronic iritis, lupus pernio (dramatic lupus-like skin lesions), and tracheal involvement are associated with a less favorable prognosis.

OTHER AUTOIMMUNE DISEASES

Autoimmune diseases associated with specific organ systems are covered in greater detail elsewhere, but autoantibody targets and clinical features are summarized in Table 6-21.

TABLE 6-19. **Differentiating Granulomatous Diseases by Chest X-Ray**

	SARCOIDOSIS	TUBERCULOSIS	HYPERSENSITIVITY PNEUMONITIS
Hilar adenopathy	Bilateral	Unilateral	Absent
Parenchymal infiltrate	Lower/middle fields	Localized or miliary	Diffuse
Cavity formation	Rare	Common	Rare
Pleural effusion	Unusual	Common	Absent

TABLE 6-21. Autoantibody Targets and Clinical Features of Autoimmune Diseases

Disease	Autoantibody Target(s)	Clinical Features
Systemic Autoimmune Diseases		
Systemic lupus erythematosus	Cell nucleus (ANA), double-stranded DNA, Smith, histone.	Arthritis, malar rash, nephritis, serositis, photosensitivity.
Systemic sclerosis	Centromere, topoisomerase (anti-Scl-70).	Calcinosis, Raynaud's phenomenon, esophageal dysmotility, sclerodactyly, telangiectasias.
Sjögren's syndrome	Muscarinic acetylcholine receptor (Anti-Ro, anti-La).	Xerostomia, xerophthalmia, parotid enlargement.
Reactive arthritis	Unknown.	Urethritis, conjunctivitis, arthritis, mucocutaneous lesions.
Sarcoidosis	Unknown.	Dyspnea, constitutional symptoms, incidental finding on chest X-ray.
Diseases of the Vascular System		
Vasculitis	Neutrophil cytoplasm components (C-ANCA, P-ANCA).	Hemoptysis (lung involvement), hematuria and proteinuria (renal involvement), palpable purpura (skin involvement).
Diseases of the Endocrine System		
Diabetes mellitus type I	Pancreatic islet cells, insulin.	Thirst, polyuria, hyperglycemia, retinopathy, nephropathy, neuropathy, ketoacidosis.
Graves' disease	Thyroid stimulating hormone receptor, thyroid peroxidase.	Hyperthyroidism, proptosis, pretibial myxedema.
Hashimoto's thyroiditis	Thyroid peroxidase, thyroglobulin.	Hypothyroidism.
Diseases of the Gastrointestinal System		
Celiac disease (nontropical sprue)	Tissue transglutaminase, gliadin, endomysium.	Ingestion of **gluten** causes diarrhea, steatorrhea, nausea, vomiting.
Primary biliary cirrhosis	Mitochondria.	Pruritus, jaundice, hepatomegaly, xanthelasma, transaminitis, hypercholesterolemia.
Primary sclerosing cholangitis	Neutrophil cytoplasm components (P-ANCA).	Pruritis, jaundice, hepatomegaly, **"beading" of bile ducts** on ERCP.
Autoimmune hepatitis	Smooth muscle, liver-kidney-microsome.	Jaundice, ascites, spider angiomata, esophageal varices, transaminitis.

(continues)

TABLE 6-21.   Autoantibody Targets and Clinical Features of Autoimmune Diseases *(continued)*

DISEASE	AUTOANTIBODY TARGET(S)	CLINICAL FEATURES
Diseases of the Blood		
Autoimmune hemolytic anemia	Red blood cells.	Pallor, fatigue.
Pernicious anemia	Parietal cells, intrinsic factor.	Cobalamin (vitamin B_{12}) deficiency, **megaloblastic anemia, beefy red tongue,** neuropathy, myelopathy.
Idiopathic thrombocytopenic purpura	Platelet membrane glycoproteins (e.g., glycoprotein IIb/IIIa).	Petechiae, ecchymoses, epistaxis, easy bruisability.
Diseases of the Musculoskeletal System		
Rheumatoid arthritis	Fc portion of IgG (rheumatoid factor).	Symmetric arthritis, swan-neck and boutonniere deformities, morning stiffness.
Diseases of the Skin		
Pemphigus vulgaris	Desmoglein 3.	Orapharyngeal erosions, flaccid cutaneous bullae.
Pemphigus foliaceus	Desmoglein 1.	Small flaccid cutaneous bullae.
Epidermolysis bullosa acquisita	Type VII collagen.	Tense vesicles, bullae, and erosions on extensor surfaces of hands, knuckles, elbows, knees, and ankles.
Bullous pemphigoid	BPAg1, BPAg2 (type XVII collagen).	Urticaria followed by formation of tense bullae on flexor surfaces.
Cicatricial pemphigoid	Laminin, BPAg2.	Oral and ocular lesions causing red eye, itching, and burning.
Linear IgA bullous dermatosis	BPAg2.	Vesicles and bullae on trunk and limbs, ocular lesions causing pain and discharge.
Dermatitis herpetiformis	Unknown (possibly TGase3).	Pruritic eruption on arms, knees, and buttocks (associated with celiac disease).
Diseases of the Nervous System		
Myasthenia gravis	**Postsynaptic** nicotinic acetylcholine receptors.	Facial muscle weakness that spreads to the trunk and limbs.
Lambert-Eaton myasthenic syndrome	Voltage-gated calcium channels on the **presynaptic** motor nerve terminal.	Proximal muscle weakness of the lower extremities, autonomic dysfunction (dry mouth, constipation, pupillary constriction, sweating).
Multiple sclerosis	Myelin.	Fatigue, paresthesias, tremor, optic neuritis.
Autoimmune inner ear disease	Various inner ear antigens.	Bilateral sensorineural hearing loss.

TABLE 6-21.   Autoantibody Targets and Clinical Features of Autoimmune Diseases *(continued)*

DISEASE	AUTOANTIBODY TARGET(S)	CLINICAL FEATURES
Diseases of the Renal System		
Anti-GBM disease	Glomerular basement membrane.	Oliguria, nephritic syndrome.
Diseases of the Respiratory System		
Goodpasture's syndrome	Glomerular basement membrane, pulmonary basement membrane.	Oliguria, nephritic syndrome, pulmonary hemorrhage.

C-ANCA = circulating anti-neutrophilic cytoplasmic antibody; P-ANCA = perinuclear anti-neutrophilic cytoplasmic antibody.

NOTES

Pathology

NEOPLASIA

Neoplasia is clonal proliferation of cells. These cells are unresponsive to normal regulation of cell division and continue to grow beyond the normal needs of the organism. The word **neoplasia** is derived from the Greek *neo* (new) and *plasia* (growth).

Definitions

- **Hyperplasia:** Increase in the **number** of cells (reversible). *Hyper-* = excessive.
- **Metaplasia:** Replacement of one adult cell type by another (reversible). Often secondary to irritation or environmental exposure (e.g., squamous metaplasia in the trachea and bronchi of smokers). *Meta-* = transformation.
- **Dysplasia:** Abnormal growth with loss of cellular orientation, shape, and size compared with normal tissue maturation. Commonly preneoplastic (reversible). *Dys-* = abnormal.
- **Anaplasia:** Abnormal cells that are undifferentiated and resemble primitive cells of the original tissue. *Ana-* = backward.

Cell Types

Neoplasms usually consist of cells of **epithelial** or **mesenchymal** origin. Tissues of mesenchymal origin are blood cells, blood vessels, smooth muscle, skeletal muscle, bone, and fat. Tumors derived from cells of more than one germ layer are called **teratomas.**

Nomenclature

- **Prefix:** The prefix of the term used for a neoplasm depends on the tissue type, as seen in Table 7-1.
- **Suffix, benign neoplasm:** The suffix *-oma* is generally used for benign neoplastic processes.
- **Suffix, malignant neoplasm:** Malignant neoplasms of epithelial origin end in *-carcinoma*, while those of mesenchymal origin end in *-sarcoma*.
  - **Exception:** There are a few malignant neoplasms whose names end in *-oma* (e.g., melanoma, mesothelioma, immature teratoma, lymphoma).

Neoplastic Progression

Cancerous cells pass through several stages as the disease progresses. Cells in more advanced stages are more poorly differentiated, as outlined in Figure 7-1.

Tumor Grade and Stage

GRADE

Classification system that describes the degree of differentiation of tumor cells based on histologic characteristics.

- Usually graded I–IV based on the degree of differentiation and number of mitoses per high-power field.
- Higher grade = more advanced tumor.

STAGE

- More prognostic value than grade.
- Indicates the spread of tumor in a specific patient.

KEY FACT

TNM staging, which measures the size of the **T**umor, the involvement of lymph **N**odes, and the presence of **M**etastases, is commonly used to determine prognosis.

TABLE 7-1. Tumor Nomenclature by Cell Type and Type of Neoplastic Process

CELL TYPE	BENIGN	MALIGNANT
Epithelium	▪ Adenoma ▪ Papilloma	▪ Adenocarcinoma ▪ Papillary carcinoma
Blood cells	All blood cell neoplasms are malignant	▪ Leukemia ▪ Lymphoma
Blood vessels	Hemangioma	Angiosarcoma
Smooth muscle	Leiomyoma	Leiomyosarcoma
Skeletal muscle	Rhabdomyoma	Rhabdomyosarcoma
Bone	Osteoma	Osteosarcoma
Fat	Lipoma	Liposarcoma
> 1 Cell type	Mature teratoma	Immature teratoma

- Based on the site and size of the primary lesion, spread to regional lymph nodes, and the presence or absence of metastases.
- A commonly used staging system is **TNM staging: T** for size of **T**umor, **N** for lymph **N**ode involvement, and **M** for **M**etastases.

Characteristics of Neoplastic Cells

Benign and malignant cells have features that distinguish them from each other, as seen in Table 7-2.

Metastasis

Malignant neoplasms have the potential to metastasize to distant sites. Following metastasis to regional lymph nodes, the lung, liver, brain, and bone are the most common sites.

METASTASIS TO LIVER

- Metastatic disease of the liver is much more common than primary liver tumors.
- Primary tumors that metastasize to the liver, in order of decreasing frequency:
  - Colon
  - Stomach
  - Pancreas
  - Breast
  - Lung

METASTASIS TO BRAIN

- Most common brain malignancy (approximately 50%) is metastatic disease from a primary tumor located elsewhere.

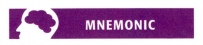
MNEMONIC

Cancer Sometimes Penetrates Benign Liver:

Colon
Stomach
Pancreas
Breast
Lung

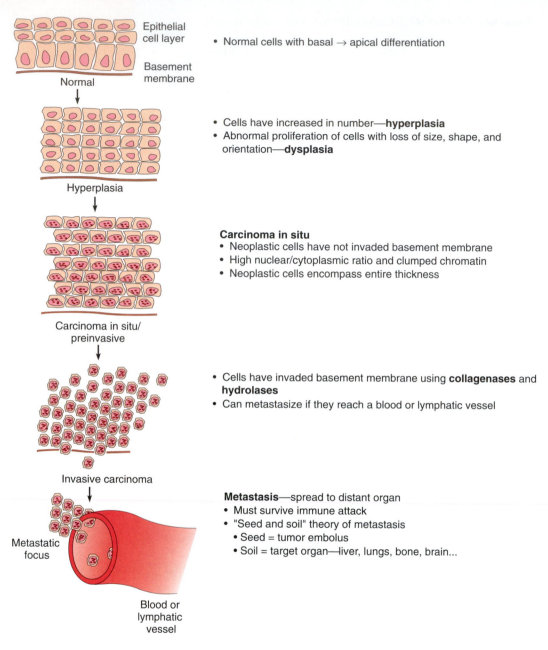

- Normal cells with basal → apical differentiation

- Cells have increased in number—**hyperplasia**
- Abnormal proliferation of cells with loss of size, shape, and orientation—**dysplasia**

Carcinoma in situ
- Neoplastic cells have not invaded basement membrane
- High nuclear/cytoplasmic ratio and clumped chromatin
- Neoplastic cells encompass entire thickness

- Cells have invaded basement membrane using **collagenases** and **hydrolases**
- Can metastasize if they reach a blood or lymphatic vessel

Metastasis—spread to distant organ
- Must survive immune attack
- "Seed and soil" theory of metastasis
  - Seed = tumor embolus
  - Soil = target organ—liver, lungs, bone, brain...

FIGURE 7-1. **Neoplastic progression.** (Modified, with permission, from McPhee S, Lingappa VR, Ganong WF, et al. *Pathophysiology of Disease: An Introduction to Clinical Medicine*, 3rd ed. New York: McGraw-Hill 2000: 84.)

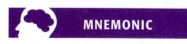

MNEMONIC

Lots of Bad Stuff Kills Glia:

Lung
Breast
Skin
Kidney
GI tract

- Primary tumors that metastasize to brain:
  - Lung
  - Breast
  - Skin (melanoma)
  - Kidney (renal cell carcinoma)
  - Gastrointestinal tract

METASTASIS TO BONE

- Metastatic disease of bone is much more common than primary bone tumors.
- The most common primary sites are breast and prostate.

TABLE 7-2. **Properties of Benign and Malignant Tumors**

PROPERTY	BENIGN	MALIGNANT
Differentiation	Well differentiated	Usually poorly differentiated
Mitotic figures	▪ Few mitotic figures ▪ No atypical mitotic figures	▪ Many mitotic figures ▪ Atypical mitotic figures
Nucleus-to-cytoplasm (N:C) ratio	Normal	Increased
Pleomorphism	Absent or minimal	Present
Hyperchromasia	Absent or minimal	Present
Circumscription and encapsulation	▪ Well-circumscribed ▪ May be encapsulated	▪ Poorly circumscribed ▪ Irregular ▪ Not encapsulated
Homogeneity	Homogeneous	May be heterogeneous
Rate of growth	Usually slow	Rapid
Metastatic potential	Does not metastasize	Can metastasize
Necrosis	No necrosis	May have necrosis/hemorrhage.
Physical examination findings	▪ Mobile ▪ Well defined	▪ Fixed ▪ Irregular; poorly defined

- Primary tumors that metastasize to bone:
  - Lungs
  - Kidney
  - Thyroid
  - Prostate
  - Testes
  - Breast

DIRECT (LOCAL) EFFECTS OF TUMOR GROWTH

- Destruction of normal architecture (**infiltration**).
  - **Nonhealing ulcers** from destruction of epithelial surfaces, such as those of the stomach, colon, mouth, or bronchus.
  - **Hemorrhage** from ulcerated areas or eroded vessels.
  - **Pain** due to involvement of any site with sensory nerve endings. Most tumors are initially painless.
  - **Seizures and increased intracranial pressure** from space-occupying brain tumors.
  - **Perforation** of a visceral ulcer can lead to **peritonitis** and **free air**.
  - **Bone involvement** can lead to pathologic fractures.
  - **Inflammation** of a serosal surface leads to **pleural effusion, pericardial effusion**, and **ascites**.

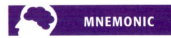

MNEMONIC

Live and Kicking Tumors Penetrate The Bone.

Lung
Kidney
Thyroid
Prostate
Testes
Breast

Alternatively: **The Kids Prefer BLT**s.

- Local neurologic deficits
    - Loss of sensory or motor function caused by nerve compression or destruction (e.g., recurrent laryngeal nerve involvement by lung or thyroid cancer results in hoarseness).
- Pressure effects on normal organs or systems (can also occur through infiltration).
    - **Obstruction:**
        - Obstructed bronchus → **pneumonia**
        - Obstructed biliary tree → **jaundice**
        - Obstructed intestines → **constipation, strangulation**
        - Obstructed venous or lymphatic drainage → **edema, superior vena cava syndrome**

Paraneoplastic Effects

Various signaling molecules may be secreted by tumors without regulation, leading to systemic effects, as seen in Table 7-3.

Carcinogenesis

Genetic damage can disturb the normal mechanisms that regulate cell proliferation and DNA repair. One genetic disruption often leaves cells vulnerable to others. Damage accumulating over time results in a process called **tumor progression**. Progression often leads to more aggressive tumor cells.

Cancer-related genes can be described under two separate categories:

TABLE 7-3. **Paraneoplastic Effects of Tumors**

NEOPLASM	MEDIATORS	EFFECT
- Squamous cell lung carcinoma. - Renal cell carcinoma. - Breast carcinoma. - Multiple myeloma. - Bone metastasis.	- Parathyroid hormone–related peptide. - TGF-α. - TNF-α. - Interleukin-2.	Hypercalcemia (most common endocrine paraneoplastic syndrome).
Small cell lung carcinoma.	ACTH or ACTH-like peptide.	Cushing's syndrome.
- Small cell lung carcinoma. - Intracranial neoplasms.	Antidiuretic hormone or atrial natriuretic peptide.	SIADH.
Renal cell carcinoma.	Erythropoietin.	Polycythemia.
- Thymoma. - Bronchogenic carcinoma.	Antibodies against. presynaptic Ca^{2+} channels at the neuromuscular junction.	Lambert-Eaton myasthenic syndrome.
- Carcinoid tumors. - Small cell lung carcinomas.	- Gonadotropin-releasing hormone. - Growth hormone.	Acromegaly.

ACTH = adrenocorticotropic hormone; SIADH = syndrome of inappropriate antidiuretic hormone secretion; TGF-α = transforming growth factor-α; TNF-α = tumor necrosis factor-α.

PROTO-ONCOGENES

- **Action:** Cause cells to grow and proliferate.
- **How they lead to cancer:** Mutations or translocations lead to **activation/overexpression** of these genes, and growth continues in an uncontrolled manner through excessive proliferation or inadequate apoptosis. Associated diseases are listed in Table 7-4.
- **Required hits:** Can cause cancerous growth with a single gene affected.

TUMOR-SUPPRESSOR GENES/ANTI-ONCOGENES

- **Action:** Regulate normal cell growth and differentiation by control of cell cycle, DNA repair, or apoptosis.
- **How they lead to cancer:** Mutations or translocations **inactivate** these genes, leading to genetic instability or unchecked cell proliferation. See Table 7-5 for associated cancers.
- **Required hits:** Usually cause cancer only if both genes are inactivated; "two-hit" hypothesis.

Carcinogenic Agents

Genetic damage can be inherited or can result from exposure to chemicals, radiation, and viruses/microbes.

- **Chemicals:** The diseases associated with chemical exposure are listed in Table 7-6.
    - **Initiators** are chemicals that lead to irreversible damage to a cell's DNA.
    - **Promoters** do not affect the DNA, but promote cell growth and differentiation by other methods; their effects are usually reversible.
- **Radiation:** Penetrant high-energy waves can directly damage DNA.
    - **Ultraviolet (UV) rays** lead to squamous cell carcinoma, basal cell carcinoma, and melanoma in the skin.
    - **UVB rays** specifically lead to the formation of **pyrimidine dimers** in DNA. Usually, the nucleotide excision repair pathway repairs these dimers, but the damage can exceed the cell's ability to repair it.
    - **Ionizing radiation** predominantly causes single- and double-strand breaks. It is associated with a variety of cancers, including **leukemia**

KEY FACT

The following can lead to cancer:
Proto-oncogenes: ON
Tumor suppressor genes: OFF

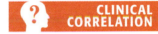

CLINICAL CORRELATION

In **xeroderma pigmentosum,** an autosomal recessive disease, the nucleotide excision repair pathway itself is dysfunctional. Those affected have very high incidence of skin cancer.

TABLE 7-4.   Proto-Oncogenes and Associated Tumor

GENE	ASSOCIATED TUMOR	ACTION
abl	Chronic myelogenous leukemia.	Signal transduction
c-myc	Burkitt's lymphoma.	Transcriptional activator
bcl-2	Follicular and undifferentiated lymphomas.	Inhibits apoptosis
erb-B2/Her-2	Breast, ovarian, and gastric carcinomas.	Growth factor receptor
ras	Colon carcinoma.	Signal transduction
L-myc	Lung tumor.	Transcriptional activator
N-myc	Neuroblastoma.	Transcriptional activator
ret	Multiple endocrine neoplasia I and II.	Growth factor receptor

TABLE 7-5. **Tumor-Suppressor Genes and Associated Tumors**

GENE	CHROMOSOME	ASSOCIATED TUMOR	ACTION
Rb	13q	▪ Retinoblastoma ▪ Osteosarcoma	Regulation of the cell cycle.
BRCA1 and 2	17q, 13q	Breast and ovarian cancer	DNA repair.
p53	17**p**	▪ Most human cancers ▪ Li-Fraumeni syndrome	Regulation of the cell cycle and apoptosis after DNA damage.
p16	9**p**	Melanoma	Cell cycle control/DNA repair.
APC	5q	Colorectal cancer	Inhibition of signal transduction.
WT1	11q	Wilms' tumor	Nuclear transcription.
NF1	17q	Neurofibromatosis type 1	Inhibition of *ras* signal transduction.
NF2	22q	Neurofibromatosis type 2	Signaling and cytoskeletal regulation.
DPC	18q	**P**ancreatic cancer	Cell surface receptor.
DCC	18q	**C**olon cancer	Cell surface receptor.

TABLE 7-6. **Chemical Carcinogens**

TOXIN	ASSOCIATED CANCER
Aflatoxins	Hepatocellular carcinoma.
Vinyl chloride	Angiosarcoma of the liver.
CCl_4	Centrilobular necrosis and fatty change of the liver.
Nitrosamines	Esophageal and gastric cancer.
Cigarette smoke	Carcinoma of the larynx and lung.
Asbestos	Mesothelioma and bronchogenic carcinoma.
Arsenic	Squamous cell carcinoma of the skin.
Naphthalene (aniline) dyes	Transitional cell carcinoma.
Alkylating agents	Leukemia.
Alcohol	Hepatocellular carcinoma.
Benzene	Acute leukemia.
Diethylstilbestrol (DES)	Clear cell adenocarcinoma of the vagina in offspring of mothers given the drug during pregnancy.

in those exposed to atomic blasts, **thyroid cancers** in those who have had previous head and neck radiation, and **osteosarcoma** in watch-dial workers who are exposed to radium.

- **Viruses and microbes:** Can cause cellular or direct DNA damage and thus predispose to cancer, as seen in Table 7-7.

Tumor Immunity

Affected cells often display tumor antigens that can stimulate the immune system. Tumor antigens may be specific (tumor-specific antigens; **TSAs**) if expressed only in tumor cells or associated (tumor-associated antigens; **TAAs**) if expressed in both normal and tumor cells. These antigens may also be used clinically to confirm the diagnosis, monitor for tumor recurrence, and to monitor response to therapy (see Table 7-8). **Cytotoxic T lymphocytes** and **natural killer cells** can destroy the neoplastic cells. The cells can escape the immune system through many mechanisms, including:

- Selection for cells that do not express tumor-specific antigens (TSAs), tumor-associated antigen (TAAs), human leukocyte antigen (HLA), or costimulatory receptors.
- Immunosuppression or immune shielding.

Epidemiology

Cancer is the second leading cause of death in the United States after heart disease. For this reason, it is important to understand the epidemiology of cancer.

TABLE 7-7.   Viruses and Microbes, Associated Cancers, and Mechanisms

VIRUS/MICROBE	ASSOCIATED CANCER	MECHANISM
HPV 16,18	Cervical, vulvar, penile, and anal carcinoma	E7 inactivates *Rb*; E6 disables *p53*.
HTLV-1	Adult T-cell leukemia	The *tax* gene leads to a high rate of proliferation of T cells, which are subsequently vulnerable to mutations and translocations.
HBV, HCV	Hepatocellular carcinoma	Causes chronic liver injury and regenerative hyperplasia, which can increase vulnerability to transformation.
EBV	▪ Burkitt's lymphoma ▪ Nasopharyngeal carcinoma	Leads to proliferation of B cells; high rate of mutations and translocations.
HHV-8	▪ Kaposi's sarcoma ▪ B-cell lymphoma	Common in immunocompromised patients.
Helicobacter pylori	Gastric cancer	Chronic inflammation

TABLE 7-8.   Tumor Antigens and Associated Cancers

ANTIGEN	ASSOCIATED CANCER
Prostatic acid phosphatase	▪ Prostatic carcinoma ▪ Used for screening
Carcinoembryonic antigen	▪ Colorectal, pancreatic, gastric, and breast cancers ▪ Nonspecific
α-fetoprotein	▪ Hepatocellular carcinomas ▪ Nonseminomatous germ cell tumors of the testis (ex-yolk sac tumor)
β-hCG	▪ Hydatidiform moles ▪ Choriocarcinomas ▪ Gestational trophoblastic tumors
CA-125	Ovarian malignant epithelial tumors
S-100	▪ Melanoma ▪ Neural tumors ▪ Astrocytomas
Alkaline phosphatase	▪ Metastases to bone ▪ Obstructive biliary disease ▪ Paget's disease of bone
Bombesin	▪ Neuroblastoma ▪ Lung and gastric cancer
Tartrate-resistant acid phosphatase	Hairy cell leukemia

β-hCG = β-human chorionic gonadotropin.

Common cancers (in order of greatest to least):

▪ **Males:** Prostate, lung, and colorectal.
▪ **Females:** Breast, lung, and colorectal.

Highest mortality rate (in order of greatest to least):

▪ **Males:** Lung, prostate.
▪ **Females:** Lung, breast.

Note: Lung cancer deaths are decreasing in males, but increasing in females.

While these cancers are common in the population at large, others are associated with particular diseases, as shown in Tables 7-9 and 7-10.

CELL DEATH

Two major forms of cell death include **apoptosis** and **necrosis.** Apoptosis occurs physiologically, but either type of cell death can occur in pathologic situations. Each type results in a distinct morphologic appearance.

TABLE 7-9. Diseases and Associated Neoplasms

CONDITION	NEOPLASM
Down's syndrome	▪ Acute lymphoblastic leukemia ▪ Acute myelogenous leukemia
Albinism	▪ Melanoma ▪ Basal and squamous cancer of the skin
▪ Chronic atrophic gastritis ▪ Pernicious anemia ▪ Postsurgical gastric remnants	Gastric adenocarcinoma
Tuberous sclerosis	▪ Astrocytoma ▪ Cardiac rhabdomyoma
Actinic keratosis	Squamous cell carcinoma of the skin
Barrett's esophagus/chronic gastroesophageal reflux	Esophageal adenocarcinoma
Plummer-Vinson syndrome	Squamous cell carcinoma of the esophagus
Cirrhosis (alcoholic; hepatitis B or C)	Hepatocellular carcinoma
Ulcerative colitis	Colonic adenocarcinoma
Paget's disease of bone	▪ Osteosarcoma ▪ Fibrosarcoma
Immunodeficiency	Malignant lymphomas
AIDS	▪ Aggressive malignant lymphomas (non-Hodgkin's) ▪ Kaposi's sarcoma
Autoimmune disease (e.g., Hashimoto's thyroiditis, myasthenia gravis)	Benign and malignant thymomas
Acanthosis nigricans	Visceral malignancy (stomach, lung, breast, uterus)
Dysplastic nevus	Malignant melanoma

Apoptosis

Apoptosis is also known as **programmed cell death.** Intracellular enzymes are activated to degrade DNA and proteins. The cell is ultimately phagocytosed, so the cell contents are not released, and therefore, does *not* result in an **inflammatory response.**

CAUSES

Apoptosis may be physiologic, usually induced by specific activation of death receptors or loss of growth factors:

TABLE 7-10. Inherited Diseases Associated With Cancers

Syndrome	Inheritance	Associated Cancer
Retinoblastoma	Autosomal dominant.	Retinoblastoma.
Familial adenomatous polyposis coli	Autosomal dominant.	Colon adenocarcinoma.
Multiple endocrine neoplasia	Autosomal dominant.	■ I: Thyroid, parathyroid, adrenal cortex, pancreas, pituitary. ■ II: Pheochromocytoma, medullary carcinoma of the thyroid. ■ III: Pheochromocytoma, medullary carcinoma, mucocutaneous neuromas.
Neurofibromatosis	Autosomal dominant.	■ Neurofibromas. ■ Pheochromocytomas. ■ Wilms' tumor. ■ Rhabdomyosarcoma. ■ Leukemia.
Von Hippel–Lindau syndrome	Autosomal dominant.	■ Hemangioblastoma. ■ Adenomas. ■ Renal cell carcinoma.
Xeroderma pigmentosa	Autosomal recessive (DNA repair).	■ Melanoma. ■ Squamous and basal cell carcinoma of the skin.
Ataxia-telangiectasia	Autosomal recessive (DNA repair).	Lymphomas (sensitivity to ionizing radiation).
Bloom syndrome	Autosomal recessive (DNA repair).	Leukemia/lymphoma.
Fanconi's anemia	Autosomal recessive (DNA repair).	Myelodysplastic syndrome/leukemia (sensitivity to mitomycin C).
Hereditary nonpolyposis colon cancer syndrome	Autosomal recessive (DNA repair).	Colon, breast, and ovarian cancers.

- **Programmed destruction** during embryogenesis.
- Tissue loss in an adult, usually hormone-dependent.
- **Cell turnover**, as in intestinal epithelia.
- Death of a host cell after its function has been fulfilled (i.e., the end of an immune response).
- Lymphocyte selection.
- Death induced by cytotoxic T cells.

Apoptosis can also occur pathologically, usually resulting from more mild injuries in which fewer cells are injured. The following are common causes:

- **DNA damage** from radiation or cytotoxic drugs.
- Certain viral infections (hepatitis).
- Pathologic atrophy.
- Tumor cell regression or turnover.

MORPHOLOGY

Distinctive features of apoptotic cells allow for easily identification by electron microscopy. These include:

- **Cell shrinkage** with dense cytoplasm.
- **Condensation of chromatin** at the periphery of the nuclear membrane.
- Membrane **cytoplasmic blebs** and cellular fragmentation into apoptotic bodies.
- **Phagocytosis** of apoptotic cells or bodies.

Typically, the plasma membrane remains intact and prevents the cellular contents from damaging adjacent tissue or stimulating an inflammatory response. On histologic section, apoptotic cells appear **strongly eosinophilic** with dense chromatin, and are generally found in small groups, as seen in Figure 7-2.

MECHANISMS OF APOPTOSIS

Cells characteristically undergo protein cleavage and DNA breakdown. **Caspases**, a family of cysteine proteases, are activated and cleave the cellular proteins which form the cytoskeleton. They also activate DNAses, which fragment the nuclear DNA into 50- to 300-kilobase pieces. This is seen as a **DNA ladder** when extracted DNA is run on agarose gel electrophoresis. Apoptotic cells also flip **phosphatidylserine** from the inner to the outer layer of their plasma membrane, which aids in recognition by macrophages.

Apoptosis can be induced by two separate pathways, as seen in Figure 7-3: Extrinsic (death receptor–initiated) or intrinsic (mitochondrial).

- The **extrinsic pathway** is activated when **death receptors**, such as the type 1 tumor necrosis factor receptor, or Fas, on the cell surface are stimulated. Cross-linking of these death receptors leads to signaling that activates caspase-8. This pathway of apoptosis is blocked by a protein called FLIP.
- The **intrinsic pathway** involves the release of proteins, including **cytochrome c**, from a leaky mitochondrion. These proteins activate caspase-9. Intrinsic apoptosis is regulated by a balance between proapoptotic cellular molecules Bak, Bax, and Bim, and anti-apoptotic molecules Bcl-2 and Bcl-x.

Both of these pathways converge on the same cascade of activated caspases. Each caspase exists as a zymogen, or inactive proenzyme, and is activated through cleavage by the previous caspase in the cascade. Caspases, including

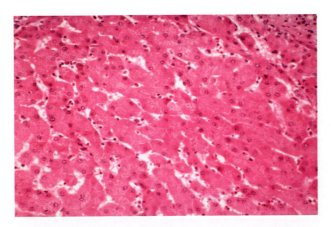

FIGURE 7-2. **Apoptosis.** Photomicrograph of liver taken from a patient with hepatitis B, showing apoptotic cells. (Image courtesy of PEIR Digital Library [http://peir.net].)

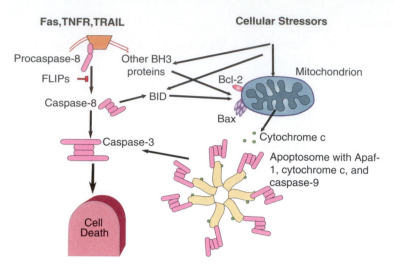

FIGURE 7-3.   Two major pathways of apoptosis. Both the intrinsic (mitochondrion-based) and extrinsic (death receptor) signaling pathways are shown. (Modified, with permission, from Lichtman M, Beutler E, Kipps T, et al. *Williams Hematology,* 7th ed, New York: McGraw-Hill, 2006: 153.)

caspase-3 and caspase-6, function as executioners and promote protein cleavage and DNA breakdown within the cell.

Necrosis

Necrosis is degradation of cells in a living tissue following a lethal injury. The plasma membrane is often disrupted, so the cellular contents leak into the surroundings, resulting in tissue damage and an inflammatory response. Debris is enzymatically digested and ultimately phagocytosed. If necrotic cells are not removed, they promote mineral deposition, leading to **dystrophic calcification.**

CAUSES

Necrosis is generally considered to be due to irreversible exogenous injury. This can have many forms.

- **Ischemia/hypoxia** is the most common type of cell injury.
- **Ischemia/reperfusion injury** can occur when blood flow returns to ischemic tissue.
- Chemical injuries.

MORPHOLOGY

The appearance of damaged cells lies on a continuum between reversibly injured and necrotic cells. Several hallmarks are visible on histologic sections.

- Increased eosinophilia
- **Myelin figures** replace dead cells.
- Breakdown of nuclear DNA leads to **karyolysis,** or loss of chromatin basophilia (in Figure 7-4).
- Alternatively, DNA may condense into a shrunken mass, seen as **pyknosis.**
- A pyknotic nucleus may fragment, known as **karyorrhexis**; ultimately, the nucleus disappears.

MECHANISMS OF NECROSIS

Can take multiple forms, based on the type of injured tissue and mechanism of injury.

KEY FACT

Irreversible injuries occur when the cell cannot reverse the disturbances in mitochondrial and membrane function.

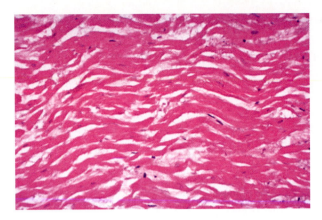

FIGURE 7-4. **Necrosis.** Photomicrograph of cardiac myocytes following an infarction. Necrotic cells with some karyolysis are visible. (Image courtesy of PEIR Digital Library [http://peir.net].)

- **Coagulative necrosis** is thought to occur when injury causes acidosis and denatures degradative enzymes. The outline of the cell is maintained. Most common type.
- Bacterial and some fungal infections cause **liquefactive necrosis.** Cell outlines are lost due to enzymatic digestion. Also follows hypoxic injury to central nervous system (CNS) cells.
- **Caseous necrosis** is usually found in granulomas following infection with tuberculosis. The appearance is often described as white and cheesy. Cells are amorphous, and tissue architecture is completely degraded.
- **Fat necrosis** is not really a morphologic pattern of necrosis, but refers to necrotic destruction of large areas of fat. Usually due to acute pancreatitis, in which activated pancreatic enzymes degrade fat cells. Released fat cells combine with calcium, resulting in **fat saponification.**

Any form of necrosis can result in the release of cellular contents, with subsequent inflammation.

INFLAMMATION

Inflammation is the complex response of vascular tissue to harmful agents or damaged cells. This response includes **vascular and cellular reactions**, involves the **secretion of mediators**, and is followed by attempted repair of the tissue.

Vascular Reaction

Changes in the vasculature allow immune cells and mediators to travel to the site of injury and escape from vessels into the damaged tissue. Changes occur in the following order:

- **Vasodilation** in the arterioles and capillary beds mainly due to the action of histamine and nitric oxide on vascular smooth muscle. This results in increased blood flow to the injured area (causing redness and heat).
- **Increased permeability** of the vessel wall results in loss of protein-rich fluid into the extracellular tissues (causing swelling).
- Loss of fluid results in increased cellular concentrations in the blood, so flow is slowed, causing **stasis.**
- Stasis allows for increased leukocyte migration through the endothelium.

KEY FACT

Remember the five cardinal signs of inflammation:
Rubor = Redness
Tumor = Swelling
Calor = Heat
Dolor = Pain
Function laesa = Loss of function

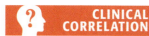

CLINICAL CORRELATION

Defects in leukocyte function compromise the immune response. **Chronic granulomatous disease** is a congenital disorder in which leukocytes cannot generate superoxide, which is required for bacterial killing. This disease results from defects in the genes encoding NADPH oxidase.

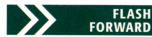

CLINICAL CORRELATION

Leukocyte-induced injury is responsible for both acute diseases (such as septic shock and vasculitis) and chronic diseases (including arthritis).

FLASH FORWARD

Many drugs target mediators of inflammation, including antihistamines and nonsteroidal anti-inflammatory drugs.

Cellular Reaction

Leukocytes, particularly neutrophils and macrophages, are responsible for the removal of offending agents and damaged tissue. At the site of injury, leukocytes must travel from the blood vessel lumen to the interstitial tissue in a process called **extravasation**. This has three steps:

- **Margination**, **rolling**, and **adhesion** to the endothelium. Endothelium is specially activated to bind cells in inflammatory states.
- **Transmigration (diapedesis)** across the vessel wall.
- **Migration** within the interstitial tissue to the site of injury.

Upon arrival, leukocytes attempt to remove the microbe or other agent via **phagocytosis** and the release of substances such as lysosomal enzymes, reactive oxygen intermediates, and prostaglandins. These mediators can damage the endothelium and surrounding tissues. Many acute and chronic human diseases result from an excessive inflammatory response.

Chemical Mediators of Inflammation

Mediators are produced in response to microbial products or host proteins activated by microbes or damaged tissues. These chemicals can be activated from precursors in plasma or may be newly produced by cells. Mediators are generally short-lived once they are activated, which helps limit the damage caused by inflammation. They fall into several categories, described in Table 7-11.

The roles of these mediators in the major reactions in inflammation are summarized in Table 7-12.

Acute Inflammation

Acute inflammation is rapid vascular and cellular response to an agent causing tissue damage. Onset occurs in seconds or minutes, and the reaction lasts for several hours or days.

STIMULI

Acute inflammatory responses can have multiple causes.

- Microbial infections or toxins.
- Tissue necrosis from any cause (e.g., hypoxia).
- Physical (trauma, frostbite) or chemical damage.
- Foreign bodies.
- Hypersensitivity reactions.

MAJOR CELLS INVOLVED

Neutrophils are recruited to the site of injury and are responsible for clearing the area. Other cell types produce mediators.

MORPHOLOGIC FEATURES

There are four patterns of acute inflammation.

- **Serous inflammation** is marked by a thin fluid, similar to that seen in a blister, surrounding the injured area.
- **Fibrinous inflammation** results from more serious injuries that allow the larger molecule fibrin to pass through the vessel wall. The fibrinous exudates may organize to form scar tissue if not removed by macrophages. This pattern is characteristic of inflammation of body cavity linings, such as the pericardium, pleura, and meninges.

TABLE 7-11. **Inflammatory Mediators**

COMPOUND	SOURCE	FUNCTION
Histamine/serotonin	Stored preformed in mast cells, platelets, and enterochromaffin cells.	▪ Dilate arterioles ▪ Increase permeability of venules.
Complement cascade (C3a, C5a)	Plasma.	▪ Functions in innate and adaptive immunity. ▪ Increases vascular permeability.
Coagulation system	Thrombin found in plasma.	Promotes vascular permeability and leukocyte migration.
Kinin system	Plasma.	Release of bradykinin causes contraction of smooth vessel and dilation of blood vessels.
Prostaglandins/leukotrienes	Many cells.	Contribute to pain and fever during inflammation.
Cytokines	Many cells.	Systemic acute-phase responses (e.g., fever, loss of appetite, neutrophilia).
Nitric oxide	Constitutively expressed or induced by cytokine activation.	▪ Potent vasodilator. ▪ Reduces platelet aggregation. ▪ Microbicidal.
Lysosomal enzymes	Leukocytes.	▪ Microbicidal. ▪ Destructive to endothelium and surrounding tissues.
O_2-derived free radicals	Leukocytes (NADPH oxidative system).	▪ Microbicidal. ▪ Destructive to endothelium and surrounding tissues.

▪ **Purulent inflammation** is marked by the production of pus, an exudative fluid containing neutrophils and necrotic cells. A contained area of purulent inflammation is referred to as an **abscess** (see Figure 7-5). This is common in bacterial infections.

TABLE 7-12. **Functions of Chemical Mediators in Inflammation**

SIGN	REACTION	MEDIATORS
Redness	Vasodilation	Histamine, prostaglandins, nitric oxide (NO).
Heat	Vasodilation, fever	Histamine, prostaglandins, NO, interleukin-1, tumor necrosis factor (TNF).
Swelling	Increased vascular permeability	Histamine, serotonin, bradykinin, leukotrienes.
Pain	Release of mediators	Prostaglandins, bradykinin.
Loss of function	Tissue damage	NO, lysosomal enzymes, O_2-derived free radicals.

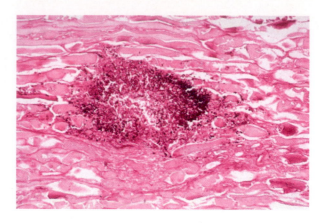

FIGURE 7-5. **Acute inflammation.** Photomicrograph of an abscess within skeletal muscle. Note the neutrophilic infiltrate. (Image courtesy of PEIR Digital Library [http://peir.net].)

- When a sufficient amount of necrotic inflammatory tissue is removed from the surface of an organ, a local defect known as an **ulcer** results. These are usually found in the mucosa of the gastrointestinal or genitourinary tract or subcutaneously in patients with impaired circulation.

OUTCOMES

Acute inflammation has three possible outcomes:

- **Progression** to chronic inflammation.
- **Resolution**, resulting in clearance of the harmful stimulus and rebuilding of injured tissue. The tissue regains its normal function.
- **Fibrosis**, in which the damaged tissue is replaced with scar tissue. The tissue loses its function permanently.

Chronic Inflammation

Inflammation, tissue destruction, and tissue repair proceed simultaneously for a longer duration.

STIMULI

The major causes of chronic inflammation are summarized below.

- **Persistent microbial infection**, characteristically tuberculosis, syphilis, or particular viral, fungal, or parasitic infections. Organisms evoke a delayed type hypersensitivity reaction from the host. Incomplete clearance of the organism leads to chronic inflammation.
- **Ongoing exposure to a toxic agent.** May be exogenous, as in silicosis due to long-term inhalation of silica, or endogenous, such as the reaction to plasma lipids in atherosclerosis.
- **Autoimmune diseases**, in which the inflammatory response to autoantigens results in tissue damage.

MAJOR CELLS INVOLVED

Chronic inflammation is marked by infiltration of mononuclear cells, especially **macrophages.** Macrophages promote fibrosis and angiogenesis through their production of growth factors and cytokines but also cause tissue damage by releasing reactive oxygen species and proteases. Lymphocytes, plasma cells, eosinophils, and mast cells may also be involved.

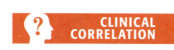

CLINICAL CORRELATION

The delayed type hypersensitivity reaction in tuberculosis is the basis for the PPD skin test.

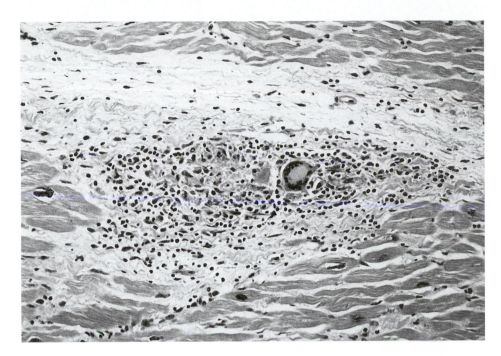

FIGURE 7-6. **Sarcoidosis.** Photomicrograph shows a noncaseating granuloma with a multinucleated giant cell (H&E, ×40) (Reproduced, with permission, from Fuster V, Alexander RW, O'Rourke RA. *Hurst's The Heart*, 11th ed. New York: McGraw-Hill, 2004: 1963.)

MORPHOLOGIC FEATURES

Generally, chronic inflammation is characterized by the presence of mononuclear cells, damaged tissue, and tissue repair. Repair is visible as fibrosis (formation of connective tissue) and angiogenesis (growth of new blood vessels).

Granulomatous inflammation is a distinctive type of chronic inflammation seen in tuberculosis, leprosy, cat-scratch disease, and several other conditions. It is characterized by the formation of granulomas, focal sites of inflammation consisting of **central caseous necrosis** surrounded by macrophages, some of which form giant cells with multiple nuclei at the periphery (Langhans-type giant cells), as seen in Figure 7-6. The periphery of the granuloma is surrounded by lymphocytes and the occasional plasma cell. Granulomas can also form without caseous necrosis, usually in response to foreign bodies or in sarcoidosis. In these cases, giant cells have nuclei scattered throughout the cell (foreign body–type giant cell).

> **KEY FACT**
>
> Caseous necrosis indicates an infectious disease, prototypically tuberculosis.

OUTCOMES

Chronic inflammation causes fibrosis, with resultant loss of function.

CELL ADHESION

The inflammatory response requires leukocytes in the blood to interact with each other and with the vessel endothelium. This occurs through specific adhesion molecules within the **selectin**, **integrin**, **mucin-like glycoprotein**, and **immunoglobulin families.** Surface expression and avidity of these molecules can be modulated by chemical mediators, such as cytokines.

The different families are involved in distinct steps of the leukocyte response (see Figure 7-7).

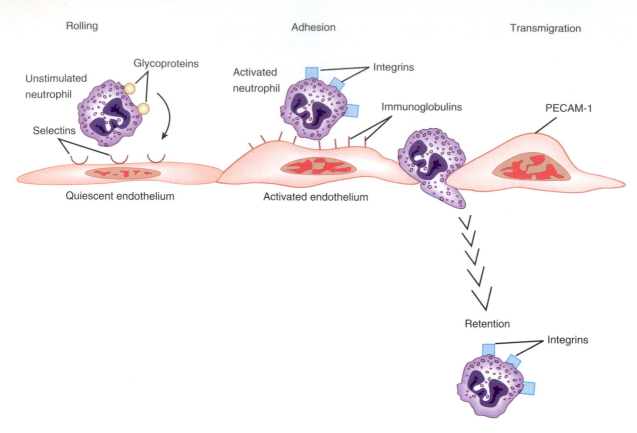

FIGURE 7-7. Molecules involved in leukocyte-endothelium adhesion.

- **Rolling:** Leukocytes migrate to the vessel periphery and move along the endothelium.
  - The endothelium increases expression of **selectins.**
  - Bound with low affinity by leukocyte **Sialyl-Lewis X glycoproteins.**
- **Adhesion:** Leukocytes bind firmly to endothelial cells.
  - The endothelium expresses immunoglobulin members **VCAM-1** and **ICAM-1.**
  - Bound with high affinity by **integrins** on the leukocyte surface.
- **Transmigration:** Leukocytes pass through the endothelium into tissue.
  - Immunoglobulin **platelet endothelial cell adhesion molecule (PECAM-1) or CD31** in the interendothelial space facilitates movement.
- **Retention in tissue:** Leukocytes remain in the extracellular space.
  - **Integrins** on the leukocyte surface bind to matrix proteins at the site of inflammation.

HLA ASSOCIATIONS

Major histocompatibility complex (MHC) alleles associated with autoimmune diseases are primarily located within the classical MHC II loci. MHC II presents antigen to CD4+ T cells, which in turn activate B cells to produce antibody. Therefore, the binding specificities of these alleles are directly linked to the capacity of MHC II to bind self-antigen and initiate an autoimmune disease.

Some alleles seem to predispose to many autoimmune diseases, whereas others can be associated with incidence and severity. In a sibling set in which

TABLE 7-13. **HLA-Associated Diseases**

HLA Type	Disease Association
B8	- Graves' disease - Celiac sprue
B27	- Ankylosing spondylitis - Reactive arthritis - Reiter's syndrome - Acute anterior uveitis - Psoriasis - Inflammatory bowel disease
DR2	- Goodpasture's syndrome - Multiple sclerosis - Narcolepsy - SLE - Hay fever - *Protective* in type 1 diabetes mellitus (type 1 DM)
DR3	- Celiac disease - Myasthenia gravis - SLE - Graves' disease - Type 1 DM - Idiopathic Addison's disease
DR4	- Rheumatoid arthritis - Type 1 DM - Pemphigus vulgaris
DR5	- Hashimoto's thyroiditis - Pernicious anemia
DR7	Steroid-responsive nephritic syndrome
DR11	- Hashimoto's thyroiditis - Celiac disease
Dw3	Sjögren's syndrome
Dw4	Rheumatoid arthritis

SLE = systemic lupus erythematosus.

one sibling has diabetes mellitus type 1 (type 1 DM), an HLA-identical sibling has a 20% risk of also developing type 1 DM. However, a sibling who shares only one HLA allele carries a 5% risk of disease. An HLA-nonidentical sibling has less than a 1% chance. There are a few alleles that predispose to multiple autoimmune diseases. The most common is the combination of DR3/DQ2 (see Table 7-13).

Autoantibodies are antibodies targeted to self; they generally bind portions of nucleic acid and protein. These antibodies can be used to **establish a diagnosis** of an autoimmune disease, **classify the disease**, or **indicate its prognosis or activity.** For example, one criterion for the diagnosis of systemic lupus erythematosus (SLE) is the presence of antinuclear antibody (ANA). However, this antibody is also seen in Sjögren's syndrome, systemic sclerosis, and rheumatoid arthritis. Therefore, more specific antibodies, such as anti-dsDNA and anti-Smith, are used to verify the diagnosis of SLE.

Autoantibodies are also used to classify disease. For instance, drug-induced SLE is almost uniformly associated with the presence of anti-histone antibodies in the peripheral blood.

Finally, autoantibodies may be used as prognostic factors and indicators of disease activity. The presence of antibodies to cyclic citrullinated peptide in rheumatoid arthritis indicates a high likelihood of developing the more severe, erosive form of the disease. In active disease, increased levels of circulating rheumatoid factor (RF) are seen, hence RF allows for an indirect measurement of the disease activity. For more information on autoantibodies and their specific disease associations, see Table 7-14.

TABLE 7-14. **Autoantibodies and Their Associations**

DISEASE	ANTIBODY	OF NOTE...
Autoimmune hemolytic anemia	Anti-RBC	Rh and I antigens are the targets.
Celiac disease	▪ Anti-gliadin ▪ Anti-tissue transglutaminase	
Crohn's disease	Anti-desmin	
Goodpasture's syndrome	Anti-basement membrane	Antigen is type IV collagen, which is also found in the lungs.
Graves' disease	Anti-thyroid stimulating hormone receptor	▪ Crosses placenta. ▪ Antibody is stimulatory at the receptor.
Hashimoto's thyroiditis	▪ Anti-thyroid peroxidase ▪ Anti-thyroglobulin	
Multiple sclerosis	Anti-myelin	
Myasthenia gravis	Anti-acetylcholine	▪ Crosses placenta. ▪ Antibody is inhibitory at the nicotinic ACh-receptor.
Pemphigus vulgaris	Anti-desmoglein-3	Crosses placenta.
Pernicious anemia	▪ Anti-intrinsic factor ▪ Anti-parietal cell	Results in vitamin B_{12} deficiency.

TABLE 7-14.   **Autoantibodies and Their Associations** *(continued)*

DISEASE	ANTIBODY	OF NOTE...
▪ Polymyositis ▪ Dermatomyositis	Anti-Jo 1	
Primary biliary cirrhosis	▪ Anti-mitochondrial ▪ Anti-actin	
Rheumatoid arthritis	Anti-IgG (rheumatoid factor)	Also found in 30% of SLE.
Scleroderma	Anti-centromere	Associated with CREST syndrome.
	Anti-Scl-70	Diffuse, specific.
SLE	Anti-nuclear	Thought to be microbially induced.
	▪ Anti-dsDNA ▪ Anti-Smith	Specific and diagnostic.
	Anti-histone	Only seen in drug-induced cases.
Thrombocytopenic purpura	Anti-platelet	Crosses placenta.
Type 1 diabetes mellitus	▪ Anti-islet cell ▪ Anti-insulin	
Vasculitis	Anti-neutrophil	
Miscellaneous	Anti-microsomal	Found in SLE, rheumatoid arthritis, Sjögren's syndrome, and Hashimoto's thyroiditis, among others.

SLE = systemic lupus erythematosus.

NOTES

General Pharmacology

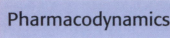

Pharmacodynamics

Pharmacodynamics describes the mechanism of action and the effects of a drug. In other words, what the drug does and how it does it.

AGONISTS AND ANTAGONISTS

With respect to their action at a target site or receptor, drugs can be broadly classified as agonists or antagonists. A single drug can have multiple actions; it may act as an agonist at one receptor and an antagonist at another.

Agonist

Binds to receptor and stabilizes it in an active conformation.

- **Full agonist:** Produces a maximum response after binding to the receptor.
- **Partial agonist:** Produces a less than maximum response after binding to the receptor.

When both full agonists and partial agonists are present in a system, the overall response may be less than the response to full agonists. Partial agonist molecules may bind to receptors and prevent full agonists from binding to the same receptors and exerting a maximum response. Thus, partial agonists may also be called **partial antagonists** or **mixed agonist-antagonists.**

Antagonist

Binds to receptor but does not activate it. Antagonists can bind to a receptor at either the active site or an allosteric site. The **active site** is where agonists bind to produce a response. **Allosteric sites** are sites other than the active site that are involved in receptor activation. In both cases, binding of the antagonist prevents agonists from activating the receptor; antagonist binding to the active site prevents agonist binding, whereas antagonist binding to an allosteric site prevents receptor activation without preventing agonist binding. Antagonists are classified into three categories based on their mechanism of action.

COMPETITIVE ANTAGONIST

- Binds reversibly to the active site of a receptor.
- By occupying the active site, the competitive antagonist blocks agonists from binding and activating the receptor.
- Similar to the mechanism of partial agonists, except that partial agonists produce a reduced response, whereas antagonists produce no response.
- Called "competitive" antagonists because they compete with agonists for the same sites.
- Antagonist effect can be overcome by flooding the system with another molecule (i.e., an agonist) that binds to the same site, thereby outnumbering and outcompeting the competitive antagonist.

NONCOMPETITIVE ANTAGONIST

- Binds to an allosteric site on the receptor.
- Exerts effect by changing the conformation of the receptor such that agonists cannot activate the receptor, even if they can bind to the active site.
- Effect cannot be overcome by flooding the system with an agonist molecule.

IRREVERSIBLE ANTAGONIST

- Binds irreversibly to either the active site or to an allosteric site on the receptor.
- Binds to the site with very high affinity; their antagonist effect cannot be overcome either by saturating the system with an agonist molecule or by washing the antagonist out of the system.

DOSE RESPONSE

Dose-response curves represent the elicited response as a function of drug dose.

Affinity

- A measure of how tightly a drug binds to a receptor.
- Inversely related to K_d, the dissociation constant for the drug-receptor complex.

Potency

- Measured by the concentration of drug required for 50% or half-maximal response.
- Drug A is more **potent** than drug B if a lower concentration of drug A is required for a 50% response.

Efficacy

- Measured by the **maximal response** that can be achieved by the drug.
- Two drugs are equally efficacious if they can achieve the same maximal response at the highest possible doses.

Figure 8-1 shows the dose-response curve of an agonist alone and when an agonist is combined with a competitive antagonist and a noncompetitive antagonist, respectively. The X-axis is a log scale of agonist dose and the Y-axis is the percent response at each dose of agonist.

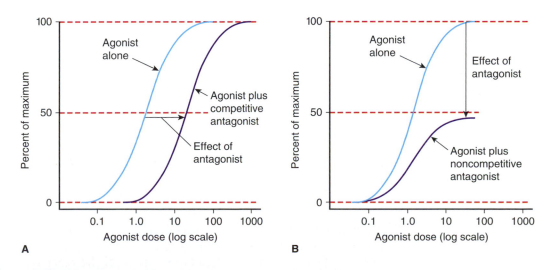

FIGURE 8-1. **Dose-response curve with antagonists.** (Modified, with permission, from Katzung BG, Trevor AJ. *Pharmacology: Examination & Board Review*, 5th ed. Stamford, CT: Appleton & Lange, 1998: 13 and 14.)

Competitive Antagonism

- Antagonist binds reversibly to the same site as the agonist (**active site**).
- The maximum response is the same as with the agonist alone.
- Produces a right shift of the curve, such that the agonist dose needed to achieve a certain response is higher in the presence of a competitive antagonist (decreased potency).
- **Summary:** A higher dose of the agonist is needed to achieve a given response (decreased potency, increased Kd), but the maximum response is unchanged (same efficacy).

Noncompetitive Antagonism

- Antagonist binds to a site other than the active site that reduces the function of the receptor (**allosteric site**).
- The maximum response in the presence of the antagonist is less than with the agonist alone.
- The agonist dose needed to achieve a certain percentage of the maximum response does not change in the presence of a noncompetitive antagonist (no change in potency), but the maximum response is reduced (decreased efficacy).
- **Summary:** The dose needed to achieve a certain percentage of the maximum response is unchanged (same potency, same Kd), but the maximum response is reduced (decreased efficacy). Noncompetitive antagonism cannot be overcome by increasing the agonist dose.

Table 8-1 shows a comparison of competitive antagonists, noncompetitive antagonists, and partial agonists.

Spare Receptors

- This is the concept that that not all receptors have to be occupied for maximal response.
- In the presence of spare receptors, maximal response occurs at a lower agonist dose than that required for receptor saturation.
- Less than 50% of receptors need to be bound to achieve half-maximal response, such that potency < Kd.

> **FLASH FORWARD**
>
> In myasthenia gravis, there are fewer spare nicotinic acetylcholine (nACh) receptors in the eyelid muscles than elsewhere in the body, and so a reduction in the number of nACh receptors initially manifests clinically as eyelid droop.

TABLE 8-1. Properties of Drug-Receptor Interaction Antagonists

Antagonist Type	Effect on Potency	Effect on Efficacy	Reversibility
Competitive antagonist.	Decreased	No change.	Reversible by adding agonist.
Noncompetitive antagonist.	No change	Decreased.	Cannot be reversed by adding agonist.
Partial agonist (mixed agonist-antagonist).	Decreased	Decreased or no change.	May or may not be reversible by adding full agonist, depending on relative binding affinities and concentrations of the full and partial agonists.

Therapeutic Index

- The therapeutic index is an important clinical tool that measures the dose-related toxicity of a drug.
- TD_{50} is the drug dose at which 50% of patients experience **adverse effects.**
- ED_{50} is the drug dose at which 50% of patients experience **desired therapeutic effects.**
- The **therapeutic index** is the ratio of the drug dose at which 50% of patients experience side effects to the drug dose at which 50% of patients experience therapeutic effects.
- **High therapeutic index** drugs achieve therapeutic dose well before causing toxicity and are relatively safe.
- Drugs with a **low or narrow therapeutic index** have a smaller dosing margin that separates desired effects from toxicity.
- Therefore, drugs with a low therapeutic index must be used precisely and serum levels should be monitored closely.

KEY FACT

Therapeutic index = TD_{50}/ED_{50} = median toxic dose/median effective dose

Pharmacokinetics

Pharmocokinetics describes the movement and metabolism of drugs into, out of, and within the body. In other words, how the body processes the drugs that enter it.

KEY FACT

Pharmacodynamics is what a drug does to the body. **Pharmacokinetics** is what the body does to a drug.

INPUT

A drug can enter the body by one of several different routes.

- Enteral (oral): PO
- Parenteral: By injection
    - Intravenous/intra-arterial
    - Intramuscular
    - Subcutaneous
    - Intrathecal: Into the subarachnoid space
- Across a mucous membrane: For example, sublingual, rectal, vaginal
- Transdermal: Across the skin

Each of these routes of administration has advantages and disadvantages in terms of cost, convenience, pain, risk of infection, rate of onset, and the ability of drugs to cross the barrier. Table 8-2 compares the two most common routes of administration: Oral and parenteral.

Bioavailability

- The fraction of the administered drug that reaches the systemic circulation and ultimately, the target organ.
- By definition, intravenous drugs are administered directly into the circulation and have a bioavailability of 1.
- Other routes of administration may have incomplete absorption or undergo first-pass metabolism, in which case bioavailability < 1.

KEY FACT

The bioavailability of drugs administered intravenously is 1.0 or 100%.

First-Pass Metabolism

- Orally administered drugs enter the gastrointestinal (GI) system: GI → portal circulation → liver → hepatic vein → inferior vena cava → heart → systemic circulation → target organs.
- All ingested drugs are first metabolized by the liver before they enter the systemic circulation; this is called **first-pass metabolism.**

KEY FACT

Orally administered drugs are subject to first-pass metabolism.

TABLE 8-2. Oral versus Parenteral Administration

ATTRIBUTE	ORAL	PARENTERAL
Convenient	Yes	No
Risk of infection	No	Yes
Bioavailability	Generally < 1	1
GI absorption required	Yes	No
First-pass metabolism	Yes	No
Onset of action	Generally slow	Generally fast

GI = gastrointestinal.

- First-pass metabolism is important to keep in mind when calculating drug dosage.
- Drugs that are not administered orally are not subject to first-pass metabolism.

DISTRIBUTION

- Once a drug reaches the systemic circulation, it has easy access to nearly every target organ in the body.
- The exceptions are the brain and the testes, which are relatively protected from the general systemic circulation by physiologic barriers.
- The drug can then spread or distribute from the bloodstream into nonvascular organs and tissues, such as muscle, fat, and bone.
- The extent to which a drug distributes among the various compartments in the body depends on multiple factors including the chemical nature of the drug, the volume of the individual compartments, and the number of drug receptors in those compartments.

Volume of Distribution

- A theoretical calculation of the fluid volume that would be needed to contain the total amount of absorbed drug at the concentration of drug found in the plasma at steady state.
- Drugs that are largely taken up by nonvascular compartments, such as fat, have a low plasma concentration and a high volume of distribution. The volume of distribution may be many times the fluid volume in the body.
- Nonvascular tissues must usually be saturated before the plasma concentration reaches steady state. Therefore, drugs with a large volume of distribution often require a higher initial dose to achieve a therapeutic concentration than drugs with a small volume of distribution.

Protein Binding

- Binding to plasma proteins keeps drugs in the vascular compartment, thus reducing the ability of the drug to diffuse from the blood into the tissues.
- Drugs can interact with their target receptors only when they are free or unbound.
- Protein-bound drugs are inactive.
- Drugs that are highly protein bound have a low volume of distribution.
- **Albumin** is the most important plasma-binding protein.

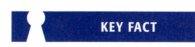

KEY FACT

Volume of distribution (Vd) = Amount of drug in body / Plasma drug concentration

KEY FACT

Only free or unbound drugs are active.

- When plasma drug levels are measured, the measurement is usually of the total drug concentration, which includes both free and protein-bound components.
- Theoretically, competition for binding sites on albumin and other proteins can produce drug-drug interactions. However, no such clinically relevant examples have been documented.

OUTPUT

Just as drugs can enter the body via several different routes, they can also be excreted by the body in several ways.

Renal Excretion

- **Urinary/renal excretion** is the most common mechanism of drug elimination.
- Drugs that are eliminated via this route are **hydrophilic** or water soluble.
- Renal excretion is affected by factors such as the glomerular filtration rate (GFR), the amount of protein binding of the drug, and urine pH.
  - For **weak acids**, alkalinize urine with bicarbonate to increase clearance.
  - For **weak bases**, acidify urine with ammonium chloride to increase clearance.
- Because most drugs are cleared by the kidneys, renal function is an important consideration when administering drugs.

Biliary Excretion

- Hepatic or biliary excretion is an important route of elimination for lipophilic drugs.
- Because drugs that are cleared by the liver must travel through the intestines, they can be reabsorbed by the gut into the enterohepatic circulation and reenter the systemic circulation.

Clearance

Clearance = Rate of elimination of drug / Plasma drug concentration

Rate of Elimination

- See Figure 8-2.

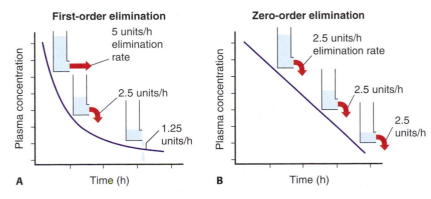

FIGURE 8-2.   Drug elimination rates. (A) First-order elimination and (B) Zero-order elimination. (Modified, with permission from Katzung BG, Trevor AJ. *Pharmacology: Examination & Board Review*, 5th ed. Stamford, CT: Appleton & Lange, 1985: 5.)

TABLE 8-3. **Percentage of Steady State as a Function of Half-life**

Number of Half-lives	1	2	3	3.3	4
Concentration	50%	75%	87.5%	90%	93.75%

- **Zero-order elimination**
  - A **constant amount** of drug is eliminated per unit time.
  - Concentration decreases linearly with time.
  - Examples: Ethanol, phenytoin, aspirin at high doses.
- **First-order elimination**
  - A **constant proportion** of drug is eliminated per unit time.
  - Concentration decreases exponentially with time.
  - Examples: Most drugs.

HALF-LIFE

- Half-life is defined as the time required for the plasma drug concentration to decrease by 50% during elimination (reduction) or constant infusion (addition).
- A drug that is constantly infused reaches 94% of its steady-state plasma concentration after four half-lives (see Table 8-3).
- Half-life is determined by the volume of distribution and clearance of the drug.

DOSAGE CALCULATIONS

Patients with impaired hepatic or renal function often receive the same loading dose but a reduced maintenance dose.

Loading Dose

- **Loading dose = $C_p \times V_d / F$**, where C_p = target plasma concentration, V_d = volume of distribution, and F = bioavailability.
- In urgent situations or when administering drugs with long half-lives, a large loading dose may be used to rapidly reach therapeutic plasma levels.

Maintenance Dose

- **Maintenance dose = $C_p \times CL / F$**, where C_p = target plasma concentration, CL = clearance, and F = bioavailability.
- To maintain a therapeutic concentration, the maintenance dose must be given to ensure that input = output.

Toxicology

Table 8-4 lists in alphabetical order the most common toxic drugs, nondrug toxins, and their antidotes. For adverse reactions associated with drugs, see Table 8-6 in the next section.

TABLE 8-4. Common Toxic Drugs, Nondrug Toxins, and Antidotes

DRUG OR TOXIN	ANTIDOTE
Acetaminophen	*N*-acetylcysteine.
Anticholinergics	Physostigmine.
Anticholinesterases, organophosphates	Atropine, pralidoxime.
Arsenic, mercury, gold	Dimercaprol.
Aspirin	Sodium bicarbonate, alkalinization of urine, dialysis.
Benzodiazepines	Flumazenil.
β-Blockers	Glucagon, calcium gluconate, dextrose-insulin therapy.
Carbon monoxide	100% O_2, hyperbaric O_2.
Copper	D-Penicillamine.
Cyanide	Amyl nitrite, sodium thiosulfate, hydroxocobalamin.
Digitalis/digoxin	Antidigoxin Fab antibodies.
Ethylene glycol (antifreeze), methanol	Fomepizole, ethanol.
Heparin	Protamine.
Iron	Deferoxamine.
Isoniazid (INH)	Pyridoxine (vitamin B_6).
Lead	EDTA, dimercaprol.
Methemoglobinemia (drugs causing)	Methylene blue.
Opioids	Naloxone/naltrexone.
Quinidine	Hypertonic sodium bicarbonate, lidocaine, magnesium sulfate.
Strychnine	Benzodiazepines, neuromuscular blockade.
Theophylline	β-Blockers, benzodiazepines.
Tissue plasminogen activator (tPA)	Aminocaproic acid.
Tricyclic antidepressants (TCAs)	Sodium bicarbonate, benzodiazepines.
Warfarin	Vitamin K, fresh frozen plasma.

CARBON MONOXIDE

MECHANISM

Binds to hemoglobin with much higher affinity than O_2, thereby inhibiting O_2 transport.

EFFECTS

Headache, confusion, seizures, death.

ANTIDOTE

100% O_2, hyperbaric O_2.

CYANIDE

MECHANISM

Reacts with iron in cytochrome oxidase in mitochondria, thereby inhibiting electron transport and ATP formation.

EFFECTS

Tachycardia followed by brachycardia, hypotension, lactic acidosis, seizures, coma, and rapid death. O_2 utilization is diminished at the tissue level, and so venous O_2 concentration is elevated. Venous blood appears bright red.

ANTIDOTE

Amyl nitrite and sodium nitrite prevents and reverses binding of cyanide to cytochrome oxidase. Sodium thiosulfate accelerates detoxification of cyanide to thiocyanate. Hydroxocobalamin chelates cyanide, forming cyanocobalamin.

ETHANOL

MECHANISM

Poorly understood. May exert effects at GABA receptors or by modifying ion channels in biologic membranes. Figure 8-3 illustrates the metabolism of ethanol.

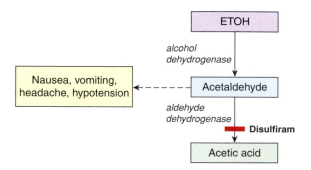

FIGURE 8-3.   **Metabolism of ethanol.**

EFFECTS

Euphoria, disinhibition, sedation, respiratory depression, pancreatitis, hepatitis, Wernicke-Korsakoff syndrome, gynecomastia, testicular atrophy, fetal alcohol syndrome.

ANTIDOTE

Benzodiazepines are used for acute withdrawal. Thiamine is used for prevention of Wernicke's disease. Disulfiram is used to treat chronic alcoholism.

METHANOL

MECHANISM

Metabolized by alcohol dehydrogenase to formaldehyde, which is metabolized by aldehyde dehydrogenase to formic acid. Formic acid accumulation causes retinal toxicity.

EFFECTS

Blindness, metabolic acidosis, and death.

ANTIDOTE

Ethanol acts as a competitive substrate for alcohol dehydrogenase; fomepizole inhibits alcohol dehydrogenase.

HEAVY METALS

See Table 8-5.

STRYCHNINE

MECHANISM

Competitive antagonist of glycine in central nervous system (CNS), leading to loss of normal inhibitory tone and subsequent excitation.

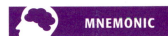

MNEMONIC

Clinical manifestations and treatment of LEAD poisoning:

Lead **L**ines on gingivae and epiphyses of long bones
Encephalopathy and **E**rythrocyte basophilic stippling
Abdominal pain and microcytic **A**nemia
Drops—wrist and foot drop from neuropathy. **D**imercaprol, **D**imercaptosuccinic acid and E**D**TA

TABLE 8-5.   **Heavy Metals (Arsenic, Cadmium, Iron, Lead, Mercury)**

HEAVY METAL	MECHANISM OF TOXICITY	CLINICAL MANIFESTATIONS	ANTIDOTE
Arsenic	Interferes with oxidative phosphorylation.	*Early:* Garlic breath, bloody diarrhea. *Late:* Hair loss, neuropathy, hyperpigmentation, lung cancer.	Dimercaprol, dimercaptosuccinic acid, D-penicillamine.
Cadmium	Complexes with metallothionein.	Metallic taste, GI corrosive, renal and pulmonary disease.	Dimercaptosuccinic acid.
Iron	Direct GI corrosive; forms reactive oxygen species; disrupts oxidative phosphorylation.	Bloody diarrhea, coma, leukocytosis, hyperglycemia.	Deferoxamine.
Lead	Inhibits heme synthesis.	Anemia, abdominal pain, lead lines, motor neuropathy, encephalopathy.	Dimercaprol, EDTA, dimercaptosuccinic acid.
Mercury	Inhibits multiple enzyme processes.	Acute renal failure, pneumonitis, tremor, irrational behavior.	Dimercaptosuccinic acid, dimercaprol.

EFFECTS

Seizure with contraction of all voluntary muscles, resulting in full extension of limbs and vertebrae (opisthotonos).

ANTIDOTE

Benzodiazepines and neuromuscular blockade.

COMMON DRUG SIDE EFFECTS

Table 8-6 presents some commonly tested drug adverse effects and causative agents by organ system. This list is not comprehensive. Please refer to each organ system in the text for more details.

TABLE 8-6. Common Drug Reactions

SYSTEM	ADVERSE REACTION	DRUG	MNEMONIC
Neurologic	Cinchonism	Quinidine, quinine, aspirin.	
	Parkinsonism	Haloperidol, chlorpromazine, reserpine, MPTP.	
	Tardive dyskinesia	Antipsychotics, metoclopramide.	
	Extrapyramidal side effects	Chlorpromazine, thioridazine, haloperidol.	
	Seizures	Imipenem, antipsychotics, tricyclic antidepressants, lithium.	
Cardiovascular	Cardiac toxicity	Doxorubicin, daunorubicin.	
	Torsades de pointes	Class III (sotalol), class IA (quinidine) antiarrythmics.	
	Coronary vasospasm	Cocaine.	
Pulmonary	Pulmonary fibrosis	**N**itrofurantoin **B**leomycin **B**usulfan **A**miodarone	**N**ot **B**eneficial for **B**reathing **A**ir
	Cough	ACE inhibitors.	
Gastrointestinal	Hepatitis	**H**alothane **Is**oniazid	Hepatit**Is**
	Focal to massive hepatic necrosis.	**V**alproic acid **A**cetaminophen **H**alothane **A**manita mushroom	**V**ariable **A**rea **H**epatic **A**ssassin
	Pseudomembranous colitis	Broad-spectrum antibiotics, e.g., clindamycin.	
	Gingival hyperplasia	Phenytoin.	

TABLE 8-6. **Common Drug Reactions** *(continued)*

SYSTEM	ADVERSE REACTION	DRUG	MNEMONIC
Renal	Lactic acidosis	Metformin, nucleoside reverse transcriptase inhibitors.	
	Tubulointerstitial nephritis	Sulfonamides, furosemide, methicillin, rifampin, NSAIDs (except aspirin).	
	Diabetes insipidus	Lithium, demeclocycline.	
	Fanconi's syndrome	Expired tetracyclines, heavy metals.	
Heme	Hemolysis in G6PD-deficient individuals	**S**ulfonamides **I**soniazid **P**rimaquine, **P**yrimethamine, **I**buprofen, **N**itrofurantoin **A**spirin **D**apsone, **C**hloramphenicol	**SIPPIN' A D**iet **C**oke
	Thrombosis	Oral contraceptives: Estrogens, progestins.	
	Agranulocytosis	**C**lozapine, **C**arbamazepine, **C**olchicine, propylthiouracil.	3 **C's**
	Aplastic anemia	**C**hloramphenicol **S**ulfonamides **N**SAIDs gold salts **B**enzene **C**hlorpromazine	**C**an't **S**ynthesize **N**ormal **B**lood **C**ells
Endocrine	Adrenocortical insufficiency	Glucocorticoid withdrawal.	
	Hot flashes	Tamoxifen	
	Gynecomastia	**S**pironolactone **D**igitalis **C**imetidine **E**strogen Chronic **A**lcohol abuse **K**etoconazole	**S**ome **D**rugs **C**reate **E**xtremely **A**wesome **K**nockers
	Hyperprolactinemia	Tricyclic antidepressants, methyldopa, reserpine, phenothiazine.	
	SIADH	ACE inhibitors, SSRIs, vincristine, cyclophosphamide, carbamazepine, chlorpromazine.	
	Hypothyroidism	Lithium.	

(continues)

TABLE 8-6. Common Drug Reactions (continued)

SYSTEM	ADVERSE REACTION	DRUG	MNEMONIC
Dermatologic	Photosensitivity	**S**ulfonamides **A**miodarone **T**etracyclines	**SAT** for a photo
	Cutaneous flushing	**V**ancomycin (red man syndrome) **A**denosine **N**iacin **C**alcium channel blockers	**VANC**
	Stevens-Johnson syndrome	**L**amotrigine **E**thosuximide **S**ulfonamides	**LES**
	Gray baby syndrome	Chloramphenicol.	
Musculoskeletal	Tendonitis, tendon rupture, and cartilage damage	Fluoroquinolones.	
	Osteoporosis	Corticosteroids, heparin.	
Multiple	Ototoxicity and nephrotoxicity	Aminoglycosides, loop diuretics, cisplatin.	
	Neurotoxicity and nephrotoxicity	**Poly**myxi**Ns**	Toxic to **Poly Ns:** Neuro/nephrotoxic
Systemic	Anaphylaxis	Penicillin and many other drugs.	
	SLE-like syndrome	**H**ydralazine **I**soniazid **P**rocainamide, **P**henytoin **P**enicillamine Chlorpromazine, methyldopa, quinidine	It's not **HIPPP** to have lupus
	Disulfiram-like reaction	Some **C**ephalosporins **P**rocarbazine **S**ulfonylureas **Metro**nidazole	Can't **P**ound **S**hots on the **Metro**
	Atropine-like side effects	Tricyclic antidepressants.	

ACE = angiotensin-converting enzyme; G6PD = glucose-6 phosphate dehydrogenase; NSAID = nonsteroidal anti-inflammatory drug; SLE = systemic lupus erythematosus; SSRIs = selective serotonin reuptake inhibitors.

CYTOCHROME P-450 SYSTEM

- A superfamily of enzymes found mainly in the smooth endoplasmic reticulum of hepatocytes.
- In the liver, these enzymes catalyze the metabolism of both exogenous drugs and toxins and endogenous compounds.
- Hydrophobic drugs are metabolized in a two-phase reaction.

Phase I Reaction

■ Enzymes add or unmask a polar moiety in the drug to make it more soluble.

Phase II Reaction

■ Conjugation reactions add more soluble moieties to the polar moiety from phase I to make the drug metabolite more soluble, and thus able to be renally excreted.

■ Drugs are usually detoxified after phase II, although in some cases metabolites are more toxic than the parent compound. Acetaminophen is one such example.

In addition to being metabolized by the cytochrome P-450 system, many drugs also either induce or inhibit the system. This in turn affects the metabolism of other drugs and forms the basis for many clinically important drug-drug interactions. Table 8-7 lists some commonly tested drugs that induce and inhibit the cytochrome P-450 system. As with the Common Drug Reactions table, this list is not meant to be comprehensive.

TABLE 8-7. P-450 Inducers and Inhibitors

INDUCERS	INHIBITORS
Barbiturates	Isoniazid
Phenytoin	Sulfonamides
Cigarette smoke	Cimetidine
Ethanol	Ketoconazole
Rifampin	Erythromycin
Griseofulvin	Ritonavir
Carbamazepine	Grapefruit juice
Omeprazole	Amiodarone
Gemfibrozil	Fluoxetine
Doxorubicin	Verapamil
Nefazodone	Quinidine
Valproic acid	Disulfiram
Zileuton	Metronidazole
	Ciprofloxacin

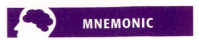

MNEMONIC

P-450 inducers: Barb uses Phen-phen, Cigarettes, and Ethanol but Refuses Greasy Carbs—

Barbiturates
Phenytoin
Cigarette smoke
Ethanol
Rifampin
Griseofulvin
Carbamazepine

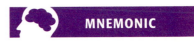

MNEMONIC

P-450 inhibitors: Inhibitors Stop Cyber-Kids from Eating Ripe Grapefruits And Flying Very Quickly to Distant Metropolis City—

Isoniazid
Sulfonamides
Cimetidine
Ketoconazole
Erythromycin
Ritonavir
Grapefruit juice
Amiodarone
Fluoxetine
Verapamil
Quinidine
Disulfiram
Metronidazole
Ciprofloxacin

NOTES

INDEX

A

About the Senior Editors

Tao Le, MD, MHS

Tao has been a well-recognized figure in medical education for the past 15 years. As senior editor, he has led the expansion of *First Aid* into a global educational series. In addition, he is the founder of the *USMLERx* online test bank series as well as a cofounder of the *Underground Clinical Vignettes* series. As a medical student, he was editor-in-chief of the University of California, San Francisco *Synapse*, a university newspaper with a weekly circulation of 9000. Tao earned his medical degree from the University of California, San Francisco in 1996 and completed his residency training in internal medicine at Yale University and allergy and immunology fellowship training at Johns Hopkins University. At Yale, he was a regular guest lecturer on the USMLE review courses and an adviser to the Yale University School of Medicine curriculum committee. Tao subsequently went on to cofound Medsn and served as its chief medical officer. He is currently pursuing research in asthma education at the University of Louisville.

Kendall Krause, MD

This is Kendall's second tour of duty with *First Aid*—she cut her teeth as a junior editor for *First Aid Cases for the USMLE Step I*. After graduating from Northwestern University, she studied public health care delivery in Madagascar and taught adaptive skiing in her home state of Colorado. She then migrated further east to attend the Yale School of Medicine. During medical school, Kendall performed research on high-altitude illness with the Colorado Altitude Research Center. Kendall was an articles editor for the *Yale Journal for Health Policy, Law, and Ethics*, and is a writer for the ABC News Medical Unit. She recently completed her internship at the Harvard Affiliated Emergency Medicine Residency, and is currently pursuing a career in international public health and humanitarian aid.

About the Editors

Elizabeth Eby

Elizabeth is a fourth-year medical student at Vanderbilt planning a residency in pediatrics. She worked as junior editor for this USMLERx project during a research year she spent in the lab of Dr. Terry Dermody. Outside of school, Elizabeth enjoys running marathons, cooking, and volunteering at the Nashville Humane Society.

Justin P. Fox, MD

Justin is currently a resident in the Wright State University general surgery program. He began working on First Aid and USMLERx.com projects as an editor while a fourth-year medical student at the Uniformed Services University of the Health Sciences.

Danielle Guez

Danielle is currently a sixth year MD/PhD student at Yale. Due to the abundance of both rats and cocaine available for study in Baltimore, Danielle decided to join the NIH Graduate Partnerships Program, and is now studying addiction at the National Institute on Drug Abuse. Danielle loves playing broomball, going to concerts, traveling, and cooking/eating Indian and Middle Eastern food. Danielle has become an expert East coast driver since she loves spending time with her family, friends, and fiancé.

M. Kennedy Hall

M. Kennedy is a fourth year student at the Albert Einstein College of Medicine pursuing Emergency Medicine, renaissance medical education, international health, and research. While serving as editor for the Einstein team he is exploring rural health in Uganda and a research fellowship in optic nerve ultrasonography. He balances academia with cello and guitar, rock climbing, running, thematic gardening, sailing, photography, and all things creative—his best Halloween costume to date is "I've got bigger fish to fry."

Sandy Mong

Sandy Mong hails from Harvard Medical School. She was a recent Howard Hughes Medical Institute Fellow, having conducted research on the role of NF2 (merlin) in wound healing in Andrea McClatchey's laboratory. In her spare time, she performs with Longwood Symphony Orchestra (an orchestra comprised of medical professionals dedicated to performing for healthcare related causes) and recently returned from a tour of London dedicated to raising money for cancer research. She will hopefully be entering otolaryngology residency in summer 2009.

Konstantina M. Vanevski, MD

Konstantina is a native of the Republic of Macedonia, where she obtained her Medical Doctorate degree at the Faculty of Medicine, University of Ss. Cyril and Methodius, followed by postgraduate and postdoctoral/clinical training mainly focused on developmental endocrinology/neuroimmunology. She joined the USMLERx/First Aid family in early 2006. Presently, she is a senior fellow with the Department of Obstetrics and Gynecology at the Uniformed Services University of the Health Sciences (USUHS). Her greatest passions are medical education and mentoring, which are coupled with pursuit of her hobbies, including writing, reading, cooking, and traveling, swimming and skiing in her spare time.

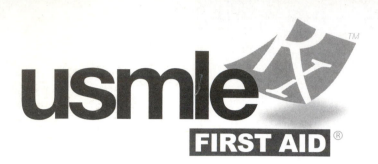
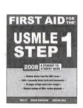
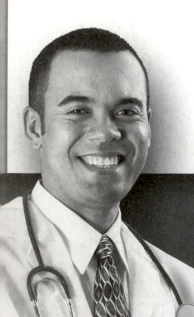